AF710022

October 3, 1993

For Dr. Richard Martin –

Here is what you taught me about soft tissue sarcomas at M.D. Anderson. Many, many thanks!

With highest regards and all best wishes –

John Raaf

Soft Tissue Sarcomas

Diagnosis and Treatment

John H. Raaf, M.D., D.Phil.
Chairman, Department of Surgery
Meridia Huron Hospital
Cleveland, Ohio

Mosby

St. Louis Baltimore Boston Chicago London Philadelphia Sydney Toronto

Mosby
Dedicated to Publishing Excellence

Sponsoring Editor: Susan Gay
Assistant Editor: Sandra Clark
Assistant Director, Manuscript Services: Frances M. Perveiler
Production Supervisor: Carol A. Reynolds
Proofroom Manager: Barbara M. Kelly

Copyright © 1993 by Mosby–Year Book, Inc.
A Year Book Medical Publishers imprint of Mosby–Year Book, Inc.

Mosby–Year Book, Inc.
11830 Westline Industrial Drive
St. Louis, MO 63416

All rights reserved. No part of this publication may be reproduced, stored in a retrieval system, or transmitted, in any form or by any means, electronic, mechanical, photocopying, recording, or otherwise, without prior written permission from the publisher. Printed in the United States of America. Permission to photocopy or reproduce solely for internal or personal use is permitted for libraries or other users registered with the Copyright Clearance Center, provided that the base fee of $4.00 per chapter plus $.10 per page is paid directly to the Copyright Clearance Center, 21 Congress Street, Salem, MA 01970. This consent does not extend to other kinds of copying, such as copying for general distribution, for advertising or promotional purposes, for creating new collected works, or for resale.

1 2 3 4 5 6 7 8 9 0 BI MV 97 96 95 94 93

Library of Congress Cataloging-in-Publication Data

Soft tissue sarcomas : diagnosis and treatment / [edited by] John H.
Raaf.
p. cm.
Includes bibliographical references and index.
ISBN 0-8151-7003-3
1. Soft tissue tumors. 2. Sarcoma. I. Raaf, John H.
[DNLM: 1. Sarcoma—diagnosis. 2. Sarcoma—therapy. 3. Soft
Tissue Neoplasms—diagnosis. 4. Soft Tissue Neoplasms—therapy.
WD 375 S681103]
RC280.S66S64 1992 92-49182
616.99' 4—dc20 CIP
DNLM/DLC
for Library of Congress

To the authors of the chapters in this book, who generously shared their time and expertise.

To professional colleagues, particularly those at Meridia Huron Hospital, for their friendship and counsel,
the patients, who present challenging problems,
the residents, who ask good questions, and
the staff, who care and provide solutions.

To my family, who cheerfully endured this writing project:
Dad and Mother, for inspiration and encouragement,
Heather, pathologist, detective, and editor,
Jennifer, physician to patients large and small,
John, intrepid explorer of mountains and seas, and
Sabrina, artist, writer, and photographer.

Sarcoma is a malignant tumor composed of cells of connective-tissue type. This definition is based on the morphology of the tumor-cells and on their histogenesis.

James Ewing, M.D.
Pathologist

I do not need to recognize different cell types. They all look the same in a Waring blender.

James Bonner, Ph.D.
Biochemist

What is known about medical science is like a speck of dust in the corner. Everything else in the room awaits discovery.

Robert A. Good, M.D., Ph.D.
Immunobiologist

What has become clear to you since we last met?

Ralph Waldo Emerson
Poet

Why, a four-year-old child could understand this. Someone get me a four-year-old child!

Groucho Marx
Actor

The physician needs a clear head and a kind heart.

Sir William Osler
Professor of Medicine

CONTRIBUTORS

J. Bradley Aust, M.D., Ph.D.
The Dr. Witten B. Russ Professor and Chairman
Department of Surgery
The University of Texas
Health Science Center at San Antonio
San Antonio, Texas

Laurence H. Baker, D.O.
Professor and Director
Division of Hematology and Oncology
Wayne State University
Detroit, Michigan

Thomas W. Bauer, M.D., Ph.D.
Staff Pathologist
Department of Anatomic Pathology
The Cleveland Clinic Foundation
Cleveland, Ohio

Oliver H. Beahrs, M.D.
Professor of Surgery Emeritus
Mayo Medical School
Department of Surgery
Mayo Clinic
Rochester, Minnesota

Richard S. Benua, M.D. (Deceased)
Chief of Nuclear Medicine
Nuclear Medicine Service
Memorial Sloan-Kettering Cancer Center
Professor of Radiology and Medicine
Cornell Medical College
New York, New York

John W. Bolen, M.D.
Pathologist, Virginia Mason Clinic
Seattle, Washington

José Botet, M.D.
Associate Attending Radiologist
Department of Radiology
Memorial Sloan-Kettering Cancer Center
New York, New York

Henry A. Briele, M.D.
Associate Professor of Surgery
Division of Surgical Oncology
University of Illinois at Chicago
Chicago, Illinois

Ted Chaglassian, M.D.
Chief, Plastic Surgical Service
Department of Surgery
Memorial Sloan-Kettering Cancer Center
New York, New York

Daniel Coit, M.D.
Assistant Attending Surgeon
Gastric and Mixed Tumor Service
Memorial Sloan-Kettering Cancer Center
New York, New York

John M. Daly, M.D.
Chief, Division of Surgical Oncology
Jonathan E. Rhoads Professor of Surgery
University of Pennsylvania School of Medicine
Philadelphia, Pennsylvania

Melinda L. Estes, M.D.
Staff Pathologist
Department of Pathology
The Cleveland Clinic Foundation
Cleveland, Ohio

Hollon W. Farr, M.D.
Attending Surgeon Emeritus
Head and Neck Service
Memorial Sloan-Kettering Cancer Center
New York, New York

Arlan F. Fuller, Jr., M.D.
Director, Gynecologic Oncology
Massachusetts General Hospital
Associate Professor
Obstetrics, Gynecology and Reproductive Biology
Harvard Medical School
Boston, Massachusetts

Harold V. Gaskill III, M.D.
Associate Professor
Department of Surgery
The University of Texas Health Science Center at San Antonio
San Antonio, Texas

John A. Greager, M.D.
Associate Professor of Surgery
Division of Surgical Oncology
University of Illinois at Chicago
Chicago, Illinois

Tapas K. Das Gupta, M.D.
Professor and Head
Division of Surgical Oncology
University of Illinois at Chicago
Chicago, Illinois

John H. Healey, M.D.
Chief of Orthopaedic Surgery
Memorial Sloan-Kettering Cancer Center
New York, New York

Herbert C. Hoover, M.D.
Chief, Surgical Oncology Research
Massachusetts General Hospital
Boston, Massachusetts

Kamal G. Ishak, M.D.
Chairman, Department of Hepatic Gastrointestinal Pathology
Armed Forces Institute of Pathology
Washington, D.C.

Constantine P. Karakousis, M.D., Ph.D.
Chief, Soft Tissue-Melanoma and Bone Service
Surgical Oncology Department
New York State Department of Health
Roswell Park Cancer Institute
Buffalo, New York

Jae Ho Kim, M.D., Ph.D.
Chairman, Department of Radiation Oncology
Henry Ford Hospital
Detroit, Michigan

Stephen A. Kramer, M.D.
Consultant, Section of Pediatric Urology
Mayo Clinic and Mayo Foundation
Professor of Urology
Mayo Medical School
Rochester, Minnesota

Bruce G. Kulander, M.D.
Pathologist, Laboratory of Pathology of Seattle
The Swedish Hospital Medical Center
Seattle, Washington

Joseph M. Lane, M.D.
Chief, Orthopaedic Surgery
Memorial Sloan-Kettering Cancer Center
New York, New York

Walter Lawrence, Jr., M.D.
Professor and Chairman
Division of Surgical Oncology
Medical College of Virginia
Richmond, Virginia

Michael M. Lieber, M.D.
Professor of Urology
Department of Urology
Mayo Clinic and Mayo Foundation
Rochester, Minnesota

William F. Lindsey, M.D.
General Surgeon
Oneida Surgical Group
Chief of Staff
Oneida City Hospital
Oneida, New York

Ronald A. Malt, M.D.
Professor of Surgery
Department of Surgery
Harvard Medical School
Chief of Gastrointestinal Surgery
Chief of Liver, Biliary and Pancreas Center
Massachusetts General Hospital
Boston, Massachusetts

Henry J. Mankin, M.D.
Chief of Orthopaedic Service
Edith M. Ashley Professor of Orthopaedic Surgery
Department of Orthopaedic Surgery
Massachusetts General Hospital Cancer Center
Harvard Medical School
Boston, Massachusetts

Oliver J. McAnena, M.Ch.
Consultant Surgeon/Senior Lecturer
The Royal London Hospital
London, England

Charles M. McBride, M.D., C.M. (Deceased)
Department of General Surgery
The University of Texas M.D. Anderson Cancer Center
Houston, Texas

Theodore R. Miller, M.D.
Clinical Professor of Surgery
University of Medicine and Dentistry of New Jersey
Piscataway, New Jersey

Clifton F. Mountain, M.D.
Professor of Surgery
Department of Thoracic Surgery
The University of Texas M.D. Anderson Cancer Center
Houston, Texas

James H. Muchmore, M.D.
Surgical Oncologist
Department of Surgery
Tulane University Medical Center
New Orleans, Louisiana

George F. Muschler, M.D.
Surgeon, Section of Musculoskeletal Oncology
Department of Orthopaedic Surgery
The Cleveland Clinic Foundation
Cleveland, Ohio

Patricia L. Myskowski, M.D.
Associate Attending Physician
Department of Dermatology
Memorial Sloan-Kettering Cancer Center
New York, New York

James P. Neifeld, M.D.
Professor of Surgery
Division of Surgical Oncology
Medical College of Virginia
Richmond, Virginia

Donald Patterson, M.D.
Assistant Clinical Professor
University of Missouri Hospital and Clinics
Columbia, Missouri

Richard Pazdur, M.D.
Assistant Professor
Division of Medical Oncology
The University of Texas M.D. Anderson Cancer Center
Houston, Texas

Joseph Pober, M.D.
Attending Plastic Surgeon
St. Luke's Roosevelt Hospital
Columbia University College of Physicians and Surgeons
Clinical Instructor for Plastic Surgery
College of Medicine
State University of New York Health Sciences Center
Manhattan, New York

Karl H. Proppe, M.D.
Chief of Pathology
Department of Pathology
Salem Hospital
Salem, Massachusetts

Heather N. Raaf, M.D.
Forensic Pathologist
Deputy Coroner
Cuyahoga County Coroner's Office
Cleveland, Ohio

John H. Raaf, M.D., D.Phil.
Chairman, Department of Surgery
Meridia Huron Hospital
Cleveland, Ohio

Bijan Safai, M.D.
Attending Physician
Department of Dermatology
Memorial Sloan-Kettering Cancer Center
New York, New York

David S. Shimm, M.D.
Associate Professor
Department of Radiation Oncology
The University of Arizona Health Sciences Center
Tucson, Arizona

Susan B. Shurin, M.D.
Chief, Division of Pediatric Hematology-Oncology
Rainbow Babies and Children's Hospital
Associate Professor of Pediatrics
Case Western Reserve University
School of Medicine
Cleveland, Ohio

Peter P. Sordillo, M.D., Ph.D.
Associate Professor of Medicine
Mount Sinai School of Medicine
Lenox Hill Hospital
New York, New York

Paul H. Sugarbaker, M.D.
Medical Director, Washington Hospital
Cancer Center Institute
Washington Hospital Center
Washington, D.C.

Herman D. Suit, M.D.
Andres Soriano Director of Cancer Management
Department of Radiation Medicine
Massachusetts General Hospital Cancer Center
Harvard Medical School
Boston, Massachusetts

Joel Tepper, M.D.
Professor and Chair
Department of Radiation Oncology
University of North Carolina School of Medicine
Chapel Hill, North Carolina

Taiji Tsukamoto, M.D.
Department of Urology
Mayo Clinic and Mayo Foundation
Rochester, Minnesota

Michael J. Walker, M.D.
Associate Professor of Surgery
Ohio State University Hospital
Columbus, Ohio

Richard E. Wilson, M.D. (Deceased)
Professor of Surgery
Chief, Surgical Oncology
Brigham and Women's Hospital
Dana-Farber Cancer Institute
Department of Surgery
Harvard Medical School
Boston, Massachusetts

Donald K. Wood, M.D.
Associate Professor of Surgery
Division of Surgical Oncology
University of Illinois at Chicago
Chicago, Illinois

William C. Wood, M.D.
Joseph Brown Whitehead Professor and Chairman
Department of Surgery
Emory University School of Medicine
Clinical Director
Winship Cancer Center
Atlanta, Georgia

Samuel D.J. Yeh, M.D.
Attending Physician
Nuclear Medicine Service
Memorial Sloan-Kettering Cancer Center
Associate Professor of Medicine
Cornell Medical College
New York, New York

PREFACE

Soft tissue sarcomas are a diverse group of malignant tumors that for decades has intrigued surgeons, radiotherapists, and medical and pediatric oncologists. Sarcomas challenge physicians because of their rarity and their pathologic and anatomic variability. Clinical sophistication is required to provide optimal multi-disciplinary treatment for each of these neoplasms.

This book is a multi-authored, multi-institutional discussion of this rare group of tumors, representing a variety of views and treatment philosophies. It is intended to be of particular value to clinicians, but the book also contains new and in-depth information on the biology, pathology, and staging of these tumors. The volume is uniquely comprehensive since it examines not only sarcomas of the extremities, but also those arising in other soft tissues such as the breast, heart, great vessels, gastrointestinal tract, and genitourinary system. Very rare sarcomas are discussed, such as Askin tumor, PNET, cystosarcoma phyllodes, and dermatofibrosarcoma protuberans.

Current knowledge regarding the cytogenetics and molecular biology of sarcomas is summarized in Chapter 1. The remainder of the book is divided into five sections. Section 1 concerns methods of diagnosis, pathology, and staging. In Section 2, specific sarcomas and anatomic sites are presented. Sections 3 through 5 contain discussions of treatment approaches using surgery, radiation therapy, and chemotherapy respectively, focusing throughout on multidisciplinary integration of the different modalities. Limb-sparing and other techniques employed by general, orthopedic, thoracic, and plastic surgeons, including methods of amputation, are presented through detailed anatomic illustrations. New approaches undergoing clinical evaluation such as brachytherapy, hyperthermia, and cryotherapy are also described. Points of controversy and confusion are addressed; for example, the difference in pathological identification and treatment of fibromatosis *versus* desmoid fibrosarcoma. Results of recent clinical trials are presented, some of which confirm the benefit of new techniques (e.g., limb-sparing surgery plus radiotherapy), while other methods have yet to be proved of value (e.g., adjuvant chemotherapy for adult soft tissue sarcomas).

I thank my teachers and colleagues in surgery for helping me define my own approach to patients with soft tissue sarcomas. At the Massachusetts General Hospital, these individuals include Drs. Leslie Ottinger, Paul Russell, Claude Welch, Ronald Malt, and W. Gerald Austen. Dr. Richard G. Martin, former Chief of Surgery at M. D. Anderson Cancer Center, was an exemplary mentor and senior partner during my first years of managing sarcoma patients. Other colleagues at M. D. Anderson were Drs. Marvin Romsdahl, John Murray, Ted Copeland, and Robert Hickey. At Memorial Sloan-Kettering Cancer Center I was privileged to practice surgical oncology with, and gain knowledge from, Drs. Man Shiu, William Knapper, Joseph Fortner, Alan Turnbull, Lemuel Bowdin, Robert Booher, Charles McPeak, Hollon Farr, Jerome DeCosse, Ted Beattie, John Daly, and Murray Brennan.

I particularly thank Drs. Jerome DeCosse and Ronald Malt who gave consistent encouragement to me during this writing effort. Others also provided strong support. Outstanding secretarial assistance was given by Abby Vance, Kathy Porcen-Robinson, Michelle Toll, Mary Anne James, and Richard Lyon. Shannon Henry and Jo Gambosi performed excellent copyediting, an activity about which I have learned much from my editorial colleagues Mr.

James McCarthy and Dr. Heather Raaf. Keith Stincic and Katherine Van Bolt, librarians at Meridia Huron Hospital, provided critical help in checking the accuracy of references.

Finally, it has been a pleasure working with Ms. Susan Gay, Mr. Daniel Doody, Mr. Edward Wickland, Ms. Kelly Ricci, Ms. Fran Perveiler, and many others from the publisher, Mosby–Year Book, whose interest and efforts made this book possible.

John H. Raaf, M.D., D.Phil.

CONTENTS

PART 4 TREATMENT: RADIATION THERAPY

PART 5 TREATMENT: CHEMOTHERAPY

Chapter 1

Overview and Etiology

John H. Raaf

DEFINITION AND HISTORY

Soft-tissue sarcomas are a diverse group of malignant neoplasms that arise in supporting connective tissue at all sites of the body, other than bone or cartilage. The word "sarcoma" is derived from the Greek *sarc* (fleshy) and *oma* (tumor). The first such tumor to be written about accurately enough to be recognized, a myxosarcoma, was described by Marcus Severinius (1580–1637).[1] Morgagni (1688–1772) described tumors found at autopsy, one of which was a liposarcoma.[2] The history of early studies and attempts to categorize soft-tissue sarcomas has been well reviewed by Hajdu[3] and by Sears.[4]

In the United States there are now approximately 7,800 newly diagnosed sarcomas of all types and 4,350 deaths due to sarcomas per year.[5] Five thousand and eight hundred of these tumors and 3,300 of the deaths are due to sarcomas of soft connective tissue. The remaining tumors are of bony or cartilaginous origin (e.g., osteosarcoma, chondrosarcoma, Ewing's sarcoma). Sarcomas arising in bone or cartilage are diagnosed and treated in a somewhat different manner from soft-tissue sarcomas and will not be discussed in this book.

Soft-tissue sarcomas comprise 0.5% of all new cancer cases in the United States each year, although they constitute 6.5% of all neoplasms in children under the age of 15 years.[6] These tumors can arise anywhere in the body. Sixty percent occur in the extremities, two thirds of these in the lower extremity. The most common soft-tissue sarcomas are malignant fibrous histiocytoma, liposarcoma, rhabdomyosarcoma, leiomyosarcoma, tendosynovial sarcoma, and fibrosarcoma.

Most soft-tissue sarcomas develop in mesodermal tissues (Fig 1–1), although neurosarcomas and primitive neuroectodermal tumors (PNETs) are of ectodermal origin. Soft-tissue sarcomas occur in all age groups, although the various histological types predominate at different ages. Rhabdomyosarcoma peaks in childhood, liposarcoma and leiomyosarcoma during middle age, and malignant fibrous histiocytoma (MFH) in elderly patients (Fig 1–2). The anatomical distribution of sarcomas is also different for the histological subtypes. There is no overall sexual or racial preponderance for these neoplasms.

The collection of tumors known as soft-tissue sarcomas represents a spectrum of biological patterns and behavior that ranges from a relatively nonaggressive mass of well-differentiated cells to a pleomorphic tumor that rapidly metastasizes to distant sites. A primary sarcoma

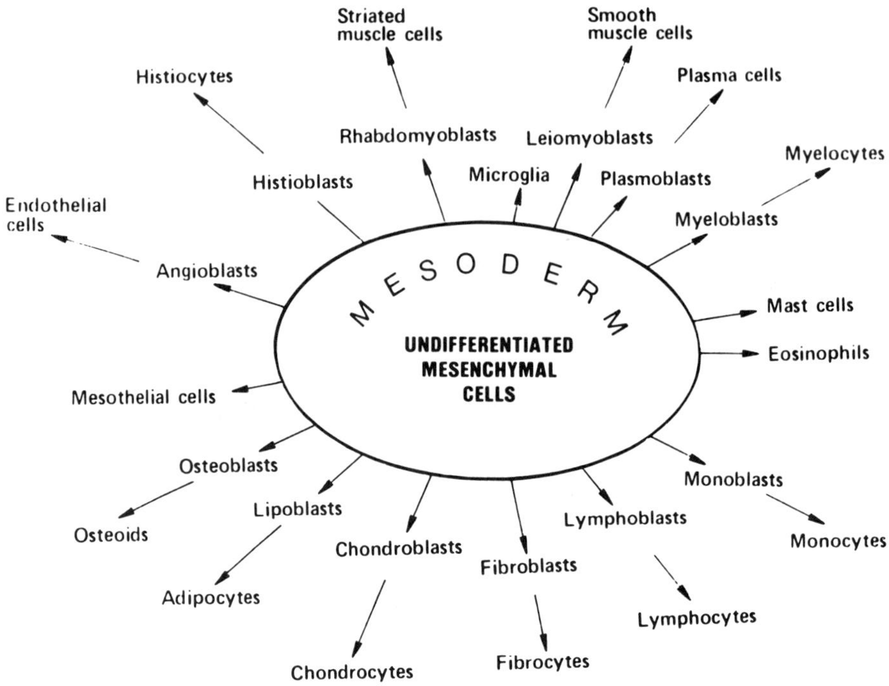

FIG 1–1.
Primitive mesenchymal cells and their derivatives. (From Hajdu SI: *Pathology of Soft Tissue Tumors.* Philadelphia, Lea & Febiger, 1979. Used by permission.)

may be relatively homogeneous histologically or may have different histological patterns within a single neoplasm, suggesting tumor heterogeneity and several different pathways or degrees of differentiation.[7, 8] For this reason, the cell of origin of a soft-tissue sarcoma is thought to be a multipotential, undifferentiated primitive cell.[9]

Soft-tissue sarcomas demonstrate a wide morphological range, reflecting the complexity of the mesenchymal tissues from which they arise. During the 20th century the modern classification of sarcomas has evolved through the study and writings of many pathologists, including Ewing,[10] Stout,[11] Stewart and Treves,[12] Enzinger and Weiss,[13] and Hajdu.[3]

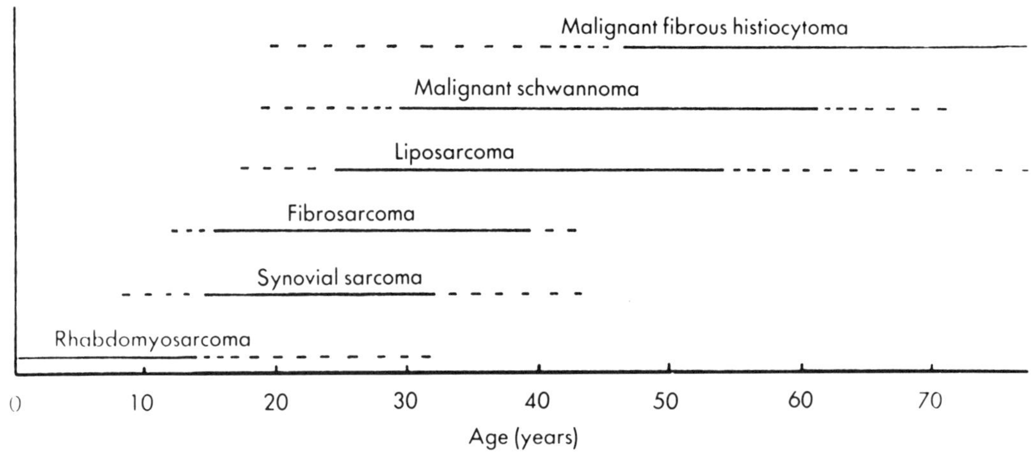

FIG 1–2.
Relationship of age to the incidence of various histological types of sarcoma. (From Enzinger FM, Weiss SW: *Soft Tissue Tumors,* ed 2. St. Louis, C. V. Mosby, 1988. Used by permission.)

TABLE 1–1.
Prognostic Factors for Soft-Tissue Sarcomas*

Factor	Prognosis: Favorable	Prognosis: Unfavorable
Grade	Low	High
Size	<5 cm	>5 cm
Primary site	Superficial	Deep
Surgical margin	Clear	Involved

* *After Hajdu SI:* Pathology of Soft Tissue Tumors. *Philadelphia, Lea & Febiger, 1979.*

Histological grade is the most important prognostic factor, whereas histological type is of little prognostic importance. High-grade sarcomas are characterized by poor differentiation, hypercellularity, minimal stroma, hypervascularity, extensive necrosis, and more than five mitoses per ten high-power fields. High-grade sarcomas metastasize hematogenously and early to the lungs (or in the case of retroperitoneal sarcomas, to the liver), whereas lymphatic spread to nodes is rare. Low-grade sarcomas are locally invasive but rarely spread to distant sites. Survival is worse if tumor size is greater than 5 cm, or the location in an extremity is deep rather than superficial (Table 1–1).[14]

ETIOLOGY

In his famous text (p. 274), *Neoplastic Diseases: A Treatise on Tumors,*[10] James Ewing wrote: "Of the specific etiology of sarcoma, little is definitely known." This is still true, although some associations are now apparent for a minority of these tumors. Putative agents contributing to the pathogenesis of soft-tissue sarcomas include environmental factors, chemical carcinogens, oncogenic viruses, immunological factors, and genetic factors.

For two centuries there has been varying certainty that soft-tissue sarcomas may be of traumatic origin. The frequent association of trauma and sarcoma is suggestive, yet in most cases trauma appears to be an event that simply calls attention to an underlying soft-tissue neoplasm. Occasionally there is sufficient evidence to suggest a causal relationship, such as dermatofibrosarcoma protuberans arising in a burn scar, or fibrosarcoma at a fracture site. Although foreign bodies readily induce sarcomas in experimental animals, this event occurs only rarely in humans.[15] Jennings and co-authors[16] reviewed 9 cases of angiosarcoma and 40 cases of sarcoma of other histological types associated with foreign material in humans. They found the latency period to vary from 4 months to 63 years.

A role for chemical carcinogens has stronger support. In laboratory animals, sarcomas have been produced by subcutaneous injection of polycyclic hydrocarbons. These animal tumors are rapidly growing, poorly differentiated sarcomas that have no specific human correlate, although rodents bearing such tumors are often used as experimental subjects.[17–19] A variety of human sarcomas has been associated with prior exposure to alkylating agents. Polyvinyl chloride may play a role in the pathogenesis of hepatic angiosarcoma. Asbestos is an important environmental carcinogen that is associated with the development of pleural and peritoneal mesotheliomas. Contained in herbicides, 2,3,7,8-tetrachlorodibenzo-*p*-dioxin (TCDD) may be an etiological agent for soft-tissue sarcomas.[20] So far, case control studies have not found a significant association between exposure to Agent Orange (a defoliating agent contaminated with dioxin) and development of sarcomas.

Radiation therapy is associated with the appearance of various soft-tissue sarcomas in the radiation therapy field, from 2 to 25 years after exposure. Such tumors are malignant fibrous histiocytoma, extraskeletal osteosarcoma, fibrosarcoma, mixed mesodermal sarcomas of the uterus, and mesothelioma.[21–23] Lymphangiosarcoma can arise in a chronically lymphedematous extremity in a woman treated for breast cancer by mastectomy and axillary node dissection (Stewart-Treves syndrome).[12] Sixty percent had also received radiotherapy, although the tumor developed outside the field of radiation in most patients. Angiosarcoma in the breast has developed in seven patients following partial mastectomy and external beam radiation therapy to the remaining ipsilateral breast tissue, an average of 8.6 years following the administration of radiotherapy.[24] Angiosarcoma has also been reported in the edematous skin of the breast after tylectomy and axillary dissection *without* radiation to the breast.[25]

Genetic factors play a role in the pathogenesis of a few types of sarcoma. Patients with neurofibromatosis (von Recklinghausen's disease) have a 7% to 10% lifetime risk of developing malignant neurofibrosarcoma. Patients with Gardner's syndrome may develop a desmoid fibrosarcoma of the mesentery, which can cause life-threatening bowel obstruction or invasion of other viscera. Osteosarcoma is associated with familial retinoblastoma. The Li-Fraumeni cancer

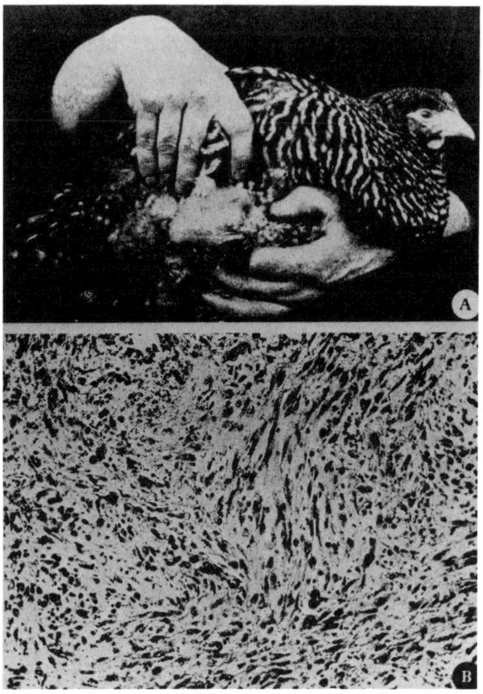

FIG 1–3.
Original illustrations by Peyton Rous of the gross, **A**, and histological, **B**, appearance of the Rous sarcoma in the Plymouth Rock fowl. [From Rous P: A transmissible avian neoplasm (sarcoma of the common fowl). *J Exp Med* 1910; 12:696–705; reprinted in Hajdu SI: *Pathology of Soft Tissue Tumors.* Philadelphia, Lea & Febiger, 1979. Used by permission.]

family syndrome is manifested by susceptibility to breast cancer, sarcomas, brain tumors, leukemia, adrenocortical carcinoma, and possibly other cancers in children and young adults.[26] Inherited mutations in the *p53* tumor suppressor gene have been recognized in some, but not all, families with this syndrome.[27] Mutations in the *p53* gene have also been found in primary and metastatic rhabdomyosarcoma[28] and in radiation-induced sarcomas.[29] There is a correlation between decreased expression of the retinoblastoma-susceptibility suppressor gene (*Rb*) and increased biological aggressiveness of human sarcomas.[30]

Studies of sarcoma biopsy specimens and cell lines grown in tissue culture have revealed receptors for estrogen and androgen,[31] glucocorticoids,[32] and insulin-like growth factor II (IGF-II).[33] Insulin-like growth factor II may act as an autocrine growth factor in human rhabdomyosarcoma, an autocrine loop that can be interrupted in vitro by the drug suramin.[34] Results of future in vivo experiments with suramin may have important therapeutic implications.

Peyton Rous demonstrated in 1911 that a filterable agent could be used to transmit a malignant sarcoma in birds (Fig 1–3),[35, 36] a discovery for which he received the Nobel prize in 1966, over half a century later. The Rous sarcoma virus, an RNA retrovirus, is now known to contain the *src* oncogene, which is expressed despite non–site-specific integration into the avian cell genome.[37]

Many sarcomas in mice, monkeys, cats, and birds are now well documented to have a viral etiology or association. It is unclear, however, what the role of oncogenic viruses might be in causing soft-tissue sarcomas in humans. Patients with acquired immunodeficiency syndrome (AIDS) can develop a generalized form of Kaposi's sarcoma. Therefore it has been suggested that the human immunodeficiency virus type 1 [HIV-1; or human T cell leukemia/lymphoma virus type III (HTLV-III)] may be oncogenic, although others have suggested that cytomegalovirus is the responsible agent. Viral particles have often been seen by electron microscopy in human soft-tissue tumors, but their role in carcinogenesis, if any, is unknown.

CYTOGENETICS

Knowledge of the cytogenetics of soft-tissue tumors is expanding rapidly. Some karyotypic abnormalities specific for certain sarcomas have been described (Table 1–2).[38–42] For example, a characteristic translocation occurs in synovial sarcoma t(X;18) (p11.2;q11.2),[43] in both biphasic and monophasic types as well as in poorly differentiated synovial sarcoma.[44] More than 50% of alveolar rhabdomyosarcomas demonstrate a t(2;13) (q37;q14) abnormality,[45] whereas a t(1;13) (p36;q14) variant has been described in very young patients.[46]

Myxoid liposarcomas have a characteristic translocation t(12;16) (q13;p11) (Figs 1–4 and 1–5),[47, 48] and benign lipomas also exhibit translocations involving 12q13–15.[49] Malignant fibrous histiocytomas (MFH) often demonstrate complex karyotypic abnormalities.[50] A 19p+ marker chromosome in MFH signals an increased relapse rate.[51]

Both extraskeletal Ewing's sarcoma and peripheral neuroepithelioma (a form of primitive neuroectodermal tumor) have a similar translocation, t(11;22) (q24;q12), providing evidence that extraskeletal Ewing's sarcoma has a neural

TABLE 1–2.
Cytogenetic Patterns in Soft-Tissue Sarcomas*

Histological Condition and Characteristics	Cytogenetic Abnormality
Uterine leiomyosarcoma	t(12;14) and 7q−
Rhabdomyosarcoma	Expression of the *MYOD1* muscle-specific gene
Alveolar	t(2;13) (q37;q14) and variant t(1;13) (p36;q14)
Embryonal	Deletion of 11p15
Synovial sarcoma	t(X;18) (p11.2;q11.2) and variants involving 18q11.2
Osteosarcoma	13q14 (loss of the retinoblastoma tumor suppressor gene)
Malignant fibrous histiocytoma	Characterized by abnormalities at diverse sites including 1q11, 3p12, 11p11, and 19p13
Liposarcoma	t(12;16) (q13;p11)
Myxoid liposarcomas and solitary lipomas	Rearrangements of chromosome 12 with chromosome 16 and other autosomes
Malignant peripheral nerve sheath tumors	17p13 in the region of the *p53* tumor suppressor gene, also 17q11 in the vicinity of the neurofibromatosis 1 gene
Ewing's sarcoma/PNET†	t(11;22) (q24;q11.2–12)
Mesothelioma	1p−, 3p−; both characteristic but nonspecific

* *After Mazanet KH, Antman KH: Sarcomas of soft tissue and bone.* Cancer *1991; 68:463–473.*
† *PNET = primitive neuroectodermal tumor.*

crest origin. This hypothesis is strengthened by the finding that these two tumors have indistinguishable patterns of expression of the protooncogenes c-*myc*, N-*myc*, c-*myb*, c-*mil*/*raf*-1, c-*fes*, and c-*sis*.[52] Osteosarcomas have a 13q− abnormality, which has also been observed in retinoblastoma. This deletion may be responsible for lack of expression of the retinoblastoma-susceptibility tumor suppressor gene (*Rb*) in these tumors.

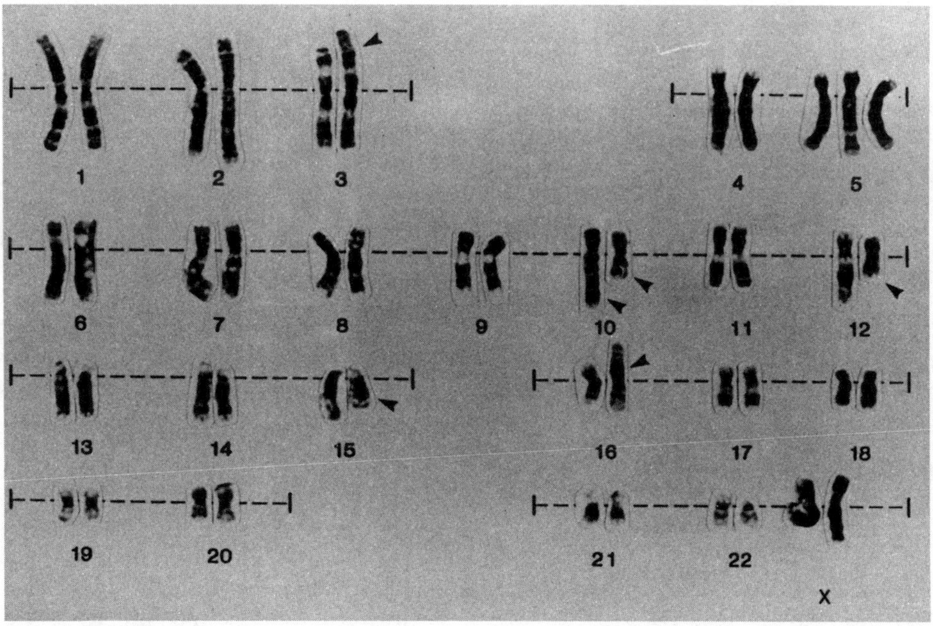

FIG 1–4.
G-banded representative karyotype from myxoid liposarcoma showing the typical t(12;16) (q13;p11) translocation, and other chromosomal rearrangements. (From Sreekantaiah C, Karakousis CP, Leong SPL, et al: Cytogenetic findings in liposarcoma correlate with histopathologic subtypes. *Cancer* 1992; 69:2484–2495. Used by permission.)

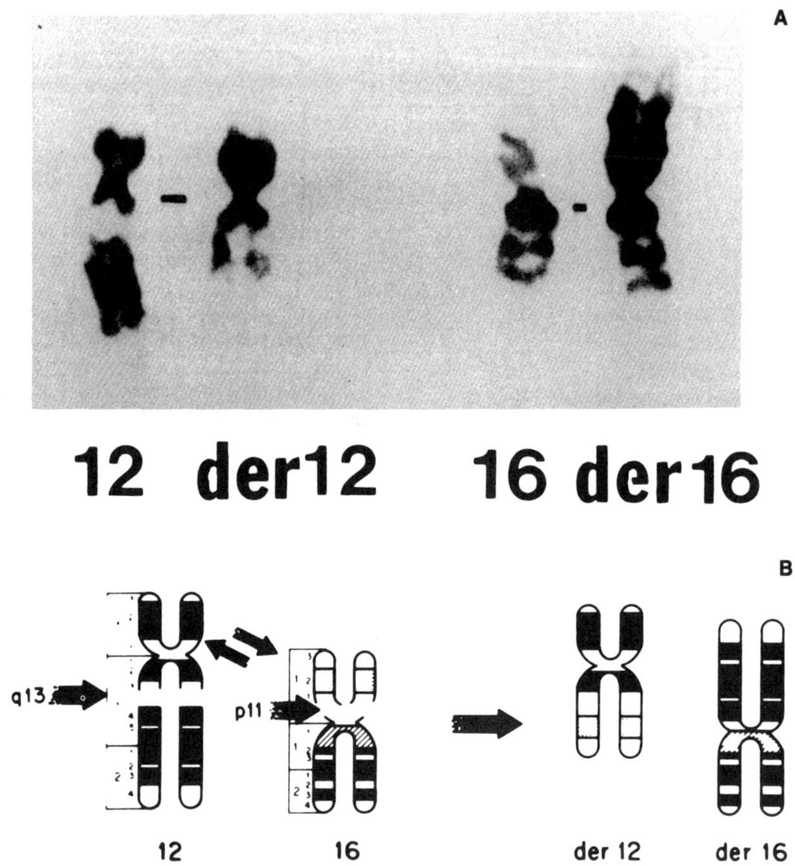

FIG 1–5.
Partial karyotype, **A,** and diagram, **B,** of the translocation t(12;16) (q13;p11) associated with myxoid liposarcoma. (From Dal Cin P, Sandberg AA: Chromosome changes in soft tissue tumors: Benign and malignant. *Cancer Invest* 1989; 7:63–76. Used by permission.)

Of great potential diagnostic interest, Scrable and colleagues[53] found that a muscle-specific gene, *MYOD1,* is expressed in both embryonal and alveolar rhabdomyosarcoma, but not in other pediatric small round cell tumors (Fig 1–6). Furthermore, the embryonal karyotype can be distinguished from that of the alveolar form, because chromosome 11 is homozygous in embryonal rhabdomyosarcoma whereas alveolar rhabdomyosarcoma carries a t(2;13) translocation.

TREATMENT OVERVIEW

Soft-tissue sarcomas are among the most challenging human tumors to treat, because a combination of treatment modalities is often preferred over to a single therapeutic method (Table 1–3). Many clinical trials have attempted to establish optimum treatments for sarcomas of different histological types and in different anatomical locations. In all patients, except perhaps those with widespread metastases, complete surgical excision of the primary sarcoma (resulting in "local control") is highly desirable. Simple excision of the primary tumor (i.e., "shelling out" the sarcoma in the plane of its pseudocapsule) is not acceptable, because local recurrence is then virtually guaranteed. On the other hand, extremely radical resection of all muscles within an anatomical compartment from origin to insertion, or major amputations as described by Pack and Ariel in their classic text on soft-tissue tumors,[54] reduce local recurrence but result in functional impairment.

Although amputation is still best for some patients, current treatment now focuses on

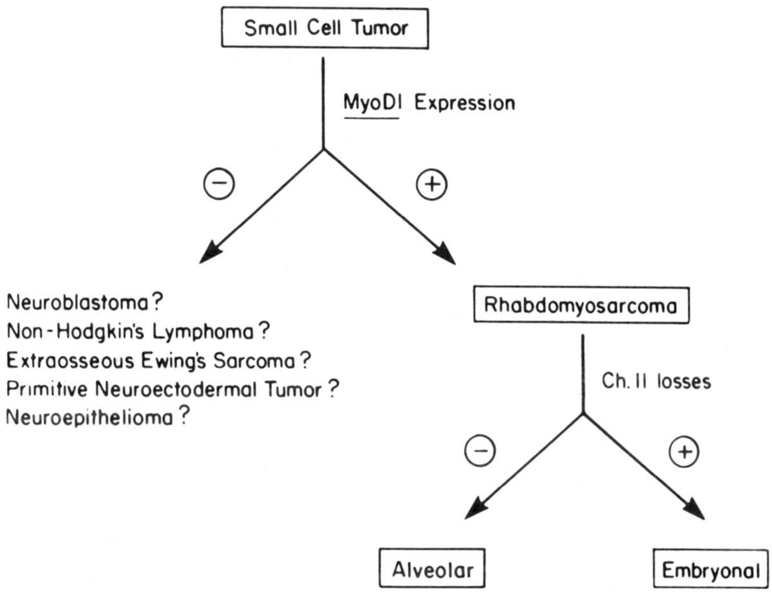

FIG 1–6.
Molecular and cytogenetic methods for diagnosing rhabdomyosarcoma and its subtypes. (From Scrable H, Witte D, Shimada H, et al: Molecular differential pathology of rhabdomyosarcoma. *Genes Chromosomes Cancer* 1989; 1:23–35. Used by permission.)

limb-sparing operations in which the tumor, together with a 2- to 5-cm margin of normal surrounding tissue, is resected. In these en bloc procedures, the surgeon should never "see" the tumor during resection. Postoperative radiation therapy may be directed to the tumor bed to eradicate microscopic residual disease. This is facilitated by intra-operative placement of radiopaque clips at the peripheral and deep margins of the resection. Local tumor control with this type of combined modality therapy should exceed 80%.

Rosenberg and colleagues[55] at the National Cancer Institute (NCI) (Bethesda, MD) per-

TABLE 1–3.
Multimodal Treatment Options for Soft-Tissue Sarcomas

Time of Treatment	Option
Pre-operative	External beam radiation therapy
	Systemic chemotherapy
	Regional (intra-arterial) chemotherapy
Intra-operative	Wide en bloc surgical excision (limb sparing)
	Limb amputation
	Intra-operative radiation therapy
	Brachytherapy (afterloading catheters for iridium 192)
Postoperative	External beam radiation therapy
	Systemic chemotherapy
	Palliative care, including pain control
	Physical therapy and rehabilitation
	Psychosocial counseling for patient and family

TABLE 1–4.
Randomized Trials of Adjuvant Chemotherapy for High-Grade Soft-Tissue Sarcomas*,†

Institute	Anatomical Site	Drugs	Number of Patients	DFS (%)			S (%)		
				−	+	*P*	−	+	*P*
EORTC		A, C, V, D	468	61	61	NS	68	74	NS
	Extremities		233	52	67	NS	74	79	NS
Bordeaux		A, C, V, D	59	16	57	<0.01‡	53	87	<0.01
	Extremities		36	NA	NA	NA	NA	NA	NA
Mayo Clinic		A, V, D, Ad	61	68	65	NS	70	70	NS
	Extremities		48	67	88	0.08	83	63	NS
M. D. Anderson		A, C, V, Ad	47	83	76	NS	NA	NA	NS
	Extremities		43	35	54	<0.05	46	65	NS
NCI	Nonextremity/nonretroperitoneal	A, C, M	31	49	77	0.075	58	68	NS
	Trunk		22	47	92	<0.01	61	82	NS
	Retroperitoneal		15	NA	NA	NA	100	47	0.06§
	Extremities		67	28	54	<0.05	60	54	NS
Scandinavia		A	181	56	62	NS	70	75	NS
	Extremities		155	NS	NS	NS	NS	NS	NS
Pooled DFCI/MGH, ISSG,		A	168	53	66	NS	65	68	NS
ECOG	Extremities		72	64	79	NS	70	79	NS
GOG		A	156	47	59	NS	52	60	NS
UCLA	Extremities	A	119	54	56	NS	74	78	NS
Rizzoli	Extremities	A	77	45	73	<0.05	70	91	<0.05

* *From Mazanet KH, Antman KH: Sarcomas of soft tissue and bone.* Cancer *1991; 68:463–473. Used by permission.*
† *DFS = disease-free survival; S = survival; − = without chemotherapy; + = with chemotherapy; EORTC = European Organization for the Research and Treatment of Cancer; DFCI/MGH = Dana Farber Cancer Institute/Massachusetts General Hospital; ISSG = Intergroup Sarcoma Study Group; ECOG = Eastern Cooperative Oncology Group; GOG = Gynecologic Oncology Group; UCLA = University of California at Los Angeles; NCI = National Cancer Institute; A = doxorubicin; V = vincristine; Ad = dactinomycin; C = cyclophosphamide; D = dacarbazine; M = high-dose methotrexate; NA = not available; NS = not significant.*
‡ *Authors reported metastasis-free survival.*
§ *Two-year survival inferior in chemotherapy arm.*

formed a randomized prospective clinical trial comparing amputation with limb-sparing surgery plus radiation therapy. Both groups received adjuvant chemotherapy. No difference in disease-free or overall survival was found. Interestingly, postoperative quality of life assessments of the patients treated at the NCI by amputation or limb-sparing procedures showed few differences between the two.[56] Therefore, surgeons should not hesitate to recommend amputation to patients for whom attempted limb salvage is unlikely to give a satisfactory result.

New treatment approaches under evaluation include brachytherapy using iridium 192 to control locally invasive or recurrent sarcoma[57–59]; intraoperative radiation therapy[60, 61] or photodynamic therapy[62] for retroperitoneal sarcomas; and pre-operative chemotherapy for high-grade sarcomas greater than 5 cm in diameter.[63] Mohs' micrographic surgery is being evaluated for very low-grade sarcomas, such as dermatofibrosarcoma protuberans,[64] but wide en bloc resection is clearly the standard therapy for high-grade tumors.[65, 66]

Despite local control at the primary sarcoma site, 40% to 60% of patients presenting with localized high-grade lesions will die from metastatic disease.[67] Great effort has been made to develop effective adjuvant chemotherapy protocols to decrease the incidence of distant metastatic disease and improve survival, but a review of results from all published trials suggests that no drug regimen tested to date, with the exception of that for childhood rhabdomyosarcoma, is effective as a postoperative adjuvant for soft-tissue sarcomas (Table 1–4).[39, 67, 68] Adjuvant chemotherapy for adult soft-tissue sarcomas should, therefore, be confined to clinical trials.

CONCLUSION

Soft-tissue sarcomas are a diverse group of malignant tumors arising in connective tissue. The etiology of these neoplasms is largely unknown. New studies of their biological properties, particularly cytogenetics, are yielding exciting new information regarding genetic deletions and translocations that may alter the function of oncogenes and tumor suppressor genes.

Treatment of soft-tissue sarcomas is challenging and requires a multimodal approach to eradicate the primary tumor completely and achieve good extremity function, without compromise of patient survival. Emphasis is placed on limb-sparing surgery, with the addition of radiation therapy to the tumor bed if microscopic tumor is suspected of being left behind after surgical resection. This multidisciplinary treatment approach serves as a model for other malignant solid tumors, although effective adjuvant chemotherapy to decrease the incidence of locally recurrent or metastatic soft-tissue sarcoma in adults is not yet available.

REFERENCES

1. Marco Aurelio Severinius: *De Acedita Abscessum. Natura Libri Octo.* Naples, Beltranus, 1632.
2. Morgagni GB: *The Seats and Causes of Disease Investigated by Anatomy,* letter 39, vol 2 (translated by Benjamin Alexander). London, Millen & Cadell, 1769, pp 364–376.
3. Hajdu SI: *Pathology of Soft Tissue Tumors.* Philadelphia, Lea & Febiger, 1979.
4. Sears HF: Soft tissue sarcoma: A historical perspective. *Semin Oncol* 1981; 8:129–132.
5. Boring CC, Squires TS, Tong T: Cancer statistics, 1991. *CA* 1991; 41:19–36.
6. Chang AE, Rosenberg SA, Glatstein EJ, et al: Sarcomas of soft tissues, in *Cancer: Principles and Practice of Oncology,* ed 3. Philadelphia, J. B. Lippincott, 1989, pp 1345–1398.
7. Okabe T, Suzuki A, Hirono M, et al: Establishment of different clonal strains from a human sarcoma of the stomach: Tumorigenic heterogeneity in athymic nude mice. *Cancer Res* 1983; 43:5456–5461.
8. Donhuijsen K, Budach V, Van Beuningen D, et al: Instability of xenotransplanted soft tissue sarcomas: Morphologic and flow cytometric results. *Cancer* 1988; 61:68–75.
9. Snover DC, Sumner HW, Dehner LP: Variability of histologic pattern in recurrent soft tissue sarcomas originally diagnosed as liposarcoma. *Cancer* 1982; 49:1005–1015.
10. Ewing J: *Neoplastic Diseases: A Treatise on Tumors.* ed. 4, Philadelphia, W. B. Saunders, 1940.
11. Stout AP: Tumors of the musculoskeletal system, in *Atlas of Tumor Pathology,* ed II, Fasc 5. Washington, D.C., Armed Forces Institute of Pathology, 1953.
12. Stewart FW, Treves N: Lymphangiosarcoma in post-mastectomy lymphedema. *Cancer* 1948; 1:64–81.
13. Enzinger FM, Weiss SW: *Soft Tissue Tumors,* ed 2. St. Louis, C. V. Mosby, 1988.

14. Gaynor JJ, Tan CC, Casper ES, et al: Refinement of clinicopathologic staging for localized soft tissue sarcoma of the extremity: A study of 423 adults. *J Clin Oncol* 1992; 10:1317–1329.
15. Moore GE: Foreign body carcinogenesis. *Cancer* 1991; 67:2731–2732.
16. Jennings TA, Peterson L, Axiotis CA, et al: Angiosarcoma associated with foreign body material: A report of three cases. *Cancer* 1988; 62:2436–2444.
17. DuBois GC, Appella E, Law LW, et al: The soluble antigens of BALB/c sarcoma Meth-A: A relationship between a serologically defined tumor-specific surface antigen (TSSA) and the tumor-associated transplantation antigen (TATA). *Transplant Proc* 1981; 13:1765–1773.
18. Wang N, Yu SH, Liener IE, et al: Characterization of high- and low-metastatic clones derived from a methylcholanthrene-induced murine fibrosarcoma. *Cancer Res* 1982; 42:1046–1051.
19. Tanooka H, Tanaka K: Evidence for single-cell origin of 3-methylcholanthrene-induced fibrosarcomas in mice with cellular mosaicism. *Cancer Res* 1982; 42:1856–1858.
20. Fingerhut MA, Halperin WE, Marlow DA, et al: Cancer mortality in workers exposed to 2,3,7,8-tetrachlorodibenzo-p-dioxin. *N Engl J Med* 1991; 324:212–218.
21. Otis CN, Peschel R, McKhann C, et al: The rapid onset of cutaneous angiosarcoma after radiotherapy for breast carcinoma. *Cancer* 1986; 57:2130–2134.
22. Laskin WB, Silverman TA, Enzinger FM: Post-radiation soft tissue sarcomas: An analysis of 53 cases. *Cancer* 1988; 62:2330–2340.
23. Wiklund TA, Blomqvist CP, Raty J, et al: Postirradiation sarcoma: Analysis of a nationwide cancer registry material. *Cancer* 1991; 68:524–531.
24. Edeiken S, Russo DP, Knecht J, et al: Angiosarcoma after tylectomy and radiation therapy for carcinoma of the breast. *Cancer* 1992; 70:644–647.
25. Benda JA, Al-Jurf AS, Benson AB: Angiosarcoma of the breast following segmental mastectomy complicated by lymphedema. *Am J Clin Pathol* 1987; 87:651–655.
26. Garber JE, Goldstein AM, Kantor AF, et al: Follow-up study of twenty-four families with Li-Fraumeni syndrome. *Cancer Res* 1991; 51:6094–6097.
27. Li FP, Fraumeni JF Jr: Predictive testing for inherited mutations in cancer-susceptibility genes. *J Clin Oncol* 1992; 10:1203–1204.
28. Felix CA, Kappel CC, Mitsudomi T, et al: Frequency and diversity of p53 mutations in childhood rhabdomyosarcoma. *Cancer Res* 1992; 52:2243–2247.
29. Brachman DG, Hallahan DE, Beckett MA, et al: p53 gene mutations and abnormal retinoblastoma protein in radiation-induced human sarcomas. *Cancer Res* 1991; 51:6393–6396.
30. Cance WG, Brennan MF, Dudas, ME, et al: Altered expression of the retinoblastoma gene product in human sarcomas. *N Engl J Med* 1990; 323:1457–1462.
31. Chaudhuri PK, Walker MJ, Beattie CW, et al: Distribution of steroid hormone receptors in human soft tissue sarcomas. *Surgery* 1981; 90:149–153.
32. Walker MJ, Lim C, Das Gupta TK, et al: Effects of glucocorticoids on the growth of human fibrosarcoma cell line HT-1080. *Cancer Res* 1986; 46:4927–4932.
33. El-Badry OM, Minniti C, Kohn EC, et al: Insulin-like growth factor II acts as an autocrine growth and motility factor in human rhabdomyosarcoma tumors. *Cell Growth Differ* 1990; 1:325–331.
34. Minniti CP, Maggi M, Helman LJ: Suramin inhibits the growth of human rhabdomyosarcoma by interrupting the insulin-like growth factor II autocrine growth loop. *Cancer Res* 1992; 52:1830–1835.
35. Rous P: A transmissible avian neoplasm (sarcoma of the common fowl). *J Exp Med* 1910; 12:696–705.
36. Rous P: A sarcoma of the fowl transmissible by an agent separable from the tumor cells. *J Exp Med* 1911; 13:397–411.
37. Lerner TL, Skalka AM, Hanafusa H: Integration of Rous sarcoma virus DNA into chicken embryo fibroblasts: No preferred proviral acceptor site in the DNA of clones of singly infected transformed chicken cells. *J Virol* 1981; 40:421–430.
38. Fletcher JA, Weidner N, Corson JM: Laboratory investigation and genetics in sarcomas. *Curr Opinion Oncol* 1990; 2:467–473.
39. Mazanet KH, Antman KH: Sarcomas of soft tissue and bone. *Cancer* 1991; 68:463–473.
40. Sandberg AA, Turc-Carel C, Gemmill RM: Chromosomes in solid tumors and beyond. *Cancer Res* 1988; 48:1049–1059.
41. Becher R, Wake N, Gibas Z, et al: Chromosome change in soft tissue sarcomas. *J Natl Cancer Inst* 1984; 72:823–831.
42. Dal Cin P, Sandberg AA: Chromosome changes in soft tissue tumors: Benign and malignant. *Cancer Invest* 1989; 7:63–76.

43. Turc-Carel C, Dal Cin P, Limon J, et al: Translocation X;18 in synovial sarcoma. *Cancer Genet Cytogenet* 1986; 23:93.
44. Dal Cin P, Rao U, Jani-Sait S, et al: Chromosomes in the diagnosis of soft tissue tumors. I. Synovial sarcoma. *Mod Pathol* 1992; 5:357–362.
45. Shapiro DN, Valentine MB, Sublett JE, et al: Chromosomal sublocalization of the 2;13 translocation breakpoint in alveolar rhabdomyosarcoma. *Genes Chromosomes Cancer* 1992; 4:241–249.
46. Douglass EC, Rowe ST, Valentine M, et al: Variant translocations of chromosome 13 in alveolar rhabdomyosarcoma. *Genes Chromosomes Cancer* 1991; 3:480–482.
47. Limon J, Turc-Carel C, Dal Cin P, et al: Recurrent chromosome translocations in liposarcoma. *Cancer Genet Cytogenet* 1986; 22:93–94.
48. Sreekantaiah C, Karakousis CP, Leong SPL, et al: Cytogenetic findings in liposarcoma correlate with histopathologic subtypes. *Cancer* 1992; 69:2484–2495.
49. Sreekantaiah C, Leong SPL, Karakousis CP, et al: Cytogenetic profile of 109 lipomas. *Cancer Res* 1991; 51:422–433.
50. Mandahl N, Heim S, Willen H, et al: Characteristic karyotypic anomalies identify subtypes of malignant fibrous histiocytoma. *Genes Chromosomes Cancer* 1989; 1:9–14.
51. Rydholm A, Mandahl N, Heim S, et al: Malignant fibrous histiocytomas with a 19p+ marker chromosome have increased relapse rate. *Genes Chromosomes Cancer* 1990; 2:296–299.
52. McKeon C, Thiele CJ, Ross RA, et al: Indistinguishable patterns of protooncogene expression in two distinct but closely related tumors: Ewing's sarcoma and neuroepithelioma. *Cancer Res* 1988; 48:4307–4311.
53. Scrable H, Witte D, Shimada H, et al: Molecular differential pathology of rhabdomyosarcoma. *Genes Chromosomes Cancer* 1989; 1:23–35.
54. Pack GT, Ariel IM: *Tumors of the Soft Somatic Tissues: A Clinical Treatise.* New York, Hoeber-Harper, 1958.
55. Potter DA, Kinsella T, Glatstein E, et al: High-grade soft tissue sarcomas of the extremities. *Cancer* 1986; 58:190–205.
56. Sugarbaker PH, Barofsky I, Rosenberg SA, et al: Quality of life assessment of patients in extremity sarcoma clinical trials. *Surgery* 1982; 91:17–23.
57. Shiu MH, Turnbull AD, Nori D, et al: Control of locally advanced extremity soft tissue sarcomas by function-saving resection and brachytherapy. *Cancer* 1984; 53:1385–1392.
58. Brennan MF, Hilaris B, Shiu MH, et al: Local recurrence in adult soft-tissue sarcoma: A randomized trial of brachytherapy. *Arch Surg* 1987; 122:1289–1293.
59. Schray MF, Gunderson LL, Sim FH, et al: Soft-tissue sarcoma: Integration of brachytherapy, resection, and external irradiation. *Cancer* 1990; 66:451–456.
60. Kinsella TJ, Sindelar WF, Lack E, et al: Preliminary results of a randomized study of adjuvant radiation therapy in resectable adult retroperitoneal soft tissue sarcomas. *J Clin Oncol* 1988; 6:18–25.
61. Willet CG, Suit HD, Tepper JE, et al: Intraoperative electron beam radiation therapy for retroperitoneal soft tissue sarcoma. *Cancer* 1991; 68:278–283.
62. Nambisan RN, Karakousis CP, Holyoke ED, et al: Intraoperative photodynamic therapy for retroperitoneal sarcomas. *Cancer* 1988; 61:1248–1252.
63. Pezzi CM, Pollock RE, Evans HL, et al: Preoperative chemotherapy for soft-tissue sarcomas of the extremities. *Ann Surg* 1990; 211:476–481.
64. Singh B, Sherry JEH II, Lanza JT: Mohs' micrographic surgery in the management of soft tissue sarcomas of the extremities. *Surgery* 1992; 111:718.
65. Shiu MH, Hajdu SI: Management of soft tissue sarcoma of the extremity. *Semin Oncol* 1981; 8:172–179.
66. Lawrence W Jr, Donegan WL, Natarajan N, et al: Adult soft tissue sarcomas: A pattern of care survey of the American College of Surgeons. *Ann Surg* 1987; 205:349–359.
67. Delaney TF, Yang JC, Glatstein E: Adjuvant therapy for adult patients with soft tissue sarcomas. *Oncology* 1991; 5:105–118.
68. Eilber FR, Huth JF, Mirra J, et al: Progress in the recognition and treatment of soft tissue sarcomas. *Cancer* 1990; 65:660–666.

PART 1

Diagnosis

Chapter 2

Radiological Techniques

José Botet

Evaluation of soft-tissue tumors requires a basic knowledge of the capabilities and limitations of the available radiological diagnostic tools. It is, therefore, important for clinicians, surgeons, and therapists to become familiar with these techniques. Some of these tools are extremely complex; detailed explanations of the principles involved are outside the scope of this chapter.

RADIOGRAPHIC STUDIES

Radiographic studies, with and without contrast material, have been the mainstay diagnostic tools of soft-tissue tumors for the past 60 years.[1]

Plain Radiography

Tissues with similar X-ray attenuation cannot be distinguished on plain radiographs; this lack of contrast limits the usefulness of plain X-rays in detecting soft-tissue tumors. Certain characteristics, however, can be observed, such as mass effect, periosteal reaction, and/or involvement of adjacent bony structures.

Plain Tomography

Thin sections of the area of involvement can be studied to look for extension of tumor, bone involvement, or cross-over into another body compartment. This can be seen to some extent with plain tomography, which is especially helpful in the area of the head and neck as well as in closed spaces such as shoulders, ribs, and spine.

Contrast-Enhanced Studies

The oral use of barium as a contrast medium significantly increases the effectiveness of plain radiographs in the evaluation of the gastrointestinal tract by outlining the tumor directly or showing displacement of hollow organs.

The use of intravenous contrast material allows evaluation of the genitourinary tract via plain radiographs. The selective use of tomography significantly increases the yield of this study.

Prior to the advent of computed tomography (CT) and magnetic resonance (MR) imaging, arteriography was the most useful study for these lesions; it is still useful to evaluate extension of tumor, involvement of vessels (arteries and veins), and vascularity, which allows some characterization of the tumors.[2] Selective contrast-enhanced vascular studies allow a comprehensive evaluation of the blood supply of the tumor as well as evidence of invasion of adjacent structures or organs.

ULTRASOUND

Initial clinical work with ultrasound was performed by Wild and Reid in 1956.[3] Since then great advances in the field have occurred, especially with high-resolution small-parts scanner and real-time sonography. Briefly, ultrasound images fluids; the greater the fluid content of the tissue the better the image obtained. Body components lacking water and containing materials such as air, fat, and bone are imaged poorly. Tissues or systems containing fluids, for example bladder, gallbladder, bile ducts, and blood vessels, are demonstrated well. The above statement is a gross simplification, but it gives an idea of the imaging capabilities of ultrasound.

For studying soft tissue, the major advantage of ultrasonography is the ability to differentiate between solid and cystic masses and to give excellent information on the internal structure of these masses. In peripheral studies, the relationship of tumor to neurovascular structures can be demonstrated. In the abdomen and pelvis, involvement of major vessels or adjacent organs can be well demonstrated; due to its multidirectional capabilities, ultrasound enables excellent discrimination of interfaces that is superior to CT. Unfortunately, the interposition of significant amounts of air, such as that present in bowel loops, fat in heavy patients, or bony structures, especially ribs, can all degrade the images significantly. As in many other diseases, the combination of diagnostic modalities, rather than individual studies, allows the correct diagnosis to be made.

COMPUTED TOMOGRAPHY

The development of computed tomography (CT) in the early 1970s provided the radiologist with a new tool that allows imaging of the human body by sectional sequential analysis.[4–6] In contrast to conventional plain radiography, CT allows spatial resolution of the organs and soft-tissue components. By using a highly collimated X-ray beam, scattered radiation is significantly reduced. This together with high-sensitivity, low-noise detectors provides a significant increase in contrast, allowing differentiation of tissues with similar X-ray attenuation values. Further contrast can be obtained by using oral and intravenous contrast media.

In the specific case of soft-tissue tumors, contrast enhancement after administration of intravenous contrast material is directly related to the vascularity of the tumor. In many cases of soft-tissue masses next to hollow organs, the oral administration of iodinated or thin barium solutions provides better discrimination between bowel loops and tumor.

At the present time, CT offers a high degree of spatial resolution, on the order of 1 to 2 mm for most modern scanners. From a practical point of view, tumors as small as 1 to 2 cm can be easily detected using CT, depending on the differential attenuation between tumor and surrounding soft tissues.

Newer scanning techniques, such as dynamic scanning, allow the study of an area of interest during the arterial capillary and venous phases. This sophisticated technique gives greater diagnostic information than conventional CT.

Computed tomography is advantageous in areas that are difficult to evaluate by other diagnostic modalities, especially the head and neck, thoracic and abdominal wall, mesentery, and retroperitoneal and pelvic spaces, where the extension of tumor is not readily appreciated by more conventional diagnostic modalities.

In planning limb-sparing surgery, intravenous contrast-enhanced CT remains the most accurate diagnostic modality to determine the extent of disease and involvement, if any, of neurovascular structures.

Eglund et al.[7] and Neifeld et al.[8] point out that the extent of disease may be overestimated on CT. This is ascribed to lymphatic blockage by the tumor and is more commonly seen in tumors of the extremities. In our experience, we are more concerned with underestimation of the extent of disease. It is important for the surgeon to realize this limitation while planning surgical excision of these tumors.

MAGNETIC RESONANCE IMAGING

Magnetic resonance (MR) imaging is based on the physical principle of nuclear magnetic resonance, which has been used in both organic and inorganic chemistry for the past three decades. This diagnostic modality does not use ionizing radiation and provides multiplanar image reconstruction through any plane (axial, coronal, sagittal, and oblique) in the body for complete definition of surgical anatomy. Lauterbur[9] in 1973 was first able to obtain three-dimensional images of the proton distribution of an object. Since then great advances in computer imaging, mainly derived from research in CT, have been applied extensively to MR imaging, allowing rapid production of two-dimensional images from the magnetic resonance signal.

Imaging protocols are far more complicated in MR than in any other diagnostic procedure. The same area of interest may have to be imaged two or three times using different parameters to obtain the desired information.

Magnetic resonance imaging is an excellent tool for imaging soft-tissue tumors, because it gives superior resolution of muscle, fat, fibrous tissue, and adjacent blood vessels (Fig 2–1).[10, 11] Tumors involving soft tissue typically show different T_1 and T_2 values, allowing them to be imaged at a different gray-scale level. Magnetic resonance can also be used to discriminate adequately between fibrous scar tissue and other soft tissues. It should prove extremely helpful in the evaluation of patients for recurrence at sites of previous surgical procedures. Currently, however, MR does not provide the degree of spatial resolution offered by CT. This is especially true in body imaging; in cases requiring resolution of small lesions, CT may still be superior. With further improvements in equipment, it should not be long before MR replaces CT as the primary mode of evaluating soft-tissue tumors.[12, 13]

PERCUTANEOUS BIOPSY

Percutaneous biopsy of soft-tissue masses is a well-accepted technique.[14] Using fluoroscopy, ultrasound, or CT localization, specimens can be easily and safely obtained and sent for cytological or histological studies. Cytology has an important advantage because results are generally available within a few hours. Most of these procedures are currently done on an outpatient basis.

However, many soft-tissue sarcomas are quite pleomorphic and should be graded histologically according to the area of tumor showing the most aggressive undifferentiated pattern. It is rather common to find large, low-grade tumors with small foci of a much higher grade. In our opinion, percutaneous biopsy of the primary site may produce a false sense of security because the specimen may not represent the true malignancy of the lesion. This is not the case in evaluating suspected recurrences or metastases, because in these cases there is already a representative specimen of the primary site that can be compared with the new tissue samples.

THE TUMOR

Sarcomas arise from mesenchymal cells, which are present in most organs and systems. These cells continue to proliferate throughout life and, in contrast to more differentiated tissues, have a potential to undergo differentiation into a variety of cell lines. Some sarcomas demonstrate easily recognizable origins, such as liposarcomas arising from fat cells or leiomyosarcomas arising from smooth muscle cells. In others, the origin is less recognizable, such as in Kaposi's or Ewing's sarcomas. These tumors can also present with various degrees of differentiation and cell lines within the same tumor. Tumors may range from teratoma, which can be composed of smooth muscle, fat, vessels, cartilage, and/or bone, to a more uniform, less variegated tumor, such as fibrosarcoma. Thus, from a radiological point of view, predicting a specific pathological diagnosis is difficult, although certain types of soft-tissue tumors have a combination of findings that allow the possibility of a more specific diagnosis, especially if multiple imaging tools are used.

RADIOLOGICAL EVALUATION OF PRIMARY SOFT-TISSUE SARCOMAS

Sarcomas of Smooth Muscle

Benign smooth muscle tumors, mainly leiomyomas, are common and are usually found in the uterus, less commonly in the gastrointestinal tract and lung, and rarely in other systems and organs. There are two main malignant varieties, the leiomyosarcoma (Figs 2–2 and 2–3) and the malignant leiomyoblastoma. Both are much rarer than their benign counterparts. These two tumors can be readily differentiated histologically.

The usual presentation is a palpable mass. Plain radiographic evaluation may show a mass effect, which in rare instances shows calcification. This is not a distinctive characteristic because many other varieties of soft-tissue tumors may show calcifications. In cases of tumors arising intra-abdominally or in portions of the gastrointestinal tract, the use of oral or rectal contrast material may prove extremely helpful in delineating the extent of tumor or invasion of the hollow structures. Both leiomyosarcoma and malignant leiomyoblastoma involving the gastrointestinal tract show three main forms of involvement: (1) intraluminal, presenting as polypoid masses that can be sessile and/or pedunculated, (2) intramural, showing thickening of the wall with or without associated ulcerations of the mucosa, and (3) extraluminal, projecting from the serosal surface. In the head and neck regions, as well as in the thorax, the use of conventional tomography is quite helpful, because the area of interest can be studied in minute detail, and evidence of invasion of adjacent bony structures can be easily evaluated.

Angiography tends to show these tumors as hypervascular masses with areas of lucency where necrosis might have occurred. The degree of vascularity does not necessarily correlate with the histological grade of malignancy. The method of choice is CT, which would demonstrate the primary tumor and also evaluate the

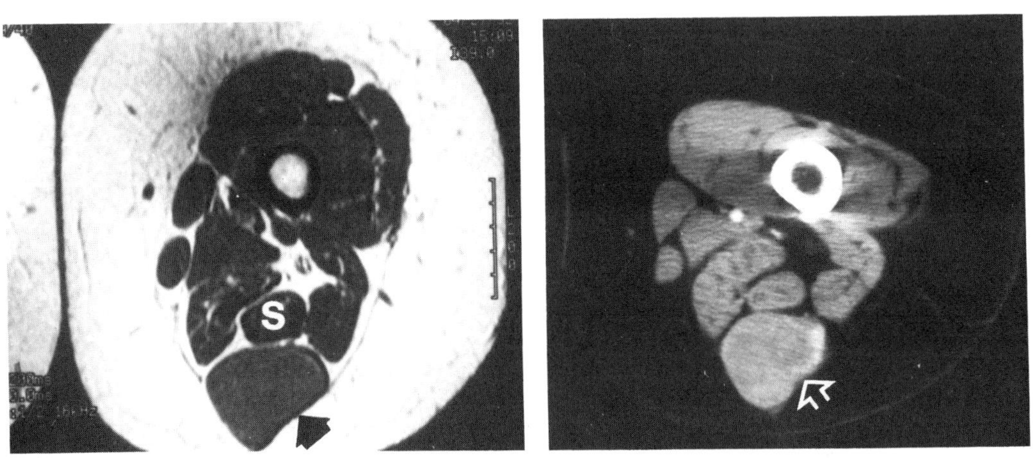

A B

FIG 2–1.
A 47-year-old female with a growing mass in the left posterior thigh. **A,** T1 weighted image demonstrates a soft tissue mass (arrowhead) posterior to the semitendinosus muscle (S). The mass has the same signal intensity as the surrounding striated muscle. **B,** Contrast enhanced CT demonstrates similar findings as the MRI. Note the slightly increased enhancement in the lateral aspect of the tumor (arrowhead).

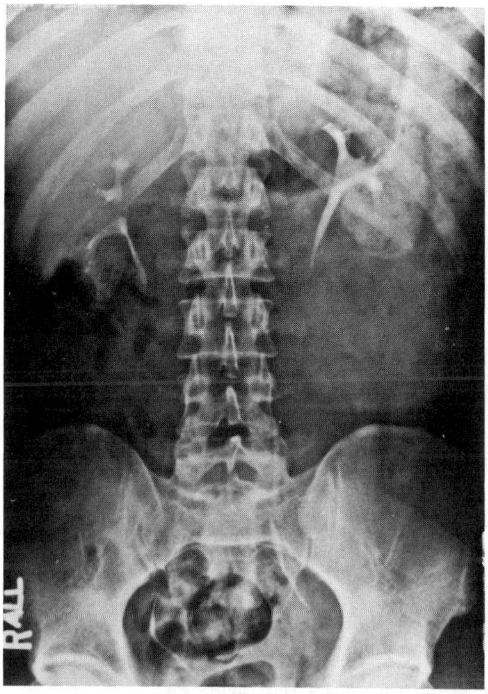

FIG 2–2.
A 29-year-old male with back pain. Intravenous urography shows a large retroperitoneal mass displacing the left ureter medially. Pathological findings: leiomyosarcoma.

metastatic involvement of other organs or lymph nodes. This is especially true in smooth muscle tumors that tend to metastasize readily.

Sarcomas of Striated Muscle

Rhabdomyosarcoma is a rather common form of sarcoma arising in a striated muscle (Figs 2–4 to 2–6). Two general forms with multiple subtypes are recognized. The juvenile form shows a distinct predilection for the urogenital tract as well as head and neck; the adult type shows a predilection for the muscle bundles of the external soft tissues.

Radiological features are similar to those of their smooth muscle counterparts. The water density masses can occasionally calcify nonspecifically, going from a powdery, diffuse appearance to large, amorphous masses that may be central, peripheral, or eccentric.

These tumors commonly involve either the bladder or prostate, and often the initial study is intravenous urography, or cystography for related symptoms. This form of diagnosis has become obsolete with the advent of CT, because the true pelvic extension of these masses and commonly associated lymphadenopathy are not detected by conventional studies. In the adult form, with its predilection for the integuments, the evaluation of surrounding bony structures should be an integral part of diagnosis.

Sarcomas of the Adipose Tissue

Liposarcomas are malignant tumors arising from adipose tissue (Fig 2–7); in our experience, they are by far the most common form of malignant sarcoma. Generally, they affect an older age group, although they do occur in children. Most commonly these sarcomas involve areas such as the thigh, pelvis, and gluteal region.

Compared with other soft tissues, fat is relatively lucent radiographically. Thus, in a thin part of the anatomy, such as an extremity, fatty tumors that are large enough show up as a lucent mass on conventional radiographs. This holds true for benign lipomas; however, liposarcomas vary in relative lucency and cover the whole spectrum from almost total fat to dense tissue, with or without associated calcifications. A lucent mass seen on conventional radiographs does not exclude the diagnosis of liposarcoma, because there can be large areas of benign-appearing fat with a focus or foci of malignant cells. Angiography has been used extensively in the past in the evaluation of these tumors, because typically benign fatty tumors are avascular, whereas their malignant counterparts show mild to moderate hypervascularity.

One important characteristic of liposarcoma is the presence of a pseudocapsule, which tends, in many cases, to give it a benign appearance. Its true nature, however, is best revealed by CT, which shows the true extension of disease as well as involvement of surrounding structures. This is especially helpful in the retroperitoneum, where deep-seated structures are not amenable to evaluation by more conventional studies.

Magnetic resonance imaging is also quite useful in the evaluation of the true extension of these tumors. Recent reports[15–18] suggest that MR provided better definition of tumor, fibrous tissue, and blood vessels than CT.

The radiological differential diagnosis of liposarcomas includes three main entities: teratoma, angiomyolipoma, and fat necrosis. Teratomas, according to the predominant tissue

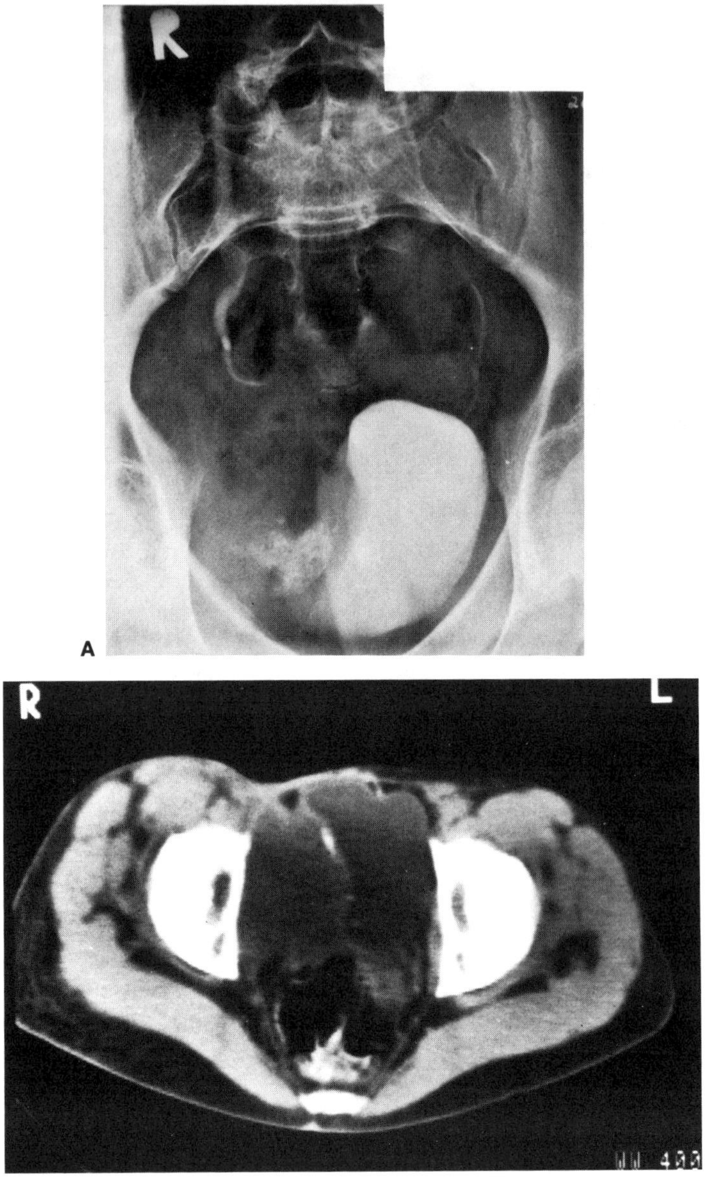

A

B

FIG 2–3.
Recurrent leiomyosarcoma. **A,** intravenous pyelogram. **B,** computed tomography.

component, can present as lucent fatty tissue with areas of increased soft-tissue density and calcifications; thus, mimicking the appearance of the more aggressive liposarcoma, they tend to occur in a younger age group and can involve practically any compartment, including the central nervous system. Angiomyolipomas contain three components, mainly vessels, smooth muscle, and fat. Two main forms are recognized. The infiltrating angiolipoma, which although not metastasizing is locally invasive, shows hypervascularity on angiography and poor definition of margins on CT, suggesting its infiltrating capabilities. It tends to recur if not totally excised. The noninfiltrating variety tends to be better defined, well encapsulated, and generally found in the subcutaneous tissues. Fat necrosis can present as a soft-tissue mass that may have

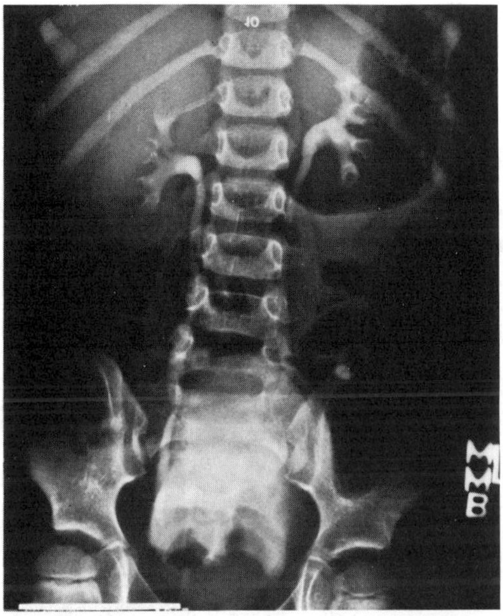

FIG 2–4.
A 3-year-old male with a pelvic mass. Intravenous urography shows elevation of bladder by enlarged prostate. Pathological findings: embryonal rhabdomyosarcoma.

amorphous calcifications similar to phleboliths. There is usually a history of trauma or injection, especially in the gluteal region.

Sarcomas of Vascular Origin

Two main forms of sarcoma, hemangiopericytoma and angiosarcoma, arise from the blood vessel cells.

Hemangiopericytoma (Fig 2–8) arises from the pericytes surrounding the capillaries. This rare tumor can occur in most body compartments, including the central nervous system, although most reported cases occur in the extremities. Plain radiographic evaluation is for the most part useless, because these tumors tend to be rather deep seated; occasionally, like other forms of soft-tissue sarcoma, they may show calcification and can show invasion of adjoining bone structures. These tumors tend to have a distinctive angiographic picture of tortuous vessels that lack the normal tapering. There is very early venous filling, mimicking an arteriovenous malformation, although the soft-tissue enhancement of the tumor persists late

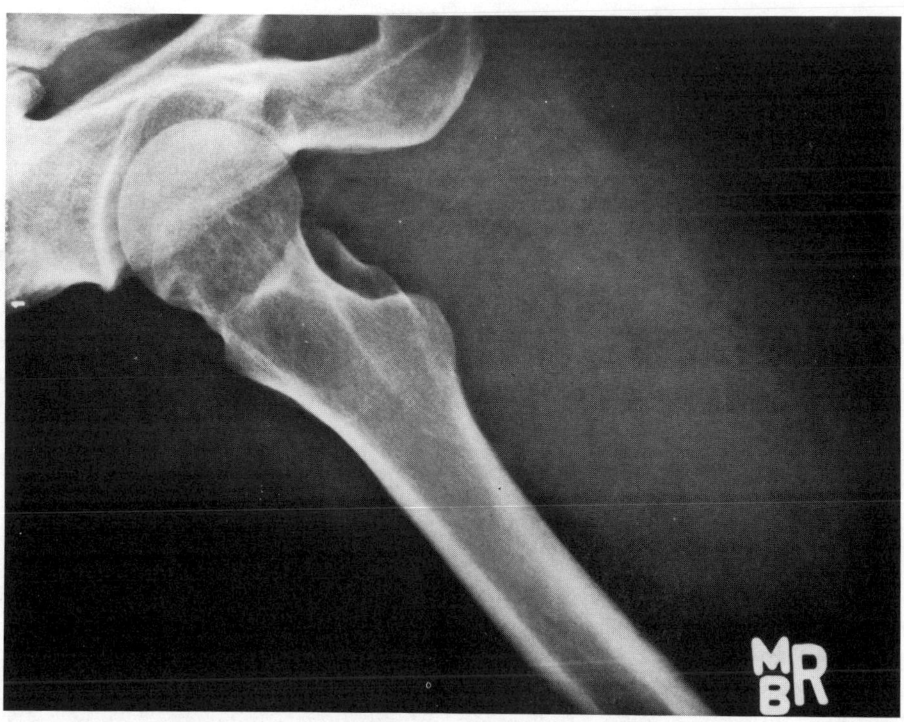

FIG 2–5.
A 37-year-old male with a mass in the medial portion of the right upper thigh. Plain radiograph shows mass with loss of fat planes. Pathological findings: embryonal rhabdomyosarcoma.

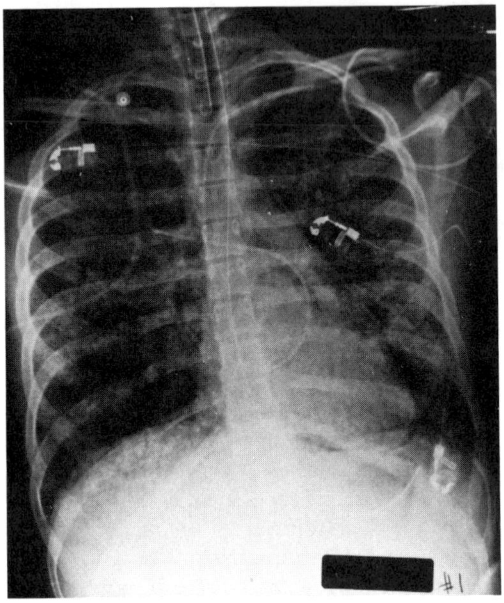

FIG 2–6.
Opportunistic infection by cytomegalovirus in an immunosuppressed patient with embryonal rhabdomyosarcoma of the prostate.

into the venous phase. Computed tomography and MR can define the extent of these tumors to a better degree than the other diagnostic modalities.

Angiosarcoma (Fig 2–9) and hemangioendothelioma are quite rare and, although they can occur in both soft tissue and bone, they are more commonly seen in the former. Conventional radiographic examinations are rarely useful because these tend to be deep-seated tumors. In the extremities, given the nearness of the neurovascular package to the bone, they are occasionally detected radiographically by their invasion of the adjacent bone. Arteriographically they show marked tortuousity of the arteries and veins, with pooling of contrast material and occasional encasement of vessels. Computed tomography and MR are useful, especially in evaluating marrow invasion of the adjacent bones. It is well to remember that smooth muscle sarcomas can arise from the walls of vessels.

Lymphangiosarcoma (Fig 2–10) is a rare tumor that arises in areas of chronically obstructed lymph drainage, such as in postmastectomy patients. Its presence is usually detected by ultrasound or CT. To our knowledge, none of these tumors has been imaged by MR.

Sarcomas of Nerve Sheath

There are two main types of nerve sheath sarcomas: malignant neurilemmoma and malignant schwannoma (Fig 2–11). They are relatively rare tumors.

As in sarcomas of vascular origin, the nearness of the neurovascular package to the bones, especially in the axial appendicular skeleton, makes it relatively easy for these tumors to invade the adjoining bony structures. Such invasion can be detected by conventional radiographs. However, evaluation of the true extent of the tumor, as well as invasion of the spinal canal, requires the use of both myelography and either CT or MR.

Sarcomas of Fibrous Tissues

Sarcomas of fibrous tissues can originate from both bone and soft tissue and tend to spread to involve adjacent structures. They include fibrosarcoma (Fig 2–12), malignant fibrous histiocytoma (Figs 2–13 and 2–14), and desmoid tumors.

Fibrosarcoma

Fibrosarcomas are often aggressive tumors that tend to invade surrounding structures. On conventional radiographs, they generally appear as a vague soft-tissue mass that may show destruction of surrounding bony structures. Angiographically, they tend to be hypervascular; as in other soft-tissue sarcomas, the degree of vascularity roughly correlates with the histological grade, that is, the greater the vascularity, the higher the grade of malignancy. Computed tomography and MR are quite helpful in defining extension into other compartments as well as into bone marrow.

Malignant Fibrous Histiocytoma

Like the fibrosarcoma, the malignant fibrous histiocytoma arises from bone and soft tissues. Malignancy can range from the benign fibrous histiocytoma to the fully malignant, highly metastatic variant. Like fibrosarcoma, it tends to occur in an older age group, although its presence in a younger population is not uncommon. The radiological features are essentially the same as for fibrosarcoma, which should always be included in the differential diagnosis.

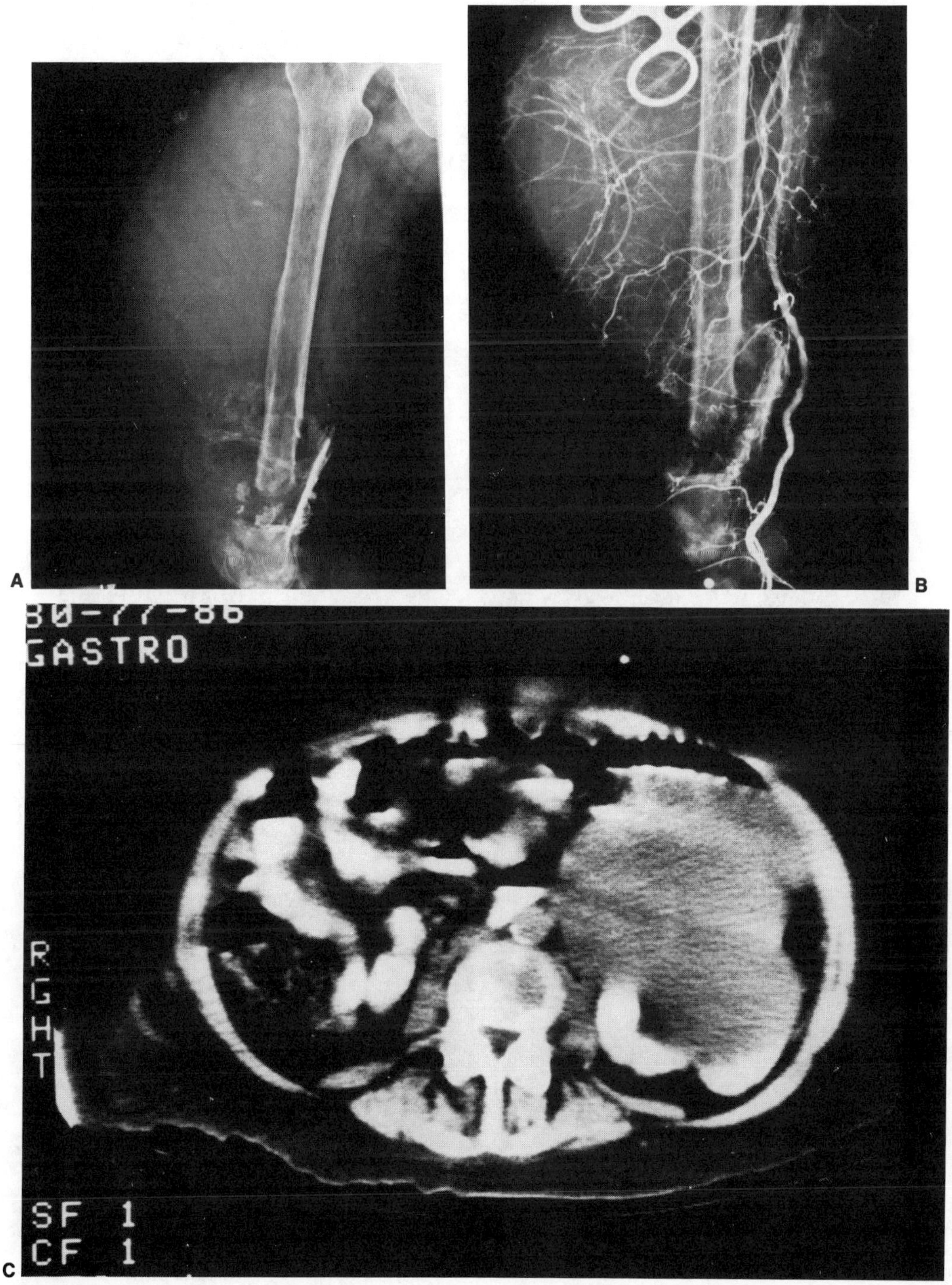

FIG 2–7.
A 61-year-old female with a large mass in the right femur. **A,** the plain radiograph shows a large dense mass with multiple calcifications; note bone involvement with fracture. **B,** the angiogram shows moderate hypervascularity. **C,** computed tomography shows abdominal metastases. Pathological findings: liposarcoma.

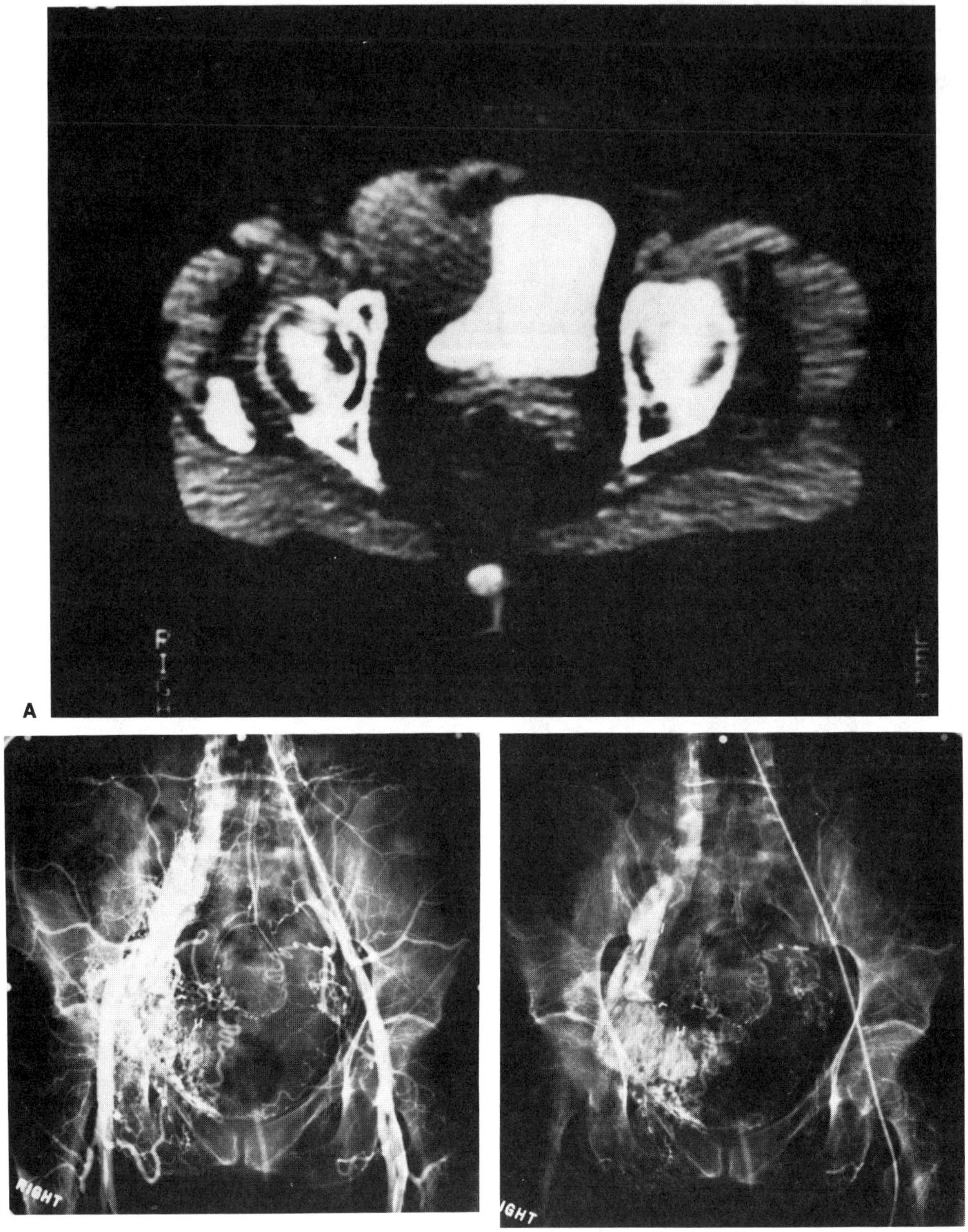

FIG 2–8.
A 59-year-old female with a pelvic mass. **A,** computed tomography shows a mass displacing the bladder. On angiography, **B**, the arterial phase shows a highly vascular soft-tissue tumor, and **C**, the early venous phase shows gross arteriovenous shunting. Pathological findings: hemangiopericytoma.

Desmoid Tumor

A desmoid tumor is a rare, locally invasive tumor. Occurrence can be both intra-abdominal and extra-abdominal. Rarely, it can arise from bone. Desmoid tumor is commonly associated with Gardner's syndrome of multiple polyposis, or it can be of primary origin. In either case, it is aggressive and can recur. Rarely, there is malignant degeneration. Conventional radiographic examination is, for the most part, use-

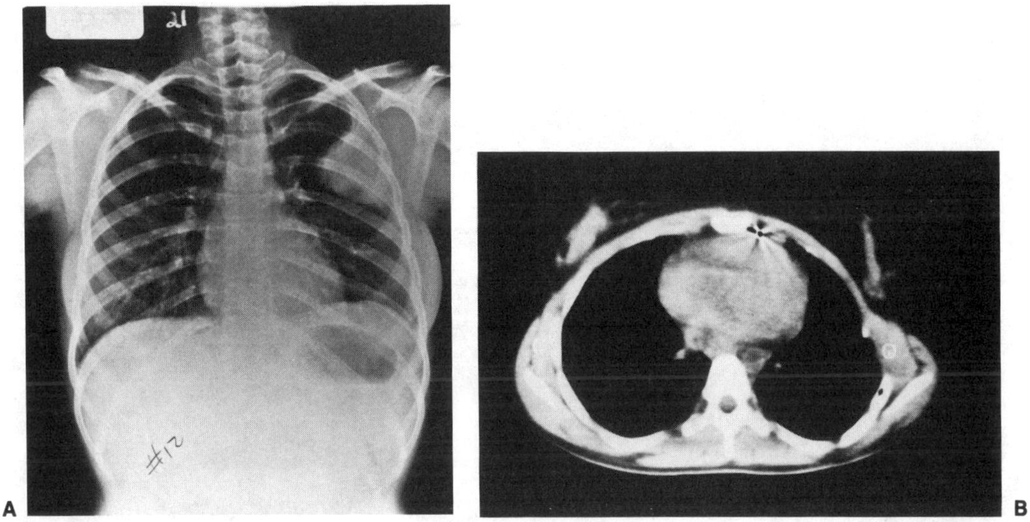

FIG 2–9.
A 13-year-old female with a mass in the left chest wall. **A,** the plain radiograph shows a large soft-tissue mass with minimal rib destruction. **B,** computed tomography 1 year after surgical resection shows recurrent tumor. Pathological findings: angiosarcoma of the chest wall.

less. Computed tomography and, to a lesser degree, ultrasound are used to evaluate the size and extension of these masses. Angiography typically shows extensive splaying of vessels with a faint blush at the end of the capillary phase. The tumor can be massive, displacing adjacent structures. In this case, tumor presence may be documented by conventional barium examinations.

Soft-Tissue Sarcoma of Bone, Cartilage, and Synovial Tissue

Extraosseous osteogenic sarcoma and chondrosarcoma are quite rare. The presence of a soft-tissue mass is the common radiological feature. The calcification pattern reflects the origin and allows a better differentiation among osteoid, chondroid, and the fleck calcifications that are seen in some synovial sarcomas.

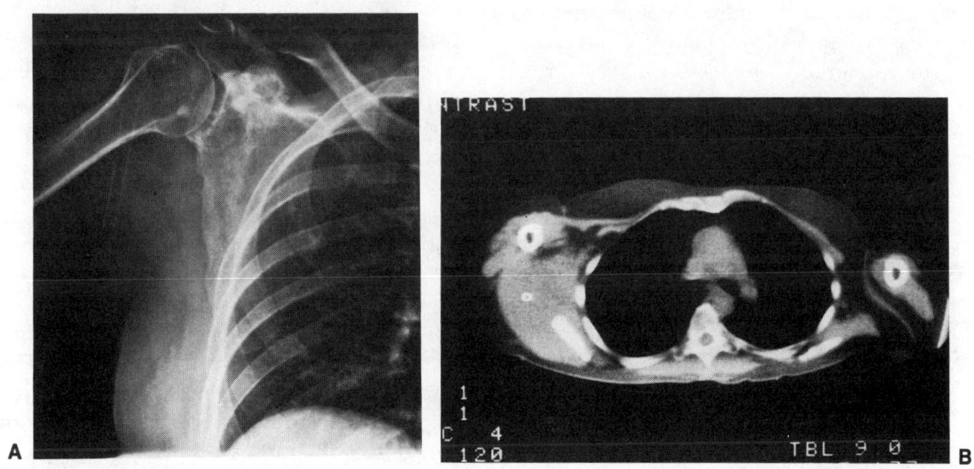

FIG 2–10.
A 54-year-old female with a right axillary mass. **A,** the plain radiograph shows a soft-tissue mass with destruction of the right scapula. **B,** computed tomography shows a large soft-tissue mass involving the right scapula. Pathological findings: lymphangiosarcoma.

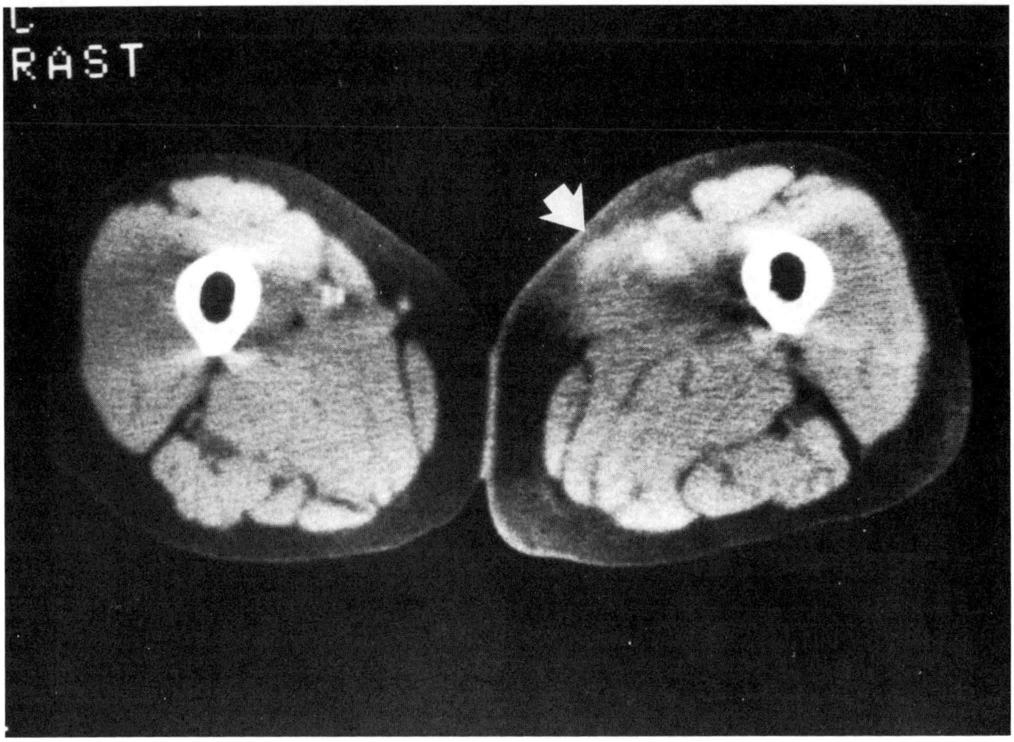

FIG 2–11.
A 70-year-old female with a left medial thigh mass. Computed tomography with intravenous contrast material shows a mildly enhancing lesion surrounding the neurovascular package. Pathological findings: malignant schwannoma.

Angiographic evaluation shows hypervascularity in both osteogenic and synovial sarcoma. The rare case of juxtacortical osteogenic sarcoma, as well as chondrosarcoma, tends to show a lesser degree of vascularity. In all cases, the relative degree of hypervascularity correlates well with the pathological grading.

Computed tomography and MR are helpful in evaluating the true extension of the tumor as well as involvement of adjacent structures.

RADIOLOGICAL EVALUATION OF RECURRENCE AND METASTASES FROM PRIMARY SOFT-TISSUE SARCOMA

The diagnostic work-up in patients with soft-tissue sarcoma must include a careful search for evidence of metastasis. This is a crucial step in the pretreatment evaluation of these patients. Major decisions on the therapeutic approach depend on finding the primary site and the presence or absence of metastatic involvement.

Most of these tumors tend to metastasize distally. Multiple pathways are available, the most common being hematogenous. Other pathways include the lymphatic system and the portal venous system in the case of primary soft-tissue sarcoma of the gastrointestinal tract. A less common pathway is metastasis to the central nervous system via cerebrospinal fluid circulation. Given the multitude of pathways, the site of origin and primary system are major factors in the evaluation of metastatic involvement.

Once the primary tumor has been removed or treated, examination follow-up is an essential part of patient management. Both local recurrence or metastatic involvement and chemotherapy or radiotherapy response must be evaluated. The diagnostic tools employed in these cases are essentially the same as those used for the evaluation of the primary site.

A

B

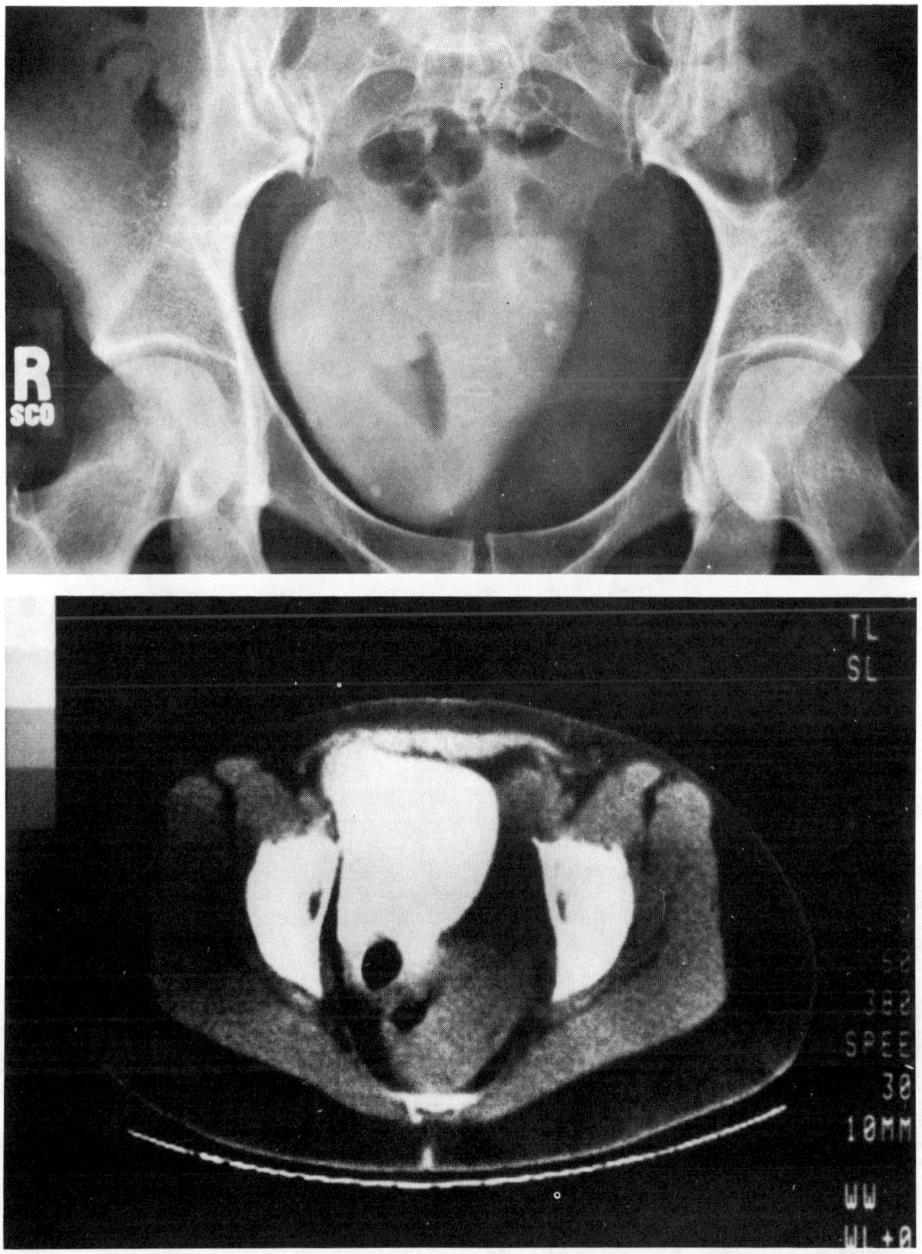

FIG 2–12.
A 38-year-old female with a pelvic mass. **A,** intravenous urography shows displacement of the bladder by a pelvic soft-tissue mass. **B,** computed tomography demonstrates a large mass following the neurovascular package into the left sciatic notch. Pathological findings: neurofibrosarcoma.

Thoracic Metastases

Metastatic spread in the thorax can involve any of the anatomical structures present; the most usual sites are lung parenchyma, pleura, mediastinum, and bone structures.

Plain radiography of the chest allows detection of involvement of lung parenchyma at a relatively early stage; however, information on involvement of either pleura or mediastinum is suboptimal. Computed tomography and MR are

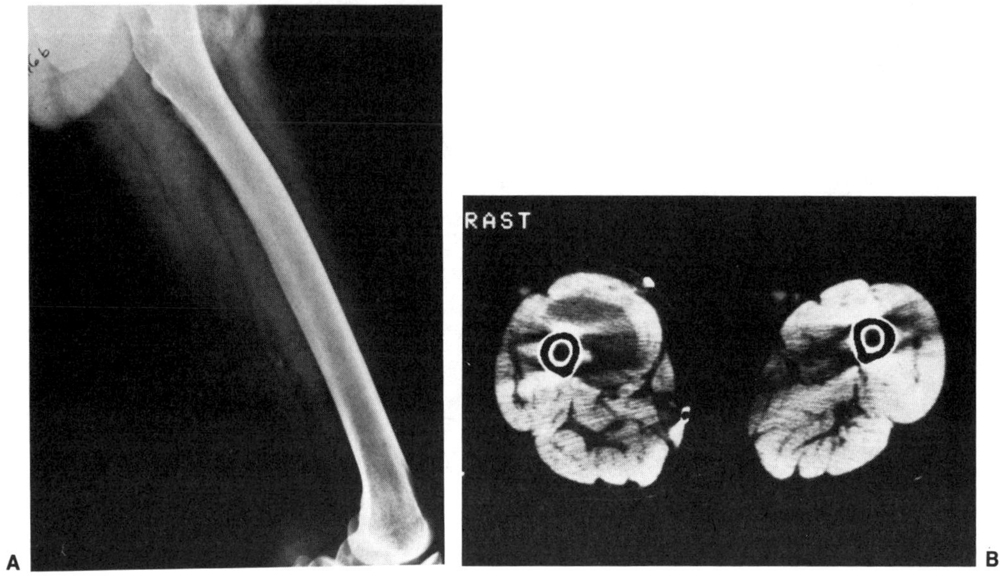

FIG 2–13.
A 58-year-old male with a palpable mass in the right lower thigh. **A,** the plain radiograph suggests a soft-tissue mass. **B,** computed tomography demonstrates the mass and its relationship to the neurovascular package. Pathological findings: malignant fibrous histiocytoma.

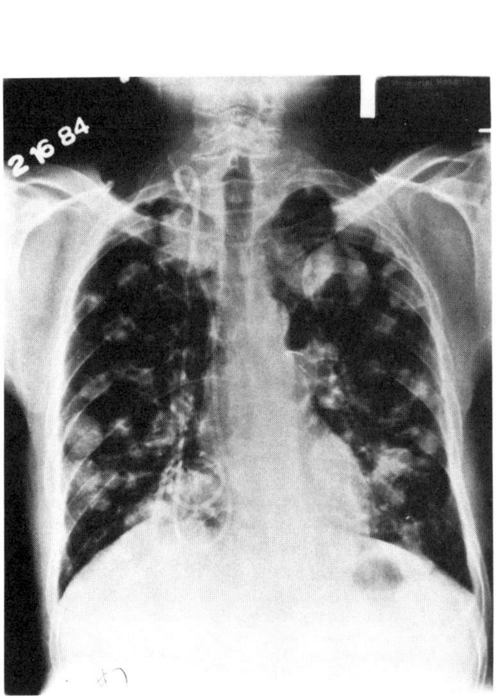

FIG 2–14.
A 58-year-old male with metastatic malignant histiocytoma.

the methods of choice in evaluating these structures. Radionuclide bone-scanning procedures are far more sensitive, although less specific, in the evaluation of early bone involvement.

Central Nervous System Involvement

Patients with CNS involvement may or may not be symptomatic. The current state of the art allows relatively easy evaluation of the central nervous system via CT or MR. These modalities can detect small lesions in both brain and meninges as well as the calvarium. In cases of suspected involvement of the spinal canal, myelography is extremely helpful in the evaluation of localized or generalized disease.

Abdominal and Pelvic Metastases

The site of metastatic involvement in the abdomen and pelvis is dependent on the location of the primary site; an example is hepatic and mesenteric involvement in primary gastrointestinal sarcoma.

The abdomen can be studied in its entirety by both CT and MR. In MR imaging, there is some degradation of the image quality close to the diaphragm due to respiratory motion; in most instances, respiratory gating is required to evaluate structures close to the diaphragm.

Ultrasound is helpful in the evaluation of major abdominal organs. The quality of the ultrasound study is to a great degree dependent on patient characteristics such as intestinal gas. However, ultrasound is a viable alternative in the evaluation of liver, spleen, kidneys, and pelvic organs.

Lymphatic Metastases

Evaluation of lymphatic involvement is not easy. Two main methods are available, lymphangiography and either CT or MR.

Lymphangiography demonstrates only the lymphatics and nodes draining the subcutaneous tissues of the extremities; however, there is good demonstration of the internal architecture of the nodes, and metastatic replacement can be diagnosed even in normal-sized nodes. The main disadvantage is lack of visualization of the lymphatics draining the internal organs.

Computed tomography and MR demonstrate changes in the size of nodes. This information is nonspecific because inflammation, postsurgical changes, or non-neoplastic processes may account for this enlargement. Lymph nodes are considered abnormal when they exceed a diameter of 3 cm in the pelvis and 1.5 cm in the para-aortic paracaval space, or mediastinum. Computed tomography and MR offer no information regarding the internal architecture of the lymph nodes.

CONCLUSION

The importance of adequate pretreatment evaluation must be stressed, including evaluation of the primary site as well as a careful search for evidence of metastatic involvement. The acquisition of reproducible baseline studies is also important to evaluate development of metastases, recurrences, and response to therapy.

REFERENCES

1. Lindell MM, Wallace S, deSantos LA, et al: Diagnostic technique for the evaluation of the soft tissue sarcoma. *Semin Oncol* 1981; 8:160–171.
2. Hudson TM, Hass G, Enneking WF, et al: Angiography in the management of musculoskeletal tumors. *Surg Gynecol Obstet* 1975; 141:11–21.
3. Wild JJ, Reid JM: Intraluminal sonogram in the rectum. *Br J Phys Med* 1956; 19:248.
4. deSantos LA, Goldstein HM, Murray JA, et al: Computed tomography in the evaluation of musculoskeletal neoplasms. *Radiology* 1978; 128:89.
5. Barlow RE, Goldman ML: Computed tomography of the skeletal system. *Comput Tomogr* 1978; 2:27–35.
6. Bulcke JA, Termote JL, Palmers Y, et al: Computed tomography of the human skeletal muscular system. *Neuroradiology* 1979; 17:127–136.
7. Eglund NO, Egund N, Ekelund L, et al: CT of soft tissue tumors. *AJR* 1981; 137:725.
8. Neifield JP, Walsh JW, Lawrence W: Computed tomography in the management of soft tissue tumors (Abstract). *Radiology* 1983; 147:911.
9. Lauterbur PC: Image formation by induced local interactions: examples employing NMR. *Nature* 1973; 242:190.
10. Crooks L, Arakawa M, Hoenninger J, et al: Nuclear magnetic resonance whole-body imager operating at 3.5 KGauss. *Radiology* 1982; 143:169–174.
11. AMA Council on Scientific Affairs: Musculoskeletal applications of magnetic resonance imaging. *JAMA* 1989; 262:2420–2427.
12. Chang AE, Matory YL, Dwyer AJ, et al: Magnetic resonance imaging *versus* computed tomography in the evaluation of soft tissue tumors of the extremities. *Ann Surg* 1987; 205:340–348.
13. Bland KI, McCoy DM, Kinard RE, et al: Application of magnetic resonance imaging and computed tomography as an adjunct to the surgical management of soft tissue sarcomas. *Ann Surg* 1987; 205:473–480.
14. Akerman M, Idvall I, Rydholm A: Cytodiagnosis of soft tissue tumors and tumor-like conditions by means of fine needle aspiration biopsy. *Arch Orthoped Traum Surg* 1980; 96:61–67.
15. Herrlin K, Ling LB, Petterson H, et al: Gadolinium-DTPA enhancement of soft tissue tumors in MRI. *Acta Radiol* 1990; 31:233.

16. Sundaraman M, McGuire MH, Herbold DR: Magnetic resonance imaging of soft tissue masses: an evaluation of fifty-three histologically proven tumors. *Mag Res Imag* 1988; 6:237.
17. Fletcher BD, Hanna GL: Musculoskeletal neoplasms: dynamic Gd-DTPA enhanced MRI. *Radiology* 1990; 177:287.
18. Erlemann R, Reiser MF, Vasallo P: Musculoskeletal neoplasms: static and dynamic Gd-DTPA-enhanced MR imaging. *Radiology* 1989; 171:767.

Chapter 3

Radionuclide Imaging of Soft-Tissue Sarcomas

Samuel D. J. Yeh

Richard S. Benua

Soft-tissue sarcomas are relatively uncommon tumors that involve a great variety of mesenchymal tissues and show various degrees of malignancy. Because radionuclide procedures are simple, sensitive, and rapidly performed, it is logical to use them as ancillary tools to study the biological nature, monitor the clinical course, and assist in the early diagnosis of sarcomas. Reports of radionuclide studies in soft-tissue sarcomas are scarce and consist largely of case reports, probably due to the relatively low incidence and diverse histological types of the tumor. The sensitivity and specificity of radionuclide studies in soft-tissue sarcomas need better definition, and it is also necessary to compare the merits and difficulties of various imaging modalities. This chapter discusses studies of the primary lesion, work-up for metastatic disease, monitoring of therapeutic response, and assessment of complications encountered during therapy.

STUDIES OF THE PRIMARY TUMOR

There are several reports demonstrating tumor uptake of bone-seeking radionuclides[1–5] or citrate Ga 67[6–8] in primary soft-tissue sarcomas. The uptake in the area of tumor can be correlated with findings on conventional radiological examinations and on computed tomograms. Computed tomography (CT) readily distinguishes soft-tissue lesions from surrounding structures. In the future, magnetic resonance (MR) images, which show alteration in proton concentration and prolongation of T_1 and T_2 relaxation times in tumor tissues, may to some degree replace radionuclide studies. The uptake of citrate Ga 67 is probably related to the degree of soft-tissue involvement, and uptake of bone-seeking radiopharmaceuticals such as methylene diphosphonate (MDP) Tc 99m is primarily related to bony involvement. Different histological subtypes do not have specific features in Ga 67- or Tc 99m-labeled MDP images. To the best of our knowledge, there is no tumor-localizing radiopharmaceutical suitable for early detection of soft-tissue sarcoma or any agent that allows differentiation of one subtype from another.

With the expansion of radioimmunodetection procedures and production of large varieties of specific antibodies, attempts have also been made to produce monoclonal antibody to soft-tissue sarcoma. Cytotoxic antibody to human leiomyosarcoma has been successfully produced.[9] It remains to be seen whether radio-

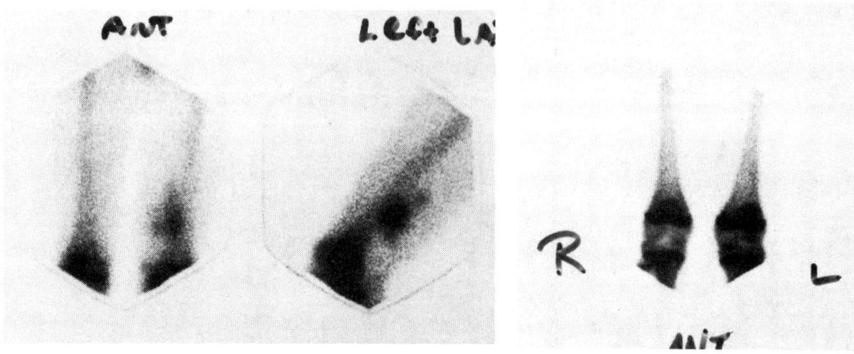

A B

FIG 3–1.
A, Gallium and **B,** MDP bone scans from a patient with spindle cell sarcoma in the left thigh.

immunodetection with specific antibodies to soft-tissue sarcoma will be as useful in sarcoma patients as it has been in patients with colorectal carcinoma,[10] melanoma,[11] ovarian tumor,[12] germ-cell tumor,[13, 14] thyroid carcinoma,[15] and renal cell carcinoma.[16]

In our institute, N 13-labeled amino acids have been successfully synthesized and studied in patients with various tumors, including soft-tissue sarcoma.[17–19] We have demonstrated tumor uptake of N 13-labeled glutamate, methionine, and the nonmetabolized α-aminoisobutyric acid (AIB), and uptake of ammonia N 13 has been demonstrated by ourselves and others.[20] Whether such uptake represents an increased nitrogen pool, increased blood flow, or alteration in protein or amino acid metabolism of the tumor tissue is presently unknown.

The tumor-to-nontumor ratios in N 13-labeled amino acid studies, however, are quite comparable with those noted in the gallium studies. Specificity and sensitivity of the amino acid uptake scans are not better than those of the gallium scans. There was no case in which the gallium scan was negative while the labeled amino acid image was unquestionably positive. It is possible that amino acid studies would provide further understanding of tumor behavior, but they do not assist in early detection or contribute to the differential diagnosis of the various histological types.

Figure 3–1 shows abnormal uptake of gallium but normal uptake of MDP in a midthigh mass of a 15-year-old patient with spindle cell sarcoma. The tumor-to-muscle ratio 72 hours after injection of citrate Ga 67 was between 20 to 1 and 34 to 1. Figure 3–2 illustrates the gradual worsening of a lesion in the right thigh of a patient with malignant fibrous histiocytoma. The initial high uptake of gallium was in contrast to relatively normal MDP uptake in the region of tumor. Figure 3–3 shows a scan of a patient with giant cell-type malignant fibrous histiocytoma in the right groin. Uptake of both citrate Ga 67 and methionine N 13 was found. Increased gallium uptake was noted in the region of local recurrences in most of our patients. Figure 3–4 compares MDP and Ga 67 in another patient with malignant fibrous histiocytoma who had little response to chemotherapy during a period of 3 months; although the bone scan shows increased uptake in the distal femur and proximal tibia, uptake in the tumor area was minimal. The tumor readily concentrates the citrate Ga 67.

WORK-UP FOR METASTATIC DISEASE

It is known that fibromatous tumors have a low local recurrence rate whereas desmoid tumors have a high local recurrence rate.[21] After local excision of desmoid tumors, there is approximately a 64% recurrence rate and death in 11% due to local extension into vital organs.[22] Synovial sarcoma commonly metastasizes to regional lymph nodes, bone, and lungs.[23] Malignant fibrous histiocytoma, a rather common soft-tissue sarcoma, tends to recur locally or metastasize to the lungs, but rarely to the regional nodes, liver, bones, or mesentery.[24] Liposarcoma usually presents as a bulky and infiltrating tumor that invades skin, blood vessels, nerve, and bone. In about 12% of patients with liposarcoma, a second primary sarcoma can be found in colon, breast, lungs, or ovaries.[25] Leiomyosarcoma usually is well circumscribed or pseudoencapsulated, has a low to moderate degree of malignancy, and involves primarily the uterus

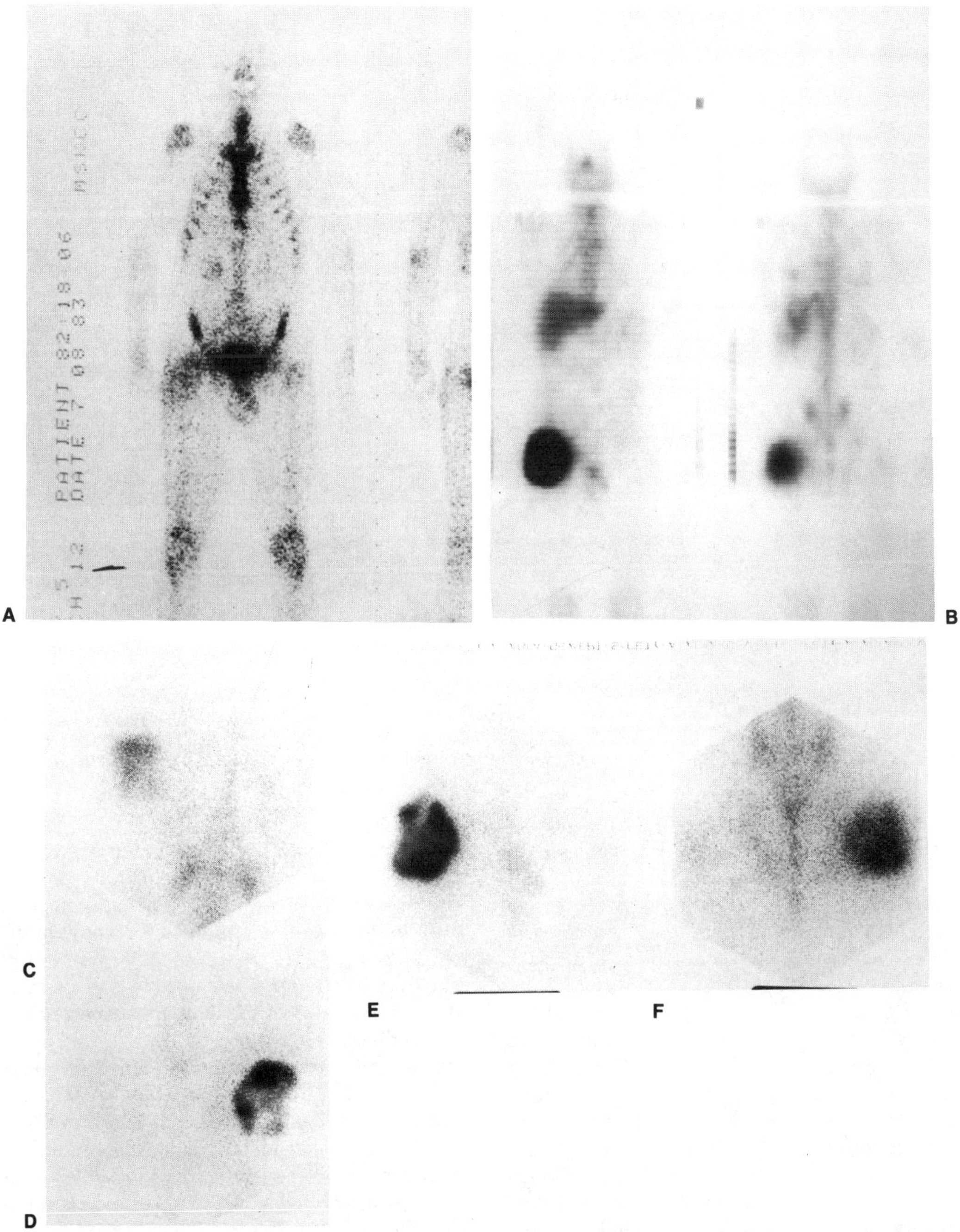

FIG 3–2.
A, Total body MDP and **B,** gallium scans of a patient with malignant fibrous histiocytoma in the right thigh. Camera views of gallium study (**C,** anterior and **D,** posterior) showed more uptake in the right buttock. Camera images 1 month later (**E,** anterior and **F,** posterior) showed more intense uptake over a wider area.

or the gastrointestinal tract. Metastases can occur in the lungs and lymph nodes.[26] Embryonal rhabdomyosarcoma arises from undifferentiated mesoderm rather than from more differentiated muscle precursors. It is common in children and represents about 4% to 9% of all malignant tumors in patients under 15 years of age. Embryonal rhabdomyosarcoma is prone to occur where striated muscle is not usually found. Visceral metastases are common.[27] Hem-

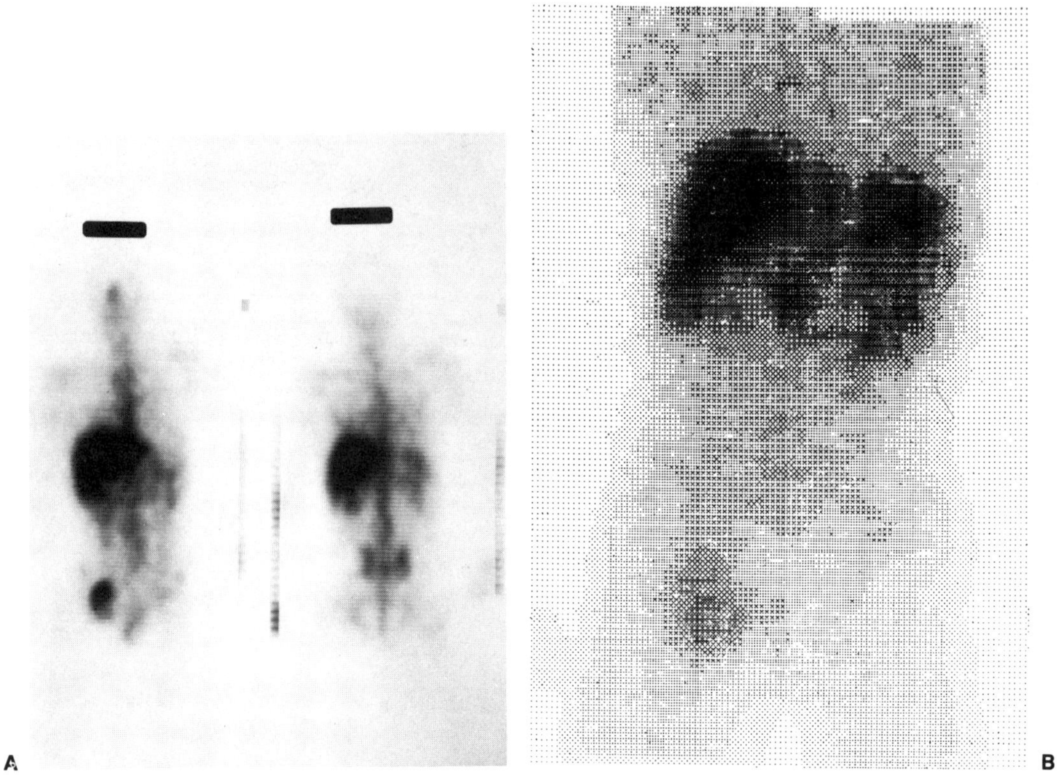

FIG 3–3.
A, Gallium and **B,** methionine N 13 studies of a patient with giant cell-type malignant fibrous histiocytoma.

angiosarcoma has a local recurrence rate of about 36%, metastasizes in 81% of cases, and causes death in 79% of patients in the first 5 years after diagnosis.[28, 29] Kaposi's sarcoma is often complicated by a second and fatal primary lesion.[30]

In general, sarcomas may spread via lymphatic or hematogenous routes to distant viscera or may extend locally by invading vital organs. Bone and liver are frequently involved and thus bone and liver scans are commonly useful in a work-up for metastasis. Despite the availability of CT, ultrasonography, and MR, the radionuclide liver scan remains the best and simplest tool for detecting space-occupying lesions of that organ. The false-positive and false-negative rates remain about 20% each and are about the same with other imaging modalities. The smallest lesion that can be detected by a radionuclide scan is about 2 cm. Sonography can detect some smaller lesions. The improvement of instrumentation and use of multiple views have not increased the accuracy of liver scans.[31] Early studies of single-photon emission tomography of the liver report greater success in demonstrating more lesions than planar examinations alone.[32] Findings on the liver scan are nonspecific, but the specificity can be improved by using multiple radionuclides to answer specific questions.[33] The liver scan should be considered as the first step if metastases to the liver are suspected because of its speed, simplicity, low risk, and operator independence. Figure 3–5 illustrates liver metastases in a patient whose leiomyosarcoma had been resected from the left atrium 6 years earlier. Because small lesions may be missed by conventional liver scans, other modalities such as CT, sonography, or peritoneoscopic examination should be considered if liver metastases are strongly suspected.

The bone scan is much more sensitive than conventional radiographs in detecting bony metastases. However, increased uptake of bone-seeking radiopharmaceuticals is nonspecific. The pattern of distribution of the abnormalities, the appearance of new foci during follow-up, and demonstration of abnormal uptake in a symptomatic region should alert physicians to

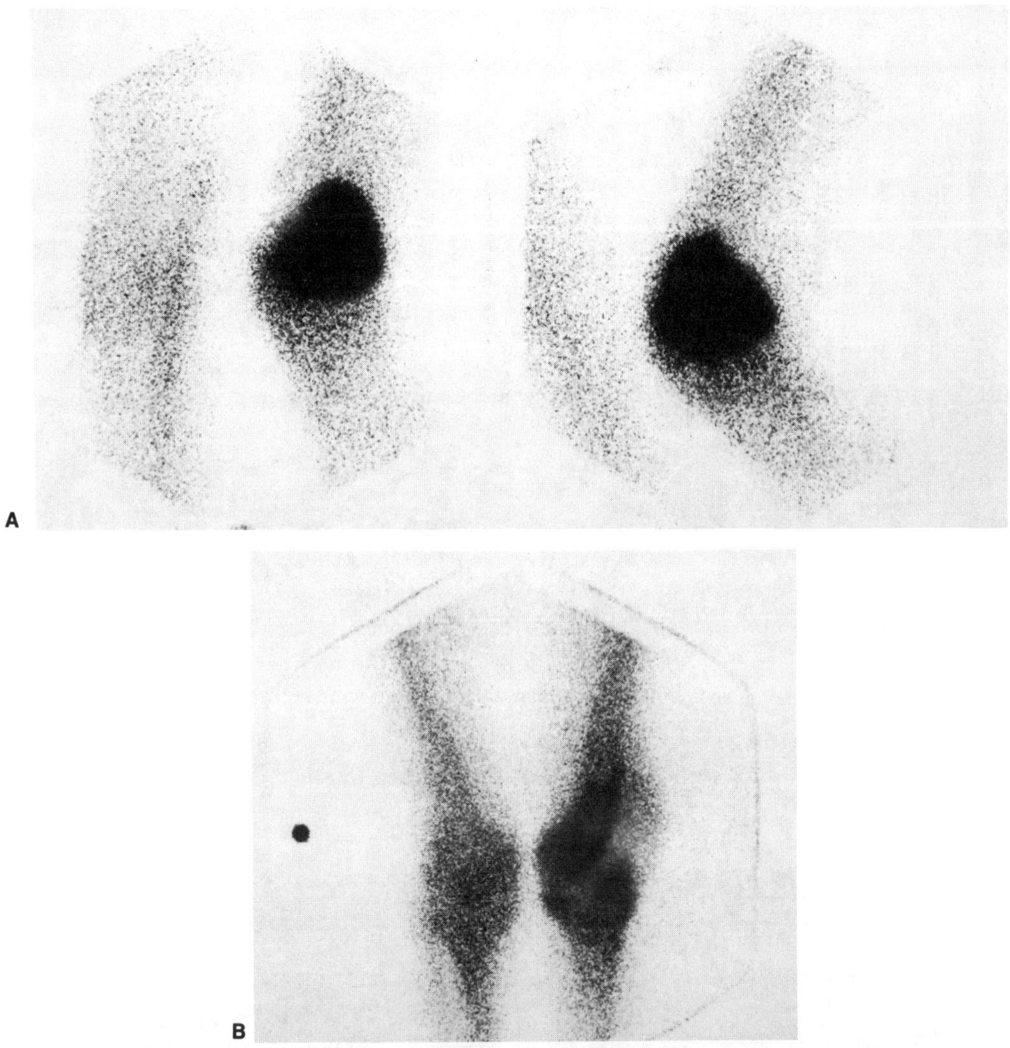

FIG 3–4.
A patient with malignant fibrous histiocytoma in the left knee area with more intense uptake of **A,** gallium than **B,** MDP.

the possible presence of skeletal metastases. With the modern, large-field gamma camera, both shoulders and the entire pelvis can be included in one view for comparison with the contralateral side. About 20 to 30 minutes is required to image the entire skeleton using total-body imagers. Single-photon emission tomography can also add information about the precise anatomical location of lesions. Figure 3–6 demonstrates bony involvement of the local area, the head of the humerus, and the right rib cage in a patient whose right arm had been partially amputated for malignant fibrous histiocytoma 20 months earlier.

Lung metastases are common in soft-tissue sarcoma. Chest radiographs, plain tomograms, and CT all may detect small pulmonary metastases. The gallium scan may add information about the activity and nature of certain lesions in the chest when they are sufficiently large. Figure 3–7 illustrates abnormal uptake of MDP and gallium in the abdomen and thorax of a patient with a recurrence of a malignant fibrous histiocytoma that had been resected about 3 years earlier. Figure 3–8 shows a young patient with abnormal uptake of gallium in a primary spindle cell sarcoma of the left thigh and metastases to the left chest wall. We have found gal-

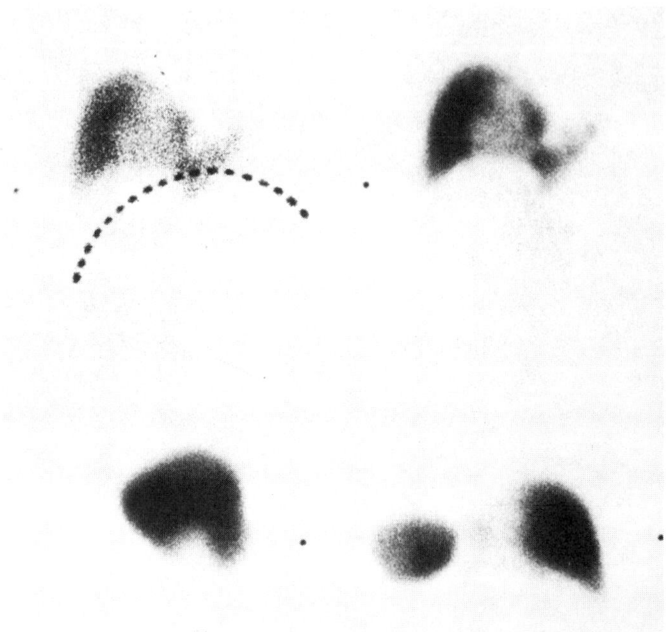

FIG 3–5.
Liver scan showing liver metastases in the left lobe in a patient who had leiomyosarcoma metastatic from the left atrium of the heart.

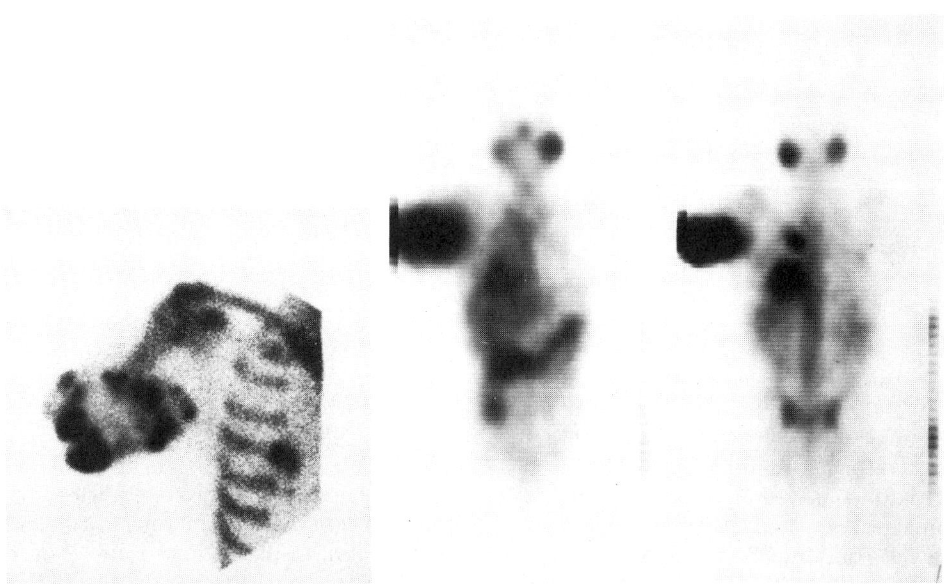

A B

FIG 3–6.
A, MDP and **B,** gallium scans from a patient who had amputation of the right arm for malignant fibrous histiocytoma. The MDP scan shows recurrence at the stump and metastases in the ribs. The gallium scan shows recurrence at the stump and metastases to the lungs.

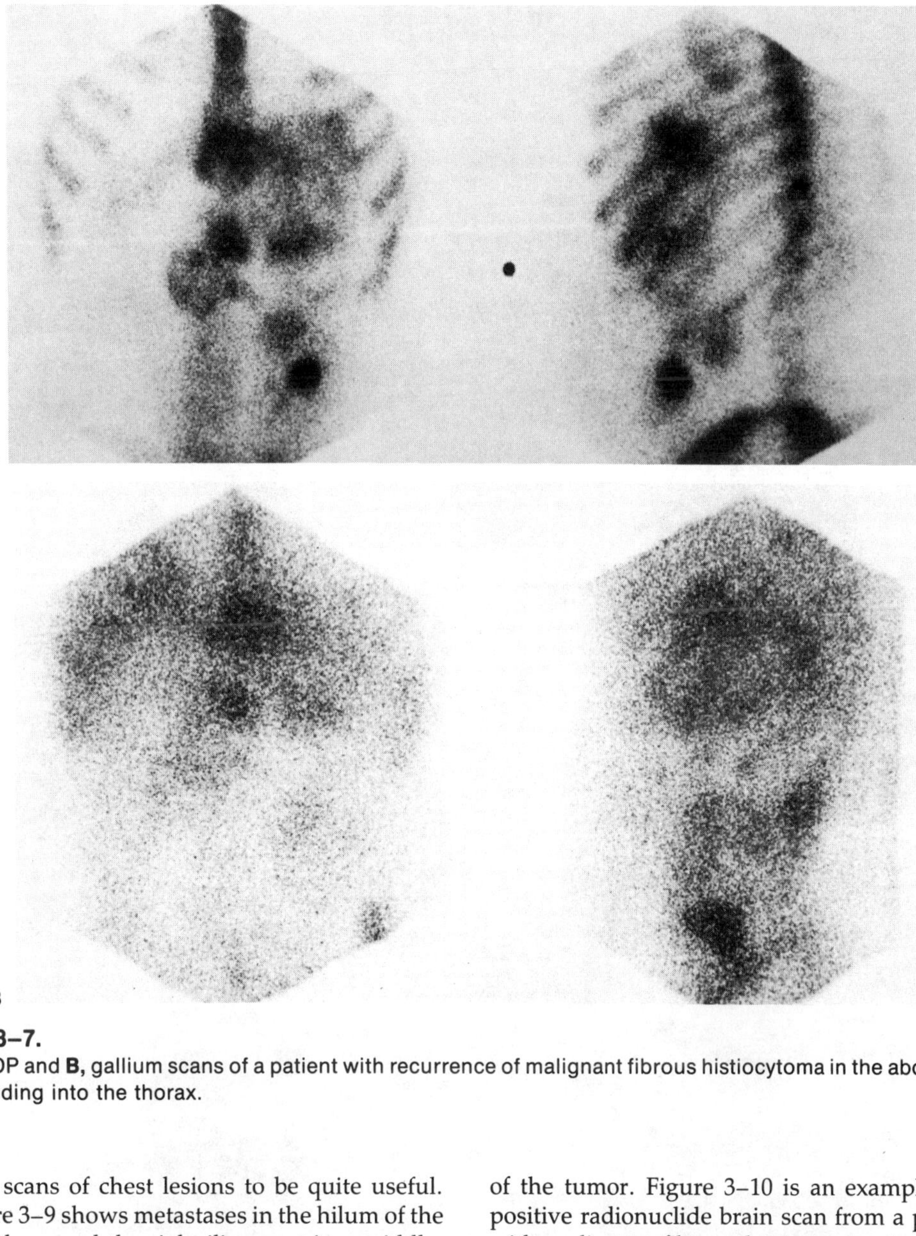

FIG 3–7.
A, MDP and **B,** gallium scans of a patient with recurrence of malignant fibrous histiocytoma in the abdomen, extending into the thorax.

lium scans of chest lesions to be quite useful. Figure 3–9 shows metastases in the hilum of the right lung and the right iliac crest in a middle-aged man whose rhabdomyosarcoma had been resected about 20 months earlier.

At the present time, radionuclide brain scans are seldom requested in a metastatic work-up. The sensitivity of the radionuclide brain scan is only slightly less than that of CT. Computed tomography does demonstrate more lesions than the radionuclide study and does provide more information, such as more precise anatomical location, the relationship to other structures, the vascularity, and even the nature of the tumor. Figure 3–10 is an example of a positive radionuclide brain scan from a patient with malignant fibrous histiocytoma in whom some mental symptoms developed. Computed tomography confirmed the presence of brain metastases. With the current interest in single-photon emission tomography and the availability of new radiopharmaceuticals, such as pH-affinity agents, neurotransmitters, receptors, and monoclonal antibodies, functional mapping of specific processes in the central nervous system should be considered.

At present, the gallium scan remains the best tool for delineating the primary soft-tissue

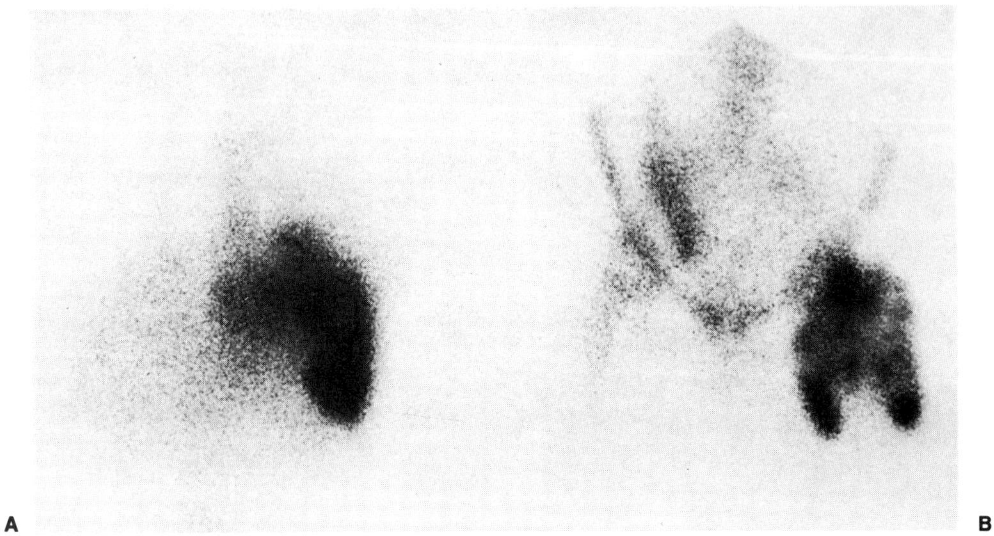

FIG 3–8.
Gallium scan of a patient with metastases to the **A,** left chest wall from spindle cell sarcoma of the **B,** left thigh.

sarcoma, its local recurrences, or metastases to lungs and other soft-tissue sites. Routine liver and bone scans are important steps to rule out involvement in these structures. The role of the gallium scan in mycosis fungoides and Kaposi's sarcoma, especially when they are associated with acquired immunodeficiency syndrome (AIDS), is less well defined and has not yet been adequately studied.

MONITORING THERAPEUTIC RESPONSE

Primary sarcomas that take up Ga 67 prior to therapy have been monitored with serial gallium scans to observe changes during chemotherapy. This technique was first used in osteosarcoma[34] as a practical application of concepts emerging from the correlation of glutamate N

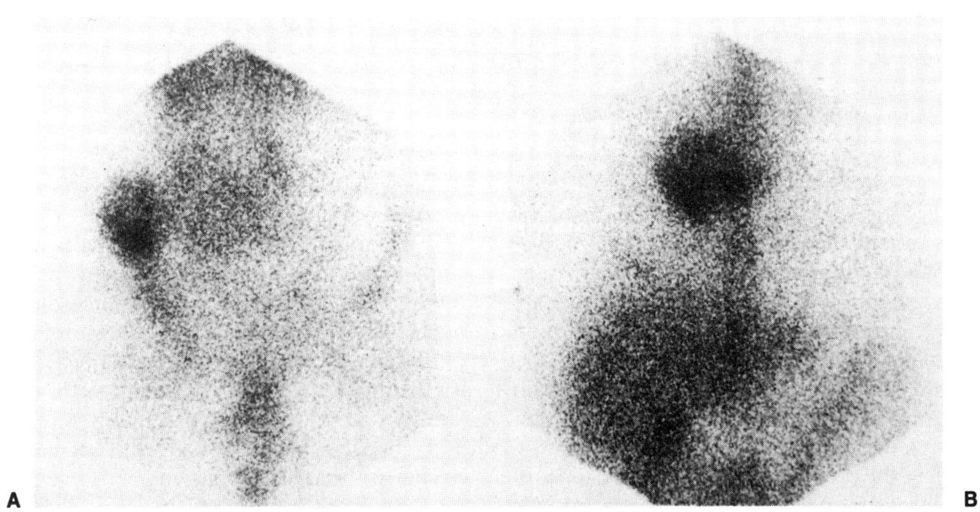

FIG 3–9.
A, Gallium scan of a patient with metastases in the right iliac crest and **B,** in the hilum of the right lung from rhabdomyosarcoma resected 20 months earlier.

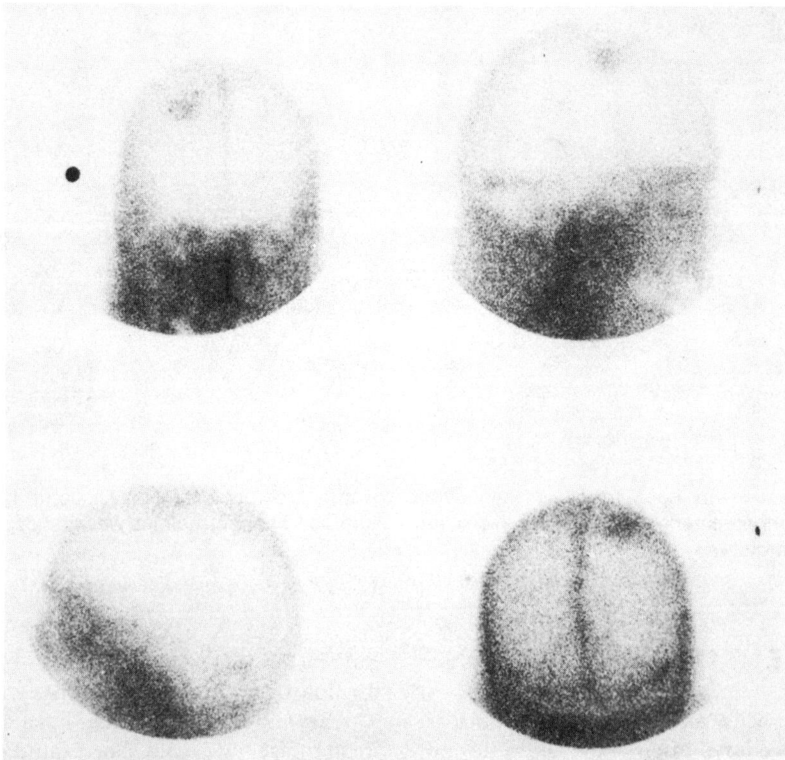

FIG 3–10.
Brain scan of a patient with malignant fibrous histiocytoma who had some mental symptoms. The right frontal lesion was seen in the radionuclide brain scan.

13 uptake in osteosarcoma with the degree of necrosis in specimens from en bloc resection after chemotherapy.[35] In a few cases of soft-tissue sarcoma, the decrease of Ga 67 uptake during therapy seems to be parallel to the clinical response of tumor size. Figure 3–11 is an example of such a patient with soft-tissue mesenchymal chondrosarcoma in the right chest wall that shows gradual improvement following chemotherapy. Increase of gallium uptake is more specific for treatment failure than is increase in MDP uptake, which may be due to healing or to increased bony erosion. The gallium scan, when positive, often gives an objective measure of tumor growth or shrinkage. Limited studies of serial gallium scans suggest that higher uptake is seen in patients with progression of disease. Decreased tumor-to-nontumor ratio occurs in some patients who show clinical and laboratory responses to chemotherapy. Because radiotherapy, iron status, and protein-binding behavior of gallium all can alter biodistribution of trace amounts of gallium, interpretation of follow-up scans often becomes quite difficult. It is too early to say whether or not decreased N 13-labeled amino acid or gallium uptake will parallel the response of soft-tissue sarcomas to chemotherapy or radiation.

In evaluating metastases that concentrate the radiopharmaceutical, the ratio of counts over the lesion to those over the contralateral anatomical sites may be taken as an index of treatment response or failure, provided the uptake in the contralateral structures was not changed by the therapy. In the case of metastases to organs such as the liver, which normally take up a scanning agent, changes in the size of the voids are readily measured. Response or lack of it may give the earliest sign of treatment effectiveness or failure and lead to timely alteration of the regimen. For lung metastases, the conventional radiograph is more sensitive than MDP or Ga 67 scans.

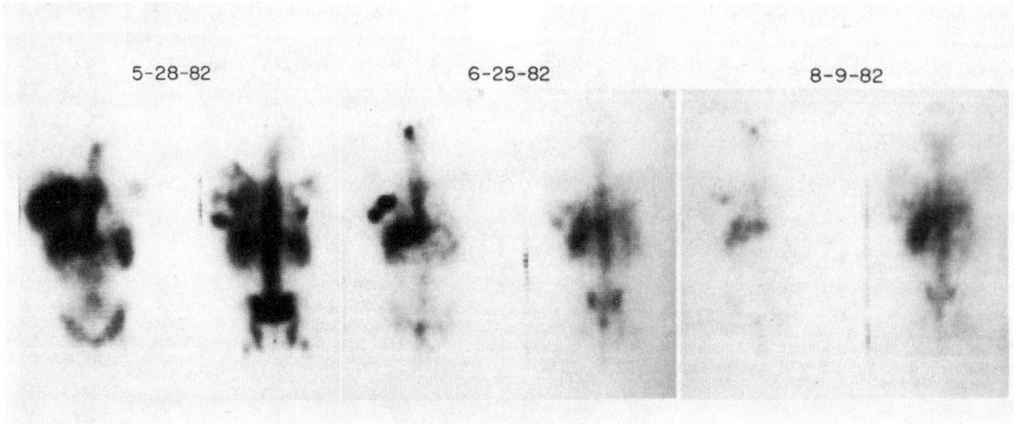

FIG 3–11.
Serial gallium scans in a patient with mesenchymal chondrosarcoma in the soft tissue of the right chest wall. Marked improvement with decrease in size and magnitude of abnormalities was first evident 1 month following chemotherapy.

ASSESSMENT OF COMPLICATIONS

The simplicity and flexibility of nuclear medicine procedures often allow us to design studies for each patient to answer specific questions about complications. For example, pericardial effusion can be easily demonstrated by blood pool imaging when the fluid accumulation has reached about 200 mL. Superior vena caval obstruction can be easily confirmed by a venous flow study with any blood pool tracer in less than 1 minute. Pulmonary embolism can be established by perfusion and ventilation studies. The precise matching of ventilation to perfusion has become easier now that Kr 81m is more readily available. Vascular supply to tumor areas can be assessed by capillary blockade scans with macro-aggregated albumin (MAA) given through arterial catheters, including those attached to an infusion pump. Pelvic lymphatic obstruction can be evaluated by lymphoscintigraphy using Tc 99m-labeled antimony colloid administered by intradermal or subcutaneous pedal injections. Infections can be studied with In 111-labeled leukocytes or citrate Ga 67.

Radionuclide cardiological studies have become a routine procedure. Adriamycin and its analogs, cyclophosphamide, and mediastinal radiation can cause cardiomyopathy and alter myocardial function. Gated blood pool studies to measure left ventricular function at rest and following exercise have become routine procedures. Changes from a baseline study may be the best guide to reducing the dose of potentially cardiotoxic antineoplastic agents.

Several interesting areas have been studied in the past few years. For example, the F 18-labeled 2-fluoro-deoxy-D-glucose utilization rate was high in high-grade soft-tissue sarcoma[36] and In 111-labeled monoclonal anti-myosin Fab fragments detected one or more lesions in 14 patients with known soft-tissue sarcoma[37]. Future developments in these areas are expected.

REFERENCES

1. Horne T, Mogle P, Finsterbush A, et al: Increased uptake of ^{99m}TC MDP in calcified synovial sarcoma. *Eur J Nucl Med* 1983; 8:75.
2. Wiss DA: Malignant fibrous histiocytoma. *J Surg Oncol* 1983; 22:228.
3. Hudson TM, Chew FS, Manaster BJ: Radionuclide bone scanning of medullary chondrosarcoma. *Am J Roentgenol* 1982; 139:1071.
4. Chew FS, Hudson TM: Radionuclide imaging of lipoma and liposarcoma. *Radiology* 1980; 136:741.
5. Enneking WF, Chew FS, Springfield DS, et al: Role of radionuclide bone scanning in determining the resectability of soft tissue sarcomas. *J Bone Joint Surg (Am)* 1981; 63A:249.
6. Bitran JD, Bekerman C, Golomb HM, et al: Scintigraphic evaluation of sarcomata in children and adults by Ga-67 citrate. *Cancer* 1978; 42:1760.

7. Kaufman JH, Cedermark BJ, Parthasarthy KL, et al: The value of ^{67}Ga scintigraphy in soft tissue sarcoma and chondrosarcoma. *Radiology* 1977; 123:131.
8. Longchampt MF, Wechsler B, Godeau P, et al: Diagnostic d'un fibrosarcome du psoas a forme febrile pure par la scintigraphie au citrate de gallium. *Nouv Presse Med* 1977; 6:3411.
9. Deng C, Terasaki PI, El-Awar N, et al: Cytotoxic monoclonal antibody to a human leiomyosarcoma. *Lancet* 1981; 1:403.
10. Mach JP, Carrel S, Forni M, et al: Tumor localization of radiolabeled antibodies against carcinoembryonic antigen in patients with carcinoma. *N Engl J Med* 1980; 303:5.
11. Larson SM, Brown JP, Wright PW, et al: Imaging of melanoma with I-131 labeled monoclonal antibodies. *J Nucl Med* 1983; 24:123.
12. Eppenetos AA, Britton KE, Mather S: Targeting of iodine 123 labelled tumor associated monoclonal antibodies to ovarian, breast, and gastrointestinal tumours. *Lancet* 1982; 2:999.
13. Halsall AK, Fairweather DS, Bradwell AR, et al: Localization of malignant germ cell tumours by external-scanning after injection of radiolabeled anti-alpha fetoprotein. *Br Med J* 1981; 283:942.
14. Goldenberg DM, Kim EE, DeLand FH, et al: Clinical radioimmunodetection of cancer with radioactive antibodies to human chorionic gonadotropin. *Science* 1980; 208:1284.
15. Fairweather DS, Breadwell AR, Watson-James SF, et al: Detection of thyroid tumours using radio-labelled antithyroglobulin. *Clin Endocrinol* 1983; 18:563.
16. Belitsky P, Ghose T, Aquino J, et al: Radionuclide imaging of primary renal cell carcinoma by I-131 labeled antitumor antibody. *J Nucl Med* 1978; 19:427.
17. Rosen G, Gelbard AS, Benua RS, et al: N-13 glutamate scanning to detect the early response of primary bone tumors to chemotherapy. *Proc Am Assoc Cancer Res* 1979; 20:189.
18. Reiman RS, Rosen G, Gelbard AS, et al: Imaging of primary Ewing sarcoma with N-13 L-glutamate. *Radiology* 1982; 142:495.
19. Sordillo P, Reiman RE, Gelbard AS, et al: Scanning with 1-^{13}N glutamate assessment of the response to chemotherapy of a patient with embryonal rhabdomyosarcoma. *Am J Clin Oncol* 1982; 5:285.
20. Schelstraete K, Simons M, Deman J, et al: Uptake of ^{13}N ammonia by human tumours as studied by positron emission tomography. *Br J Radiol* 1982; 55:797.
21. Hajdu SI: *Pathology of Soft Tissue Tumors.* Philadelphia, Lea & Febiger, 1979, p 78.
22. Hajdu SI: *Pathology of Soft Tissue Tumors.* Philadelphia, Lea & Febiger, 1979, p 125.
23. Cadman NL, Soule EH, Kelly RL: Synovial sarcoma, an analysis of 134 tumors. *Cancer* 1966; 18:613.
24. Weiss SW, Enzinger FM: Malignant fibrous histiocytoma. *Cancer* 1978; 41:2250.
25. Enzinger FM, Winslow PJ: Liposarcoma—a study of 103 cases. *Virchow's Arch Pathol Anat* 1962; 335:367.
26. Enterline HT: Histopathology of sarcoma. *Semin Oncol* 1981; 8:133.
27. Fernandez CH, Sutow WW, Merino OR, et al: Childhood rhabdomyosarcoma. *Am J Roentgenol Radiat Ther Nucl Med* 1975; 123:588.
28. Enzinger FM, Smith BH: Hemangiosarcoma. *Hum Pathol* 1976; 7:61.
29. Hajdu SI: *Pathology of Soft Tissue Tumors.* Philadelphia, Lea & Febiger, 1979, p 395.
30. O'Brien PH, Brasfield RD: Kaposi sarcoma. *Cancer* 1966; 19:1497.
31. Fee HR Jr, Prokop EK, Cameron JL, et al: Liver scanning in patients with suspected abdominal tumors. *JAMA* 1975; 230:1675.
32. Strauss L, Bostel F, Clorius JH, et al: Single-photon emission computed tomography (SPECT) for assessment of hepatic lesions. *J Nucl Med* 1982; 23:1059.
33. Yeh SDJ, Leeper RD, Benua RS: A study of filling defects in the liver and spleen with multiple radionuclides. *Clin Bull* 1977; 7:1.
34. Yeh SDJ, Rosen G, Caparros B, et al: Semiquantitative gallium scintigraphy in patients with osteogenic sarcoma. *J Nucl Med* 1983; 24:112.
35. Reiman RE, Huvos AG, Benua RS, et al: Quotient imaging with N-13 L-glutamate in osteogenic sarcoma. *Cancer* 1981; 48:1976.
36. Kern KA, Brunetti A, Norton JA, et al: Metabolic imaging of human extremity musculoskeletal tumor by PET. *J Nucl Med* 1988; 29:181.
37. Kairemo KJA, Wiklund TA, Liewendahl K, et al: Imaging of soft-tissue sarcomas with indium-111-labeled monoclonal antimyosin Fab fragments. *J Nucl Med* 1990; 31:23.

Chapter 4

Pathology of Soft-Tissue Sarcomas

Bruce G. Kulander

John W. Bolen

Management of soft-tissue sarcomas depends on assessment of clinical stage (size of the tumor, location, node status, presence or absence of distant metastasis), histological diagnosis, and histological grade. Crucial to this evaluation is the procurement of adequate tissue. The goal of any biopsy of a soft-tissue lesion should be to provide adequate material for diagnosis without compromising the ultimate definitive treatment if it should prove to be malignant. Superficial or small lesions may be diagnosed and treated via excisional biopsy; however, large or deep-seated lesions require a carefully planned incisional biopsy. Frozen sections should be restricted to determining whether representative neoplastic tissue has been obtained. Needle biopsies should be discouraged except for evaluation of recurrent or metastatic tumor in a patient with a previous diagnosis. Shelling out of a deep-seated, large, soft-tissue sarcoma that grossly may appear well demarcated or "encapsulated" should be absolutely avoided as it almost assures that the patient will have subsequent recurrence of the neoplasm.

Accurate histological diagnosis of most soft-tissue sarcomas can be done on the basis of well-prepared routine histological sections, although tissues should always be saved for electron microscopy and possible immunocytochemistry should diagnostic problems arise. A great deal of attention has been focused on the grading of sarcomas. It has been apparent for some time that within the diagnostic groups of liposarcoma and fibrosarcoma there is great variability in behavior and prognosis that can to some extent be predicted by histological appearance. Russel et al. utilized grade as the principal determinant of stage, in the report of the Soft Tissue Tumor Task Force of 1,200+ tumors.[1] The methods of grading used were discussed only in a general way. There have been several studies[2–7] that apply grading systems to groups of sarcomas that include all types. All of the studies seem to show a relationship of grade to survival. In one study, an analysis of 163 cases by Costa et al.,[2] necrosis was the single best factor among seven histological factors, with a strong predictive value of time to recurrence and survival. In their study, it was proposed that grade 1 be determined on the basis of histological type (tumors known to have an excellent prognosis if completely excised, such as well-differentiated and myxoid liposarcoma), whereas grades 2 and 3 should be separated on the basis of necrosis—grade 3 if more than 15% of the tumor is necrotic. Their results were shown to be independent of age, sex, and size and were also applicable to the first recurrence.

Histological diagnosis of type continues to be important in the management of soft-tissue sarcomas. There are no data to suggest that a grade 2 sarcoma of one type will necessarily behave or respond to therapy the same way as one of another type. In some cases, certain biological tendencies are implied by a histological classification, that is, nerve sheath tumors tend to spread along the perineurium and endoneurium of nerve sheaths, and epithelioid sarcomas and alveolar rhabdomyosarcomas have a propensity for node metastasis.

In the following sections the basic histological appearances of the more common soft-tissue sarcomas will be reviewed. It is, by necessity, an overview and not all inclusive; those readers interested in a more comprehensive discussion are referred to several excellent books.[8–10]

LIPOSARCOMA

Liposarcomas continue to be one of the most common malignant adult soft-tissue tumors, although their overall incidence is decreasing as many neoplasms previously considered to be liposarcomas are now being included with malignant fibrous histiocytomas. They are primarily lesions of adults, with the peak incidence between 40 and 60 years of age. Liposarcomas characteristically exhibit a wide spectrum of growth patterns, and clinical outcome is closely tied to their histological subclassification.[11–14] Both the myxoid and well-differentiated variants represent low-grade lesions with 5-year survival rates approaching 80%. In contrast, the more cellular and aggressive tumors classified as round cell, dedifferentiated, or pleomorphic constitute medium- to high-grade tumors with a significant risk of metastatic spread and decreased long-term survival. Liposarcomas are deep-seated tumors occurring most frequently in the extremities (particularly the thigh), retroperitoneum, inguinal region, and popliteal fossa. Less common sites include chest wall, breast, mediastinum, and the omentum.

The main approach to the treatment of liposarcomas remains surgical. There is, however, little evidence to suggest that radical excision and/or amputation offers better results than a wide en bloc resection of the tumor with documented tumor-free margins. Radiation therapy has been shown to be effective postoperatively in reducing the rate of local recurrence, and is occasionally useful pre-operatively in reducing the size of the primary tumor so that a previously unresectable tumor can be surgically excised. The role of adjuvant chemotherapy for high-grade lesions with a significant risk of metastatic spread continues to be under study.

Pathological Findings.—Well-differentiated liposarcomas consist of a variable mixture of adipose tissue composed of univacuolate adult lipocytes, chronic inflammatory cells, and fibrous connective tissue containing non–fat-storing spindle- to stellate-shaped cells arranged in a loosely fascicular pattern. Primarily located within the fibrous areas but also scattered within the adipose-rich regions are neoplastic cells with large hyperchromatic and pleomorphic nuclei (Fig 4–1). Evidence of necrosis and mitotic activity is generally absent. When these lesions become more aggressive, they show a dedifferenti-

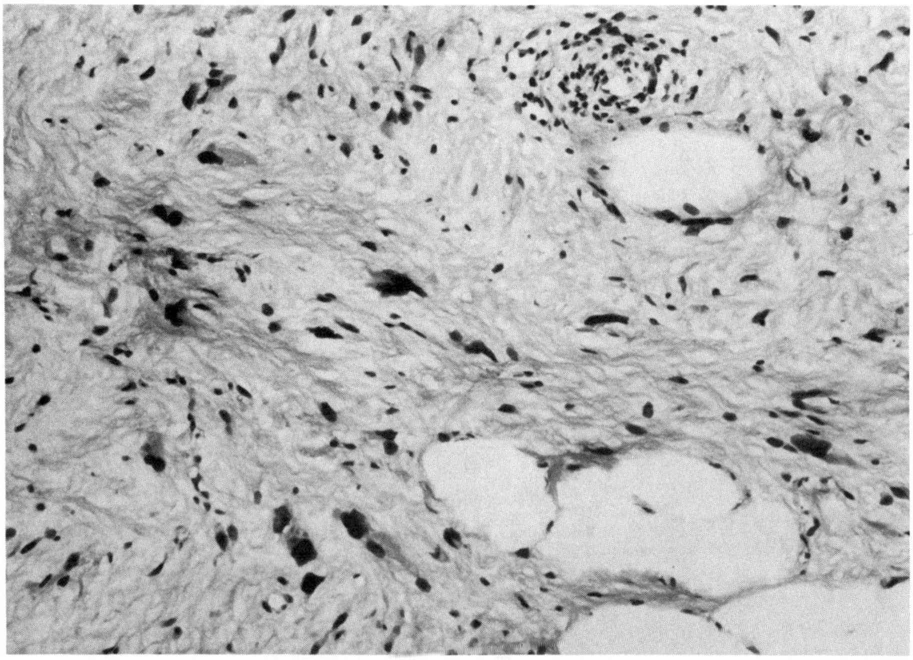

FIG 4–1.
Well-differentiated liposarcoma.

ated growth pattern consisting of a densely cellular, spindle-shaped or pleomorphic sarcoma without appreciable fat storage. These hypercellular areas often exhibit a fascicular fibrosarcoma-like growth or storiform fibrous histiocytoma-like growth.

Myxoid/round cell liposarcomas represent a continuum in relation to the degree of cellularity (Fig 4–2). The least cellular pattern is that of myxoid liposarcoma, consisting of a histologically low-grade tumor composed of small spindle- to stellate-shaped cells concentrated around a plexiform vascular pattern that stands out prominently against a background of abundant extracellular acid mucopolysaccharide (Fig 4–3,a). The neoplastic cells show marked variation in the amount of stored cytoplasmic fat, rare mitoses, and no significant necrosis. The most cellular pattern is that of a round cell liposarcoma consisting of closely packed, uniformly round to ovoid cells that fill the space between and tend to obscure the appearance of the plexiform vasculature (Fig 4–3,b). Mitotic figures are more frequent than in the less cellular areas; however, significant cellular pleomorphism is not a feature of this group of tumors. Many of these neoplasms show a spectrum of cellularity combining the features of both myxoid and round cell neoplasms.

Pleomorphic liposarcomas are quite uncommon. They represent histologically high-grade, cellular, pleomorphic sarcomas with numerous giant cells, necrosis, and a high mitotic rate. They are often histologically and ultrastructurally identical to malignant fibrous histiocytomas except for variable numbers of bizarre lipoblasts (Fig 4–4). Their prognosis is likewise similar, with an overall 5-year survival of 50% or less.

Fat stains on frozen tissue are generally of little help in diagnosing liposarcomas, as most soft-tissue sarcomas contain lipid. Ultrastructural examination may occasionally be helpful in the evaluation of a fat-storing neoplasm.[15] Such studies have demonstrated distinct difference between the major subtypes of liposarcomas. Immunoperoxidase techniques have not yet proved helpful in this area of soft-tissue pathology.

FIBROMATOSIS

The term *fibromatosis* covers a fairly wide spectrum of well-differentiated fibroblastic proliferations that are collectively defined as a nonencapsulated and usually noncircumscribed proliferation of uniform collagen-forming fi-

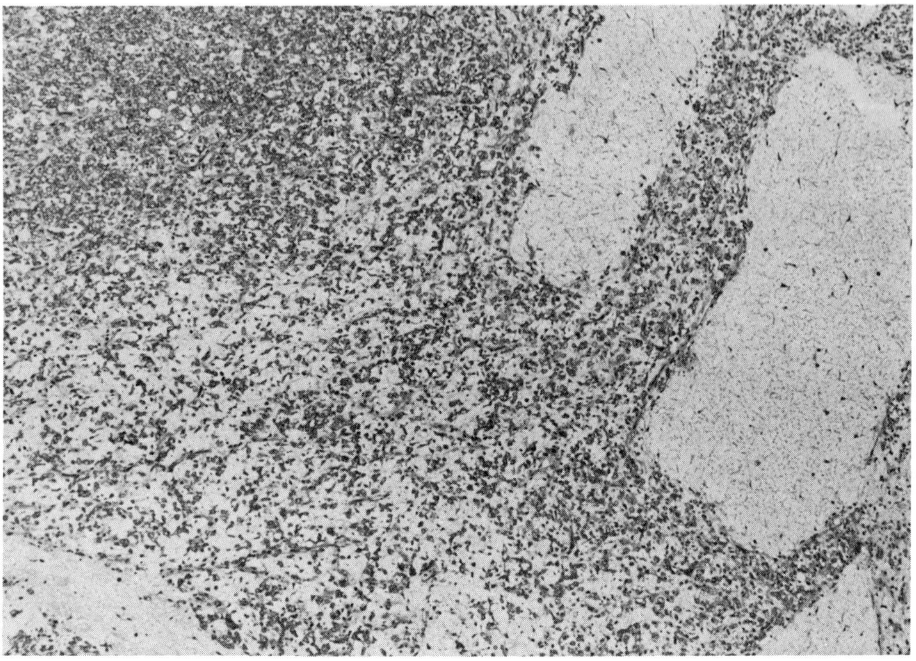

FIG 4–2.
Myxoid/round-cell liposarcoma.

broblasts, or myofibroblasts exhibiting no anaplasia and usually scant or absent mitotic activity. There are numerous subtypes, and this discussion will focus on abdominal and extra-abdominal desmoid tumors. This terminology is preferred by the authors to the usage of well-differentiated fibrosarcoma for this lesion.

The treatment of this lesion has generally been considered to be surgical, but a recent study reports the "recurrence" rate to be the

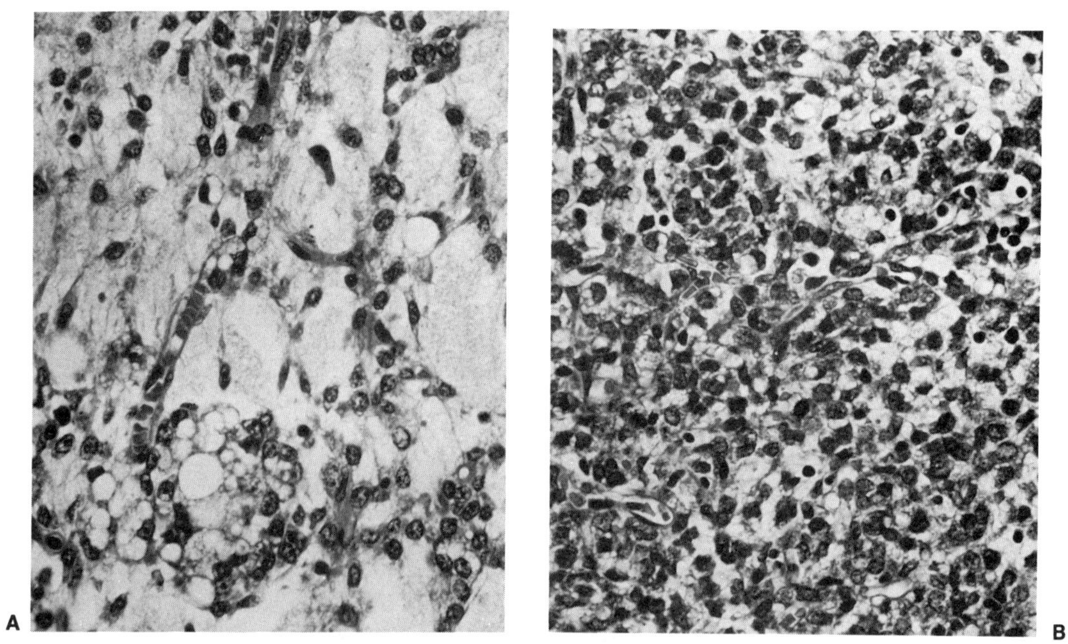

FIG 4–3.
A, myxoid liposarcoma. **B,** round-cell liposarcoma.

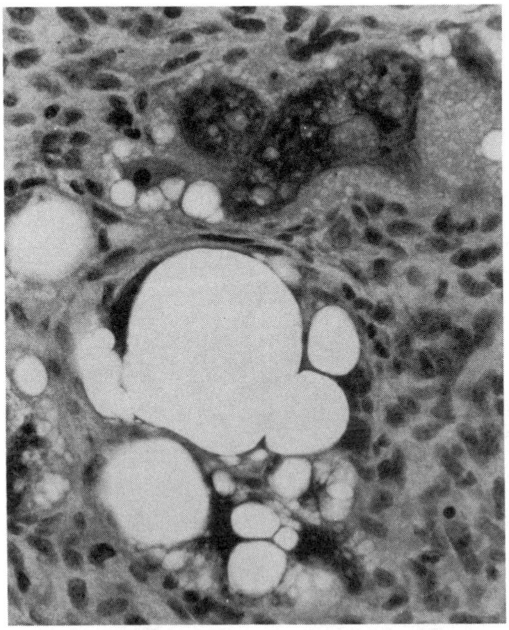

FIG 4–4.
Pleomorphic liposarcoma.

same with both complete and incomplete excision,[16] and another study reports that tamoxifen treatment may be associated with tumor regression.[17]

In addition to the well-known association with Gardner's syndrome,[18] common association with multiple skeletal anomalies (80% of cases) has been cited.[16] With rare exceptions, desmoid tumors do not metastasize, but may be life threatening due to local infiltration of vital structures.

Pathological Findings.—These tumors present as masses within the musculature of the abdominal wall or peripheral muscles, the root of the mesentery, and rarely other locations. They are firm, with a gray-white, scarlike appearance on section, and usually interdigitate with the surrounding muscle (in contrast to fibrosarcoma, which is typically pseudoencapsulated). The histological appearance is that of a well-collagenized uniform fibroblastic tumor with "bland" nuclei. It may exhibit rare mitoses and tends to infiltrate adjacent tissues such as fat and muscle (Fig 4–5). Distinction from fibrosarcoma (with metastatic potential) may be difficult, but gross circumscription, increased cellularity, nuclear anaplasia, and mitotic activity would favor a diagnosis of fibrosarcoma.

FIBROSARCOMA

Fibrosarcoma is a rare tumor, and may be defined as a neoplasm of fibroblasts capable of producing metastatic spread. To be excluded are a number of spindle cell tumors associated with collagen production, especially desmoplastic melanoma, spindle cell squamous cell carci-

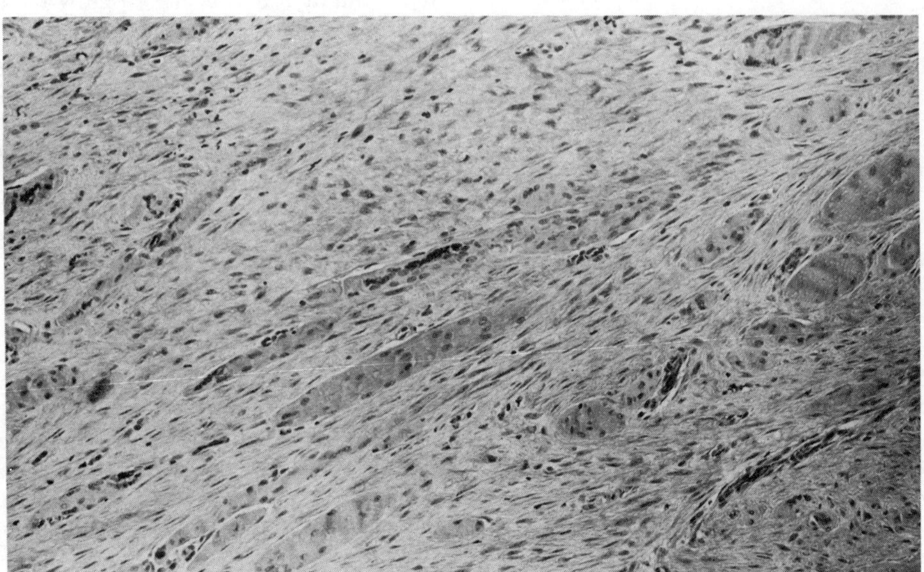

FIG 4–5.
Fibromatosis.

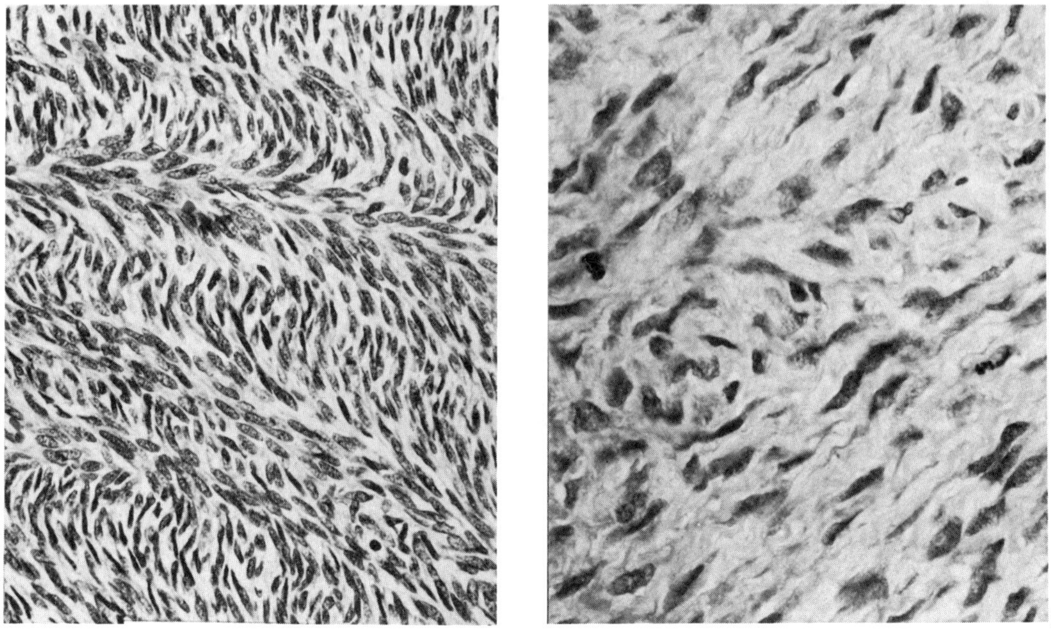

FIG 4–6.
A and **B,** fibrosarcoma.

noma, and sarcomatoid renal cell carcinoma. The most common locations include the upper and lower extremities and trunk. They are usually intramuscular or intermuscular and involve tendons, fascia, bone, or deep subcutaneous tissue. Head and neck, visceral, intrathoracic, and intra-abdominal occurrence is unusual.

Pathological Findings.—The moderate to richly cellular neoplasm is characteristically composed of fairly uniform spindle-shaped cells arranged in a herringbone or fascicular pattern (Fig 4–6). Collagen production is generally not abundant, and reticulin is usually complex rather than parallel. Mitoses are obvious in most cases, in contrast to desmoid tumors. Significant pleomorphism, palisading nuclei, storiform areas, multinucleated tumor giant cells, and myxoid areas are all absent or rare, and their presence suggests another diagnosis such as peripheral nerve sheath tumor, leiomyosarcoma, or malignant fibrous histiocytoma.

Behavior can be predicted to some extent by histological appearance. The high-grade, richly cellular lesions with minimal collagen production and high mitotic rate (more than 2/HPF (high power field)), carry a 35% chance for 5-year survival in contrast to 80% for low-grade tumors.[19, 20]

DERMATOFIBROSARCOMA PROTUBERANS

This superficial tumor of skin and subcutaneous tissue is most common on the trunk and shoulder of young to middle-aged males. It presents as a slowly growing tumor of several years' duration that begins to grow rapidly. It may be associated with a burn or surgical scar. Its appearance varies from a flat indurated area with a violaceous border, to polypoid or multinodular with surface ulceration. At the time of surgical treatment, the diameter of these tumors is often 5 cm or larger. The histogenesis is controversial. Histologically identical tumors may occur in the deep soft tissues.

The recurrence rate is in the range of 50%, but metastatic spread is unusual. Wide local excision is the treatment of choice.

Pathological Findings.—A monotonous proliferation of slender, uniform, spindle-shaped cells arranged in a radial organoid pattern referred to as storiform characterizes this neoplasm (Fig 4–7). It often shows a lacelike pattern of infiltration of the subcutaneous fat. The cells lack pleomorphism, and the mitotic rate is low. A myxoid pattern has been described,[21] which may be underdiagnosed or mis-

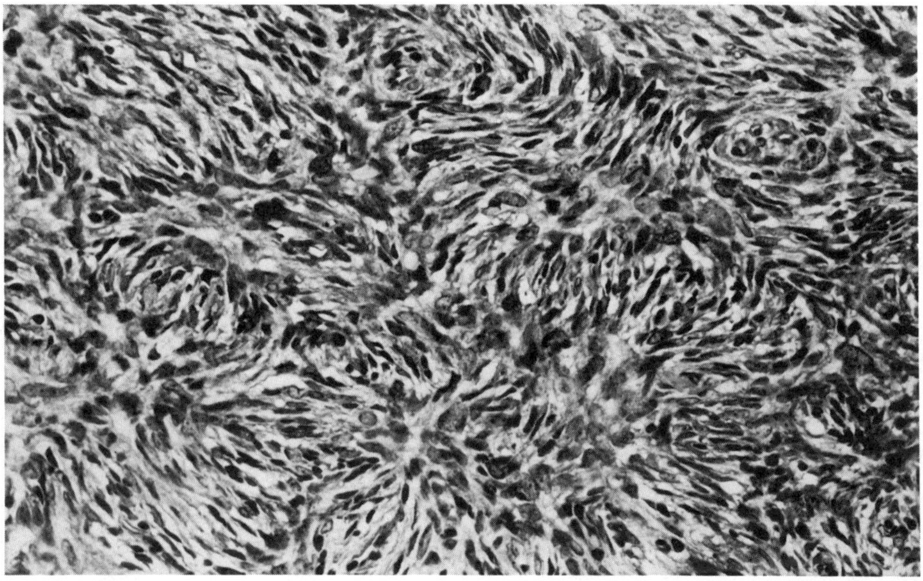

FIG 4–7.
Dermatofibrosarcoma protuberans.

diagnosed as a myxoid liposarcoma if the superficial location is not known. Some cases have reported to contain melanin, but S-100 protein has not yet been demonstrated in either pigmented or unpigmented types.[22]

MALIGNANT FIBROUS HISTIOCYTOMA

Malignant fibrous histiocytoma[23] is the most common soft-tissue sarcoma of late adult life. Its incidence is increasing, as many tumors previously diagnosed as pleomorphic rhabdomyosarcoma or liposarcoma are now reclassified in this category. Histogenesis of this tumor remains unsettled. Its name stems from cell culture work that suggested that the tissue histiocyte can become a "facultative fibroblast."[24] It typically presents as a deep-seated tumor of the extremities and is more common in males (two thirds of cases). As with most sarcomas, prognosis is closely related to depth, size, and location of the tumor and, to a lesser extent, to histological features including the presence of significant necrosis.[2] Overall, about 40% to 60% recur. The metastatic potential varies from approximately 20% in angiomatoid and myxoid variants[25, 26] to 40% to 60% in giant cell and storiform-pleomorphic tumors.[27, 28]

Pathological Findings.—This group of tumors is composed of a mixture of fibrohistiocytic cells usually arranged in a characteristic storiform growth.[29] Most have a combination of spindle and tumor giant cells separated by variable quantities of extracellular collagen and myxoid material (acid mucopolysaccharide). Areas resembling hemangiopericytoma and fibrosarcoma may be seen. Five types can be recognized: storiform-pleomorphic, myxoid, giant cell, inflammatory, and angiomatoid.[28] The first is the largest group, accounting for probably two thirds to three fourths of all cases. Its histological growth pattern varies from a relatively uniform lesion resembling dermatofibrosarcoma protuberans to a highly cellular pleomorphic tumor (Fig 4–8,a). The myxoid type accounts for 25% of all cases and is characterized by an abundance of extracellular myxoid matrix (Fig 4–8,b). It appears to have a better prognosis than the storiform-pleomorphic type.[25] The giant cell type (malignant giant cell tumor of soft parts) is so named because of the presence of numerous osteoclast-type giant cells in addition to the usual pleomorphic giant cells of malignant fibrous histiocytoma[27, 30] (Fig 4–8,c). The inflammatory type is most commonly retroperitoneal and may be associated with systemic signs such as fever and leukocytosis. It is distinguished by the presence of numerous xantho-

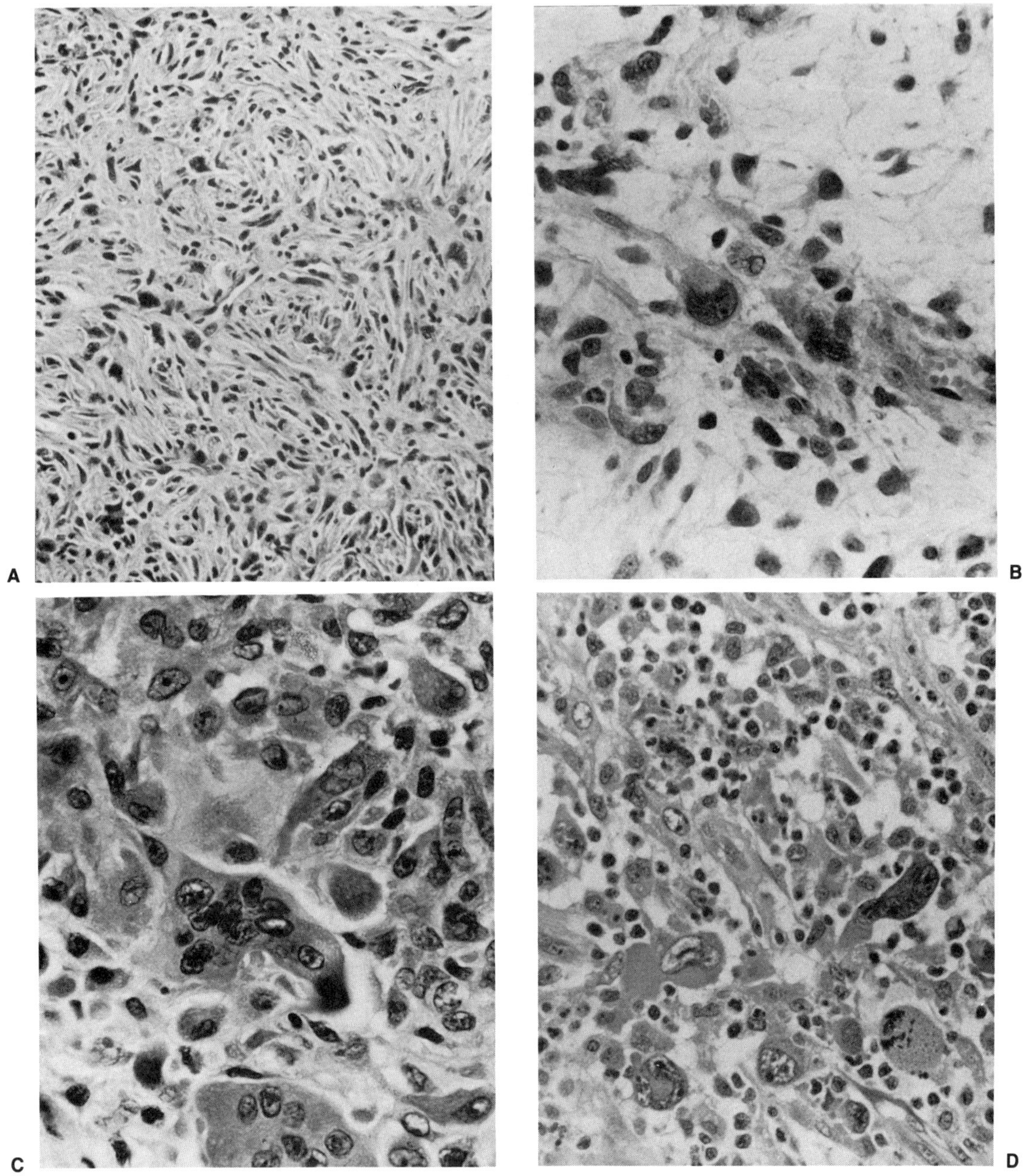

FIG 4–8.
A, malignant fibrous histiocytoma (MFH; storiform-pleomorphic type). **B,** MFH (myxoid type). **C,** MFH (giant cell type). **D,** MFH (inflammatory type).

matous histiocytes and inflammatory cells, including neutrophils[31] (Fig 4–8,d). The angiomatoid type is rare and is unique in this category of tumors in that it predominates in younger individuals. It is less aggressive clinically than other types of malignant fibrous histiocytomas, possibly reflecting its tendency to occur in superficial locations. Approximately two thirds recur locally, and one fifth metastasize, usually to the lungs.[26] Ultrastructural studies of malignant fibrous histiocytomas have shown a spectrum of cell differentiation from primitive mesenchymal cells to "fibroblastic" and "histiocytic" cells[32]; the proportion of each

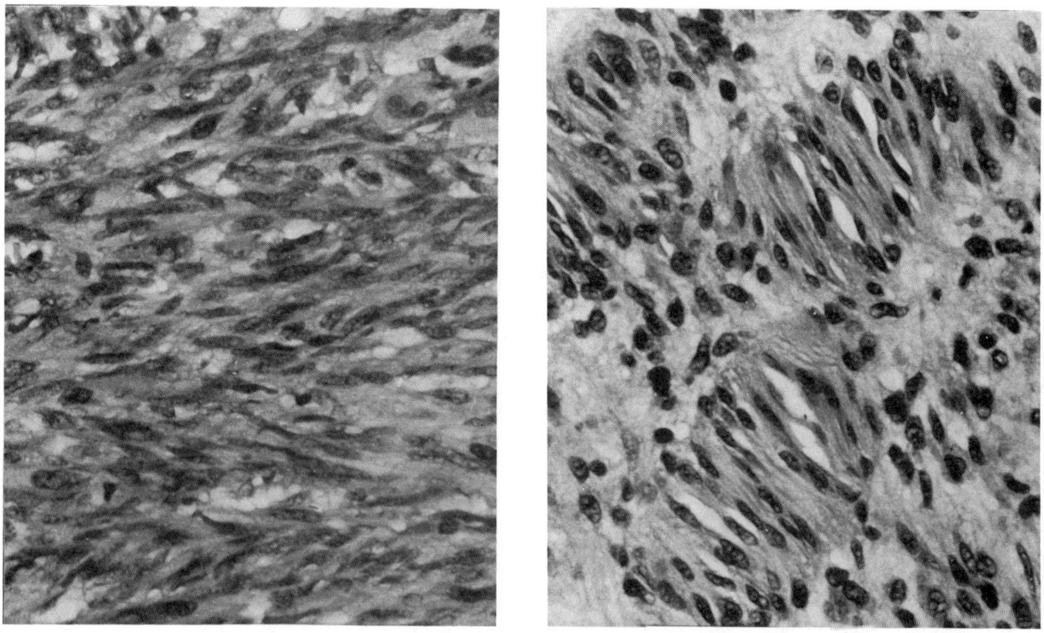

A B

FIG 4–9.
A and **B**, malignant peripheral nerve sheath tumor.

cell type varies greatly from one tumor to the next. A number of antibodies to histiocytic markers have been employed, but their utility in diagnostic pathology is somewhat limited by their lack of specificity.[33]

MALIGNANT PERIPHERAL NERVE SHEATH TUMORS

The many terms for malignant tumors of peripheral nerve sheath origin reflect the ongoing controversy regarding their histogenesis. It is generally accepted that benign *schwannomas* (*neurilemmomas*) are composed of differentiated Schwann cells, and neurofibromas represent proliferations of Schwann cells, perineurial cells, fibroblasts, and scattered axons. Most studies of *malignant peripheral nerve sheath tumors* have failed to demonstrate differentiated features of Schwann cells, and it has been argued that they more closely resemble perineurial cells. Harkin and Reed[34] suggest that perineurial and Schwann cells are closely related and represent different developmental and functional stages of a common precursor cell of neural crest origin.

Malignant peripheral nerve sheath tumors represent 10% to 15% of soft-tissue sarcomas. Those that occur in association with von Recklinghausen's disease affect younger patients than do spontaneously occurring tumors and overall have a worse prognosis. Both arise along major nerves, presenting as fusiform masses in proximal portions of the upper and lower extremities. They represent medium- to high-grade sarcomas with a marked predilection for local recurrence and metastatic spread to the lungs, liver, and bone. Their tendency to be deep seated may require amputation for complete removal, with careful attention to the nerve margin, because there is a tendency for malignant cells to spread along the nerve sheath.

Pathological Findings.—The histological growth pattern closely resembles that of fibrosarcoma. The spindle cells form sweeping, intersecting fascicles (Fig 4–9,a). Nuclei are irregularly contoured, wavy to comma shaped, and feature varying degrees of cytological atypia. Densely cellular areas may alternate with looser myxoid regions. Rudimentary tactoid differentiation (Fig 4–9,b) and nuclear palisading are occasionally seen, and there may be extensive perineural and intraneural spread. Heterologous differentiation consisting of cartilage,

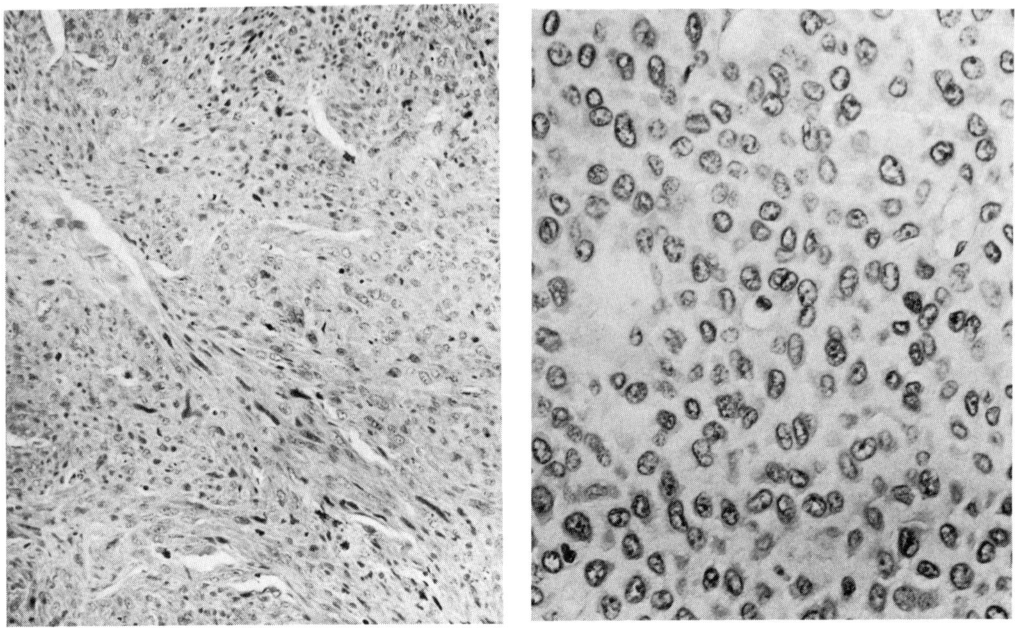

FIG 4–10.
A, leiomyosarcoma. **B,** epithelioid leiomyosarcoma.

bone, skeletal muscle, or mucin-producing glands has been described.

These tumors express a broad range of histological grade, based on mitotic rate and other criteria of malignancy, but clinical relevance has not been firmly established.

There have been several ultrastructural studies of malignant peripheral nerve sheath tumors.[35, 36] Neoplastic cells lack the differentiated features of Schwann cells but may have numerous, tangled elongate cell processes that may be partly invested by basal lamina, with primitive cell junctions. Long-spacing collagen (Luse bodies) may be present. Immunoperoxidase staining of S-100 protein has been reported to be positive in approximately 50% of malignant peripheral nerve sheath tumors,[37] and staining of other neural markers (e.g., myelin basic protein) occurs in an additional 15% to 20% of tumors.[38]

LEIOMYOSARCOMA AND EPITHELIOID LEIOMYOSARCOMA

Leiomyosarcomas account for 7% of soft-tissue tumors.[1] Among the somatic soft tissues, they can be divided into retroperitoneal/intraabdominal, cutaneous/subcutaneous, and vascular groups.[39, 40] Retroperitoneal tumors occur primarily in women and tend to be large by the time they are clinically detected. They usually prove fatal, with a high rate of local recurrence and metastatic spread.[41] Those in the peripheral soft tissues are usually subcutaneous or cutaneous and have a relatively favorable prognosis.[42, 43] The cutaneous leiomyosarcomas frequently recur locally but rarely metastasize, whereas the subcutaneous tumors have a metastatic potential. Wide excision is the most common form of management. Members of the final group, vascular leiomyosarcomas, are rare and affect primarily females. They usually involve medium-sized and major vessels, notably the inferior vena cava.[44]

Epithelioid leiomyomas and leiomyosarcomas most frequently occur in the stomach, although extragastric tumors have been described. Most examples are benign, although sizes greater than 6 cm in diameter and/or more than five mitoses per 50 HPF have been reported as indicative of malignancy.[45]

Pathological Findings.—Leiomyosarcomas have a relatively uniform structure throughout, characterized by well-defined bundles of elongate cytoplasmic cells forming sweeping, intersecting patterns (Fig 4–10,a). Hyperchromatic, blunt-ended, cigar-shaped nuclei that may be palisaded are a hallmark of this tumor. The pink-staining strappy cytoplasm is fuchsinophilic with a Masson trichrome stain, may be vacuolated, and usually contains glycogen (unlike fibrosarcoma and malignant fibrous histiocytoma). Cells seen in longitudinal profile on trichrome or phosphotungstic acid-hematoxylin (PTAH) stain may have a fine fibrillar appearance attributed to myofilaments. There may be small amounts of collagen and/or myxoid material interposed between the smooth muscle cells. Microvasculature and inflammatory cells are as a rule inconspicuous. The distinction of leiomyoma from leiomyosarcoma can be difficult, and criteria vary depending on the location. Mitoses are one of the most useful criteria. Most malignant smooth muscle tumors of the soft tissues have more than five mitoses per 10 HPF, although large tumors with relatively few mitoses may metastasize.[41] Histological grading of leiomyosarcomas has not correlated well with prognosis.[40, 41] However, location and size are of great importance to the eventual outcome.

The histological appearance of epithelioid leiomyosarcoma features cells with round outlines and pale pink-staining to clear cytoplasm that in some areas appears vacuolated (Fig 4-10,b). There are often areas of standard leiomyosarcoma, and conversely small areas of epithelioid appearance can be found in a significant proportion of leiomyosarcomas. The frequency with which differentiated features of smooth muscle cells are ultrastructurally identified varies depending on the location of the tumor. Uterine cutaneous/subcutaneous, and many retroperitoneal lesions often exhibit thin filaments with dense bodies, pinocytotic vesicles, and basal lamina typical of smooth muscle cells, whereas gastric tumors frequently lack these features.[46] Similarly, epithelioid lesions often resemble poorly differentiated mesenchymal cells without specific evidence of smooth muscle differentiation, unless extensively sampled.[47] Immunocytochemical detection of the muscle-specific intermediate filament desmin may prove helpful in the diagnosis of smooth muscle tumors.

RHABDOMYOSARCOMA

Rhabdomyosarcoma is the most common soft-tissue malignancy in children, adolescents, and young adults. It occurs more frequently in males than in females and exhibits a bimodal age distribution. The botryoid and embryonal types occur in infants and young children up to the age of 15 years and are primarily located in the head and neck area, particularly the orbit and nasal cavity, nasopharynx, genitourinary tract, and retroperitoneum. The alveolar type occurs in young adults between 10 and 25 years of age and shows a higher incidence in voluntary muscle of the upper and lower extremities.[48] It has a worse prognosis and may metastasize to regional lymph nodes or even be widely disseminated before the primary tumor is detected. A recently introduced system divides childhood rhabdomyosarcomas into monomorphous, anaplastic, and mixed types. The first two comprise 18.5% of cases and portend a poor prognosis.[49] The rare example of pleomorphic rhabdomyosarcoma occurs primarily in adults.

The prognosis for this previously fatal disease has improved dramatically with multimodality therapy.[50] Surgery is restricted to conservative resection of the lesion followed by radiation therapy and multidrug chemotherapy. Prognosis is closely related to clinical stage. Much of the improved survival is in patients with embryonal or botryoid tumors; alveolar rhabdomyosarcomas continue to be aggressive tumors less responsive to current radiation and chemotherapeutic regimens.

Pathological Findings.—Embryonal rhabdomyosarcomas closely resemble the various stages of normal skeletal muscle differentiation. The same tumor may exhibit the full range of cytodifferentiation from primitive undifferentiated mesenchymal cells to multinucleated striated rhabdomyoblasts consistent with myotube formation. Tumor cells are long, slim, and spindle shaped, with thin bipolar or stellate processes. They may be arranged in a loosely fascicular pattern alternating with less cellular myxoid zones. Rhabdomyoblasts are elongated and straplike to plump and tadpole shaped in configuration. There is only moderate nuclear pleomorphism.

The "botryoid" variant is derived from the Greek word for grapes, referring to its characteristic gross appearance. It occurs in mucous membrane-covered surfaces including the nasal cavity, vagina, urinary bladder, and nasopharynx. It presents as a polypoid to grapelike tumor that characteristically is hypocellular and edematous. Its most distinctive histological feature is the formation of a "cambium layer," a densely

A

B

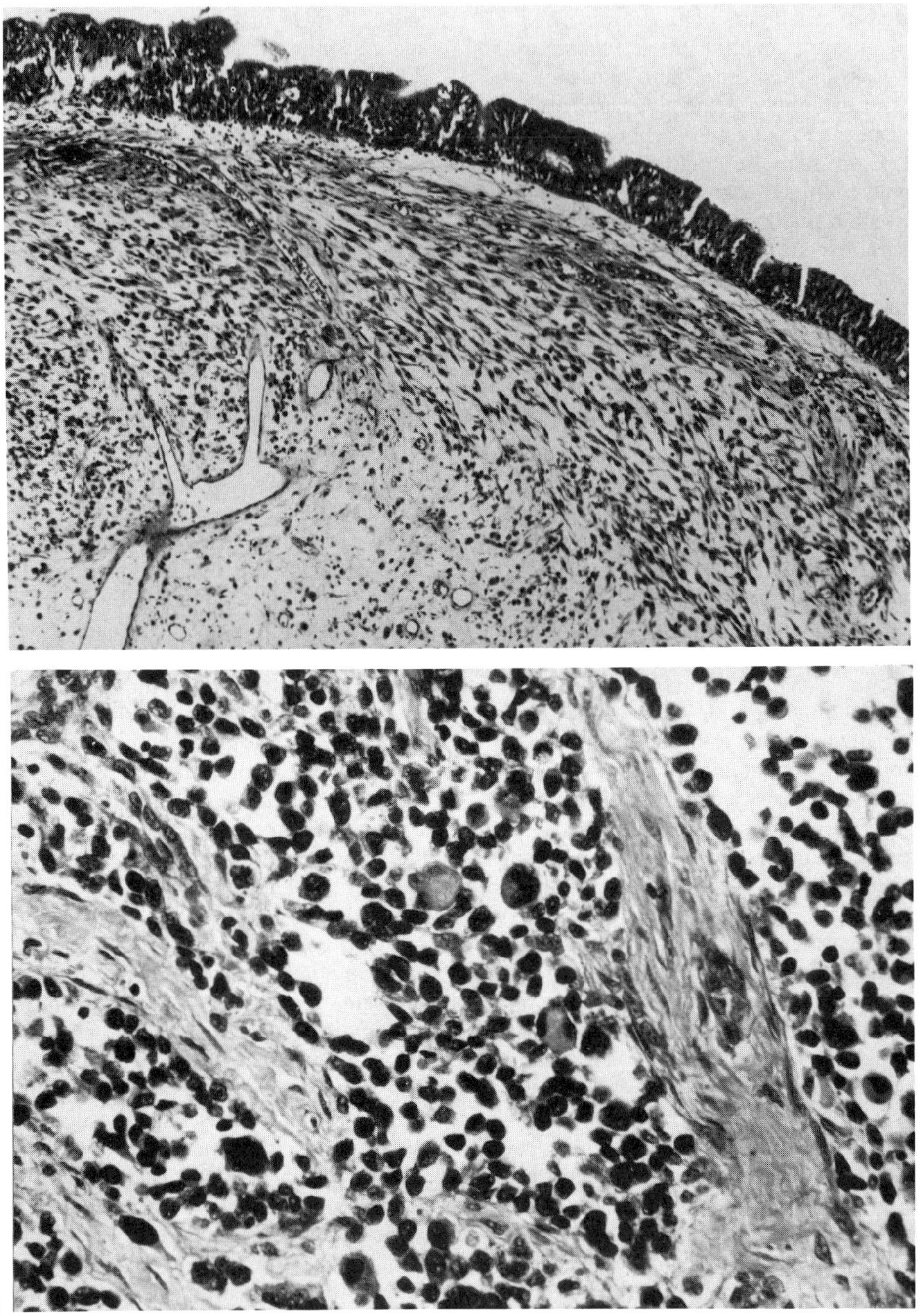

FIG 4–11.
A, botryoid rhabdomyosarcoma. **B,** alveolar rhabdomyosarcoma.

cellular compact zone of tumor cells immediately underlying the mucosal surface (Fig 4–11,a).

Alveolar rhabdomyosarcoma is characterized by aggregates of poorly differentiated round to ovoid cells divided by collagenous stromal septa (Fig 4–11,b). Cells vary from 15 to 30 μm and frequently have hyperchromatic, grooved, lobulated, or reniform nuclei with scant cytoplasm. The peripherally placed tumor cells show a distinct tendency to adhere to the fibrous septa, where they may form a single layer. The centrally placed tumor cells are more loosely arranged and frequently show degeneration and necrosis. Multinucleated cells are a common finding. Rhabdomyoblasts are seen only in 20% to 30% of cases and tend to be located along the fibrous septa. Areas of solid growth may also be present.

Pleomorphic sarcomas with definite skeletal muscle differentiation are exceedingly rare. They occur in adults and must be distinguished from more frequently occurring malignant fibrous histiocytomas and pleomorphic liposarcomas. Rhabdomyoblastic differentiation may occur as a heterologous component of other malignancies, for example, malignant mixed Müllerian tumor. All rhabdomyosarcomas are high-grade tumors.

Ultrastructural examination may demonstrate the presence of both thin and thick filaments in poorly differentiated rhabdomyosarcomas.[51, 52] Immunoperoxidase techniques may also prove helpful. Antibodies to the muscle-specific intermediate filament protein desmin, the oxygen-binding protein myoglobin, and skeletal muscle myosin have been used with varying degrees of success.[53–55]

ANGIOSARCOMA (MALIGNANT HEMANGIOENDOTHELIOMA)

Malignant endothelial vascular neoplasms form several fairly well-defined groups, including cutaneous-subcutaneous angiosarcoma, angiosarcoma of the breast, and angiosarcoma of deep soft tissues.[56, 57] These are all highly malignant tumors that tend to metastasize to the lymph nodes (except those arising in the breast) and the lungs.

Angiosarcoma of skin and subcutaneous tissue[58] has a notable tendency to occur in the scalp or face of the elderly, but also occurs many years following irradiation in a variety of sites and in areas of prolonged vascular stasis. It is well described in the lymphedematous arm in the combination postmastectomy-radiation setting (occurring about 10 years after therapy) and with chronic lymphedema, which may be either congenital or acquired. The nosologic category of lymphangiosarcoma was originally used for malignant endothelial neoplasms of this type,[59] but others argue that distinction of blood vessel and lymphatic endothelial neoplasms is difficult at best and prefer the noncommital term angiosarcoma.[57] Angiosarcoma in these sites tends to be characterized by multifocality, extending well beyond clinically apparent margins, and has a hemorrhagic, bruiselike, or blood blister-like appearance.

Angiosarcoma of the breast[60] is a rare neoplasm presenting in females during the reproductive years as a painless increase in the size of the breast with red-blue discoloration. It differs histologically from angiosarcoma of the skin-subcutaneous tissue by having large areas of vascular spaces lined by flattened endothelial cells, often producing a deceptively benign appearance. Overall, the prognosis is extremely poor, with a median survival of 22 months.[61] Two reports have suggested that small size (less than 5 cm), the absence of solid areas, and, perhaps, absence of blood lakes and necrosis histologically select a subset with a decidedly better prognosis.[62, 63] Lymph node metastases are rare. Benign vascular tumors of the breast are seemingly even rarer than angiosarcoma, but do occur, and are distinguished in part by sharp circumscription.[63]

Angiosarcomas of the deep soft tissues are usually high-grade tumors that occur in the extremities and the abdominal cavity. Maddox and Evans[56] suggest that this group resembles angiosarcomas of bone in that they have less papillary and solid growth and lower mitotic rates. Occurrence in the mediastinum and orbit has also been reported.

Pathological Findings.—The formation of vascular channels by neoplastic cells affords recognition of this neoplasm. Distinction from benign vascular processes can be made by attention to the lack of circumscription and the dissection of tissue planes by angiosarcomas, and the plump, hyperchromatic nuclei that tend to project into the lumen and form papillary projections (Fig 4–12). In addition, they lack the lobular organization of a benign vascular neoplasm. In poorly differentiated tumors, the vascular nature of the process may not be evident due to a solid pattern of epithelioid cells suggestive of carcinoma and/or of spindle cells similar to fibrosarcoma. Reticulin stains may reveal a basic vascular pattern in such cases.

Ultrastructural and immunoperoxidase techniques can be helpful in the evaluation of angiosarcomas. Intracytoplasmic lumen formation typical of early angiogenesis along with segmental basal lamina and pinocytotic vesicles can often be found, but the distinctive Weibel-Palade body is rarely, if ever, present in malig-

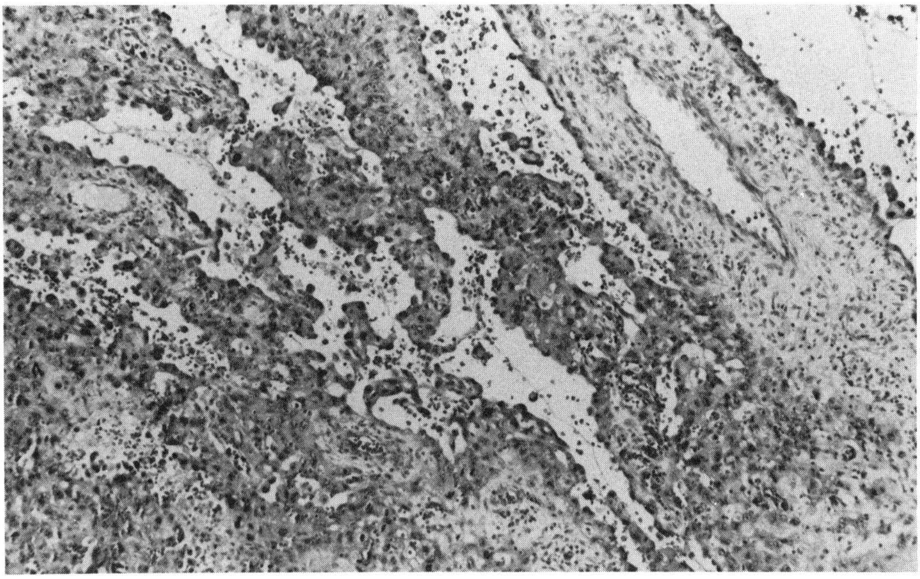

FIG 4–12.
Angiosarcoma.

nant vascular tumors. Likewise, factor VIII antigen is present only in well-differentiated lesions and is rarely helpful in difficult or poorly differentiated tumors. *Ulex europaeus* lectin is more sensitive but less specific. The absence of cytokeratin is useful in excluding carcinoma.

KAPOSI'S SARCOMA

Classical non-AIDS (acquired immune deficiency syndrome)-associated Kaposi's sarcoma is primarily a disease of males. Rarely seen in the United States, it is more common in Eastern

A 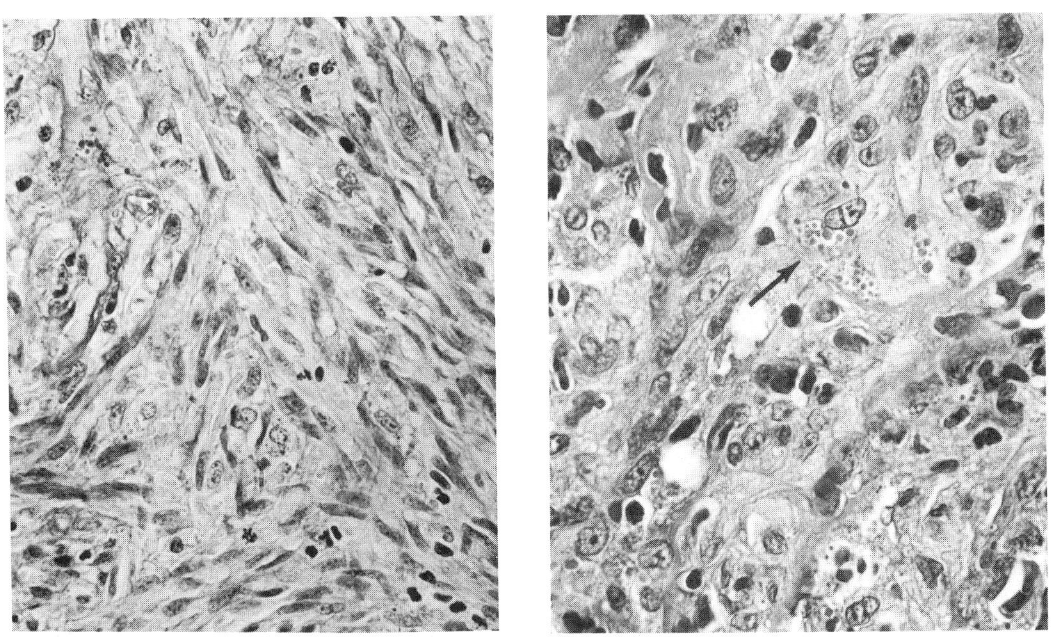 B

FIG 4–13.
Kaposi's sarcoma. **A,** characteristic "shot-through" pattern. **B,** *arrow* indicates PAS-positive bodies.

Europe and Italy and very common in equatorial Africa, where its geographical distribution is similar to that of Burkitt's lymphoma. In non-AIDS patients, it appears as a multifocal process affecting primarily the distal lower extremities and presents as elevated blue-red to hemorrhagic nodules. It may be accompanied by edema of the extremity. These nodules gradually increase in size and number, coalesce, may ulcerate, and spread proximally.[64] In contrast, the Kaposi's lesions seen in the AIDS population have a random distribution, are often small (less than 1 cm), and vary from pink to light purple. They may be round, but are often linear, following lines of cutaneous cleavage and are characterized by early, wide dissemination with a fulminating clinical course complicated by opportunistic infections.[65]

Pathological Findings.—The earliest histological manifestation of Kaposi's sarcoma can be extremely subtle. It is characterized by irregularly distributed capillaries with jagged outlines, lined by a single layer of hyperchromatic endothelial cells, with an accompanying mixed inflammatory reaction. Collections of uniform hyperchromatic spindle-shaped cells resembling fibrosarcoma or leiomyosarcoma are present in more advanced lesions, with a characteristic "shot through" pattern of extravasated red blood cells (Fig 4–13,a). Various combinations of these two patterns proliferate as the nodular form of the disease develops. The exact relationships of these cells to endothelium remains uncertain as authors have found variable staining with antibodies to factor VIII.[66, 67] Hemosiderin is usually present, as are periodic acid-Schiff stain (PAS)-positive diastase-resistant bodies ranging up to several microns in diameter[64] (Fig 4–13,b). The lesion may progress to a process indistinguishable from angiosarcoma or fibrosarcoma.[68]

HEMANGIOPERICYTOMA

In contrast to the other soft-tissue tumors discussed in this chapter, the majority of hemangiopericytomas are benign. They were first described by Stout and Murray[69] in 1942 and remain a source of diagnostic difficulty. The same histological pattern can be seen focally in other neoplasms (e.g., synovial sarcoma and fibrous histiocytoma), and diagnostic criteria have not always been strictly adhered to. The cell comprising this tumor resembles the pericyte[70] in its structure and relationship to vascular channels. It usually occurs as a deep tumor, with more than one half of the reported cases in the retroperitoneum, pelvis, and lower extremity.[71, 72] A similar, uniformly benign tumor occurs in the nasal cavity and paranasal sinuses. Size varies from a few centimeters to huge tumors that on occasion are associated with hypoglycemia. There may be clinical evidence of arteriovenous shunting. Pre-operative radiotherapy or ligation of afferent vessels reduces intra-operative bleeding.[73] Local excision appears to be adequate therapy for benign tumors, but more extensive surgery is required for the malignant forms.

Pathological Findings.—Hemangiopericytomas are circumscribed and histologically characterized by a monotonous proliferation of relatively small, slightly elongated cells with round to oval nuclei, arranged in haphazard, tortuous fashion around the myriads of capillaries that ramify through the tumor (Fig 4–14). They may abruptly empty into large, thin-walled channels, forming a "stag horn" pattern. The tumor cells are usually closely packed, but may be focally separated by varying amounts of connective tissue or mucoid material. Reticulin forms a complex arrangement around individual cells.

Ultrastructural studies have revealed elongated spindled mesenchymal cells closely apposed to capillary spaces. They may be partly invested by basal lamina and show cell membrane pinocytotic vesicles. Immunocytochemistry studies show the tumor cells to be positive for actin and vimentin but not desmin.[74–76]

Clinical behavior has been difficult to predict on the basis of pathological findings. Features associated with malignancy include size, cellularity, mitotic rate (more than four mitoses per 10 HPF), cellular pleomorphism, necrosis, and hemorrhage.[71, 72]

SYNOVIAL SARCOMA

Synovial sarcomas represent distinctive soft-tissue sarcomas of uncertain histogenesis. The name stems from their histological similarity to normal and reactive synovium and their tendency to occur in para-articular soft tissues near large joints. They may involve the tendon sheaths and bursae, but only rarely are seen in continuity with synovial membrane. Their occurrence in locations away from joints and ultrastructural features distinct from normal

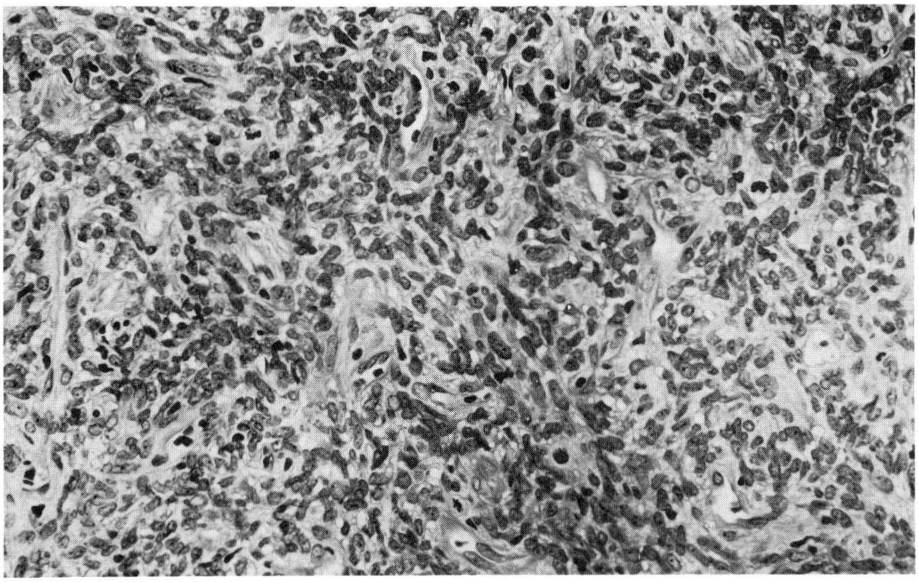

FIG 4–14.
Hemangiopericytoma.

synovial cells have cast doubt on their synovial derivation.[77]

These tumors occur primarily in adolescents and young adults and affect males more frequently than females.[78, 79] The presence of calcification may on occasion be visualized radiographically and serves as a helpful preoperative clue to the diagnosis. Despite some progress in the treatment of synovial sarcomas, the prognosis remains guarded. Postoperative radiotherapy has been effective at reducing the incidence of local recurrence, but distant metastases appear in 50% to 75% of the patients who are followed for sufficient periods of time. Clinical outcome is influenced by clinical stage at the time of presentation. Pathological features influencing prognosis include extensive calcification (82%, 5-year survival), size, and perhaps histological grade and mitotic rate.[80, 81]

Pathological Findings.—Most observers require the presence of a biphasic growth pattern to make a diagnosis of synovial sarcoma (Fig 4–15). The epithelial areas are composed of plump cuboidal to columnar cells with pale-staining cytoplasm. They form cords, nests, and glandular spaces. Intraluminal epithelial mucins are often present. The epithelial nesting pattern can often be highlighted with reticulin stains. The spindled fibrosarcoma-like areas are often the predominant pattern. They are composed of relatively uniform fasciculated spindle cells that may show focal areas of nuclear palisading and a hemangiopericytoma-like growth. Individual cells are typically surrounded by reticulin. The connective tissue matrix may be altered by areas of myxoid change, hyalinized fibrosis, calcification, and, on occasion, osteochondroid metaplasia.

The existence of a monophasic synovial sarcoma has been questioned by many. It has been suggested that calcification, proximity to a major joint, and the presence of a hemangiopericytoma-like growth pattern all favor a diagnosis of monophasic synovial sarcoma. Fibrosarcomas feature greater amounts of intercellular collagen, more elongated spindle cells in broader fascicles (often with a herringbone pattern), and a tendency for slightly greater cellular pleomorphism. The immunocytochemical detection of keratin in monophasic tumors lends further support for the separation of this lesion from the rare case of true fibrosarcoma.

Ultrastructural examination[82] of biphasic tumors confirms the mixed differentiation evident by light microscopy. The epithelial areas are invested by basal lamina and may show true lumen formation with apical microvilli, tight junctions, and laterally placed desmosomes. These findings contrast to the mesenchymal spindle-shaped fibroblasts, which are surrounded by abundant reticulin. The demonstra-

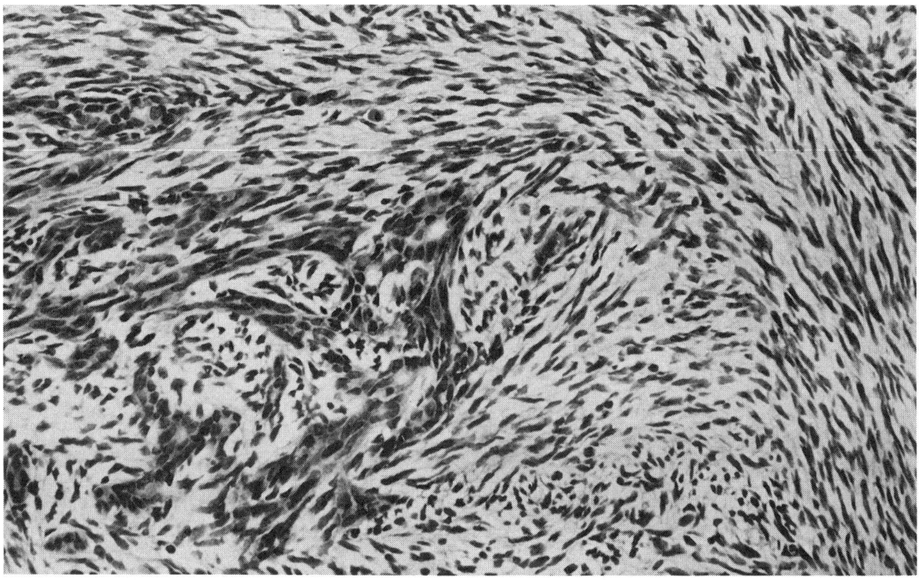

FIG 4–15.
Synovial sarcoma.

tion of cytokeratin in both biphasic and monophasic tumors[83] further contrasts these lesions to normal and reactive synovium, which do not express cytokeratin.

CLEAR CELL SARCOMA

This rare sarcoma is grouped with tendosynovial sarcomas by Hajdu,[9] but given unique status by others because of the presence of melanin in some cases. This slow-growing neoplasm typically involves tendons and aponeuroses of the extremities of young adults, seldom involves skin. In the largest published series, only 34 of 115 patients were living without disease.[84] Delayed recurrences and metastases are not uncommon, as in synovial sarcoma and epithelioid sarcoma. Radical excision or amputation with adjuvant chemotherapy has been recommended.

Pathological Findings.—Clear cell sarcoma typically presents as a circumscribed, lobulated, or multinodular tumor whose cut surface may show evidence of brown or black pigmentation in up to 20% of cases. The microscopic appearance is characterized by nests or fascicles of pale-staining elongated cells with uniform nuclei and a low mitotic rate (Fig 4–16). Although the cell groups are bordered by collagen that becomes continuous with the surrounding indigenous collagen, collagen production by individual cells does not appear common. Glycogen is present in two thirds of cases, and is partly responsible for the clear cytoplasm. Melanin stains are positive in many cases; premelanosomes may be ultrastructurally identified; and these tumors are reported to have the same immunocytochemical profile as malignant melanoma.[85] S-100 protein has been demonstrated by immunohistochemistry in most cases.[84, 86–89] Grading is presently not of value.

EPITHELIOID SARCOMA

There have been over 200 cases of epithelioid sarcoma reported since its description in the English literature in 1970.[90, 91] Despite this, its origin remains uncertain, and its distinctive growth pattern continues to be mistaken for granulomatous inflammation or metastatic carcinoma. Synovial, histiocytic, and fibroblastic origins have been suggested. It occurs most commonly on the extremities in areas having little subcutaneous fat, especially the hands and fingers (where it is the most common soft-tissue sarcoma), and is rarely seen on the trunk, head, and neck. The age prevalence is 15 to 35 years, with a 2 : 1 male-to-female ratio.[90] A slowly growing, painless nodule or multiple nodules

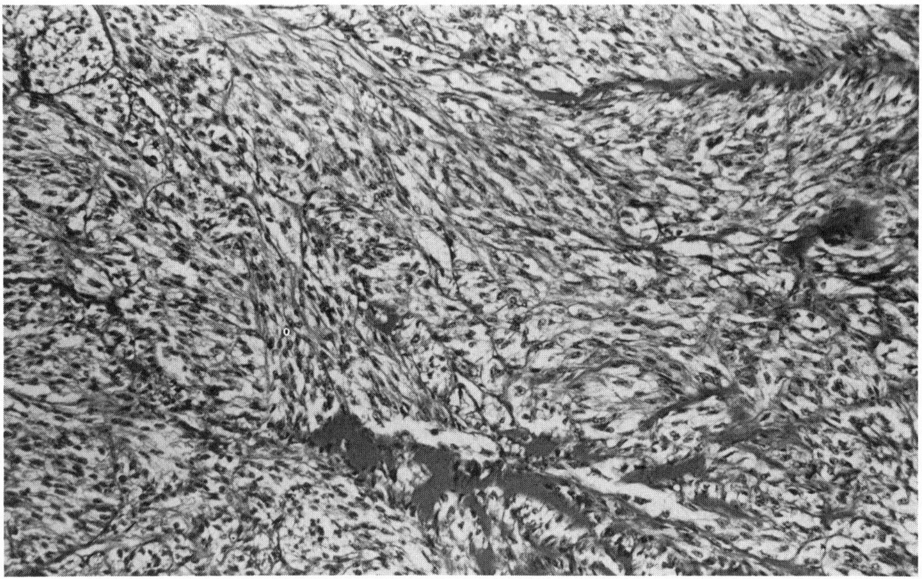

FIG 4–16.
Clear cell sarcoma.

are usually noted, which may be in the subcutaneous tissue or deeper, and may involve the skin, tendon, and aponeuroses. Size is highly variable, but many are quite small and innocent appearing. Radiographs may show calcification and/or bone erosion. Three out of four patients will develop recurrences (often multiple), some delayed by many years (in common with synovial sarcoma and clear cell sarcoma). Extension along the neurovascular bundle is a typical feature. Multiple regional and distant skin metastases tend to develop, with subsequent metastases to the lymph nodes and lung in about half the cases.[92–94] In one study female patients had an 80% 5-year survival compared to 40% for males.[95, 96]

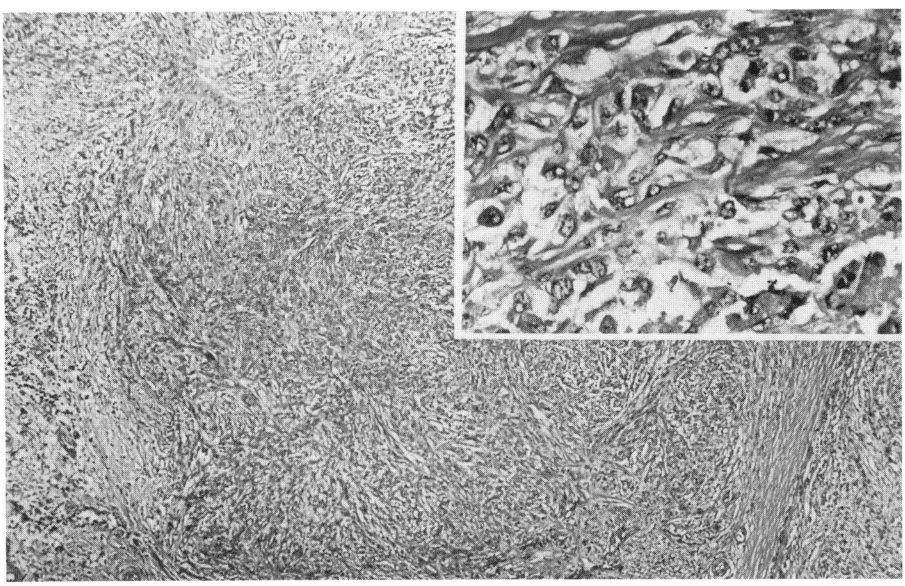

FIG 4–17.
Epithelioid sarcoma (inset: high power view of tumor).

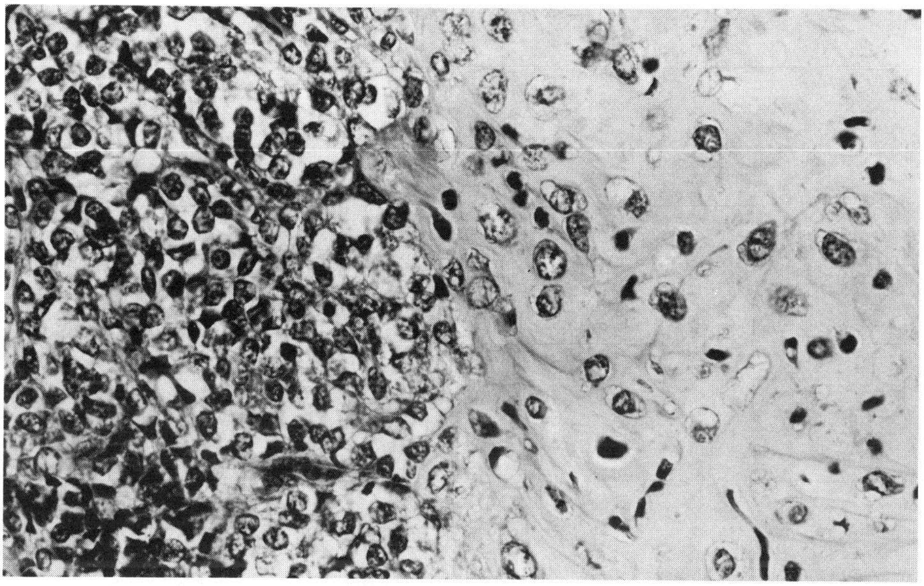

FIG 4–18.
Mesenchymal chondrosarcoma.

Pathological Findings.—The growth pattern consists of a nodular arrangement of epithelioid cells with eosinophilic cytoplasm, with necrosis in the centers of the nodules (Fig 4–17). This latter feature imparts a granulomatous appearance to the lesion. There is often a spindle cell component at the periphery of the nodules, but a biphasic pattern similar to synovial sarcoma is not seen. Epithelioid sarcomas have been shown to have intracytoplasmic cytokeratin.[97]

MESENCHYMAL CHONDROSARCOMA

Mesenchymal chondrosarcoma may occur as a tumor of soft tissue or, more commonly, bone.[98] It is a high-grade tumor composed largely of primitive "precartilage mesenchyme." The evolution of this tumor is rapid, with early metastases in most cases. It is most often encountered in the head and neck area (notably the orbit), the dura mater of brain and spinal cord, and less often the lower extremities.[99] Both radical surgery and chemotherapy are required in most cases.[100]

Pathological Findings.—The histological appearance is distinctive, with fields of relatively small, crowded cells with hyperchromatic nuclei and scant cytoplasm, showing abrupt transition to chondroid islands that may have central calcification or ossification (Fig 4–18). Richly vascular areas may bear a resemblance to hemangiopericytoma.[99] Small biopsies or poorly handled material may create confusion with other small cell tumors. Histological grading is not of value.

MYXOID CHONDROSARCOMA

Myxoid chondrosarcoma occurs primarily in the deep soft tissues of the extremities as well as in bone. It is a neoplasm of middle age and beyond, presenting as a slowly growing mass that may be painful or tender. The thigh and popliteal areas are favored sites. Slow growth with recurrence in a significant number of cases and metastases in some, often delayed, characterize this tumor.[101] Radical local excision is reported to be the treatment of choice, with consideration of adjunctive therapy in the more cellular examples.[102] Most observers feel that myxoid chondrosarcomas and the so-called "chordoid sarcoma" are the same neoplasm.[103–105]

Pathological Findings.—Myxoid chondrosarcomas are well circumscribed or encapsulated, with a lobulated cut surface made up of

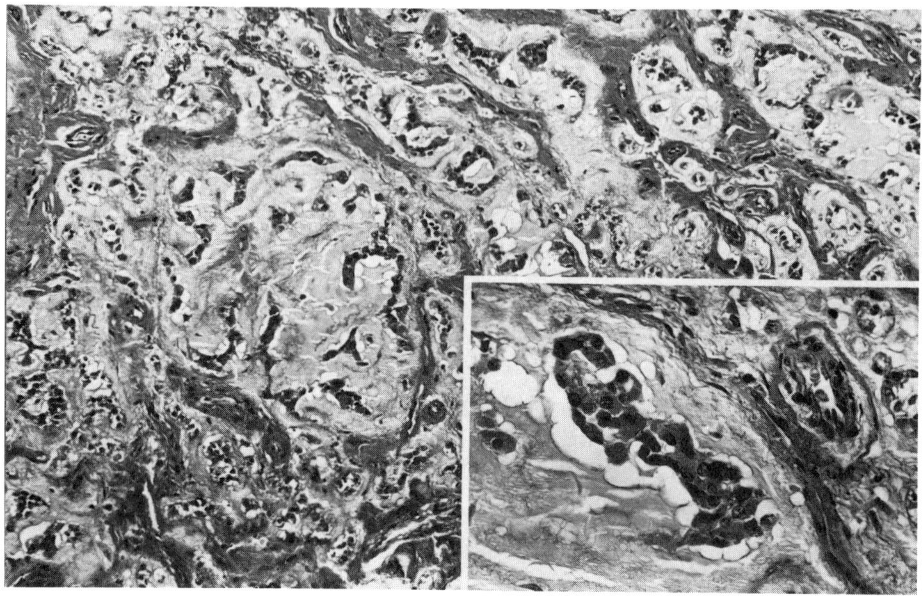

FIG 4–19.
Myxoid chondrosarcoma (inset: high power view showing cords of chondroblasts).

a gelatinous tan to brown tissue with varying degrees of hemorrhage. Histologically, each lobule is composed of cords of chondroblasts suspended in myxoic material (Fig. 4–19). Rare areas with a chondroid appearance may be seen. The individual cells are uniform, with distinctively eosinophilic cytoplasm and hyperchromatic nuclei. Mitoses are rare. The cytoplasm contains glycogen. The matrix shows characteristics of chondroid mucin, being resistant to digestion with hyaluronidase and showing metachromatic staining with toluidine blue. Enzinger and Weiss[88] report that the rate of recurrence and metastasis is closely related to cellularity and the relative amounts of myxoid material.

Ultrastructural features and S-100 protein positivity, and appropriate mucopolysaccharide content of stroma, have been cited in support of the chondroid derivation of this distinctive soft-tissue tumor.[105–108]

EXTRASKELETAL EWING'S SARCOMA

Extraskeletal Ewing's sarcoma is histologically identical to its osseous counterpart and must be distinguished from Ewing's sarcoma of bone, which may have a clinically subtle osseous component. The histogenesis is undetermined, but is thought to be a primitive mesenchymal cell.[109, 110] Soft-tissue Ewing's sarcoma typically presents as a rapidly growing deep mass in the paravertebral area, chest wall, pelvis, hip, or lower extremity of an adolescent or young adult. The tumor may be painful and may involve peripheral nerves or the spinal cord with consequent neurological deficit.

In this highly lethal tumor, early metastases to the lungs and skeleton are the rule, often being present at the time of initial diagnosis. Therapy consists of radical surgery and irradiation to control the primary site, and sequential chemotherapy for early metastatic disease.

Pathological Findings.—This highly cellular, small, round cell tumor is compartmentalized into "lobules" by interconnecting bands of delicate connective tissue. The cells are uniform with rounded nuclei possessing a smooth, delicate chromatin and scant cytoplasm that is often clear (Fig 4–20). Mitoses are relatively few. Special stains usually show the presence of cytoplasmic glycogen and the absence of reticulin within the cell sheets.[111, 112] All of these tumors are high-grade. Ultrastructural and immunoperoxidase studies have failed to show any consistent evidence of cell differentiation and are helpful in excluding other differentiated round cell tumors.[110]

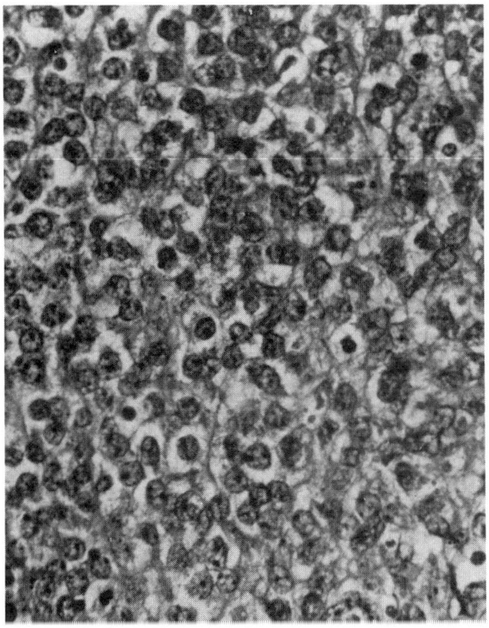

FIG 4–20.
Extraskeletal Ewing's sarcoma.

ALVEOLAR SOFT-PART SARCOMA

Alveolar soft-part sarcoma is an extremely rare neoplasm of uncertain histogenesis, commonly involving the lower extremity of young adults.[113, 114] Pulsation or bruit may be present due to rich vascularity, and operative hemorrhage may be massive. Brain or lung metastasis may be the presenting feature, or may be delayed many years. In children, head and neck location is common, notably the orbit and tongue.

This very slowly growing tumor has a poor prognosis; approximately 60% of patients survive only 5 years. Currently recommended therapy consists of radical limb-sparing surgical excision of primary and metastatic sites with radiotherapy and/or chemotherapy.

Pathological Findings.—Rounded nests of cells are circumscribed by a single layer of endothelial cells that form the lining of the intervening vascular channels. These alveolar groups are further divided into masses by coarse, fibrous trabeculae (Fig 4–21). The individual cells are large, loosely cohesive, and fairly regular, with a central or eccentric nucleus possessing a small but prominent nucleolus. Cytoplasm is moderate, eosinophilic, and granular, and in most cases has PAS-positive, diastase-resistant crystals.[115] Glycogen is also present. Mitoses are not prominent, but vascular invasion is often seen.

Distinctive membrane-bound, rod-shaped or platelike crystals are ultrastructurally found in most but not all cases of alveolar soft-part sarcoma.[115] The crystals have some similarity

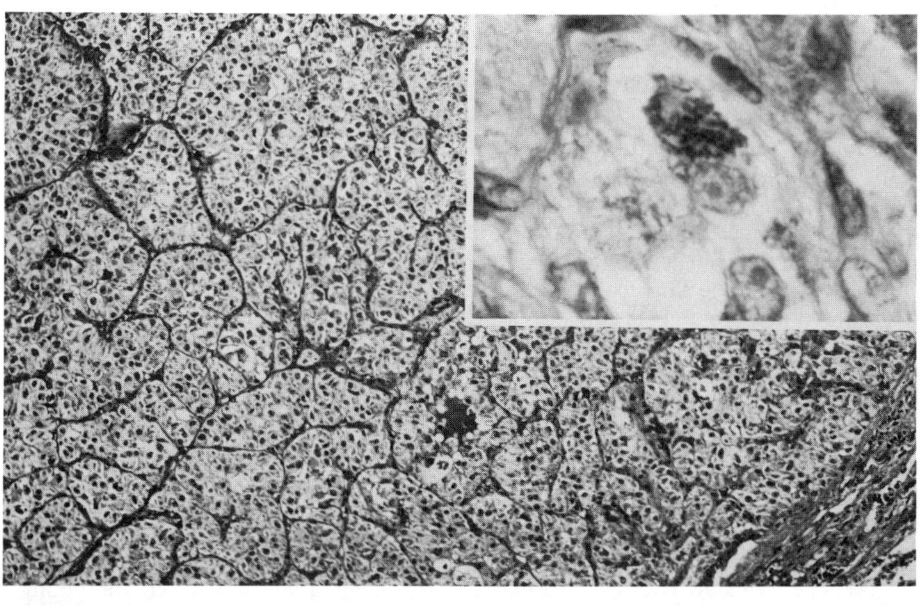

FIG 4–21.
Alveolar soft-part sarcoma (inset: high power view demonstrating PAS-positive, diastase-resistant crystals).

to those seen in rhabdomyomas and nemaline myopathy. Immunocytochemical detection of renin prompted one group of investigators to suggest a close kinship with juxtaglomerular tumors of the kidney,[116] but a subsequent study failed to confirm these findings.[117] Other immunocytochemical studies have also been conflicting, some being entirely negative when tested with multiple antibodies,[118] and others, perhaps the majority, suggesting a kinship with skeletal muscle.[119, 120]

REFERENCES

1. Russell WO, Cohen J, Enzinger F, et al: A clinical and pathological staging system for soft tissue sarcomas. *Cancer* 1977; 40:1562–1570.
2. Costa J, Wesley RA, Glatstein E, et al: The grading of soft tissue sarcomas. Results of a clinicohistopathologic correlation in a series of 163 cases. *Cancer* 1984; 53:530–541.
3. Myhre-Jensen O, Kaae S, Madsen EH, et al: Histopathological grading in soft-tissue tumors. Relation to survival in 261 surgically treated patients. *Acta Pathol Microbiol Immunol Scand* [*A*] 1983; 91:145–150.
4. Trojani M, Contesso G, Coindre JM, et al: Soft-tissue sarcomas of adults; study of pathological prognostic variables and definition of histopathological grading system. *Int J Cancer* 1984; 33:37–42.
5. Mandard AM, Petiot JF, Marnay J, et al: Prognostic factors in soft tissue sarcomas. A multivariate analysis of 109 cases. *Cancer* 1989; 63:1437–1451.
6. Tsujimoto M, Aozasa K, Ueda T, et al: Multivariate analysis for histologic prognostic factors in soft tissue sarcomas. *Cancer* 1988; 62:994–998.
7. Kulander BG, Polissar L, Yang CY, et al: Grading of soft tissue sarcomas: Necrosis as a determinant of survival. *Mod Pathol* 1989; 2:205–208.
8. Enzinger FM, Weiss SW: *Soft Tissue Tumors*, 2nd ed. St. Louis, C. V. Mosby, 1988.
9. Hajdu SI: *Pathology of Soft Tissues*. Philadelphia, Lea & Febiger, 1979.
10. Lattes R: Tumors of the soft tissues, in Hartmann WH (ed): *Atlas of Tumor Pathology*, 2nd series, fasc 1. 1982, pp 160–168.
11. Enzinger FM, Winslow DJ: Liposarcoma: A study of 103 cases. *Virchow Arch Path Anat* [*A*] 1962; 335:367–388.
12. Evans HL, Soule EH, Winkelmann RK: Atypical lipoma, atypical intramuscular lipoma, and well differentiated retroperiteonal liposarcoma. *Cancer* 1979; 43:574–584.
13. Evans HL: Liposarcoma: A study of 55 cases with a reassessment of its classification. *Am J Surg Pathol* 1979; 3:507–523.
14. Kindblom LG, Angervall L, Svendsen P: Liposarcoma: A clinicopathologic, radiographic, and prognostic study. *Acta Pathol Microbiol Scand* [*A*] 1975; (suppl 253).
15. Bolen JW, Thorning D: Liposarcoma: A histogenetic approach to the classification of adipose tissue neoplasms. *Am J Surg Pathol* 1984; 8:3–17.
16. Reitamo, JJ: The desmoid tumor. IV. Choice of treatment, results, and complications. *Arch Surg* 1983; 118:1318–1322.
17. Kinzbrunner B, Ritter S, Domingo J, et al: Remission of rapidly growing desmoid tumors after tamoxifen therapy. *Cancer* 1983; 52:2201–2204.
18. Richards RC, Rogers SW, Gardner EJ: Spontaneous mesenteric fibromatosis in Gardner's syndrome. *Cancer* 1981; 47:597–601.
19. Enzinger FM, Weiss SW: *Soft Tissue Tumors*. St. Louis, C. V. Mosby, 1983, p 114.
20. Pritchard DJ, Soule EH, Taylor WF, et al: Fibrosarcoma—a clinicopathologic and statistical study of 199 tumors of the soft tissues of the extremities and trunk. *Cancer* 1974; 33:888–897.
21. Frierson HF, Cooper PH: Myxoid variant of dermatofibrosarcoma protuberans. *Am J Surg Pathol* 1983; 7:445–450.
22. Dupree WB, Weiss SW: Pigmented dermatofibrosarcoma protuberans (Bednar tumor): A clinicopathologic, ultrastructural, and immunohistochemical study (abstract). *Lab Invest* 1983; 48:21A–22A.
23. Weiss SW, Enzinger FM: Malignant fibrous histiocytoma: an analysis of 200 cases. *Cancer* 1978; 41:2250–2266.
24. Ozzello L, Stout AP, Murray MR: Cultural characteristics of malignant histiocytomas and fibrous xanthomas. *Cancer* 1963; 16:331–344.
25. Weiss SW, Enzinger FM: Myxoid variant of malignant fibrous histiocytoma. *Cancer* 1977; 39:1672–1685.
26. Enzinger FM: Angiomatoid malignant fibrous histiocytoma: A distinct fibrohistiocytic tumor of children and young adults simulating a vascular neoplasm. *Cancer* 1979; 44:2147–2157.

27. Angervall L, Hagmar B, Kindblom LG: Malignant giant cell tumor of soft tissues: A clinicopathologic, cytologic, ultrastructural, angiographic and microangiographic study. *Cancer* 1981; 47:736–747.
28. Enzinger FM, Weiss SW: *Soft Tissue Tumors*. St. Louis, C. V. Mosby, 1983, p 171.
29. Kempson RL, Kyriakos M: Fibroxanthosarcoma of the soft tissues: A type of malignant fibrous histiocytoma. *Cancer* 1972; 29:961–976.
30. Guccion JG, Enzinger FM: Malignant giant cell tumor of soft parts: An analysis of 32 cases. *Cancer* 1972; 29:1518–1529.
31. Kyriakos M, Kempson RL: Inflammatory fibrous histiocytoma. *Cancer* 1976; 37:1584–1606.
32. Hoffman MA, Dickerson GR: Malignant fibrous histiocytoma: An ultrastructural study of eleven cases. *Hum Pathol* 1983; 14:913–922.
33. DuBoulay CEH: Demonstration of alpha 1-antitrypsin and alpha-1-antichymotrypsin in fibrous histiocytomas using the immunoperoxidase technique. *Am J Surg Pathol* 1982; 6:559–564.
34. Harkin JC, Reed RJ: Tumors of the peripheral nervous system, in Firminger HI (ed): *Atlas of Tumor Pathology*, 2nd series, fasc 3. Washington, D.C., Armed Forces Institute of Pathology, 1969.
35. Erlandson RA, Woodruff JM: Peripheral nerve sheath tumors. An electron microscopic study of 43 cases. *Cancer* 1982; 49:273–287.
36. Taxy JB, Battifora H, Trujillo Y, et al: Electron microscopy in the diagnosis of malignant schwannoma. *Cancer* 1981; 48:1381–1391.
37. Weiss SW, Langloss JM, Enzinger FM: Value of S100 protein in the diagnosis of soft tissue tumors with a particular reference to benign and malignant Schwann cell tumors. *Lab Invest* 1983; 49:299–308.
38. Wick MR, Swanson PE, Scheithauer BW, et al: Malignant peripheral nerve sheath tumor. An immunohistochemical study of 62 cases. *Am J Clin Pathol* 1987; 87:425–433.
39. Enzinger FM, Weiss SW: *Soft Tissue Tumors*. St. Louis, C. V. Mosby, 1983, p 298.
40. Wile AG, Evans HL, Ramsdahl MM: Leiomyosarcoma of soft tissue: A clinicopathologic study. *Cancer* 1981; 48:1022–1032.
41. Shmookler BM, Lauer DH: Retroperitoneal leiomyosarcoma: A clinicopathologic analysis of 36 cases. *Am J Surg Pathol* 1983; 7:269–280.
42. Dahl I, Angervall L: Cutaneous and subcutaneous leiomyosarcoma: A clinicopathologic study of 47 patients. *Pathol Eur* 1974; 9:307–315.
43. Fields JP, Helwig EB: Leiomyosarcoma of the skin and subcutaneous tissue. *Cancer* 1981; 47:156–169.
44. Hajdu SI: *Pathology of Soft Tissues*. Philadelphia, Lea & Febiger, 1979.
45. Appelman HD, Helwig EB: Gastric epithelioid leiomyoma and leiomyosarcoma (leiomyoblastoma). *Cancer* 1976; 38:708–728.
46. Ming S-C: Tumors of the esophagus and stomach, in Firminger HI (ed): *Atlas of Tumor Pathology*, 2nd series, fasc 7. Washington, D.C., Armed Forces Institute of Pathology, 1973, p 210.
47. Knapp RH, Wick MR, Goellner JR, et al: Leiomyoblastomas and their relationship to other smooth-muscle tumors of the gastrointestinal tract: An electron microscopic study. *Am J Surg Pathol* 1984; 8:449–461.
48. Enzinger FM, Shiraki M: Alveolar rhabdomyosarcoma: An analysis of 110 cases. *Cancer* 1969; 24:18–31.
49. Palmer N, Foulkes M: Histopathology and prognosis in the second intergroup rhabdomyosarcoma study (IRS-II). *Proc Am Soc Clin Oncol* 1983; 3:897.
50. Maurer HM, Moon T, Donaldson M, et al: The intergroup rhabdomyosarcoma study: A preliminary report. *Cancer* 1977; 40:2015–2026.
51. Bundtzen JL, Norback DH: The ultrastructure of poorly differentiated rhabdomyosarcoma: A case report and literature review. *Hum Pathol* 1982; 13:301–313.
52. Morales AR, Fine F, Horn RC: Rhabdomyosarcoma: An ultrastructural appraisal. *Pathol Annu* 1972; 7:81–106.
53. DeJong ASH, van Raamsdonk W, van Vark M, et al: Myosin and myoglobin as tumor markers in the diagnosis of rhabdomyosarcoma; a comparative study. *Am J Surg Pathol* 1984; 8:521–528.
54. Kagnana N, Sano T, Inaba H, et al: Immunohistochemistry of myoglobin in rhabdomyosarcoma. *Acta Pathol Jpn* 1983; 33:515–522.
55. Miettinen M, Lehto VP, Badley RA, et al: Alveolar rhabdomyosarcoma: Demonstration of the muscle type of intermediate filament protein desmin as a diagnostic aid. *Am J Pathol* 1982; 108:246–251.

56. Maddox JC, Evans HL: Angiosarcoma of skin and soft tissue; a study of 44 cases. *Cancer* 1981; 48:1907–1921.
57. Enzinger FM, Weiss SW: *Soft Tissue Tumors.* St. Louis, C. V. Mosby, 1983, pp 422–437.
58. Rosai J, Sumner HW, Kostianovsky M, et al: Angiosarcoma of the skin. *Hum Pathol* 1976; 7:83–109.
59. Stewart FW, Treves N: Lymphangiosarcoma in post-mastectomy lymphedema: A report of six cases in elephantiasis chirurgica. *Cancer* 1948; 1:64–81.
60. Steingaszner LC, Enzinger FM, Taylor HB: Hemangiosarcoma of the breast. *Cancer* 1965; 18:352–361.
61. Antman KH, Corson J, Greenberger J, et al: Multimodality therapy in the management of angiosarcoma of the breast. *Cancer* 1982; 50:2000–2003.
62. Mering MJ, Carter D, Berman M: Angiosarcoma of the breast. *Am J Surg Pathol* 1983; 7:53–60.
63. Donnell RM, Rosen PR, Lieberman PH, et al: Angiosarcoma and other vascular tumors of the breast, pathologic analysis as a guide to prognosis. *Am J Surg Pathol* 1981; 5:629–642.
64. Templeton AC: Kaposi's sarcoma. *Pathol Annu* 1981; 16(part 2):315–336.
65. Gottlieb GJ, Ackerman AB: Kaposi's sarcoma: An extensively disseminated form in young homosexual men. *Hum Pathol* 1982; 13:882–892.
66. Akhtar M, Bunuan H, Ali M, et al: Kaposi's sarcoma in renal transplant recipients: Ultrastructural and immunoperoxidase studies in 4 cases. *Cancer* 1984; 53:258–266.
67. Morales AR, Nadji M, Ziegles-Weissman J, et al: Kaposi's sarcoma: Immunohistologic evidence for an endothelial origin. *Arch Pathol* 1981; 105:274–275.
68. Schwartz RA, Kardashian JF, McNutt NS, et al: Cutaneous angiosarcoma resembling anaplastic Kaposi's sarcoma in a homosexual man. *Cancer* 1983; 51:721–726.
69. Stout AP, Murray MR: Hemangiopericytoma: A vascular tumor featuring Zimmermann's pericytes. *Ann Surg* 1942; 116:26–33.
70. Zimmermann KW: Der feinere Bau der Blutcapillaren. *Z. Anat Entwicklungsg* 1923; 68:29–109.
71. Enzinger FM, Smith BH: Hemangiopericytoma: An analysis of 106 cases. *Hum Pathol* 1976; 7:62–81.
72. McMaster M, Soule EH, Ivins JC: Hemangiopericytoma: A clinicopathologic study and long-term followup of 60 patients. *Cancer* 1975; 36:2232–2244.
73. Enzinger FM, Weiss SW: *Soft Tissue Tumors.* St. Louis, C. V. Mosby, 1983, p 479.
74. Dardick I, Hammar SP, Scheithauer BW: Ultrastructural spectrum of hemangiopericytoma: A comparative study of fetal, adult, and neoplastic pericytes. *Ultrastruct Pathol* 1989; 13:111–154.
75. Hultberg BM, Daugaard S, Johansen HF, et al: Malignant haemangiopericytomas and haemangioendotheliosarcomas: An immunohistochemical study. *Histopathology* 1988; 12:405–414.
76. Mittal KR, Gerald W, Truel D: Hemangiopericytoma of the breast: Report of a case with ultrastructural and immunohistochemical staining. *Hum Pathol* 1986; 17:1181–1183.
77. Schmidt D, Mackay B: Ultrastructure of human tendon sheath and synovium: Implications for tumor histogenesis. *Ultrastruct Pathol* 1982; 3:269–278.
78. Evans HL: Synovial sarcoma: A study of 23 biphasic and 27 probably monophasic examples. in Sommers S, Rosen PP (eds): *Pathol Annu 1980,* part 2. New York, Appleton-Century Crofts, 1980, pp 309–331.
79. Krall RA, Kostinovsky M, Patchefsky AS: Synovial sarcoma: A clinical, pathological, and ultrastructural study of 26 cases supporting the recognition of a monophasic variant. *Am J Surg Pathol* 1981; 5:137–151.
80. Varela-Duran J, Enzinger FM: Calcifying synovial sarcoma. *Cancer* 1982; 50:345–352.
81. Rooser B, Willen H, Hugoson A, et al: Prognostic factors in synovial sarcoma. *Cancer* 1989; 63:2182–2185.
82. Abenoza P, Manivel JC, Swanson PE, et al: Synovial sarcoma: Ultrastructural study and immunohistochemical analysis by a combined peroxidase-antiperoxidase/avidin-biotin-peroxidase technique. *Hum Pathol* 1986; 17:1107–1115.
83. Corson JM, Weiss LM, Banks-Schlegel SP, et al: Keratin proteins in synovial sarcomas (letter to the editor). *Am J Surg Pathol* 1983; 7:107–109.
84. Enzinger FM: Clear cell sarcoma of tendons and aponeuroses: An analysis of 21 cases. *Cancer* 1968; 18:1163–1174.
85. Swanson P, Wick MR: Clear cell sarcoma. An immunohistochemical analysis of six

cases and comparison with other epithelioid neoplasms of soft tissue. *Arch Pathol Lab Med* 1989; 113:55–60.

86. Chung EB, Enzinger FM: Malignant melanoma of soft parts: A reassessment of clear cell sarcoma. *Am J Surg Pathol* 1983; 7:405–413.
87. Eckhardt JJ, Pritchard DF, Soule EH: Clear cell sarcoma: A clinicopathologic study of 27 cases. *Cancer* 1983; 52:1482–1488.
88. Kindblom LG, Lodding P, Angervall L: Clear cell sarcoma of tendons and aponeuroses: An immunohistochemical and electron microscopic analysis indicating neural crest origin. *Virchow's Arch Pathol Anat [A]* 1983; 401:109–128.
89. Mukai M, Torikata C, Iri H, et al: Histogenesis of clear cell sarcoma of tendons and aponeuroses. *Am J Pathol* 1984; 114:264–272.
90. Enzinger FM: Epithelioid sarcoma: A sarcoma simulating a granuloma or a carci noma. *Cancer* 1970; 26:1029–1041.
91. Chase DR, Enzinger FM: Epithelioid sarcoma. Diagnosis, prognostic indicators, and treatment. *Am J Surg Pathol* 1985; 9:241–263.
92. Enzinger FM, Weiss SW: *Soft Tissue Tumors.* St. Louis, C. V. Mosby, 1983, pp 787–795.
93. Prat J, Woodruff JM, Marcove RC: Epithelioid sarcoma: An analysis of 22 cases indicating the prognostic significance of vascular invasion and regional lymph node metastasis. *Cancer* 1978; 41:1472–1487.
94. Santiago H, Feinerman LK, Lattes R: Epithelioid sarcoma: A clinical and pathological study of nine cases. *Hum Pathol* 1972; 3:133–147.
95. Bos GD, Pritchard DJ, Reiman HM, et al: Epithelioid sarcoma. An analysis of fifty-one cases. *J Bone Joint Surg (am)* 1988; 70A:862–870.
96. Manivel JC, Wick MR, Dehner LP, et al: Epithelioid sarcoma. An immunohistochemical study. *Am J Clin Pathol* 1987; 87:319–326.
97. Chase DR, Enzinger FM, Weiss SW, et al: Keratin in epithelioid sarcoma: An immunohistochemical study. *Am J Surg Pathol* 1984; 8:435–441.
98. Lichtenstein L, Bernstein D: Unusual benign and malignant chondroid tumors of bone: A survey of some mesenchymal cartilage tumors and malignant chondroblastic tumors including a few multicentric ones and chondromyxoid fibromas. *Cancer* 1959; 12:1142–1157.
99. Guccion JG, Font RL, Enzinger FM, et al: Extraskeletal mesenchymal chondrosarcoma. *Arch Pathol* 1973; 95:336–340.
100. Huvos AG, Rosen G, Dabska M, et al: Mesenchymal chondrosarcoma: A clinicopathologic analysis of 35 cases with emphasis on therapy. *Cancer* 1983; 51:1230–1237.
101. Enzinger FM, Shiraki M: Extraskeletal myxoid chondrosarcoma: An analysis of 34 cases. *Hum Pathol* 1972; 3:421–435.
102. Enzinger FM, Weiss SW: *Soft Tissue Tumors.* St. Louis, C. V. Mosby, 1983, p 705.
103. Martin R, Melnick PJ, Warner NE, et al: Chordoid sarcoma. *Am J Surg Pathol* 1973; 59:623–635.
104. Robertson DI, Hogg GR: Chordoid sarcoma: Ultrastructural evidence supporting a synovial origin. *Cancer* 1980; 45:520–527.
105. Weiss SW: Ultrastructure of the so-called "chordoid sarcoma": Evidence supporting cartilaginous differentiation. *Cancer* 1976; 37:300–306.
106. Fu Y, Kay S: A comparative ultrastructural study of mesenchymal chondrosarcoma and myxoid chondrosarcoma. *Cancer* 1974; 33:1531–1542.
107. Wetzel WJ, Reuhl KR: Micro-tubular aggregates in the rough endoplasmic reticulum of a myxoid chondrosarcoma. *Ultrastruct Pathol* 1980; 1:519–525.
108. Fletcher CD, Powell G, McKee PH: Extraskeletal myxoid chondrosracoma: A histochemical and immunohistochemical study. *Histopathology* 1986; 10:489–499.
109. Dickman PS, Liotta LA, Triche TJ: Ewing's sarcoma: Characterization in established cultures and evidence for its histogenesis. *Lab Invest* 1982; 47:375–382.
110. Moll R, Lee I, Gould VE, et al: Immunocytochemical analysis of Ewing's tumors. Patterns of expression of intermediate filaments and desmosomal proteins indicate cell type heterogeneity and pluripotential differentiation. *Am J Pathol* 1987; 127:288–304.
111. Angervall L, Enzinger FM: Extraskeletal neoplasm resembling Ewing's sarcoma. *Cancer* 1975; 36:240–251.
112. Wigger HJ, Salazar GH, Blanc WA: Extraskeletal Ewing sarcoma. *Arch Pathol Lab Med* 1977; 101:446–449.
113. Lieberman PH, Foote FW Jr, Stewart FW, et al: Alveolar soft-part sarcoma. *JAMA* 1966; 198:1047–1051.

114. Christopherson WM, Foote FW Jr, Stewart FW: Alveolar soft-part sarcoma: Structurally characteristic tumors of uncertain histogenesis. *Cancer* 1952; 5:100–111.

115. Ekfors TO, Kalimo H, Rantakakko V, et al: Alveolar soft part sarcoma: A report of two cases with some histochemical and ultrastructural observations. *Cancer* 1979; 43:1672–1677.

116. DeSchryver-Kecskemeti I, Kraus FT, Engelman BA, et al: Alveolar soft-part sarcoma—a malignant angioreninoma. Histochemical, immunocytochemical, and electron-microscopic study of four cases. *Am J Surg Pathol* 1982; 6:5–18.

117. Mukai M, Iri H, Nakajima T, et al: Alveolar soft part sarcoma: A review on its histogenesis and further studies based on electron microscopy, immunohistochemistry, and biochemistry. *Am J Surg Pathol* 1983; 7:679–689.

118. Auerbach HE, Brooks JJ: Alveolar soft part sarcoma. A clinicopathologic and immunohistochemical study. *Cancer* 1987; 60:66–73.

119. Ordonez NG, Ro JY, Mackay B: Alveolar soft part sarcoma. An ultrastructural and immunocytochemical investigation of its histogenesis. *Cancer* 1989; 63:1721–1736.

120. Mukai M, Torikata C, Shimoda T, et al: Alveolar soft part sarcoma. Assessment of immunohistochemical demonstration of desmin using paraffin sections and frozen sections. *Virchows Arch Pathol Anat [A]* 1989; 414:503–509.

Chapter 5

Staging and Sarcoma Subtypes: Effect on Response and Survival

Richard Pazdur

Laurence H. Baker

Staging systems attempt to classify cancer patients according to subgroups (stages) involving a common natural history, extent of disease, and predicted response to therapy. The goal is to assign therapeutic interventions to each stage, formulate accurate prognoses, and compare treatment modalities in end-results studies.

Staging systems for soft-tissue sarcomas are still controversial: although most of these neoplasms arise in the extremities, they also appear in other areas, including the abdomen, and the head and neck, thus precluding a uniform surgical approach. In addition, the variety of histological subtypes makes definitive statements regarding biological activity difficult.[1] For example, myxoid liposarcomas and well-differentiated liposarcomas have low metastatic potential: in contrast, synovial sarcomas and rhabdomyosarcomas may display aggressive clinical behavior. Another complicating factor may be the presence of varying histopathological patterns within the same tumor; thus, the assignment of histological subtype will depend on who determined the dominant features and on the amount of tissue examined.

The *significance* of grade may vary between histological subtypes, complicating the acceptance of uniform staging systems for all soft-tissue sarcomas. The presence of a similar number of mitotic figures may correlate with differing clinical behavior in different subtypes. For example, infantile fibrosarcomas may display numerous mitotic figures; but these tumors possess low metastatic potential.

The influence of grade on the biological behavior of sarcomas was acknowledged by Quick and Cutler in 1927.[2] In their analysis of 100 cases of neurogenic sarcoma, these early investigators divided sarcomas into three grades. Grade 1 sarcomas were defined as acellular, fibrous tumors composed of large spindle cells lying in a dense stroma of hyaline fibrous material—cells were few in number and stroma abundant (low grade of malignancy). Grade 2 sarcomas were described as "cellular tumors composed of large spindle cells arranged in compact intertwining bundles, very little intercellular substance" (moderate grade of malignancy). Grade 3 sarcomas were said to be "very cellular tumors composed of small spindle cells arranged in whorls and and fasciculi growing diffusely in a loose fibrillar network" (highly malignant). Quick and Cutler correlated these grades with the subsequent development of metastases, noting that patients who developed pulmonary metastases had histological grade 2 and 3 tumors, and "in no case was pulmonary metastasis observed from the acellular fibrous type of growth" (grade 1).

Furthering these observations, Broders et al.[3] in 1939 demonstrated that survival rates for 132 fibrosarcoma patients ranged from 45% for grade 1 tumors to 6% for grade 4 neoplasms. Later, in 1965, Van der Werf-Messing and Unnik[4] correlated mitotic indices (mitotic figures per 10 high-power fields [HPF]) with the eventual development of metastases. Sarcomas with mitotic indices of 0, 1–6, 7–11, and greater than 11 eventually developed metastases in 24%, 37%, 69%, and 100% of patients, respectively.

Different staging systems use different criteria to define grade. Various systems have used mitotic indices, degree of pleomorphism, cellularity, matrix, and/or necrosis in assigning grade. Determination of grade is discussed in Chapter 4 of this book. Several authors[5–9] have concluded that tumor grade is one of the most important predictors of survival.

TNMG CLASSIFICATION

In 1968, the American Joint Committee for Cancer Staging and End Results Reporting appointed a task force to devise a staging system for soft-tissue sarcomas.[10] Over an 8-year span, 1,215 soft-tissue sarcoma cases were analyzed from 13 institutions. The resulting schema for staging is presented in Table 5–1. The task force utilized the TNMG classification, wherein "T" represented tumor size or local invasion of nerves, blood vessels or bone; "N" denoted nodal involvement; and "M" designated metastases. Grade (G) of the sarcoma was also essential to the formulation of this system. Cases were analyzed both clinically and pathologically to determine the factors useful in constructing a staging system. Sarcomas arising from hollow viscera were excluded. Histological subtypes included in this analysis were alveolar soft-part sarcoma, angiosarcoma, extraskeletal chondrosarcoma, extraskeletal osteosarcoma, fibrosarcoma, and leiomyosarcoma. Other histological subtypes included were liposarcoma, malignant fibrohistiocytoma, malignant mesenchymoma, malignant schwannoma, rhabdomyosarcoma, synovial sarcoma, and sarcoma, type not designated. Regardless of differentiation, certain subtypes were recognized as being highly malignant and designated as grade 3. These subtypes included rhabdomyosarcomas, synovial sarcomas, and certain angiosarcomas.

As delineated in Table 5–1, this system has nine stages. Fifty-three percent of the tumors originated in the extremities, with synovial sarcoma representing the predominant subtype. Rhabdomyosarcoma (34%) and malignant schwannoma (25%) were the most common tumors in the head and neck. Of the retroperitoneal sarcomas, leiomyosarcomas represented approximately half the sarcomas originating in this area.

Survival was found to be inversely correlated with stage, with use of the TNMG classification. Of the 1,215 cases, 423 had grade recorded after further examination of the histological slides; the survival data in Table 5–2 refer to these patients. Table 5–3 shows survival by stage of all patients, even without further slide reviews. As can be observed, the survival data from the cases reviewed histologically (Table 5–2) and from the entire group of patients (Table 5–3) are similar. Patients in each stage seem to represent a distinct biological group, with a defined natural history and survival.

The TNMG system of the American Joint Committee has been criticized. First, the existence of nine stages makes its clinical use cumbersome. Because determination of grade is based on the judgment of the pathologist, the use of three grades (rather than "high" or "low" grades) allows for greater discrepancies between pathologists using the system. In addition, the division of sarcomas into three grades offers little in terms of therapeutic guidance because there is no "middle" surgical procedure.[12] Also, more than 40% of cases in the TNMG analysis[10] were located in the head, neck, and retroperitoneum, which pose different management problems than do extremity sarcomas.

Surgical criticisms of the TNMG staging system address the roles of tumor size, regional lymph node involvement, and invasion of bone and neurovascular structures. Surgical decision making is not entirely dictated by tumor size; rather, anatomical setting (compartmentalization) rather than size per se has the greater impact.

Regional lymph node involvement and distant metastases carry a similar prognosis, but the former is accorded a "better" stage (IIIc) in contrast to neurovascular invasion (IVa), which may dictate a different surgical procedure, but

TABLE 5–1.
Schema for Staging Soft-Tissue Sarcoma by T N M G*,†

Code letter		Description
T		Primary tumor; T_1—tumor < 5 cm; T_2— ≥ 5 cm; T_3—tumor grossly invades bone, major vessel, or major nerve
N		Regional lymph nodes; N_0—no histologically verified metastases to regional lymph nodes; N_1—histologically verified regional lymph node metastasis
M		Distant metastasis; M_0—no distant metastasis; M_1—distant metastasis
G		Histological grade of malignancy; G_1—low; G_2—moderate; G_3—high
Stage	**Code**	
I		
Ia	$G_1T_1N_0M_0$	Grade 1 tumor < 5 cm in diameter with no regional lymph nodes or distant metastases
Ib	$G_1T_2N_0M_0$	Grade 1 tumor ≥ 5 cm in diameter with no regional lymph nodes or distant metastases
II		
IIa	$G_2T_1N_0M_0$	Grade 2 tumor < 5 cm in diameter with no regional lymph nodes or distant metastases
IIb	$G_2T_2N_0M_0$	Grade 2 tumor ≥ 5 cm in diameter with no regional lymph nodes or distant metastases
III		
IIIa	$G_3T_1N_0M_0$	Grade 3 tumor < 5 cm in diameter with no regional lymph nodes or distant metastases
IIIb	$G_3T_2N_0M_0$	Grade 3 tumor ≥ 5 cm in diameter with no regional lymph nodes or distant metastases
IIIc	Any G $T_{1-2}N_1M_0$	Tumor of any grade or size (no invasion) with regional lymph nodes but no distant metastases
IV		
IVa	Any G $T_3N_{0-1}M_0$	Tumor of any grade that grossly invades bone, major vessel, or major nerve with or without regional lymph node metastases but without distant metastases
IVb	Any GTN M_1	Tumor with distant metastases

**Adapted from Russell WO, Cohen J, Enzinger F, et al:* Cancer *1977; 40:1562–1570.*
† A more recent version of this schema has been simplified by elimination of the "T_3" designation and of stage IIIc. Stage IVa is redefined as: Any G, any T, N_1, M_0.[11]

TABLE 5–2.
TNMG Classification: Soft-Tissue Sarcoma Survival by Stage (Cases in Which the Histological Slides Were Reviewed)*

		Percent Surviving†					
Stage	Number of Cases	1 year	2 years	3 years	4 years	5 years	10 years
I	85	92	84	78	78	76	(59)
II	78	86	74	(64)	(59)	(56)	(42)
III	211	71	46	35	30	26	13
IV	49	(29)	(14)	(10)	(8)	(4)	0

**Adapted from Russell WO, Cohen J, Enzinger F, et al:* Cancer *1977; 40:1562.*
† Rates in parentheses have standard errors between 5% and 10%.

TNMG Classification: Soft-Tissue Sarcoma Survival by Stage (All Patients)*

		Percent Surviving†					
Stage	Number of Cases	1 year	2 years	3 years	4 years	5 years	10 years
I	177	91	84	79	78	75	63
II	86	87	74	(63)	(58)	(55)	(40)
III	329	71	47	37	32	29	19
IV	110	37	19	11	10	7	3

**Adapted from Russell WO, Cohen J, Enzinger F, et al:* Cancer *1977; 40:1562.*
† Rates in parentheses have standard errors between 5% and 10%.

carries the same ominous prognosis as nodal metastases.[13] Also, the initial surgical procedure may be an important prognostic factor in survival. The TNMG system did not address "initial surgical procedure" as a variable in survival analysis.

HAJDU'S SYSTEM[14]

On review of more than 2,400 patients treated for soft-tissue sarcomas at Memorial Sloan-Kettering Cancer Center from 1950 to 1974, Hajdu devised a system based on size, site, and histological grade. Four stages were formulated based on "prognostic signs."

Characteristic	Good Prognostic Signs	Bad Prognostic Signs
Size	Small (< 5 cm)	Big (> 5 cm)
Site	Superficial (not beyond superficial fascia)	Deep (beyond superficial fascia)
Grade	Low	High

Hajdu's low-grade sarcomas were defined as hypocellular tumors containing "much stroma," minimal necrosis, good maturation, and less than five mitoses per 10 HPF. High-grade tumors were hypercellular, with minimal stroma, necrosis, poor maturation, and more than five mitoses per 10 HPF.

In Hajdu's system, stage 0 tumors were defined as having three good prognostic signs; stage I sarcomas had two good prognostic signs and one unfavorable sign. Stage II tumors were characterized by one favorable and two poor prognostic features; stage III sarcomas contained tumors with all three three unfavorable signs. Stage IV was defined as tumors with evidence of metastases. Table 5–4 presents the four stages and their subdivisions.

Just as with the American Joint Commission TNMG staging system, the system devised by Hajdu is not particularly useful in assigning a definitive surgical procedure for primary management of the sarcoma. Although tumor size and site (superficial versus deep) have prognostic importance, these factors may not dictate the surgical approach.

ENNEKING'S SYSTEM[12, 15]

A third staging system, developed by Enneking emphasized three elements useful in surgical decision making: histological grade, anatomical location, and distant metastases.

This system is based on the rationale that lesions arising from and confined within the

TABLE 5–4.
Sarcoma Staging According to the System of Hajdu*

Stage	Size (cm)	Site	Grade
0	< 5	Superficial	Low
I			
A	< 5	Superficial	High
B	< 5	Deep	Low
C	> 5	Superficial	Low
II			
A	< 5	Deep	High
B	> 5	Superficial	High
C	> 5	Deep	Low
III	> 5	Deep	High
IV			
A	Metastatic soft-tissue sarcoma, regional metastases		
B	Metastatic soft-tissue sarcoma, distant metastases		

* *Adapted from Hajdu SI: History and classification of soft tissue tumors, in Hajdu SI (ed):* Pathology of Soft Tissue Tumors. *Philadelphia, Lea & Febiger, 1979, pp 45–47.*

fascia that delimits the major muscular compartments are less apt to recur than sarcomas residing in the extracompartmental fascial planes or extending beyond the compartment of origin. Enneking divided the thigh into intracompartmental and extracompartmental tissues. Intracompartmental tissues of the thigh included those contained within the three major muscular compartments, within joints, or superficial to the deep fascia. A sarcoma must be confined *entirely* within a compartment to be "intracompartmental." Extracompartmental lesions were defined as extending beyond the compartment into another compartment, into extracompartmental tissues, or arising in extracompartmental tissues. Anatomical compartments have natural barriers to occult tumor extension, such as fascial septae and tendinous origins of muscle. Interfascial spaces are not contained and do not resist tumor extension.

Enneking implemented the concept of compartmentalization along with grade and presence or absence of metastases into the following system:

Stage I:	Low grade: A—intracompartmental; B—extracompartmental
Stage II:	High grade: A—intracompartmental; B—extracompartmental
Stage III:	Any grade or site with regional or distal metastases.

General recommendations implemented by Enneking are wide excisions for stage IA sarcomas, wide amputation for stage IB, radical resection for stage IIA, and radical disarticulation for stage IIB lesions. Clinical use of this system is discussed further in Chapter 29.

In all of these staging systems, tumor grade is important. For the most part, these systems were based on results in patients treated surgically. In contrast, Suit and associates[16] analyzed results in 100 patients with soft-tissue sarcomas treated with radical dose radiation therapy alone or combined with limited surgery. This series underscores anatomical grade as the most important prognostic indicator with regard to disease-free survival. Tumor size was a less important indicator and histopathological type was "at best, a weak" prognostic indicator.[16]

A European study of 265 sarcoma patients at The Netherlands Cancer Institute in Amsterdam[17] examined the prognostic factors of histological diagnosis, age, sex, anatomical location, depth of lesion, size, mitosis, necrosis, myxoid component, and degree of differentiation. The histological subtypes analyzed were liposarcoma, malignant fibrohistiocytoma, leiomyosarcoma, fibrosarcoma, rhabdomyosarcoma, and undifferentiated sarcoma. In this series, histological type and tumor size were the best criteria for prognosis, followed by mitotic index, necrosis, and degree of differentiation. Liposarcomas and fibrosarcomas carried the best prognosis. Tumors larger than 5 cm have a worse prognosis than do smaller lesions.

Although many studies have examined prognostic factors for localized sarcomas, little information is available regarding prognostic factors in metastatic sarcomas. Yap et al.[18] reviewed the records of 331 adult patients with advanced soft-tissue sarcomas treated with several adriamycin-containing regimens at M. D. Anderson Hospital (Houston, TX). In this series with an overall 45% response rate (16% complete and 29% partial), no significant difference in response rate or survival was observed among the various histological subtypes. However, patients with rhabdomyosarcomas had the shortest median survival (only 6 months). Age, sex, race, primary site, and size were not of prognostic significance in disseminated disease. Higher grade of malignancy, poor performance status, weight loss, and low serum albumin correlated with short survival. Patients who had received less than 50 mg/m^2 of adriamycin had a response rate of 27% in contrast to a 54% response rate in patients receiving greater than 50 mg/m^2 ($p < 0.02$). Minimal versus extensive tumor involvement of the lung, liver, and abdomen influenced the complete response rate. The complete response rate for individuals with minimal lung involvement was 45% compared with 11% for extensive involvement ($p < 0.001$); for liver, 50% versus 4% ($p < 0.01$); and for intra-abdominal disease, 50% versus 12% ($p < 0.01$).

A Southwest Oncology Group (SWOG) study of advanced soft-tissue sarcoma patients was analyzed for prognostic factors.[19] In this study with a mandatory pathology review, 335 patients were randomly allocated to three adriamycin combinations: adriamycin, dacarbazine, (dimethyl-triazeno-imidazole tri-geno carboxamide, DTIC); cyclophosphamide, adriamycin, DTIC; actinomycin D, adriamycin, DTIC. No significant differences were observed in terms of response, duration of response, or survival among the three treatments.

Neither was any statistical difference observed in this SWOG study among the various histological subtypes for response rate, but an overall difference in survival ($p = 0.04$) was noted. Leiomyosarcomas and liposarcomas had the best prognosis with a median survival of 58 and 69 weeks, respectively. Rhabdomyosarcomas had the poorest prognosis, with a survival of 26 weeks. Of interest also was the influence of sexual status on survival. Although the sex of the patient did not influence response rates, the median survival for women was 57 weeks compared with 36 weeks for men ($p = 0.01$, Breslow).

Intensity of chemotherapy as manifested by myelosuppression had prognostic importance for response rates. Patients whose white cell count fell below 3,000 had a response rate of 40%, whereas in individuals without myelosuppression, the rate was 16% ($p = 0.001$). No survival advantage, however, was observed with myelosuppression ($p = 0.20$).

SUMMARY

Soft-tissue sarcomas represent a spectrum of neoplasms with differing biological behaviors arising in varied locations. A uniform staging system is difficult to construct. Different medical specialties place different requisites on staging systems. For example, the TNMG system of the American Joint Committee does not provide optimal guidance for the surgical management of soft-tissue sarcomas, whereas the staging system developed by Enneking is specifically designed for surgical decision making.

The three staging systems discussed use tumor grade as an integral factor. The TNMG system, and the staging system developed by Hajdu, recognize the prognostic importance of size. Enneking believes size "has prognostic significance that is a complex composite of anatomical setting, rate of growth, and time to physician intervention."[12] In this system, "tumor extent" is defined by anatomical setting (compartmentalization) rather than by size or invasion into neurovascular structures.

Although positive correlations with survival have been established for both the TNMG system and the staging system formulated by Enneking, both have drawbacks. A 1984 National Institutes of Health consensus on adult soft-tissue sarcomas recommended that a unified staging system be developed combining features of both systems.[20] This system should be based on reliable prognostic data and consider the effect of surgical treatment on survival.

The understanding of prognostic factors in advanced soft-tissue sarcomas and their impact on response rates to chemotherapy and survival require further investigation. Histological subtypes may influence survival as noted in the analysis of a SWOG chemotherapy study.[19] In this study, rhabdomyosarcomas had the worst prognosis, whereas liposarcomas and leiomyosarcomas allowed the most favorable survival. Further elucidation of prognostic factors is required and will serve both in future designs and comparisons of clinical trials in soft-tissue sarcoma patients.

REFERENCES

1. Enzinger FM, Lattes R, Torloni R: Histological typing of soft tissue tumors. *International Classification of Tumors,* No. 3. Geneva, World Health Organization, 1969.
2. Quick D, Cutler M: Neurogenic sarcoma. *Ann Surg* 1927; 86:810–829.
3. Broders AC, Hargrave R, Meyerding HW: Pathological features of soft tissue sarcomas. *Surg Gynecol Obstet* 1939; 69:267–280.
4. Van der Werf-Messing B, Unnik JAM: Fibrosarcoma of the soft tissues—a clinicopathological study. *Cancer* 1965; 18:1113–1123.
5. Pritchard RJ, Soule EH, Tayler WF, et al: Fibrosarcoma—a clinicopathological and statistical study of 199 tumors of the soft tissues of the extremities and trunk. *Cancer* 1974; 33:888–897.
6. Stout AP: Fibrosarcoma. *Cancer* 1948; 1:30–63.
7. Heller EL, Seiber WK: Fibrosarcoma. *Surgery* 1950;27:539–547.
8. Reszel PA, Soule EH, Coventry MB: Liposarcoma of the extremity and limb-girdles. *J Bone Joint Surg* 1966; 48:229–244.
9. Costa J, Wesley RA, Glatstein E, et al: The grading of soft tissue sarcomas. Results of a clinicohistopathologic correlation in a series of 163 cases. *Cancer* 1984; 53:530–541.
10. Russell WO, Cohen J, Enzinger F, et al: A clinical and pathological staging system for soft tissue sarcomas. *Cancer* 1977; 40:1562–1570.
11. Beahrs OH, Hensen DE, Hutter RVP, et al (eds): *Manual for Staging of Cancer,* 3rd ed. Philadelphia, J. B. Lippincott, 1988, pp 127–131.

12. Enneking WF, Spanier SS, Goodman MA, et al: Current concepts review. The surgical staging of musculoskeletal sarcoma. *J Bone Joint Surg* 1980; 62-A:1027–1030.
13. Ryan JR: Staging of soft tissue sarcomas, in Baker LH (ed): *Soft Tissue Sarcomas.* The Hague, Martinus Nijhoff, 1983, pp 49–52.
14. Hajdu, SI: History and classification of soft tissue tumors, in Hajdu SI (ed): *Pathology of Soft Tissue Tumors.* Philadelphia, Lea & Febiger, 1979, pp 45–47.
15. Enneking WF, Spanier SS, Malawer MM: The effect of anatomical setting on the results of surgical procedures for soft part sarcomas of the thigh. *Cancer* 1981; 47:1005–1022.
16. Suit HD, Russell WO, Martin RG, et al: Sarcoma of soft tissue. Clinical and histopathologic parameters and response to treatment. *Cancer* 1975; 35:1478–1483.
17. Albus-Lutter CHE: Typing and grading of soft tissue sarcomas. Experience of members of the EORTC (European Organization for Research on Treatment of Cancer). Pathology Subcommittee, *Proc. Symposium Management of Soft Tissue and Bone Sarcomas,* Utrecht, The Netherlands, June, 1984.
18. Yap BS, Rasmussen SL, Burgess MA, et al: Prognostic factors in adults with advanced soft tissue sarcomas. *Proc Am Soc Clin Oncol* Abstract #C-608, p 473, 1980.
19. Baker LH: Prognostic Factor Analysis in Disseminated Soft Tissue Sarcomas: Southwest Oncology Group (SWOG) 7613. (In preparation.)
20. National Institutes of Health Consensus Development Panel. Limb-sparing treatment of adult soft tissue sarcomas and osteosarcomas. *Cancer Treat Symp* 1985; 3:1–5.

PART 2

Approach to Specific Tumors and Anatomic Sites

Chapter 6

Sarcomas of the Head and Neck

Oliver H. Beahrs

Hollon W. Farr

Twelve percent of soft-tissue sarcomas will occur in the head and neck area. Sarcoma should be considered in the differential diagnosis of any tumor mass in this anatomical region, especially in the younger patient.

Over 80% of cancers of the head and neck area are epithelial in origin, primarily squamous cell carcinoma, so that other types of tumor might not be considered. Because the head and neck contain almost all types of body tissues from which benign and malignant tumors may occur, the evaluation of a mass in this area can be complex. Nevertheless, considering the exact anatomical location and relationship to other tissues, along with the clinical information and physical findings, the number of possible pathological types of lesions can be reduced. Biopsy or removal of the tumor with histological study of the tissue will be the only definite way to establish the diagnosis.

CLINICAL HISTORY

Because the neck is an exposed area, the occurrence of a painless lump is often noticed early by the patient or a relative. Unfortunately, evaluation of such a lump is often delayed, and concern over it occurs after it has persisted, or increased in size, or other symptoms develop. There may or may not be a history of injury or trauma to the neck area. This may be of interest, but usually is not pertinent because there is no established casual relationship between soft sarcomas and trauma. The age of the patient is an important factor, as is information regarding duration or growth of the lesion.

PHYSICAL EXAMINATION

Inspection.—Inspection of the neck, appearance of the tumor mass, asymmetry, and the exact location in relationship to other structures are factors pertinent to establishing a diagnosis. Involvement of skin is unusual unless the tumor is large or has its origin in the subcutaneous tissues. Some soft-tissue sarcomas do, however, involve the skin: for example, Kaposi's sarcoma, angiosarcoma, lymphangiosarcoma, dermatofibrosarcoma protuberans.

Palpation.—Sarcomas are rubbery and firm, although not as hard as calcified tissue. Very soft tumors are likely to be benign, such as a lipoma. The firmer the lesion, the more likely that it is malignant. Findings on palpation alone will not determine the diagnosis but may suggest the pathological condition.

Auscultation.—Soft-tissue sarcomas overlying a major vessel in the head and neck region may have a transmitted bruit. The rare tumor of vascular origin might have a bruit or pulsation because of arteriovenous shunts. A chemodectoma, usually a benign tumor, might have a bruit on auscultation.

The physical examination of any head and neck tumor must always include a thorough examination of the oral cavity, pharynx, larynx, salivary glands, and thyroid gland, as well as the skin of the scalp, face, and neck, for a possible primary cancer that could be the source of metastatic lesions in the neck.

RADIOLOGICAL STUDIES

Conventional radiography or xerography may occasionally be of help in ruling out a primary bone lesion, or they may give information regarding underlying bone or other adjacent tissue. Also, the presence of a foreign body may be ruled out. Computed tomography (CT) scanning or magnetic resonance imaging (MRI) may help in delineating the extent of a tumor in the head and neck region, but because of the ease of physical examination of this anatomical region they may not always be indicated. Arteriography usually is not necessary but might give information regarding the relationship of the tumor and vascular structures. Lymphangiography is generally not indicated.

TISSUE DIAGNOSIS

If the tumor in the head and neck is small and other primary sources for it have been ruled out, excisional biopsy of the lesion is reasonable for tissue confirmation. If the lesion proves to be a soft-tissue sarcoma, then further treatment decisions can be made. On the other hand, an incisional biopsy might be indicated because of the size of the tumor before deciding on the extent of the surgical resection and other measures to be taken. A biopsy is frequently required prior to definitive resection to give the pathologist time to establish the diagnosis.

Fine-needle aspiration cytologic study might be considered in selected cases of head and neck tumors to determine that the lesion is sarcomatous rather than carcinomatous prior to excisional or incisional biopsy. Another indication for fine-needle aspiration might be confirmation of recurrent sarcoma in a patient previously treated for a sarcoma.

Any sarcoma of the head or neck should be appropriately staged on clinical-diagnostic grounds or by postsurgical pathological study to aid in treatment decisions and final diagnosis.[1] The error rate in staging based on clinical-radiological data is about 30% when compared to all pathological data available from examination of the definitively resected specimen as well as cervical and supraclavicular lymph nodes.

SURGICAL TREATMENT

Almost all types of soft-tissue sarcomas occur in the head and neck area. In general the surgical treatment of each is about the same. If the lesion is small, after thorough clinical evaluation excisional removal of the tumor mass can be considered. On the other hand, incisional biopsy, core biopsy, or fine-needle aspiration are reasonable approaches to establish the histological diagnosis prior to proceeding with a definitive surgical resection.

While elsewhere in the body radical surgical removal of the anatomical part in which the soft-tissue sarcoma has its origin can be done (e.g., amputation of an extremity), in the head and neck region there are soft tissues and structures that must be saved in order to preserve life (e.g., the carotid artery). Certain tissues (e.g., the esophagus) can be removed and reconstructive measures used to reduce anatomical or functional morbidity. However, the problems associated with major resections are hardly acceptable unless the operation is definitive and offers the patients a chance of cure. This anatomical region is not amenable to amputation so the extent of resection is necessarily limited.

Fortunately, however, other modalities, such as radiation therapy and chemotherapy, can be used in combination with surgical resection and are proving to be of benefit in the management of soft-tissue sarcomas.

Many areas of the extracranial head and neck can be surgically removed. When severe cosmetic deformity results, reconstruction of the area can be done and this is justified if the prognosis is reasonable. If orbital exenteration has been done, a prosthesis will mask the defect. If the parotid gland has been radically removed along with the facial nerve, a free nerve graft can be inserted with an expected success rate of 70% to 90%. Sarcomas of the larynx may be treated by endoscopic excision and fulguration, or excised using a thyrotomy approach or a hemilaryngectomy if the lesion is well localized or small. On the other hand, if the tumor is relatively large, a wide-field laryngectomy is considered best, leaving a permanent tracheostomy. If the lesion requires cervical esophagectomy, a free graft of small intestine can be used to bridge the defect. For a primary sarcoma in the lateral neck or for regional cervical metastasis of tumors elsewhere in the head and neck region, a radical neck dissection can be done. In the classical neck dissection, the spinal accessory nerve is removed. If the nerve is preserved, there is little morbidity associated with neck dissection except for slight flattening of the neck. If the nerve is removed, about 20% of patients will complain of some lameness of the shoulder. Other nerves—lingual, hypoglossal, vagus, and phrenic—can also be removed if in doing so the procedure becomes definitive, albeit with some morbidity of function. Structures deep to the prevertebral fascia are best preserved, to protect major nerve trunks. Most importantly, however, the common carotid and internal carotid arteries should be preserved to prevent severe mortality and morbidity. If wide excision of overlying skin must be performed, cover of the operative area can be accomplished with a free skin graft, pedicle flap, or other type of reconstructive procedure.

A radical surgical approach to soft-tissue sarcomas in the head and neck region previously was justified with the hope that a cure could be obtained. However, with the evidence of the value of radiation treatment and chemotherapy, more conservative operations are warranted, even to the extent of leaving microscopic or even gross tumor behind, reducing surgical morbidity and depending on the other modalities to treat the residual tumor. End results of managing sarcomas in this manner are proving to be better than those using radical surgery alone.

MULTIDISCIPLINARY MANAGEMENT

Complete excision of sarcomas of the head and neck may be difficult because of anatomical limitations in the head and neck area and the intraconnecting fascial planes and proximity to high-risk structures, such as the base of the skull, the internal carotid artery, cervical esophagus, and tracheolarynx. The high recurrence rate (about 70%) and low salvage rate for sarcomas in this area provide a strong rationale for considering adjuvant radiation treatment, which is best done by individuals or teams experienced in treating head and neck tumors or who have a special interest in sarcomas.

In pediatric patients sarcomas are primarily rhabdomyosarcomas, most commonly in the head and neck, then in the extremities, trunk, and genitourinary system. This differs from sarcomas in adults in terms of the anatomical distribution and also in that less than half are surgical resectable. Surgery plus combination chemotherapy, with or without radiation, has produced excellent results. Combination chemotherapy using vincristine, actinomycin D, and cyclophosphamide (VAC) has thus far been the mainstay of these programs, but the national Intergroup Rhabdomyosarcoma Study (IRS) includes investigation of other agents and studies of variations in order and timing of the treatment modalities for various anatomical sites. Patients with this group of sarcomas should be referred to a specialty center participating in clinical trials, such as the IRS, to receive optimal therapy.[2]

The experience in management of adult soft-part sarcomas of the head and neck at Memorial Sloan-Kettering (New York) was reviewed in 1971[3] and in 1981[4] by Farr, who reported a 5-year determinate and absolute cure rate of 78 of 242 cases, or 32%. In 1990, Farhood and colleagues[5] reviewed more recent results from treatment of 176 adult patients seen at that institution and concluded that treatment failure was associated with large tumor size, positive surgical margins, bone involvement, local recurrence, metastatic spread, and high histological grade. Other series from the Mayo Clinic (Rochester, Minnesota) ,[6] M. D. Anderson,[7] University of Illinois,[8] and St. Jude Hospital[9] have been published. A registry for head and neck sarcomas was established by the Society of Head and Neck Surgeons.[10]

Specific histological types of soft-tissue sarcomas of the head and neck differ in presentation and treatment. Fibrosarcomas are prone to local recurrence, resistant to radiotherapy, and require radical excision. Invasion is direct, by extension along fascial planes; margins are ill defined and finally form bulky solid pseudoencapsulated masses, eventually involving adjacent bone and producing progressive pain and fixation. Patients in the Sloan-Kettering study[4] with fibrosarcoma had an average age of 50 years, although one patient had congenital fibrosarcoma of the tongue. In that study the average duration prior to treatment was 12 months; 80% had tumor fixation, 75% had pain, and 75% had bone attachment. The sites of origin were the maxilla in 16, neck in eight, cheek in four, and one each in the palate, tongue, and lip.

Desmoid fibrosarcoma is a histologically benign-appearing lesion with infiltrating and locally invasive behavior. Complete excision is the only effective treatment, resulting in cure in 75% of patients.[11] Radiotherapy seems to be of little value in controlling these low-grade tumors. Half the patients with local recurrence can be salvaged by re-excision.

Liposarcoma may occur in the deep structures of the neck and adjacent shoulder girdle, and may be cured by radical neck dissection or brought under control with surgery plus radiation therapy.

Juvenile (embryonal and alveolar) rhabdomyosarcoma of the head and neck is characterized by rapidity of onset, capacity for generalized metastasis, and frequent fatal outcome; it is a fulminating disease occurring most often in children, although occasionally in adults.[12] Unlike neuroblastoma, rhabdomyosarcoma is not particularly radiosensitive; furthermore, the high radiation dose needed may affect bone growth centers and soft tissue. Surgery followed by radiotherapy and chemotherapy is the treatment of choice. Cyclic chemotherapy using adriamycin, vincristine, actinomycin D, and cytoxan has shown an appreciable 5-year cure rate.

Angiosarcoma comprises malignant angioendothelioma, hemangioendothelioma, and lymphangiosarcoma; these tumors are made up of malignant endothelial structures with a common fibrosarcomatous stroma, and may contain both capillary and lymphatic elements. Angiosarcoma is aggressive, and can extend for long distances before metastasis; clinical course is relatively rapid and the patient is usually either cured by initial treatment or dies of persistent local disease within 3 years. Cure usually involves radical excision; radiation therapy is effective in some patients[13] and may be augmented by use of adriamycin.

Hemangiopericytoma is a tumor of solid connective tissue; the clinical course is prolonged, with death usually occurring within 10 years. The tumor begins as a painless, slowly enlarging firm mass, poorly encapsulated and infiltrative, and recurs frequently at the site of excision; it may be spread by blood to distant multiple organs, and regional node metastasis may occur. Radiation therapy may be used as a palliative measure.

The differential diagnosis of head and neck sarcoma includes primary neuroblastoma, which occurs primarily in childhood. Four to six months usually elapse prior to treatment, average age of onset is 5 years, and distribution between the sexes is equal. The disease is rapidly fatal; more than 50% of the young patients die within a year, although the outcome in teenagers and young adults is considerably better.

Malignant chemodectoma or carotid body tumor is extremely rare. Metastasis to regional nodes may occur, and rarely to distant sites such as bone and lung. Because carotid body tumors are locally malignant over time, early excision to preserve carotid circulation is recommended.

Esthesioneuroblastoma occurs in the olfactory bulb and neuroepithelium of the nasal cavity and is resistant to all forms of therapy. The peak incidence is in young adults, and the duration is long. Local recurrence is common and the potential of radiation damage to adjacent vital structures is high; in addition, the tumor, like all mature neural tissue tumors, is not radiosensitive. Surgical treatment involves extensive resection, including the contents of the nasal cavity, the cribriform plate, the site of origin in the frontal fossa and frontal lobe, and often orbital exenteration. This may be done in stages or in a single-stage craniomaxillary approach; common sequelae are meningitis, brain abscess, and local recurrence.

CONCLUSION

The management of soft-tissue sarcomas of the head and neck should always be by the multidisciplinary approach, because prognosis for most such lesions is much better with this approach that when treated by one modality alone. The patient will thus receive the best treatment available.

REFERENCES

1. Beahrs OH, Henson DE, Hutter RVP, et al: *American Joint Committee on Cancer; Manual*

for Staging of Cancer, 3rd ed. Philadelphia, J. B. Lippincott, 1988, pp 127–131.

2. Wilson RE: Cancer Management Course. Chicago, American College of Surgeons, 1984.
3. Farr HW: Soft part sarcomas of the head and neck. *Am J Surg* 1971; 122:714–718.
4. Farr HW: Soft part sarcomas of the head and neck. *Semin Oncol* 1981; 8:185–189.
5. Farhood AI, Hajdu SI, Shiu MH, et al: Soft tissue sarcomas of the head and neck in adults. *Am J Surg* 1990; 160:365–369.
6. Freedman AM, Reiman HM, Woods JE: Soft tissue sarcomas of the head and neck. *Am J Surg* 1989; 158:367–372.
7. Weber RS, Benjamin R, Peters LJ, et al: Soft tissue sarcomas of the head and neck in adolescents and adults. *Am J Surg* 1986; 152:386–392.
8. Greager JA, Patel MK, Briele HA, et al: Soft tissue sarcomas of the adult head and neck. *Cancer* 1985; 56:820–824.
9. Rao BN, Santana VM, Fleming ID, et al: Management and prognosis of head and neck sarcoma. *Am J Surg* 1989; 158:373–377.
10. Wanebo HJ, Koness J, McFarlane J, et al: Head and neck sarcomas—report of head and neck registry. Abstract presented at the 36th Annual Meeting of the Society of Head and Neck Surgeons, Washington, D.C., May 1990, p 148.
11. Fasching MC, Saleh J, Woods JE: Desmoid tumors of the head and neck. *Am J Surg* 1988; 156:327–331.
12. Nakhleh RE, Swanson PE, Dehner LP: Juvenile (embryonal and alveolar) rhabdomyosarcoma of the head and neck in adults; a clinical, pathologic, and immunohistochemical study of 12 cases. *Cancer* 1991; 67:1019–1024.
13. Holden CA, Spittle MF, Jones EW: Angiosarcoma of the face and scalp, prognosis and treatment. *Cancer* 1987; 59:1046–1057.

Chapter 7

Sarcomas of the Upper Extremity; Lymphangiosarcoma

John H. Raaf

James H. Muchmore

Soft-tissue sarcomas of the upper extremity constitute 14% of all soft-tissue sarcomas; they are one third as common as those of the lower extremity.[1] Clinical management is similar to that for sarcomas in the lower limb, but surgical resection is more challenging. This is because (1) there is less muscle bulk in the upper limb than the lower, making it more difficult to achieve a clear margin around a tumor, and (2) preservation of hand function is critically important.

CLINICAL PRESENTATION

For the present discussion, the upper extremity will be defined as the shoulder and axilla, upper arm, elbow and antecubital space, forearm, wrist, and hand. Soft-tissue sarcomas of the upper extremity occur in patients of all ages. In 108 patients reported by Collin et al.,[2] the most frequent location of soft-tissue sarcomas of the upper extremity was the upper arm, followed by the shoulder/axilla (Table 7–1). Distribution of histological types in Collin's series is shown in Table 7–2. The most frequently seen histology was tendosynovial sarcoma, followed by liposarcoma and fibrosarcoma.

Soft-tissue sarcomas of the upper extremity have a variety of clinical presentations.[3] A low-grade sarcoma may present as a slow-growing, painless mass; a high-grade sarcoma is often rapidly growing and may cause pain, weakness, and limitation of motion. Consistency of the tumor may vary from a soft, low-grade liposarcoma to a firm or hard, high-grade fibrosarcoma with dense cellularity. Because these tumors are frequently located within muscle bundles, their texture can depend on whether the patient is contracting the encompassing muscle or tensing the surrounding muscle fascia.

Because of its location in a tight fascial compartment, a soft-tissue sarcoma in the upper extremity may assume a discoid or fusiform shape rather than the more spherical configuration of such tumors in the lower extremity, trunk, or retroperitoneum. Sarcomas in the upper extremity are generally smaller than those of other anatomical areas due to the limited volume of upper-extremity muscle and subcutaneous spaces.

TABLE 7–1.
Location of Soft-Tissue Sarcomas of the Upper Extremity*

Location	Percentage at Location
Shoulder/scapula/axilla	23
Upper arm	34
Elbow/antecubital fossa	13
Forearm	19
Wrist/hand	9
Diffuse involvement	2

* *Adapted from Collin C, Hajdu SI, Godbold JA, et al:* Ann Surg *1987; 205:331–339.*

DIAGNOSIS

Following a careful history, the physical examination should focus on tumor characteristics (e.g., size, depth, texture, fixation), resectability, and evidence of regional or distant disease. Epitrochlear and axillary lymph nodes should be palpated, although nodal metastases from sarcomas are rare[4, 5] except for childhood rhabdomyosarcoma or by direct extension in advanced disease.

Computed tomography (CT) or magnetic resonance imaging (MRI) are routinely performed to demonstrate the size, location, and relationship of tumor to vital structures.[6, 7] Computed tomography is superior to MRI in demonstrating cortical bone erosion and tumor calcification, whereas only MRI can provide sagittal and coronal views as well as axial sections. The fatty nature of the tumor can be predicted from the MRI signal intensity, and MRI images are not distorted by streak artifacts due to metal clips that are characteristic of CT images. A chest X-ray is obtained to detect pulmonary metastases.

Soft-tissue sarcomas of the extremity rarely invade blood vessels or major nerves, but they can displace or encase them. A surgeon planning wide en bloc resection of a soft-tissue sarcoma of the upper extremity may find an arteriogram helpful.[8] This was the case for the patient described in Figure 7–1.

TABLE 7–2.
Histological types of Upper-Extremity Soft-Tissue Sarcomas*

Type	Percentage
Tendosynovial sarcoma†	21.3
Liposarcoma	19.4
Fibrosarcoma	19.4
Malignant peripheral nerve tumor‡	13.9
Malignant fibrous histiocytoma	9.3
Pleomorphic rhabdomyosarcoma	4.6
Angiosarcoma	3.7
Leiomyosarcoma	3.7
Extraskeletal osteogenic sarcoma	2.8
Embryonal rhabdomyosarcoma	1.9

* *Adapted from Collin C, Hajdu SI, Godbold JA, et al:* Ann Surg *1987; 205:331–339.*
† *Includes monophasic and biphasic tendosynovial sarcoma, epithelioid sarcoma, and clear cell sarcoma.*
‡ *Includes malignant schwannoma and neurofibrosarcoma.*

BIOPSY

Biopsy of a soft-tissue mass in an extremity should provide a representative tissue sample for histological diagnosis, and it should avoid compromising subsequent definitive resection. Although fine-needle aspiration is increasingly advocated,[9–11] most pathologists prefer a larger specimen obtained by open biopsy. This is because needle aspiration sampling of a necrotic area of the tumor, or of an area containing low-grade tumor, may lead to a missed diagnosis of high-grade sarcoma. Aspiration or core-needle biopsy may be useful in diagnosing recurrent or metastatic tumor.

Careful planning and surgical technique are critical to open biopsy of an extremity sarcoma. The complication rate of bone or soft-tissue sarcoma biopsy (including hemorrhage, wound breakdown, infection, and fracture) in one series was 17.3%.[12] The authors also report a major error in diagnosis affecting patient management in 18.2% of biopsies, and nonrepresentative or technically poor results from an additional 10.3%.

The biopsy site should be placed so it is encompassed completely in the ellipse of skin and block of soft tissue that are removed during the definitive resection. In the upper extremity, the orientation of the biopsy incision is almost always longitudinal, *not transverse.* Ideally, the surgeon who will do the definitive resection should also perform the biopsy. Both the biopsy and the resection can be done under the same general anesthetic if frozen-section diagnosis is definitive. More often, resection will follow biopsy by a few days, to permit study of permanent histological sections.

Lipoma is the benign lesion most frequently biopsied to exclude sarcoma. Most lipomas are

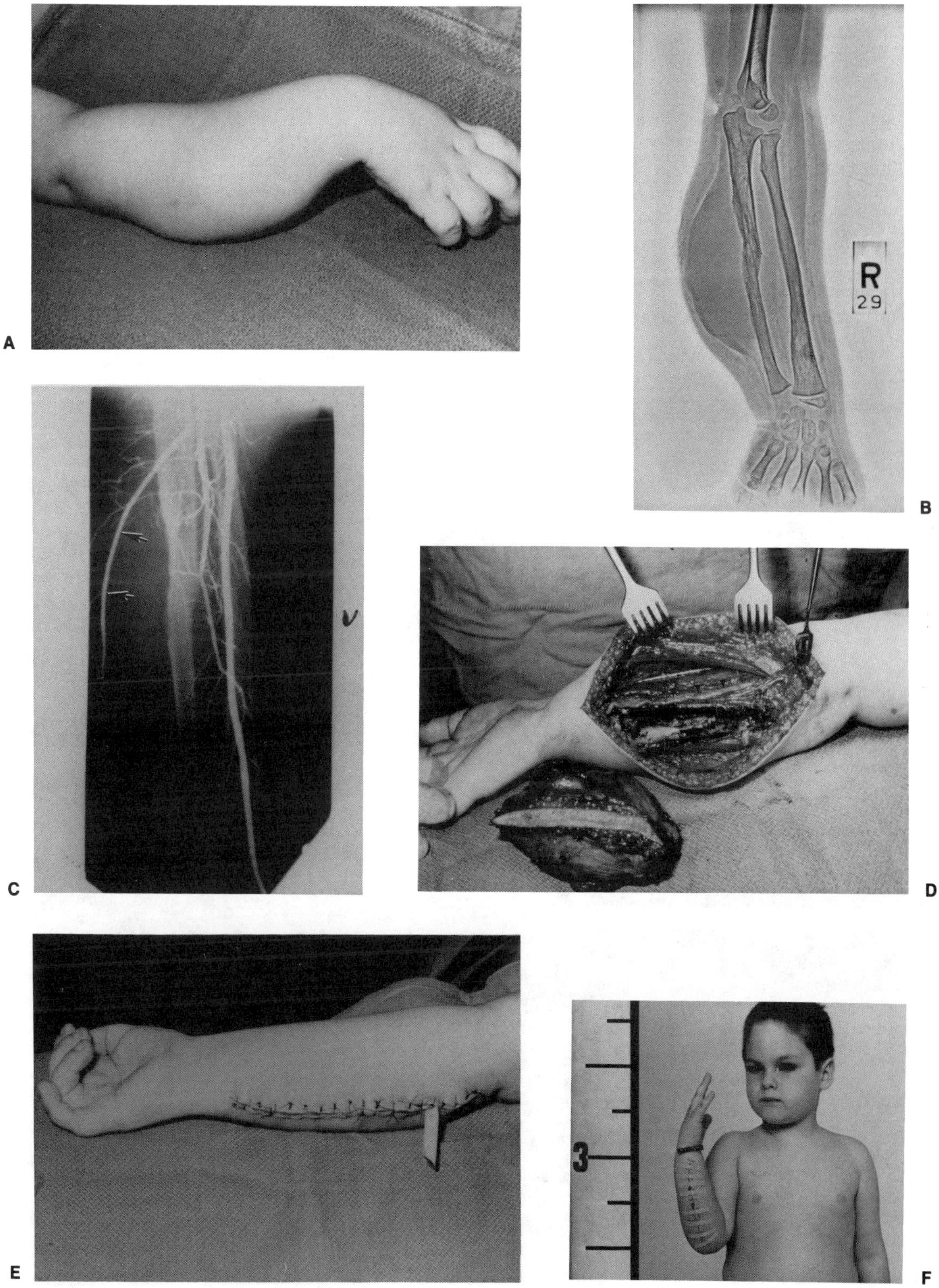

FIG 7–1.

A, a 4-year-old boy presented with a large, fixed, firm mass in the ulnar side of his right forearm. **B,** by xerogram it appeared to be associated with a healed fracture of the ulna. **C,** an arteriogram demonstrated medial displacement of the ulnar artery (*arrows*). Biopsy showed the tumor to be a grade I fibrosarcoma. **D,** the mass was resected, with sparing of the ulnar artery and nerve (*arrowheads*). **E** and **F,** complete function of the hand was preserved. Childhood fibrosarcomas such as this are locally invasive but rarely metastasize.

small, superficial, and mobile. Often they have been present for years; they may be multiple and bilaterally symmetrical. If a mass is small, mobile, and typical of lipoma, it may be safely observed. If there are uncharacteristic features such as recent appearance, change in size, fixation, firm consistency, or size greater than 3 cm in diameter, it is justified to perform excisional or incisional biopsy. An area of firmness in an otherwise soft tumor that appears to be a benign lipoma may reflect a focus of increased cellularity, which on microscopic examination will be considered low-grade liposarcoma. A mass containing such an area should be removed. Completely benign lipomas can be large and deforming and require excision for cosmetic or functional reasons, as illustrated by the patient in Figure 7–2.

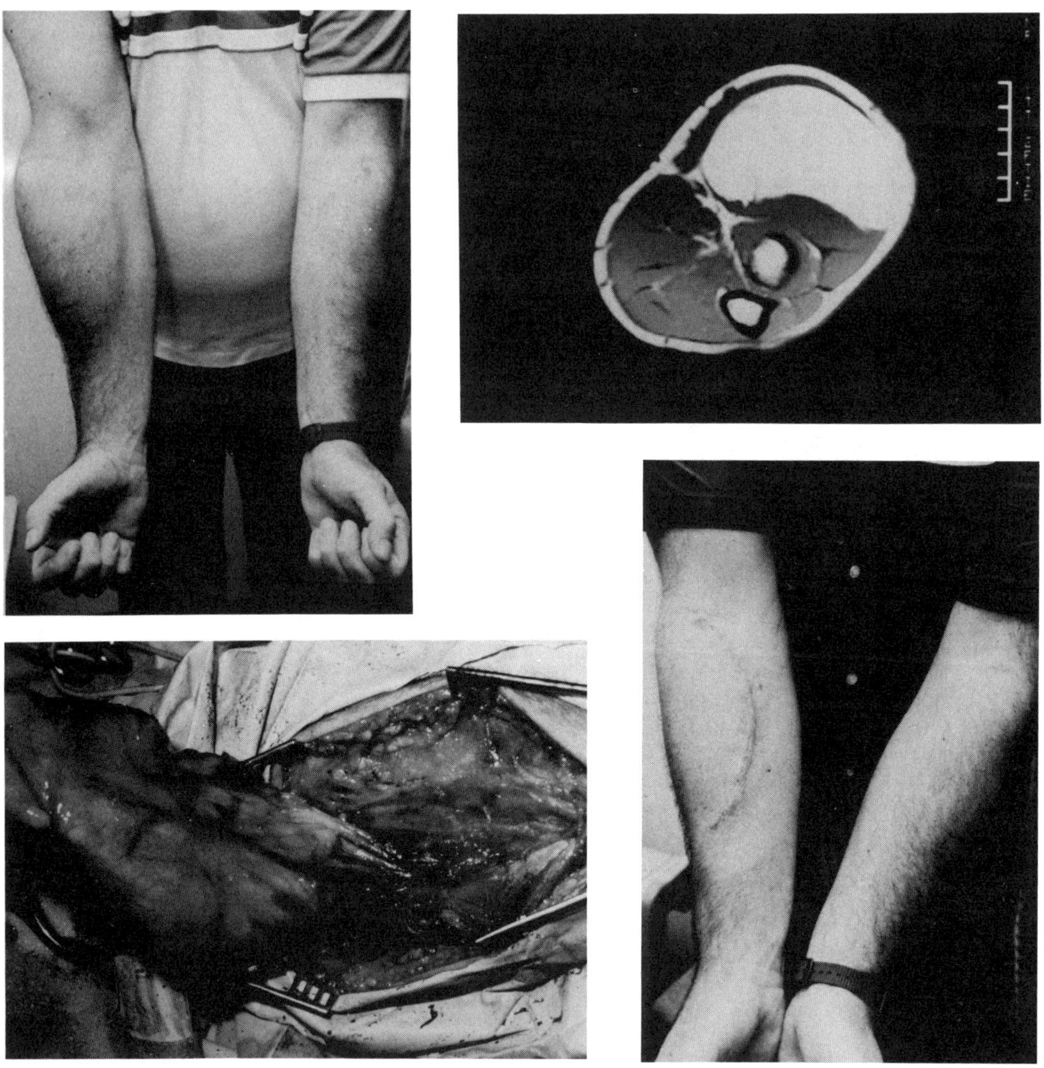

A B C D

FIG 7–2.
A, a 42-year-old homicide detective noted a recent increase in size of a large, soft mass in the right forearm that felt firm when he tensed the forearm muscles. Despite the benefit in his profession of having a powerful-appearing upper extremity, concern about a malignant tumor and difficulty in getting his forearm through shirt sleeves led him to seek medical consultation. **B,** magnetic resonance imaging demonstrated that the mass lay beneath the splayed-out brachioradialis muscle and had a high fat content. **C,** resection of this benign intermuscular lipoma was performed, sparing the radial artery and nerve. **D,** the patient's appearance and marksmanship remained satisfactory.

MULTIMODALITY TREATMENT

The goal of surgical resection of a primary or locally recurrent soft-tissue sarcoma arising in the upper extremity is complete removal of the tumor. As in the case of sarcoma in the lower extremity, surgical treatment choices are wide en bloc resection (limb-sparing surgery), or amputation. A third approach—simple excision (also termed "shelling out," enucleation, or marginal excision)—is not advisable, because this type of dissection just outside the tumor pseudocapsule results in a local recurrence rate of 40% to 90%. The pseudocapsule is not a true fascial barrier.[13] It is permeated by tumor projections, and clinically occult tumor extensions or "skip areas" may exist beyond the periphery of the primary mass, particularly for synovial sarcomas, high-grade fibrosarcomas, and liposarcomas.

Prevention of local recurrence is a particularly challenging problem in the upper extremity. Sixty-four patients treated between 1955 and 1976 at the Memorial Sloan-Kettering Cancer Center for primary or locally recurrent soft-tissue sarcomas of the wrist (4), forearm (37), or elbow (23) were reviewed by Raaf.[14] None had evidence of metastases at the time of presentation. Initially, 49 patients had their sarcomas widely resected, whereas 15 were treated by amputation. Of the 49 who had en bloc resection, 18 (37%) subsequently required amputation for locally recurrent disease. Thus, half of all patients in the series eventually had either above- or below-elbow amputation. No local stump recurrences followed amputation. Of the 49 widely resected patients, 22 had a single local recurrence, while 11 had recurrence more than once, giving an overall local recurrence rate in these patients of 67%. Adjuvant radiotherapy was rarely used in this early series.

Shiu and Hajdu[13] reviewed 194 patients with both upper- and lower-extremity sarcomas treated at Memorial Sloan-Kettering from 1949 to 1968. They found local recurrence rates for previously untreated extremity sarcomas to be higher in the upper extremity (32%) than in the lower—15% if the primary tumor was above the knee, 24% if below. Following amputation for previously untreated tumors, the local recurrence rate was 10% for upper-extremity sarcomas, and 6% and 0% for lower-extremity tumors, above and below the knee, respectively. It might appear from these data that amputation is the safest surgical method, but 5- and 10-year survival rates were actually lower in the patients receiving amputation than in those with en bloc resection, in this retrospective, nonrandomized study. These results are likely due to selection of patients for amputation who had aggressive tumors that were large at presentation or involved neurovascular structures, whereas smaller tumors were treated by wide resection.

A prospective trial for resectable, localized high-grade soft-tissue sarcomas of the extremity was performed by Rosenberg and colleagues.[15, 16] Forty-three patients were randomized to receive either amputation at or above the joint proximal to the tumor, including all involved muscle groups, or a limb-sparing resection plus adjuvant radiation therapy. In the latter patients, wide local excision was followed by 5,000 cGy to the entire anatomical area at risk for local recurrence, and 6,000 to 7,000 cGy to the tumor bed. In 27 patients who received limb-sparing resection and radiation therapy, and 16 who received amputation (randomization was 2 : 1), there were four local recurrences in the limb-sparing group and none in the amputation group. No significant differences were found in disease-free or overall survival rates between the two groups. Subsequent analysis of 211 patients seen at the National Cancer Institute (Bethesda, Maryland) with resectable soft-tissue sarcoma of the extremity showed no difference between amputation versus limb-sparing surgery plus postoperative radiotherapy in disease-free or overall survival.[17]

In patients with resectable sarcomas of the extremity, limb salvage treatment now routinely combines wide en bloc resection with either pre- or postoperative radiation therapy. If patients are properly selected, the local control rate is 70% to 90%.[18–20] A similar local control rate can be achieved by adding brachytherapy with iridium 192 implants to wide resection (Fig 7–4).[21, 22]

Despite the proven efficacy of chemotherapy for unresectable soft-tissue sarcoma, evidence supporting use of adjuvant cytotoxic drugs following resection to reduce the future risk of metastases is inconclusive. Numerous studies of adjuvant therapy for sarcomas have been conducted and reviewed by Chang et al.,[1] Antman et al.,[23] Delaney et al.,[24] and Mazanet and Antman[25] among others. Current practice is that patients rendered free of localized high-grade sarcoma are considered for entry into adjuvant clinical trials, usually coordinated by national cooperative groups.

Follow-up examination of patients who have undergone multimodality treatment for soft-tissue sarcoma of the extremity is performed every 3 months for 1 to 2 years, at 6-month intervals for another 1 to 2 years, and then annually. The excision site is meticulously examined for evidence of local recurrence, and an annual chest X-ray is obtained to screen for pulmonary metastases. A CT or MRI scan of the extremity obtained at about 3 months postoperatively can be helpful as a baseline if recurrent disease is later suspected.

Any suspicious nodule in or near the surgical scar must be considered a possible tumor growth, although in the early post-treatment period there will be wound changes associated with healing. Liberal use of biopsy will allow recurrent disease to be discovered and treated early. Attention to recurrent tumor histology may reveal a change in morphology or increase in tumor grade. If recurrent tumor is confirmed, the patient should be restaged and aggressively treated by the most appropriate multidisciplinary approaches.

LIMB-SPARING SURGERY IN THE UPPER EXTREMITY

During en bloc resection in the upper extremity, the tumor itself should never be exposed. If possible, the surgeon should resect a block of tissue containing the tumor that includes a 1 to 2-cm margin of normal tissue around the primary tumor mass, with preservation of only those nerves and vessels that are critical for limb viability and function. If tumor closely approximates bone, a section of periosteum or even a layer of cortical bone may be resected in continuity with the tumor mass.

Gross tumor should not be left behind, although small foci of microscopic tumor that re-

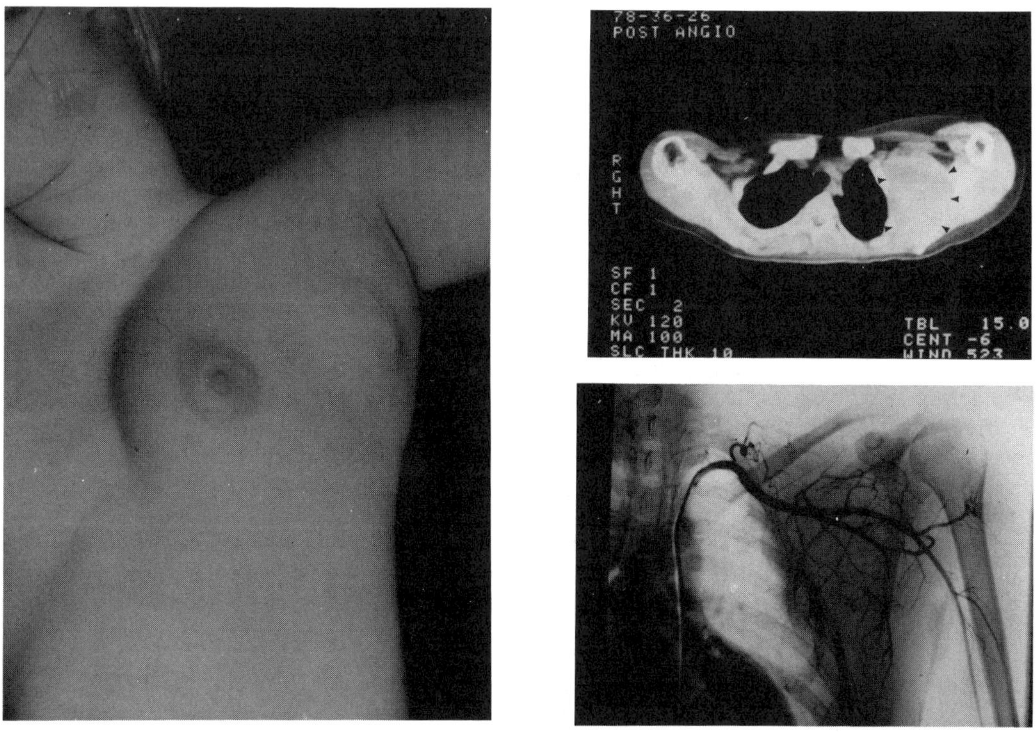

A B C

FIG 7–3.
A, a 25-year-old female presented with a mass in her left axilla. Biopsy showed it was a desmoid fibrosarcoma. **B,** computed tomography indicated involvement of both the chest wall and subscapularis muscle (*arrowheads*). **C,** an arteriogram showed that the axillary artery was displaced anteriorly by the tumor. **D,** a radical resection was performed, including a portion of the chest wall containing segments of ribs 2 through 4. **E,** the chest wall defect was repaired with Marlex mesh, leaving a window superiorly for the axillary vessels (*arrows*) and brachial plexus. Good cosmesis, **F,** and arm function, **G,** were restored.

main along major nerves or vessels may later be "sterilized" by radiation therapy. To assist the radiation oncologist in determining the extent of surgical dissection, the surgeon can place metal clips (visible in subsequent X-rays) at the periphery and deep margins of dissection just prior to wound closure, so that all exposed tissue planes will be included in the postoperative radiation therapy field.

Sarcomas of the shoulder and axilla can be large at presentation. The first symptom is often pain radiating down the arm, which is due to compression by tumor of the brachial plexus. Even if low-grade (e.g., desmoid fibrosarcoma), these tumors can be technically challenging to resect due to the difficulty of dissecting the brachial plexus and axillary artery and vein away from adjacent tumor (Figs 7–3 and 7–4). Careful planning by means of CT or MRI, and often arteriogram, is essential. If necessary, a segment of axillary artery may be resected and replaced by a vein graft (Fig 7–5). If fixation and encasement of the axillary artery is demonstrated by an arteriogram, and weakness and pain in the arm suggest invasion of the brachial plexus by a biopsy-proven, high-grade sarcoma, then in the absence of metastatic disease a forequarter (interscapulothoracic) amputation can be considered (Fig 7–6).

Reconstruction of the soft tissue of the shoulder may be accomplished by use of various myocutaneous flaps (Fig 7–7). A free-flap composite tissue transfer, performed using microvascular technique, offers a new alternative for coverage of an extensive, infected, or irradiated resection site. Krag et al.[26] believe this technique can extend the indications for limb salvage surgery and offers an alternative to amputation in selected patients.

Limb-sparing resection of a soft-tissue sarcoma located between the shoulder and elbow usually involves the biceps or triceps muscle. If

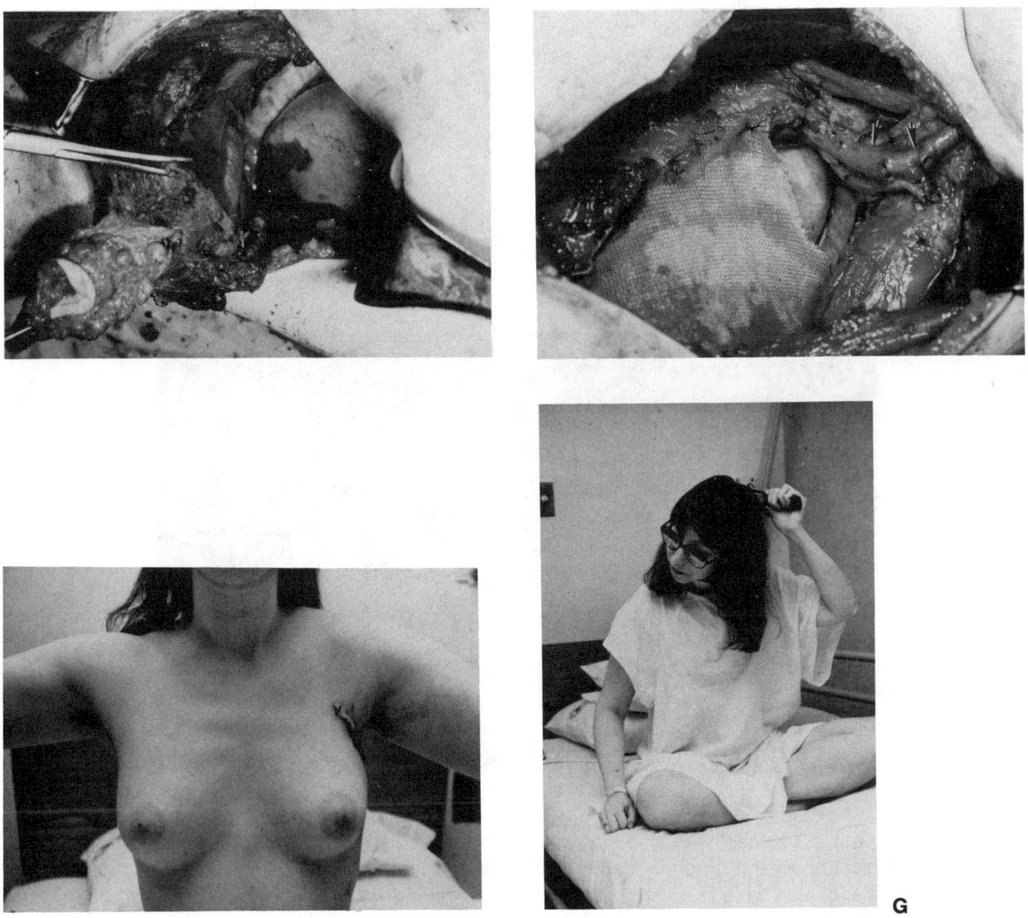

D E F G

FIG 7–3.—*Cont.*

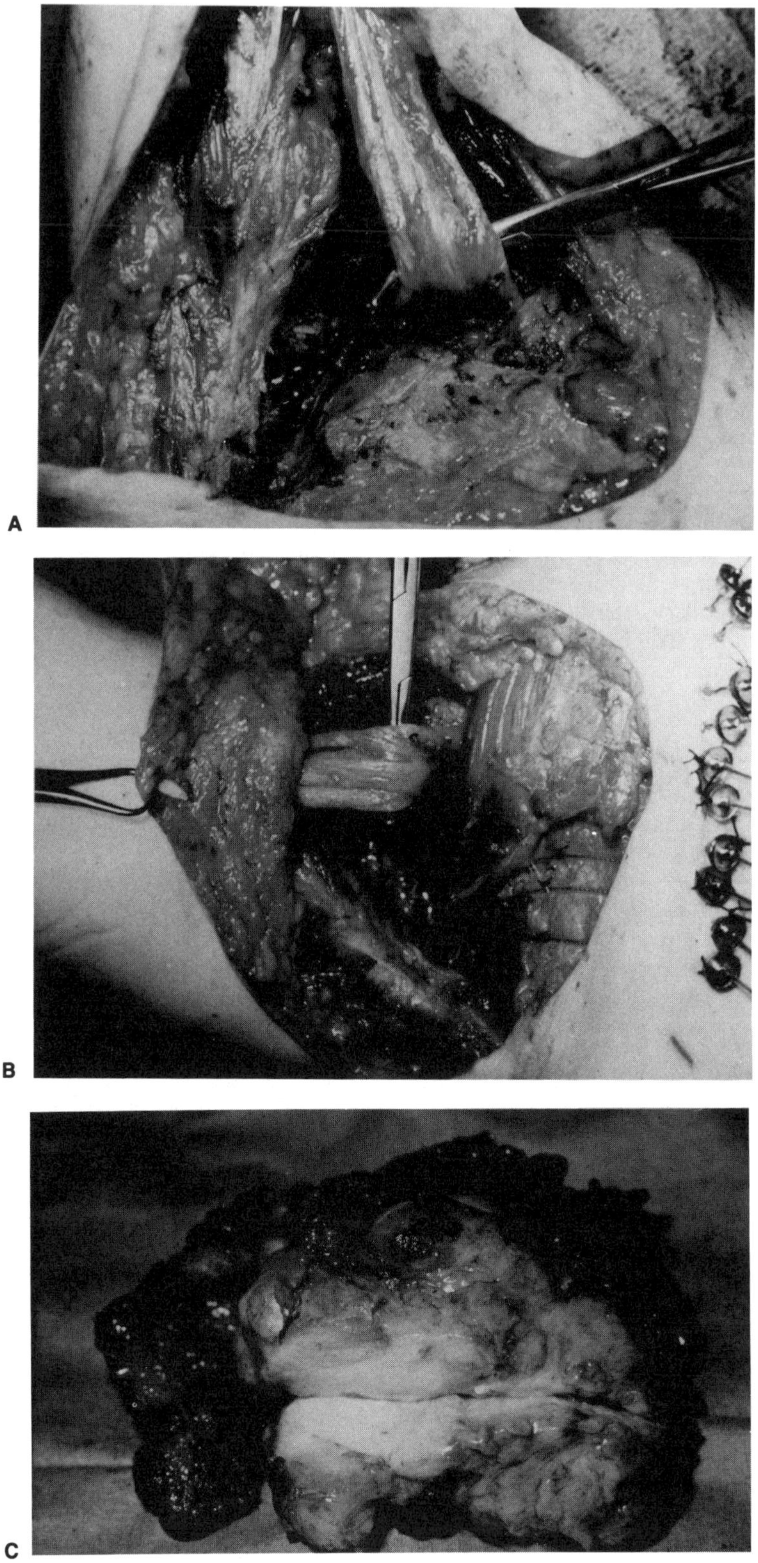

FIG 7–4.

This female patient presented with a bulky, fixed, recurrent desmoid fibrosarcoma in the left axilla. **A,** complete dissection of the brachial plexus and axillary artery was performed. The subscapularis and serratus anterior muscles were resected with the tumor, leaving histologically positive margins in a few areas. **B,** to prevent later recurrence, afterloading catheters were placed between the scapula and chest wall for iridium 192 (^{192}Ir) brachytherapy. **C,** the specimen contained typical fibrous desmoid tumor and measured 24 cm in greatest diameter.

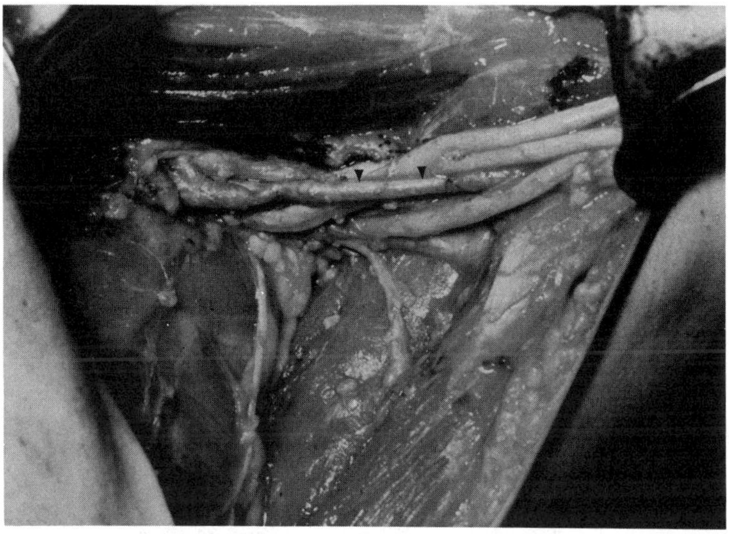

FIG 7–5.
Recurrent hemangiopericytoma was resected from the left axilla of this young woman by radical resection of the axillary contents, with complete anatomical dissection and sparing of the brachial plexus. The axillary vein and artery were encased by tumor and were resected with it. The axillary artery was reconstructed using a vein graft (*arrowheads*).

the triceps muscle is the primary tumor site, the radial nerve should be carefully dissected free and preserved (Fig 7–8). A mass in the biceps muscle must be biopsied and studied before radical surgery is undertaken, to avoid inappropriately radical treatment for benign conditions such as biceps muscle avulsion or myositis ossificans. If the diagnosis of biceps muscle tear is strongly suggested by history and physical examination, selected patients may be carefully observed without biopsy or other surgical intervention.

In patients with sarcomas in the upper extremity distal to the axilla, axillary lymphadenectomy is not indicated except when palpable, firm nodes are present. Regional node metastases are so rare[4, 5] that axillary dissection should be done only following confirmation by positive biopsy of a suspicious node. An exception is childhood embryonal rhabdomyosarcoma (ERMS), in which regional node metastases are common.[27]

Sarcomas of the hand are uncommon. Digital or ray amputation may be successful in achieving local control or even cure. In one case, we attempted to reduce the extent of resection by pre-operative intra-arterial chemotherapy, but the success of this approach was limited (Fig 7–9). Central tumor necrosis was seen following intra-arterial drug administration, but cells in the periphery of the tumor remained viable despite significant toxicity to surrounding normal tissue.

LYMPHANGIOSARCOMA

Lymphangiosarcoma (LAS) is a rare malignant tumor of the vascular endothelium that usually arises in a chronically edematous extremity. Most cases have been in patients with postmastectomy lymphedema of the upper extremity (Fig 7–10), a syndrome described by Stewart and Treves in 1948.[28] Lymphangiosarcoma appears a median of 11 years after mastectomy.

Two thirds of the 34 patients with postmastectomy LAS reported by Sordillo et al.[29] had received radiation therapy after their breast surgery on the side where their tumor occurred, although the tumors frequently originated outside the radiation field. Other sites of origin include the scalp, face, and lower extremity.[30] There have been reports of angiosarcoma developing in the breast in women following lumpectomy and radiation therapy for breast adenocarcinoma.[31, 32]

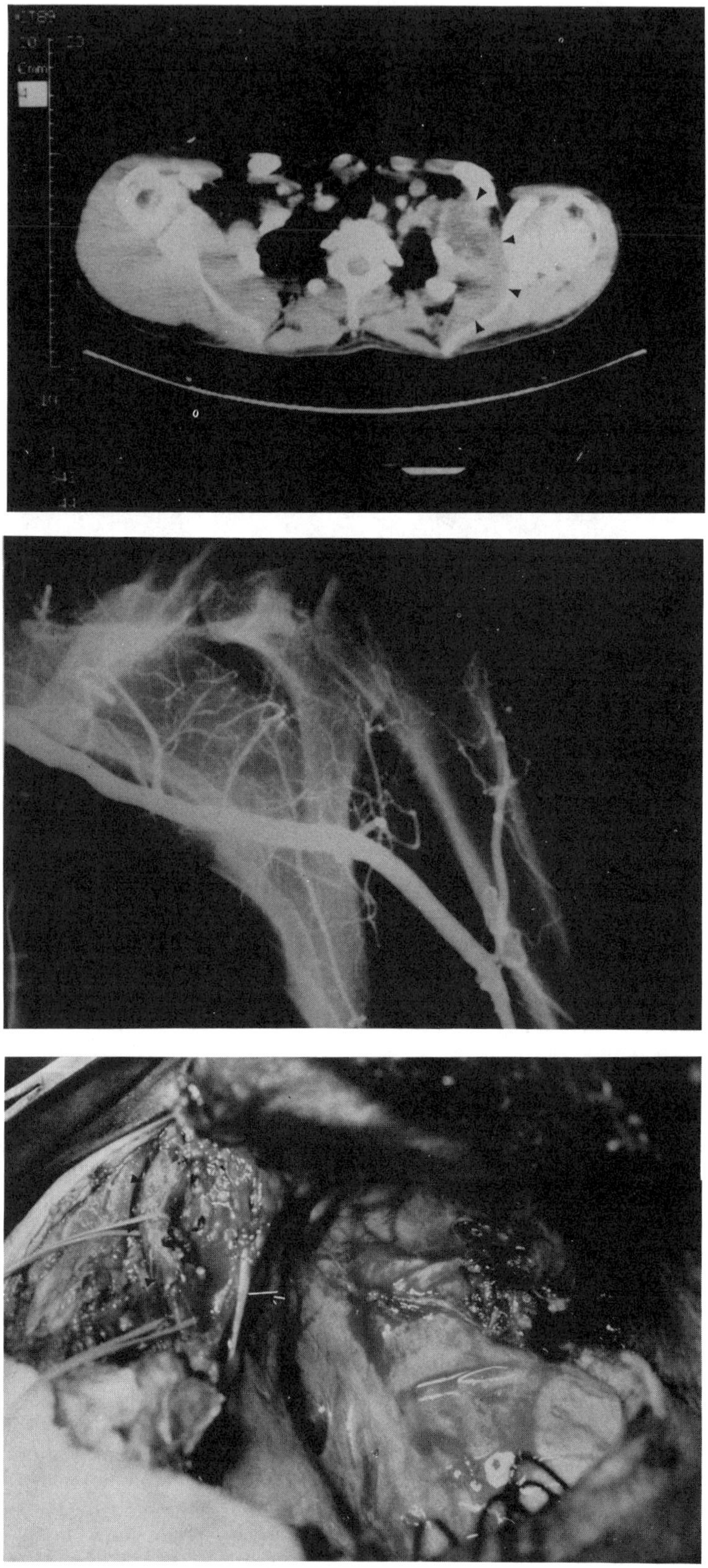

A

B

C

FIG 7–6.

This 38-year-old man developed recurrent clear cell sarcoma in both the left axilla and supraclavicular space. **A,** a CT scan showed the tumor (*arrowheads*) was closely approximating the scapula and invading the chest wall. **B,** an arteriogram demonstrated encasement of the axillary artery and presence of multiple tumor vessels. **C,** because there was no evidence of distant disease, forequarter amputation was offered and performed, including resection of a segment of chest wall. The phrenic nerve (*arrow*) and left brachiocephalic vein (*arrowheads;* held by vessel loops) were spared.

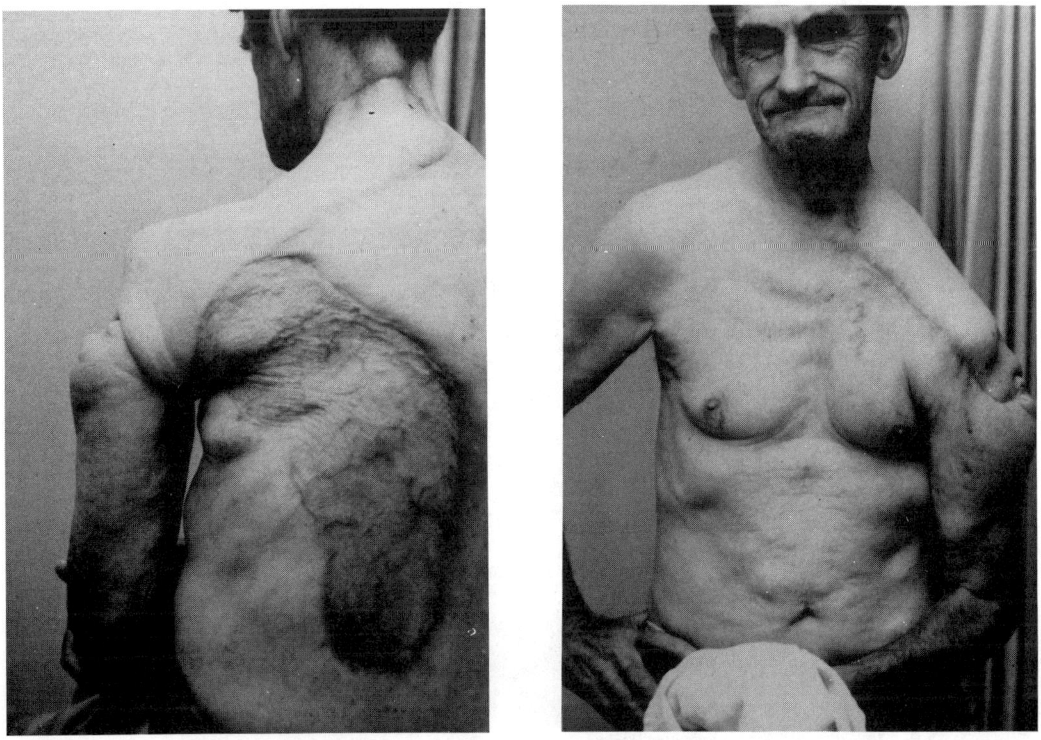

A B

FIG 7–7.
This 70-year-old man had a bulky malignant tumor of the shoulder that filled the supraclavicular space and caused a pathological fracture of his clavicle. The tumor was widely resected for cure by partial scapulectomy, claviculectomy, infra-omohyoid neck dissection, and level II and III axillary dissection. **A,** reconstruction of the defect was achieved using a latissimus dorsi myocutaneous flap. **B,** the patient had good use of his hand postoperatively.

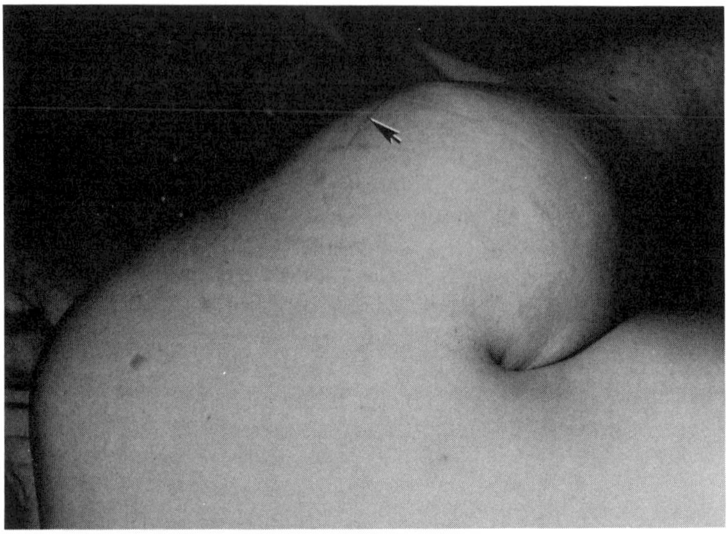

A

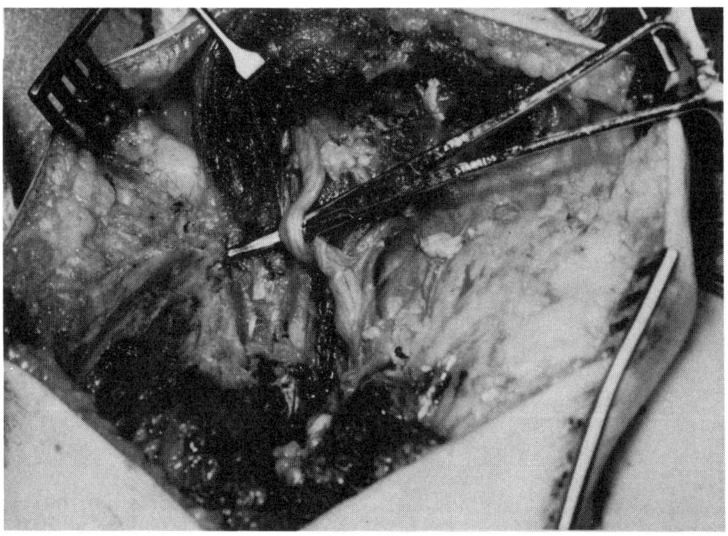

B

FIG 7–8.
A, a pleomorphic liposarcoma in the right triceps muscle was diagnosed by open, incisional biopsy (*arrow*) in this 60-year-old woman. **B,** wide en bloc resection required removal of the medial and long heads of the triceps muscle as well as portions of the deltoid and teres major muscles and the axillary nerve. The radial nerve (lifted by the hemostat) was spared. **C** and **D,** following removal of the specimen the incision was closed. **E,** upper-extremity function remained intact. Postoperative radiation therapy (6,000 cGy) was given, and the patient remained free of recurrence.

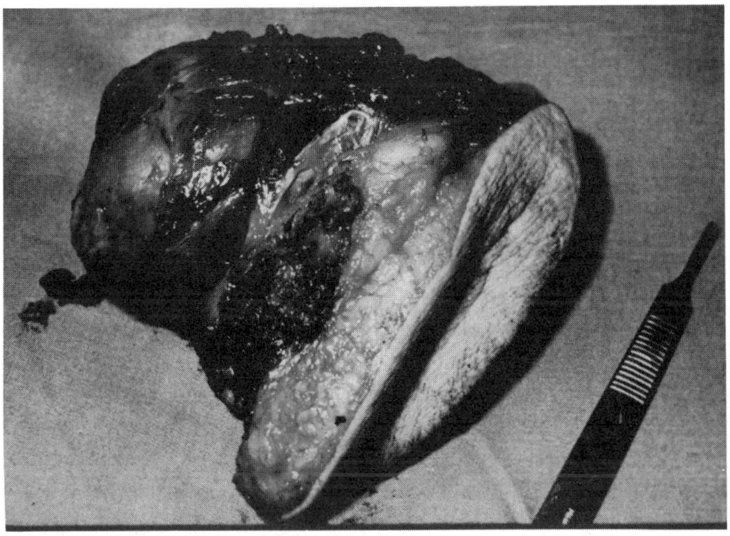

C

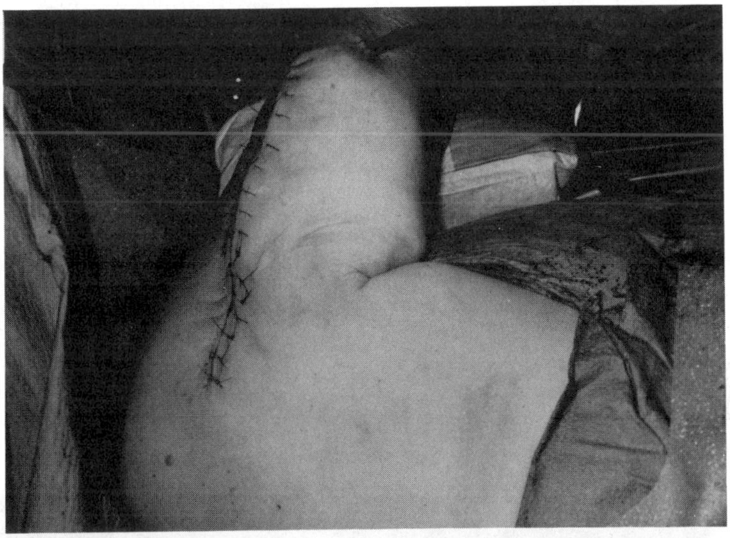

D

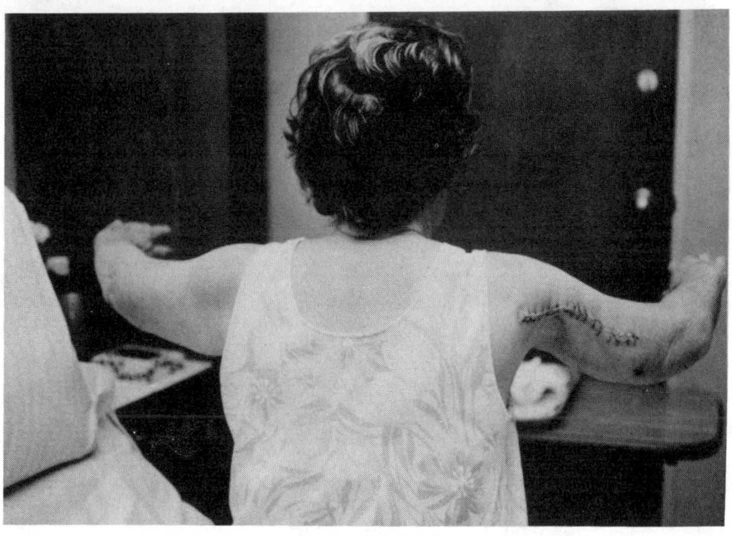

E

FIG 7–8.—*Cont.*

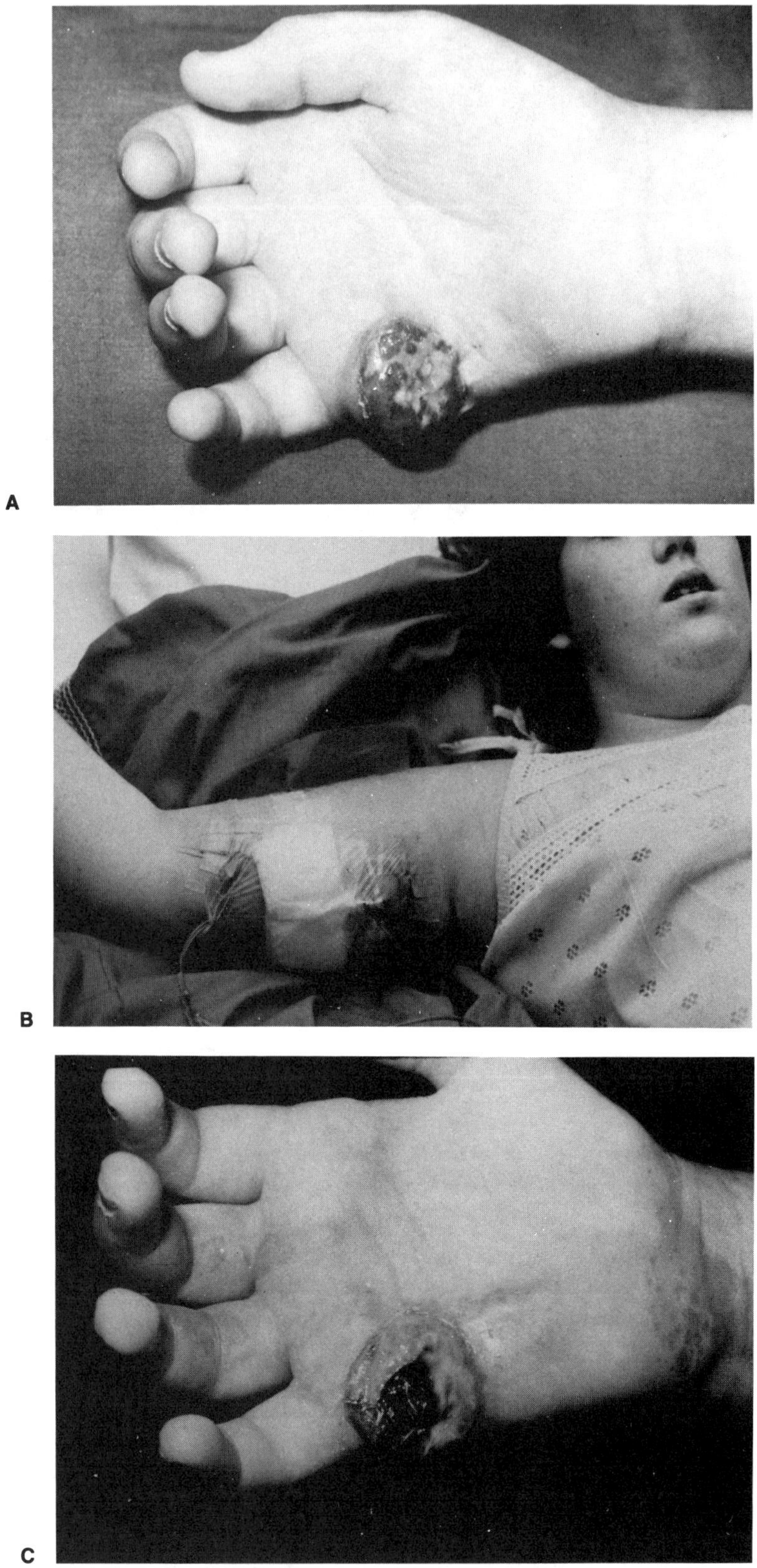

FIG 7–9.
A, A teen-age girl presented with a synovial sarcoma on the ulnar side of the palmar aspect of her right hand. Because of her desire not to have a ray amputation of the fourth and fifth digits, an attempt was made to decrease the tumor size using intra-arterial Adriamycin (doxorubicin). **B,** drug delivery was through a vascular access port and fine-tipped catheter implanted into the brachial artery. **C,** this treatment caused central tumor necrosis but no real shrinkage of the tumor, even though sufficient drug was given to cause severe erythema of the surrounding normal tissue. Ultimately a ray amputation was done.

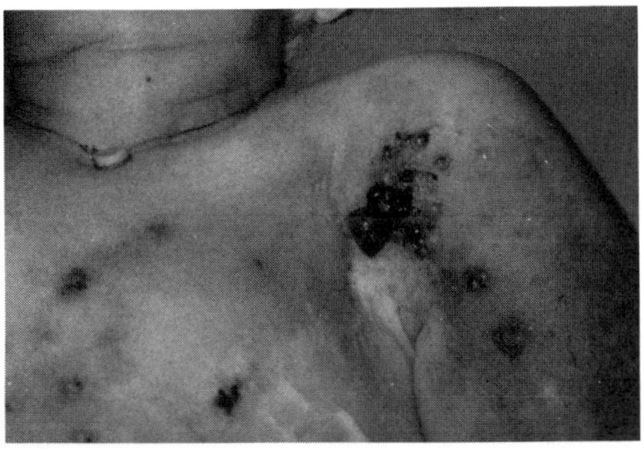

FIG 7–10.
Lymphangiosarcoma in the left arm and chest wall of a woman with longstanding arm edema following mastectomy and radiation to the axilla.

Prognosis in patients with LAS is poor, although early amputation of an affected limb seems to give the best chance of survival. The tumor is frequently multifocal at the time of presentation, so wide excision is usually followed by repeated recurrences in the arm, shoulder, and chest wall with eventual metastases to the lungs. Responses of limited duration can be achieved with radiation therapy or chemotherapy.[29, 33]

CONCLUSION

Limb-sparing surgery is technically feasible for most soft-tissue sarcomas of the upper extremity, but if used as the only mode of treatment, there is a high rate of local recurrence. Surgical judgment is critical for a successful outcome, and amputation should be considered if wide resection will leave residual gross disease.

Following limb-sparing surgery, irradiation of a tumor bed that possibly contains residual microscopic tumor will decrease the chance of local recurrence. The role of adjuvant chemotherapy is controversial and unproven. Patients should receive adjuvant chemotherapy by participation in controlled clinical trials.

REFERENCES

1. Chang AE, Rosenberg SA, Glatstein EJ, et al: Sarcomas of soft tissues, in DeVita VT, Hellman S, Rosenberg SA (eds): *Cancer, Principles and Practice of Oncology*, 3rd ed, ch 40. Philadelphia, J. B. Lippincott, 1989, pp 1345–1398.
2. Collin C, Hajdu SI, Godbold J, et al: Localized operable soft tissue sarcoma of the upper extremity: Preservation, management, and factors affecting local recurrence in 108 patients. *Ann Surg* 1987; 205:331–339.
3. Raaf JH, Ragsdale BD: Malignant tumours of soft parts: Surgical management of liposarcoma, in Fleegler EJ, Bogumill GP (eds): *Tumours of the Hand and Upper Limb*. London, Churchill-Livingstone (in press).
4. Weingrad DN, Rosenberg SA: Early lymphatic spread of osteogenic and soft-tissue sarcomas. *Surgery* 1978; 84:231–240.
5. Mazeron J-J, Suit HD: Lymph nodes as sites of metastases from sarcomas of soft tissue. *Cancer* 1987; 60:1800–1808.
6. Petasnick JP, Turner DA, Charters JR, et al: Soft tissue masses of the locomotor system: Comparison of MR imaging with CT. *Radiology* 1986; 160:125–133.
7. Neifeld JP, Walsh JW, Lawrence W Jr: Computed tomography in the management of soft tissue tumors. *Surg Gynecol Obstet* 1982; 155:535–540.
8. Lindell MM Jr, Wallace S, de Santos LA, et al: Diagnostic technique for the evaluation of the soft tissue sarcoma. *Semin Oncol* 1981; 8:160–171.
9. Kissin MW, Fisher C, Webb AJ, et al: Value of fine needle aspiration cytology in the diagnosis of soft tissue tumors: A preliminary study on the excised specimen. *Br J Surg* 1987; 74:479–480.
10. Layfield LJ, Anders KH, Glasgow BJ, et al: Fine-needle aspiration of primary soft-tissue lesions. *Arch Pathol Lab Med* 1986; 110:420–424.
11. Oland J, Rosen A, Reif R, et al: Cytodiagnosis of soft tissue tumors. *J Surg Oncol* 1988; 37:168–170.
12. Mankin HJ, Lange TA, Spanier SS: The hazards of biopsy in patients with primary bone and soft-tissue tumors. *J Bone Joint Surg* 1982; 64:1121–1127.
13. Shiu MH, Hajdu SI: Management of soft tissue sarcoma of the extremity. *Semin Oncol* 1981; 8:172–179.
14. Raaf JH: Soft tissue sarcomas of the arm: The frequent challenge of local recurrence. *ASCO Proc* 1986; 5:265.
15. Rosenberg SA, Kent H, Costa J, et al: Prospective randomized evaluation of the role of limb-sparing surgery, radiation therapy, and adjuvant chemoimmunotherapy in the treatment of adult soft-tissue sarcomas. *Surgery* 1978; 84:62–69.

16. Rosenberg SA, Tepper J, Glatstein E, et al: The treatment of soft-tissue sarcomas of the extremities: Prospective randomized evaluations of (1) limb-sparing surgery plus radiation therapy compared with amputation and (2) the role of adjuvant chemotherapy. *Ann Surg* 1982; 196:305–315.
17. Potter DA, Kinsella T, Glatstein E, et al: High-grade soft tissue sarcomas of the extremities. *Cancer* 1986; 58:190–205.
18. Kraybill WG, Emami B, Lyss AP: Management of soft tissue sarcomas of the extremities. *Surgery* 1991; 109:233–235.
19. Owens JC, Shiu MH, Smith R, et al: Soft tissue sarcomas of the hand and foot. *Cancer* 1985; 55:2010–2018.
20. Talbert ML, Zagars GK, Sherman NE, et al: Conservative surgery and radiation therapy for soft tissue sarcoma of the wrist, hand, ankle, and foot. *Cancer* 1990; 66:2482–2491.
21. Shiu MH, Collin C, Hilaris BS, et al: Limb preservation and tumor control in the treatment of popliteal and antecubital soft tissue sarcomas. *Cancer* 1986; 57:1632–1639.
22. Zelefsky MJ, Harrison LB, Shiu MH, et al: Combined surgical resection and iridium 192 implantation for locally advanced and recurrent desmoid tumors. *Cancer* 1991; 67:380–384.
23. Antman K, Suit H, Amato D, et al: Preliminary results of a randomized trial of adjuvant doxorubicin for sarcomas: Lack of apparent difference between treatment groups. *J Clin Oncol* 1984; 2:601–608.
24. Delaney TF, Yang JC, Glatstein E: Adjuvant therapy for adult patients with soft tissue sarcomas. *Oncology* 1991; 5:105–118.
25. Mazanet R, Antman KH: Sarcomas of soft tissue and bone. *Cancer* 1991; 68:463–473.
26. Krag DN, Klein H, Schneider PD, et al: Composite tissue transfer in limb-salvage surgery. *Arch Surg* 1991; 126:639–641.
27. Raaf JH, Exelby PR: Childhood tumors, in Copeland EM (ed): *Surgical Oncology*, ch 34. New York, John Wiley & Sons, 1983, pp 591–613.
28. Stewart FW, Treves N: Lymphangiosarcoma in postmastectomy lymphedema: A report of six cases in elephantiasis chirurgica. *Cancer* 1948; 1:64–81.
29. Sordillo PP, Chapman R, Hajdu SI, et al: Lymphangiosarcoma. *Cancer* 1981; 48:1674–1679.
30. Maddox JC, Evans HL: Angiosarcoma of skin and soft tissue: A study of forty-four cases. *Cancer* 1981; 48:1907–1921.
31. Givens SS, Ellerbroek NA, Butler JJ, et al: Angiosarcoma arising in an irradiated breast. *Cancer* 1989; 64:2214–2216.
32. Stokkel MPM, Peterse HL: Angiosarcoma of the breast after lumpectomy and radiation therapy for adenocarcinoma. *Cancer* 1992; 69:2965–2968.
33. Yap B-S, Yap H-Y, McBride CM, et al: Chemotherapy for postmastectomy lymphangiosarcoma. *Cancer* 1981; 47:853–856.

Chapter 8

Dermatofibrosarcoma Protuberans; Fibromatosis of the Hands and Feet; Pseudosarcomatous Lesions

Harold V. Gaskill III

J. Bradley Aust

DERMATOFIBROSARCOMA PROTUBERANS

Dermatofibrosarcoma protuberans was first described by Taylor in 1890.[1] His patient was a 43-year-old man presenting with a 15-year history of a slowly growing mass on the left shoulder. Limited surgical excision was followed by local recurrence on four occasions. This characteristic clinical presentation was associated with the distinctive histopathological appearance of the lesion as described by Darier and Ferrand in 1924.[2] The name *dermatofibrosarcoma protuberans* was proposed by Hoffman the following year.[3]

The pathophysiology of these lesions is not well understood. The only predisposing factor suggested by the literature is prior trauma reported in 12% to 17% of cases.[4, 5] There is even considerable controversy over the cell type from which they arise. Based on electron microscopic morphology, both fibroblastic-histiocytic and neural origins have been proposed.[6, 7] More recently, both tissue culture and immunohistochemical techniques have supported a combined fibroblastic-histiocytic origin.[8, 9]

Dermatofibrosarcoma protuberans is uncommon, comprising about 1% of skin tumors and 0.1% of all malignant tumors. They appear most often during the third and fourth decades, but have been reported in patients ranging from 3 to 80 years of age.[5] Most series suggest a slight male predominance.[10] There does not appear to be any racial predilection, and a series of black patients reported by Ani et al.[11] revealed no significant differences in incidence or distribution.

When first noticed, these lesions are usually small and firm with a reddish to bluish-purple color that may blanch with slight pressure.[10] Their distribution appears random, with all areas of the body affected save the palms and soles. Because small lesions are almost always painless, patients rarely seek medical attention early. More often, the lesions grow slowly for years, during which time they develop their characteristic gross morphology: a protuberant, polypoid mass 2–10 cm in diameter. Large lesions may have a bosselated or multilobular appearance, with marked skin changes around the base. Some patients may present only after ulceration has occurred, resulting in bleeding or secondary infection. Alternatively, patients may present with recurrent disease after one or more prior excisions.

Histologically, the lesion is composed of uniform spindle cells arranged in characteristic whorls and bundles (Fig 8–1). The pattern has been described most often as cartwheel or storiform and is considered pathognomonic. Burkhardt and colleagues report this pattern to be prominent in over 90% of cases and present in all.[12] Other patterns that may be seen include twisted strip and herringbone arrangements. In most cases, mitotic figures are rare. In addition to these cells, variable amounts of collagen are seen, as well as vascular spaces lined with endothelium. In larger tumors, an actively growing outer layer surrounds a less cellular central region with evidence of fibrosis. Invasion of underlying adipose tissue is common, and infiltration of fascia and muscle are seen less often.[4]

It is important to note that although metastasis is rare, it has been reported.[13, 14] These metastatic lesions, as well as some local recurrences, vary in appearance from the primary tumor and may not demonstrate the characteristic cartwheel pattern.

In view of the high incidence of recurrence, adequate treatment consists of excision with a 3- to 6-cm margin of grossly normal skin at the base. Because penetration into adipose tissue is common, the dissection should be carried to and include the underlying fascia. In most cases, an adequate resection will require coverage with a split-thickness skin graft (Fig 8–2).

Several cases treated successfully by microscopically controlled chemosurgery (Mohs technique) have been reported.[15, 16] This method may prove useful for treatment of recurrent disease, or as primary therapy in cosmetically important areas.

As might be expected with such an indolent lesion, radiotherapy does not appear to be effective.[12] Chemotherapy, for example methotrexate,[17] has been effective against metastases as well as primary tumors not amenable to complete excision.

Case Report

A 40-year-old man had a polypoid mass removed from his right arm by simple excision and closure. Recurrence was evident within 3 months and the patient sought additional treat-

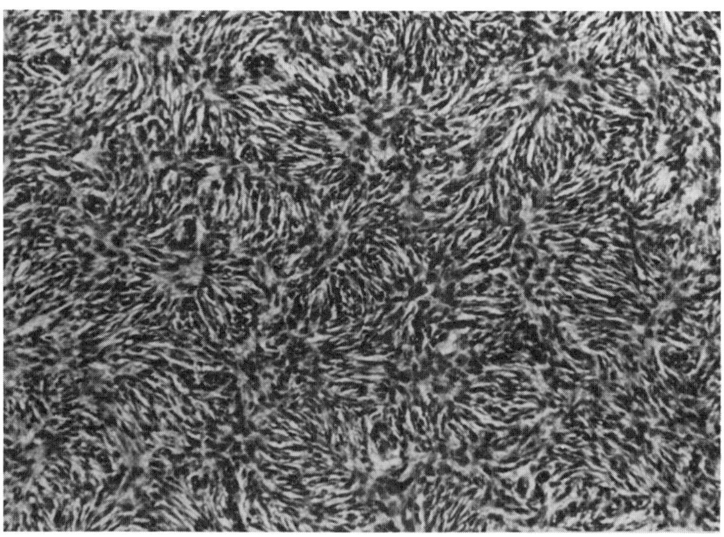

FIG 8–1.
Dermatofibrosarcoma protuberans, demonstrating the characteristic storiform or cartwheel pattern.

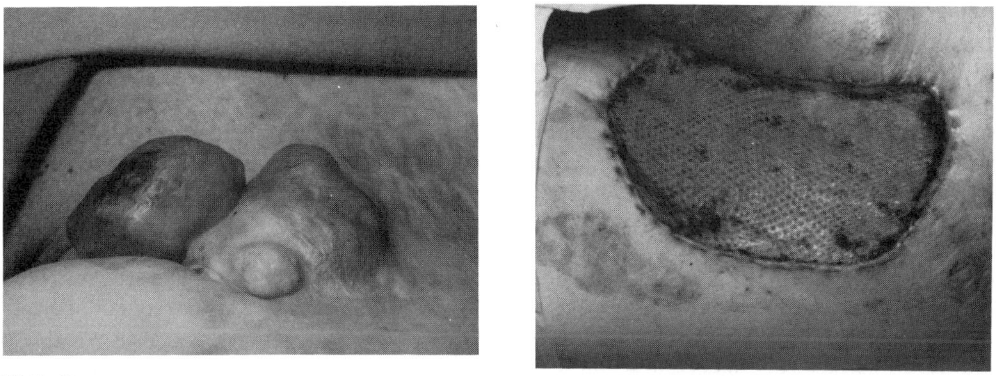

FIG 8–2.
A, recurrent dermatofibrosarcoma protuberans in the left groin. Each nodule is 3–4 cm in diameter. **B,** treatment by wide excision and meshed, split-thickness skin graft.

ment at 6 months. The lesion measured approximately 1 cm in diameter and arose from the excision scar. Skin changes in the area were evident (Fig 8–3). The lesion was excised via the Mohs technique and covered with a split-thickness skin graft. There has been no recurrence.

FIBROMATOSIS OF THE HANDS AND FEET

In 1831, Baron Guillaume Dupuytren described a patient who had developed an insidious contraction of the ring finger in both hands, apparently caused by a tense band of fibrous tissue extending down onto the palm. Although this description may not have been the first, Dupuytren's name has been inseparably associated with palmar fibromatosis since that time.[18, 19] It was known even then that these contractures were frequently accompanied by fascial thickening and nodules in other parts of the body as well.[20] Indeed, Anderson, in 1891, used the term "diathesis" to describe the course in certain patients with a predisposition for involvement of multiple sites.[21]

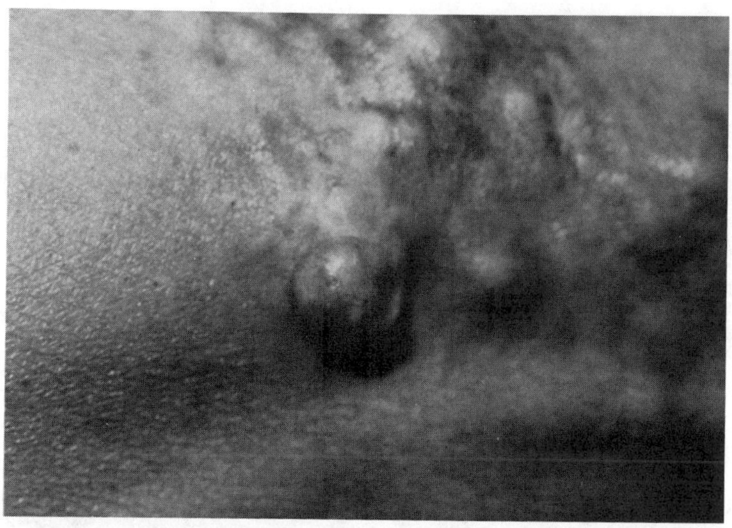

FIG 8–3.
Recurrent dermatofibrosarcoma protuberans at the site of previous excision. Changes in the surrounding skin are evident. The lesion measures approximately 1 cm across.

Remarkably little is known about the pathophysiology of this disease. One of the most popular theories has suggested that the trauma of manual labor plays a causative role.[18] Yet, although these lesions are reported as occurring from two to seven times more often in males, there does not appear to be any relationship to occupation.[22, 23] Furthermore, this theory does not account for the association with fibrous lesions on the feet and other parts of the body. Heredity does appear to be a significant factor, and from 30% to 40% of patients will have a positive family history of finger contraction. The disease is virtually unknown among blacks, Orientals, and American Indians.[22, 23] Individuals with alcoholic liver disease have been reported to have an increased incidence (as high as 66%), as have patients with epilepsy, peptic ulcer, cholecystitis, and diabetes.[22, 24]

More recently, it has been shown that collagen from the fascia of these patients differs biochemically from normal collagen. The changes observed are characteristic of those seen during normal wound healing and contraction. These include an abundance of type III collagen, with increased levels of hydroxylysine and hydroxylysinohydroxy-norleucine cross-links. Significantly, these changes are also seen in grossly and histologically normal fascia from affected patients.[25] These data suggest that fibromatosis of the hands and feet is the primary manifestation of a systemic disease characterized by a defect in collagen synthesis and maturation, with an autosomal dominant pattern of inheritance.

Histologically, both palmar and plantar fibromatosis have similar pictures and both can be confused with malignant sarcomas. Beginning as a localized fibroblastic overgrowth, they progress to form strands and bundles with loss of cell polarity and pleomorphism (Fig 8–4). They appear more malignant histologically than their clinical course warrants. Giant pacinian corpuscles may also be seen, as well as histological evidence of chronic inflammation.[26]

Despite the apparent similarity of their pathophysiology, the clinical presentation and management of palmar and plantar fibromatosis differs and each will be discussed separately.

The characteristic clinical presentation of palmar fibromatosis was first described by Plater in 1614 and by many others since then.[18] The deformity of the involved digits is so characteristic that the diagnosis is rarely in doubt (Fig 8–5). The differential diagnosis would include congenital deformity and scarring from a previous laceration or severe tenosynovitis. Although the disease has been reported in teenagers, it usually presents during the fifth or sixth decade. As mentioned earlier, males are affected more often than females, and a positive family history is obtainable in up to 40% of patients.[27] Involvement of the ring finger (64%) is most common, followed by the little finger (53%) and middle

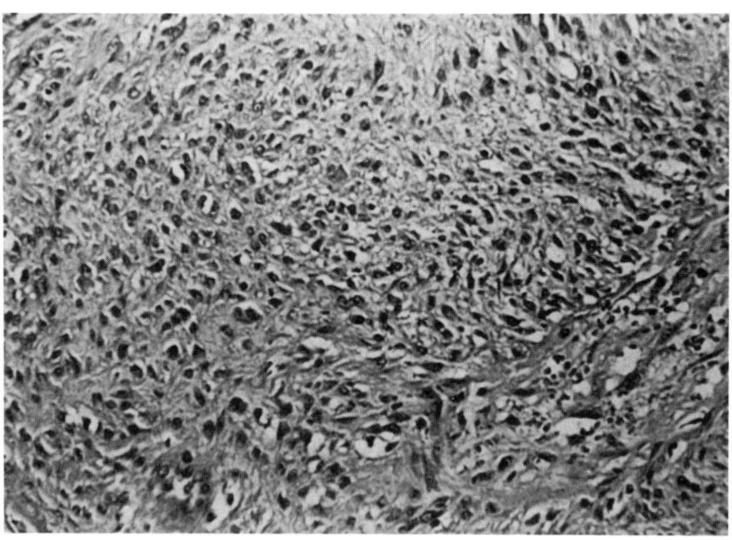

FIG 8–4.
Plantar fibromatosis. Note marked pleomorphism with loss of cell polarity.

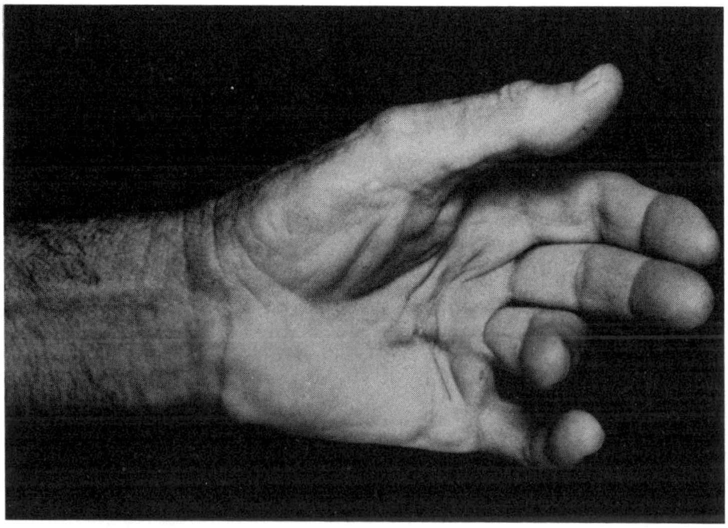

FIG 8–5.
Characteristic clinical appearance of palmar fibromatosis.

finger (24%). These figures reflect occurrence in more than one digit in some patients.[18]

The first symptom of the disease is usually a firm nodule beneath the palmar skin opposite the metacarpophalangeal joint. With progression, a definite cord extending from the nodule to the base of the affected finger appears. Over a period of months or years, the finger flexes increasingly toward the palm. McIndoe and Beare have divided this progression into four distinct clinical stages.[23] In stage I, the disease is limited to the palmar fascia only. The fingers are not yet contracted and there is no impairment of function. Stage II begins with the onset of minor contracture with dimpling of the palmar skin, while stage III exhibits major finger contracture but normal joint function. Stage IV disease is characterized by long-standing contracture with hyperextension of the terminal phalanges and fibrosis of the metacarpophalangeal joints. Once the disease has progressed to the point of actual flexion of the digit, intervention is indicated. The treatment of palmar fibromatosis is surgical and should be carried out by an individual experienced in operations on the hand. Several procedures are applicable and include fasciotomy, regional fasciectomy, and dermofasciectomy. Fasciotomy is limited to simple interruption of the fibrous band with splinting and/or an interposition graft. Its use should be limited to elderly patients or to those with minimal disability. More often, fasciotomy is extended into a regional fasciectomy of involved tissue with meticulous preservation of the digital nerves.

Extensive fasciectomy is reserved for patients with involvement of the entire palmar fascia. Currently, there is no role for the "prophylactic radical fasciectomy" advocated in the past.[28] The last procedure mentioned, dermofasciectomy, is based on the observation that palmar fibromatosis does not recur beneath a skin graft. The operation consists of excision of the skin, subcutaneous tissue, and fascia followed by coverage with full-thickness autografts. The procedure is indicated primarily in young patients with a strong family history of rapid progression, or in patients with recurrent disease.[28] Operative complications include hematoma formation, skin loss, digital nerve injury, and joint stiffness. Long-term results reflect the underlying pathology. Recurrence within 1 or 2 years is common in young patients with a strong family history, whereas in older patients progressive disease frequently develops during the ensuing decades.[29, 30]

Fibromatosis of the plantar fascia has received comparatively little attention in the literature. Although the underlying pathophysiology is similar to that of the palmar lesion, clinical presentation and management differ. First, it is much less common, being reported in fewer than two per 100,000 hospital admissions.[31] More than 60% of patients with plantar fibromatosis will also have palmar fibromatosis, with the palmar lesions most commonly antedating the plantar, occasionally by ten or more years.[32]

The clinical presentation of plantar fibromatosis differs in that contracture of the toes is not a component. The patient usually does not seek treatment until a large nodule or mass results in pain or aching on ambulation.

As with palmar fibromatosis, evaluation of the patients should begin with a family history to identify the presence of the disease in blood relatives. The physical examination should include a search for manifestations of the disease in other parts of the body, for example, palms, knuckles, and penis. Examination of the foot is facilitated by dorsiflexion of the toes, thus tensing the plantar fascia. One or more nodular swellings will be palpable, usually along the medial longitudinal area of the foot. The differential diagnosis includes scars from previous lacerations, calluses, fibrosarcoma, chondromas, and exostosis.[31, 33]

Again, the primary mode of treatment is surgical. After the neurovascular status of the foot has been carefully assessed, the patient is prepared for an operation. The plantar fascia is explored through a sigmoid incision extending from just behind the first metatarsal head, extending longitudinally down the arch, and curving anterior to the heel (Fig 8–6). The entire plantar fascia is then excised by blunt dissection with meticulous preservation of the median plantar nerve.[34] Excision of less than the entire fascia results in early recurrence in up to 70% of patients.[35] By contrast, total excision has reduced the recurrence rate to about 8%.[36] Because contracture is not a feature of the disease, extension of the incision onto the digits is not required. The wound is then dressed and splinted, with ambulation begun in 2 to 4 weeks.[37] It is most important that the clinical picture be correlated with pathological findings. The histological picture of fibromatosis has been confused with low-grade sarcoma and amputations have been reported.[32] The most common postoperative complications include hematoma, infection, and skin loss.

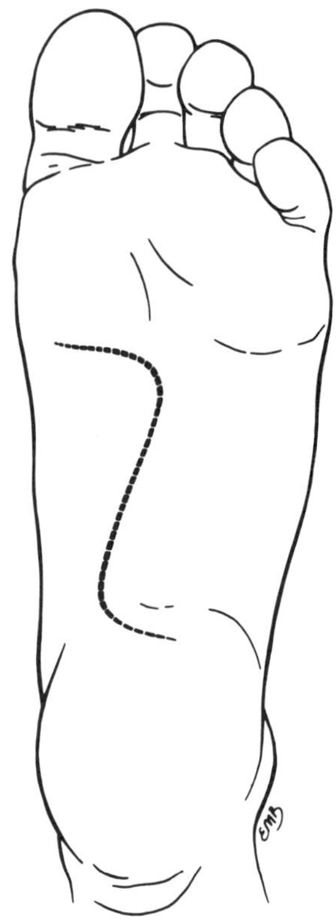

FIG 8–6.
Sigmoid incision through which the plantar fascia is excised, leaving minimal vascular compromise.

PSEUDOSARCOMATOUS PROLIFERATIVE LESIONS OF SOFT TISSUE

Over the last 30 years, a number of lesions have been recognized that, despite many clinical and histological characteristics similar to those of sarcomas, exhibit a predictably benign course. Thus, the term "pseudosarcoma" has been applied to a variety of benign reactive lesions sharing this common behavioral thread. Because in most cases they are cured by local excision alone, early recognition is crucial if unnecessarily mutilating surgical procedures are to be avoided.

More recently, it has been suggested that these lesions may be considered as a similar histological expression by a spectrum of soft-tissue types. Four varieties are well defined: lesions occurring in (1) dermis (atypical fibroxanthoma), (2) fibrous septa of subcutaneous fat and fascia (proliferative fasciitis), (3) fascia (nodular fasciitis), and (4) muscle (proliferative myositis).[38–41]

Atypical Fibroxanthoma

Atypical fibroxanthoma presents most often as a small, firm nodule on the head or neck. Individuals affected are usually older and may have a significant history of previous sun exposure. The first series of 20 patients was reported by Helwig[42] in 1963, and the term *atypical fibroxanthoma* was used because of the xanthomatous appearance of some of the bizarre cells present. The benign clinical course of these lesions was immediately recognized.[42] Since that time, the atypical fibroxanthoma has been well characterized through large series collected by Fretzin, Helwig, Dahl, and others.[41, 43, 44]

The lesion is not common. Kroe and Pitcock identified only ten cases out of 260,000 surgical specimens.[45] It occurs twice as often in males as in females. Seventy-five percent of these lesions are located on the head and neck, with a predilection for the ears and nose. The remainder are scattered throughout the trunk and limbs. There is a bimodal age distribution, with the peak incidence of head and neck lesions occurring at age 70, whereas trunk and limb lesions are seen most often during the third and fourth decades.[41] Caucasians are affected almost exclusively although several cases have been reported in blacks.

The patient presents most often with a single nodule less than 2 cm in diameter, which is usually firm and nontender with a smooth surface. Some lesions, however, may range up to 10 cm in diameter, or present with ulceration and bleeding. Most are slow growing and will have been present for several years at the time of diagnosis. Several predisposing factors are suggested, including sun exposure, acute or chronic trauma, and prior therapeutic irradiation.[41]

The clinical presentation of these lesions is highly suggestive of the more common basal cell carcinoma, and correct diagnosis almost always depends on recognition of the characteristic histological picture. The lesion arises in the dermis and extends to the epidermis. Although there is considerable variation from lesion to lesion, they are usually highly cellular without apparent organization. Most tumors contain a mixture of spindle cells interspersed with large polygonal cells with prominent nucleoli and frequent mitotic figures (Fig 8–7). Bizarre multinucleated giant cells may also be present. Tumor cells are seen to surround capillaries and telangiectatic vessels. The margin is usually demarcated by a thin band of collagen with areas of lymphocytic infiltration. Dermal appendages are either surrounded by the lesion or pushed aside. A zone of epidermal hyperplasia may be seen surrounding the lesion (Fig 8–8.)[45] Vascular invasion is extremely uncommon and has been associated with metastasis in one case.[41]

Once the correct diagnosis has been made, treatment is limited to simple excision with clear margins and routine follow-up. Although recurrence is rare, it should probably be treated by a more aggressive excision of the previous operative site as well as a margin of surrounding tis-

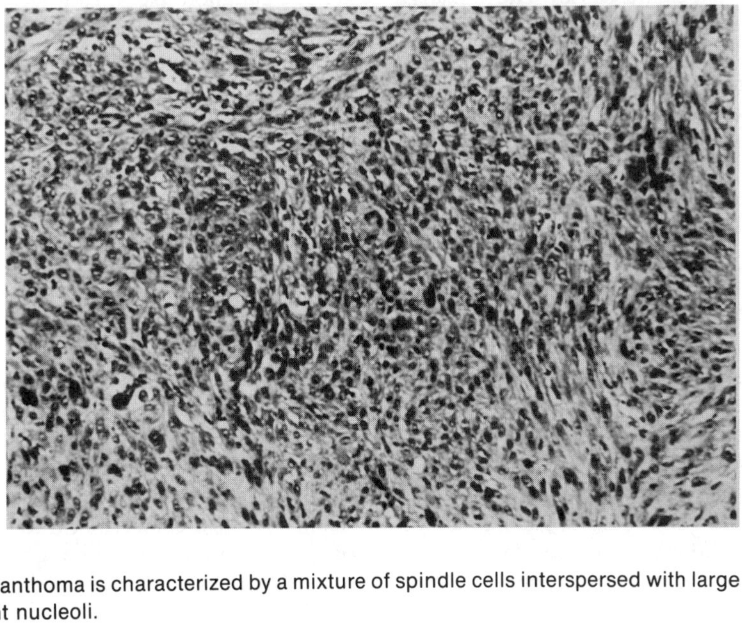

FIG 8–7.
Atypical fibroxanthoma is characterized by a mixture of spindle cells interspersed with large polygonal cells with prominent nucleoli.

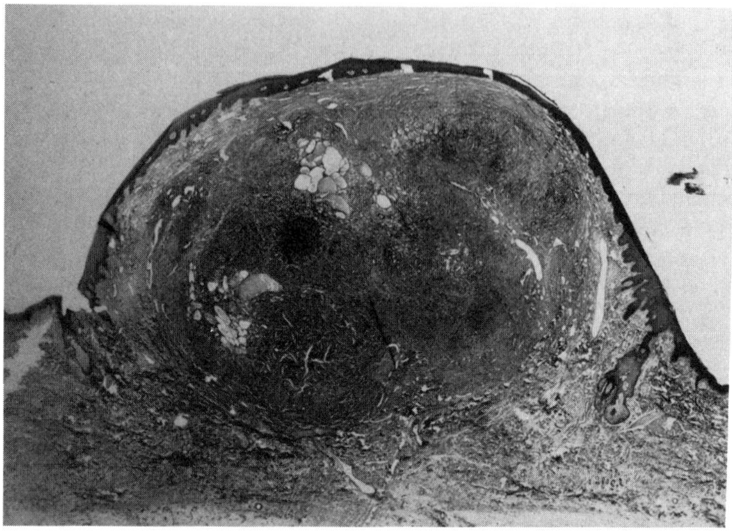

FIG 8–8.
Atypical fibroxanthoma compressing and pushing aside dermal elements. The lesion measured approximately 8 mm across.

sue. One such case was also treated by local irradiation. It should be noted, however, that primary lesions have shown no response to radiotherapy.[43, 44]

Proliferative Fasciitis

The term *proliferative fasciitis* is most correctly used to describe a pseudosarcomatous process involving the fascia and the interlobular fibrous septa of subcutaneous fat. The first large series of patients was reported by Chung and Enzinger in 1975.[39] These authors emphasized that this lesion is distinct from the more common *nodular fasciitis* (see the next section).

Proliferative fasciitis occurs most often during the fourth, fifth, and sixth decades. Males and females are equally affected and it has been reported in both blacks and whites. No cases have been reported in children. The disease presents as a firm, mobile, subcutaneous nodule 1–5 cm in diameter. Pain and tenderness are common. Most lesions will have been present for several weeks at the time of diagnosis, some for as long as 1 year. Three fourths are located on the extremities, with the remainder occurring on the head and trunk.

Histologically, proliferative fasciitis is characterized by a mixture of large, basophilic "giant" cells and fibroblast-like spindle cells surrounded by a myxoid matrix. The giant cells may resemble either mature ganglion cells or rhabdomyoblasts. Binucleated forms are seen and mitotic figures are common. The fibroblastic component may be arranged in fascicles, bundles, or in a twisted storiform pattern. Similarity to the picture seen in proliferative myositis suggests that proliferative fasciitis may be a subcutaneous variant of the same entity. It is differentiated from the more common nodular fasciitis by its multifocal nature as well as by the characteristic ganglion-like "giant" cells. Multinucleated giant cells, although present, are seen less often than in nodular fasciitis.[39]

Treatment consists of simple excision with clear margins. Indeed, some cases have been reportedly "cured" by biopsy alone, with less than complete excision. One case of recurrent disease was treated successfully by a second limited excision. Metastases have not been reported.

Nodular Fasciitis

In 1955, Konwaler et al.[38] described a series of patients presenting with subcutaneous nodules characterized by a benign clinical course despite a histological picture suggestive of malignancy. These lesions were less than 2 cm in diameter, and most were excised within 2 weeks of their appearance. Although half were reexcised widely on the basis of the histological findings, none recurred. These authors proposed the name *subcutaneous pseudosarcomatous fibromatosis* for this entity. The term *nodular fasciitis,* first proposed by Price et al.,[46] has since gained widespread acceptance.

Nodular fasciitis is the most common of all the pseudosarcomatous lesions.[47] Although it has been reported in patients as young as 17 months, it occurs most frequently during the third, fourth, and fifth decades of life.[48] Males and females are equally affected. Approximately half of these lesions are found in the upper extremities, with the remainder equally distributed between the trunk and the rest of the body. In younger patients, head and neck lesions are most common.[49] The lesion has also been reported to occur in the breast, parotid, and skeletal muscle.[50, 51] The hands and feet are spared.

The patient usually presents with a small subcutaneous nodule that is rapidly increasing in size. Pain and tenderness may be minimal or absent. As with other pseudosarcomatous lesions, there may be a history of previous trauma. Most are less than 2 cm in diameter at the time of diagnosis, and multiple lesions are rare.[48]

Histologically, nodular fasciitis consists of plump fibroblasts with large, pale nuclei and frequent mitotic figures. The cells are surrounded by variable amounts of collagen and myxoid ground substance. The overall picture is one of haphazard bundles of fibroblasts with a characteristic feathery pattern (Fig 8–9). Although these lesions are usually well circumscribed, they may appear to invade into surrounding fat and muscle, suggesting a more invasive fibrosarcoma. In some cases, an extremely bizarre cellular pattern is seen (Fig 8–10). Nodular fasciitis also contains some elements in common with other pseudosarcomatous lesions. It is usually possible to identify some of the large binucleate cells more characteristic of proliferative fasciitis. Another unusual finding in some specimens is evidence of bone formation, occasionally reported with proliferative myositis[52] (see the next section).

As with all pseudosarcomatous lesions, an accurate diagnosis is prerequisite to proper management. Although this is accomplished most often by incisional or excisional biopsy, several authors have reported successful diagnosis by needle aspiration cytology.[51, 53] Excision with clear margins is curative in most cases. Several cases have been cured with less than complete excision and in one instance spontaneous regression has been reported.[54] One lesion with a duration of 3 years was reported to have invaded through the sternum into the marrow. Despite this aggressive behavior, simple excision was curative.[55]

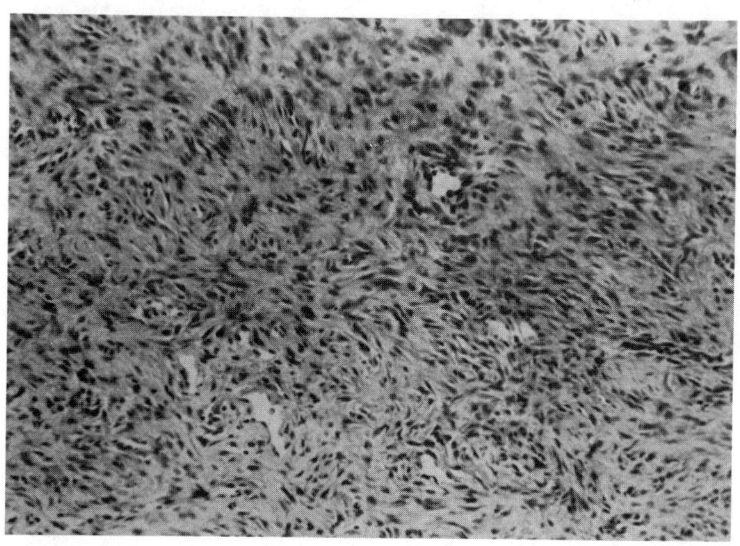

FIG 8–9.
Nodular fasciitis with feathery bundles of fibroblasts in a myxoid ground.

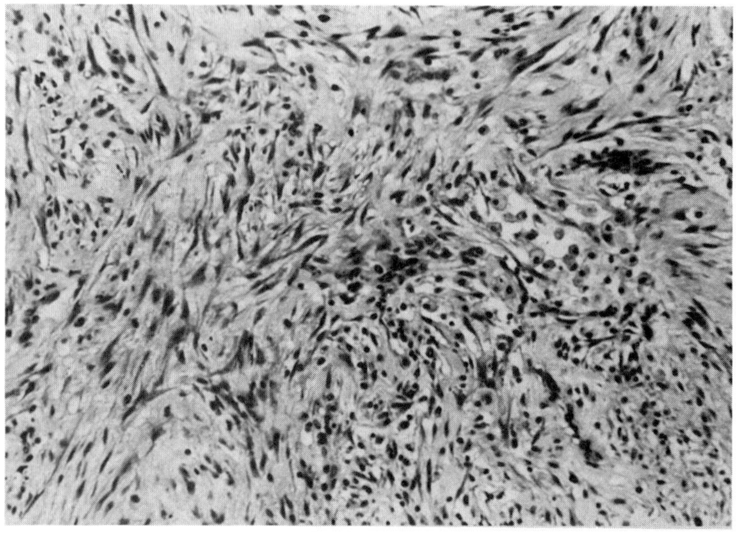

FIG 8–10.
Nodular fasciitis demonstrating a more bizarre cellular pattern.

Proliferative Myositis

The first series of patients with proliferative myositis was reported by Kern in 1960.[40] This lesion is much less common than those discussed previously. Reported cases range from the early twenties in age, with a mean of 50 years. More than two thirds occur in the pectoralis, latissimus dorsi, or serratus anterior muscles. The clinical history is typically that of a rapidly growing lesion, with most patients presenting within a few weeks of onset. The chief complaint is usually a tender mass 3–5 cm in diameter within the affected muscle. About 25% of these patients will relate a history of previous trauma, but severe trauma is not characteristic.

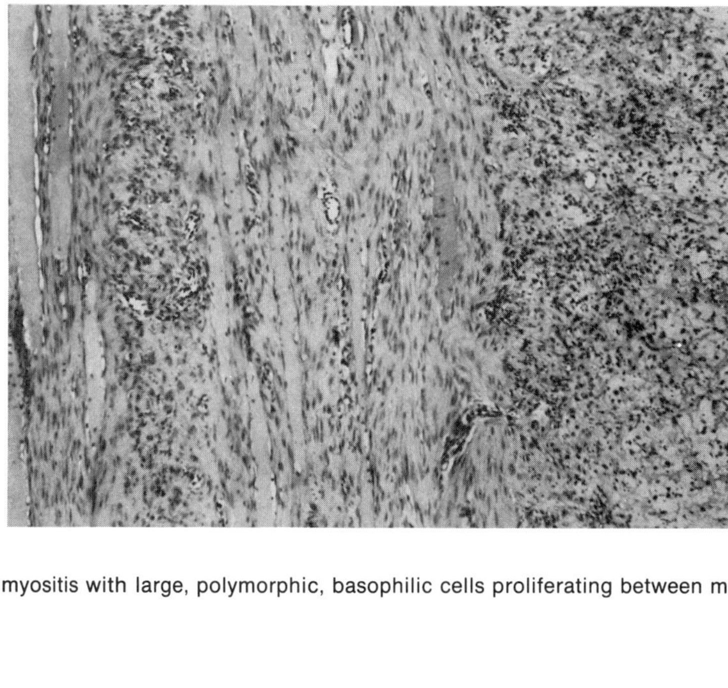

FIG 8–11.
Proliferative myositis with large, polymorphic, basophilic cells proliferating between muscle bundles.

Histologically, proliferative myositis consists of a diffuse fibrosing process. Large, polymorphic, basophilic cells are seen to proliferate between the fascia and the muscle. Deposits of fibrinous material are common (Fig 8–11). Also seen are the large plump ganglion-like cells common to proliferative fasciitis. In some lesions, there is evidence of osteoid formation. Indeed, transition to a histologic picture characteristic of myositis ossificans is possible.[40]

Treatment consists of simple excision. To date, there have been no reports of invasive lesions or metastasis. As with all pseudosarcomatous lesions, the key to proper management is recognition of the benign nature of the lesion despite a generally ominous histological pattern.

CONCLUSION

The lesions described in this chapter are all characterized by distinct clinical presentations and well-described histological patterns. Dermatofibrosarcoma protuberans requires the most aggressive surgical approach, with excision of a margin of apparently normal skin and soft tissue. Fibromatosis of the hands or feet is usually a slow-growing tumor. Treatment consists of surgical excision with particular attention to preservation of function. Fibromatosis is probably associated with a hereditary defect in collagen metabolism, and co-existing lesions in other parts of the body should be sought. The crucial element in management of pseudosarcomas is recognition of their benign nature. With rare exceptions, simple excision is curative.

REFERENCES

1. Taylor RW: Sarcomatous tumors resembling in some respects keloid. *J Cutan Genito-Urin Dis (NY)* 1890; 8:384.
2. Darier PJ, Ferrand M: Dermatofibromes progressifs et récidivants ou fibrosarcomes de la peau. *Ann Derm Syph* 1924; 6:545.
3. Hoffman E: Über das knollentreibende Fibrosarkom der Haut (Dermatofibrosarkom protuberans). (Knobby fibrosarcoma of skin.) *Dermat Zeitschr* 1925; 43:1.
4. Doms SR, Goldberg MK, Yungst PG, et al: Dermatofibrosarcoma protuberans. *J Am Podiatry Assoc* 1982; 72:63.
5. Martin RG: Dermatofibrosarcoma protuberans, in Freitag SB, Culhane DL (eds): *Neoplasms of the Skin and Malignant Melanoma.* Chicago, Year Book Medical Publishers, 1976, pp 243–250.
6. Fisher ER, Vuzevski VD: Cytogenesis of Schwannoma (neurilemoma), neurofibroma, dermatofibroma, and dermatofibrosarcoma as revealed by electron microscopy. *Am J Clin Pathol* 1968; 49:141.
7. Hashimoto K, Brownstein MH, Jakobiec FA: Dermatofibrosarcoma protuberans. *Arch Dermatol* 1974; 110:874.
8. Ozzelo L, Hamels J: The histiocytic nature of dermatofibrosarcoma protuberans. *Am J Clin Pathol* 1976; 65:136.
9. Kindblom LG, Jacobsen GK, Jacobsen M: Immunohistochemical investigations of tumors of supposed fibroblastic-histiocytic origin. *Hum Pathol* 1982; 13:834.
10. McPeak CJ, Cruz T, Nicastri AD: Dermatofibrosarcoma protuberans: An analysis of 86 cases—five with metastasis. *Ann Surg* 1967; 166:803.
11. Ani AN, Attah EB, Ajayi OO: Dermatofibrosarcoma protuberans: Analysis of eight cases in an African population. *Am Surg* 1976; 42:934.
12. Burkhardt BR, Soule EH, Winkelmann RK, et al: Dermatofibrosarcoma protuberans. *Am J Surg* 1966; 111:638.
13. Brenner W, Schaefler K, Chhabra H, et al: Dermatofibrosarcoma protuberans metastatic to a regional lymph node. *Cancer* 1975; 36:1897.
14. Ishii T, Koide O: An autopsy case of metastasizing protuberant dermatofibrosarcoma. *Acta Pathol Jpn* 1975; 25:503.
15. Peters W, Hanke CW, Pasarell HA, et al: Dermatofibrosarcoma protuberans of the face. *J Dermatol Surg Oncol* 1982; 8:823.
16. Hobbs ER, Wheeland RG, Bailin PL, et al: Treatment of dermatofibrosarcoma protuberans with Mohs micrographic surgery. *Ann Surg* 1988; 207:102–107.
17. Mendoza CB Jr, Gerwig WH Jr, Watne AL: Dermatofibrosarcoma protuberans with metastases treated with methotrexate. *Am J Surg* 1970; 120:119.
18. Skoog T: Dupuytren's contraction. *Acta Chir Scand [Suppl]* 1948; 139:1.
19. Cooper AP: *A Treatise on Dislocations and on Fractures of the Joints.* London, Logmans, Hurst, Rees, Dome, and Browne, 1822.
20. Dupuytren G: *Leçons Orales de Clinique Chirurgicale, Faites a Hôtel-Dieu de Paris. Recueil-*

lies et Publiées par Brierre de Boismont et Marx. Paris, Bailliere, 1839, p 500.

21. Anderson W: Lectures on contractures of the fingers and toes: Their varieties, pathology, and treatment. *Lancet* 1891; 2:1.
22. Pojer J, Radivojevic M, Williams TF: Dupuytren's disease. *Arch Intern Med* 1972; 129:561.
23. McIndoe A, Beare RL: The surgical management of Dupuytren's contracture. *Am J Surg* 1958; 95:197.
24. Wolfe SM, Summerskill WH, Davidson CS: Thickening and contraction of the palmar fascia (Dupuytren's contracture), associated with alcoholism and hepatic cirrhosis. *N Engl J Med* 1956; 255:559.
25. Brickley-Parsons D, Glimcher MJ, Smith RJ, et al: Biochemical changes in the collagen of the palmar fascia in patients with Dupuytren's disease. *J Bone Joint Surg* 1981; 63-A:787.
26. Hajdu S: *Pathology of Soft Tissue Tumors.* Philadelphia, Lea & Febiger, 1979, pp 72–73.
27. Early PF: Population studies in Dupuytren's contracture. *J Bone Joint Surg* 1962; 44B:602.
28. Hueston JT: Dupuytren's contracture, in Flynn JE (ed): *Hand Surgery.* Baltimore, Williams & Wilkins, 1982, pp 797–823.
29. Hueston JT: The control of recurrent Dupuytren's contracture by skin replacement. *Br J Plast Surg* 1969; 22:152.
30. Hueston JT: Limited fasciectomy. *Plast Reconstr Surg* 1961; 27:569.
31. Pickren JW, Smith AG, Stevenson TW, et al: Fibromatosis of the plantar fascia. *Cancer* 1951; 4:846.
32. Allen RA, Woolner LB, Ghormley RK: Soft-tissue tumors of the sole. *J Bone Joint Surg* 1955; 37-A:14.
33. Kashuk KB, Pasternack WA: Aggressive infiltrating plantar fibromatosis. *J Am Podiatry Assoc* 1980; 71:491.
34. Wiseman GG: Multiple recurring plantar fibromatosis and its surgical excision. *J Foot Surg* 1983; 22:121.
35. Burns AE, Harvey CK: Plantar fibromatosis. *J Am Podiatry Assoc* 1983; 73:141.
36. Aviles E, Arlen M, Miller T: Plantar fibromatosis. *Surgery* 1971; 69:117.
37. Kates M, Cohen S, Reese HW, et al: A clinical conference on plantar fibromatosis. *J Am Podiatry Assoc* 1974; 64:427.
38. Konwaler BE, Keasbey L, Kaplan L: Subcutaneous pseudosarcomatous fibromatosis (fasciitis). *Am J Clin Pathol* 1955; 25:241.
39. Chung EB, Enzinger FM: Proliferative fasciitis. *Cancer* 1975; 36:1450.
40. Kern WH: Proliferative myositis; a pseudosarcomatous reaction to injury. *Arch Pathol* 1960; 69:209.
41. Fretzin DF, Helwig EB: Atypical fibroxanthoma of the skin. *Cancer* 1973; 31:1541.
42. Helwig EB: Atypical fibroxanthoma. *Taxas J Med* 1963; 59:664.
43. Dahl I: Atypical fibroxanthoma of the skin. *Acta Pathol Microbiol Scand* 1976; 84:183.
44. Kempson RL, McGavran MH: Atypical fibroxanthomas of the skin. *Cancer* 1964; 17:1463.
45. Kroe DJ, Pitcock JA: Atypical fibroxanthoma of the skin. *Am J Clin Pathol* 1969; 51:487.
46. Price EB, Silliphant WM, Shuman R: Nodular fasciitis. *Am J Clin Pathol* 1961; 35:122.
47. Dahl I, Jarlstedt J: Nodular fasciitis in the head and neck. *Acta Otolaryngol* 1980; 90:152.
48. Bernstein KE, Lattes R: Nodular (pseudosarcomatous) fasciitis, a nonrecurrent lesion. *Cancer* 1982; 49:1668.
49. Enzinger FM: Recent trends in soft tissue pathology, in Cumley RW, McCay J, Beane DA (eds): *Tumors of Bone and Soft Tissue.* Chicago, Year Book Medical Publishers, 1965, pp 315–332.
50. Stout AP: Pseudosarcomatous fasciitis in children. *Cancer* 1961; 14:1216.
51. Fritsches HG, Muller EA: Pseudosarcomatous fasciitis of the breast. *Acta Cytol* 1983; 27:73.
52. Dahl I, Angervall L: Pseudosarcomatous proliferative lesions of soft tissue with or without bone formation. *Acta Pathol Microbiol Scand* 1977; 85:577.
53. Dahl I, Akerman M: Nodular fasciitis. *Acta Cytol* 1981; 25:215.
54. Majumdar B: Spontaneously regressing nodular fasciitis of the neck. *J Laryngol Otol* 1983; 97:973.
55. Toker C: Pseudo-sarcomatous fasciitis. *Ann Surg* 1971; 174:994.

Chapter 9

Cystosarcomas of the Breast

Herbert C. Hoover

Primary breast sarcomas are rare, constituting 0.5% to 3% of all malignant breast tumors in most series.[1] Their rarity, combined with the lack of agreement among pathologists concerning nomenclature, makes a review of this subject difficult. For discussion purposes, breast sarcomas will be divided into three broad categories: cystosarcoma phyllodes, angiosarcoma, and mammary stromal sarcomas.

CYSTOSARCOMA PHYLLODES

Although Chelius described a "cystic hydatid" of the breast in 1828,[2] it was Müller[3] who 10 years later gave the first full description of cystosarcoma phyllodes. He did not use the term *sarcoma* to imply malignancy but to describe the fleshy appearance of the tumor. He, in fact, considered these tumors to be totally benign. His description is considered a classic in this field and is worthy of quotation in part:

> The tumor forms a large firm mass, with a more or less uneven surface. The fibrous substance which constitutes the greater part of it is a greyish white color, extremely hard, and as firm as fibro-cartilage. Large portions of the tumor are made up entirely of this mass, but in some parts are cavities or clefts not lined with a distinct membrane. These cavities contain but little fluid; for either their parietes, which are hard like fibro-cartilage, and finely polished, be in close opposition with each other, or a number of firm, irregular laminae sprout from this mass, and form the walls of the fissures; or excrescences of a foliated or wart-like form sprout from the bottom of the cavities and fill up their interior. These excrescences are perfectly smooth on their surface, and never contain cysts or cells. The laminae lie very irregularly, and project into the cavities and fissures like the folds of the psalterium in the interior of the third stomach of ruminant animals. Tumors of this kind attain an enormous size, hitherto the author has seen them only in the breast, nor are they even there of frequent occurrence. They are decidedly innocent, occur earlier than it is usual for cancer in the mamma to develop itself, and sometimes they appear even in youth; they have but little tendency to grow to the skin or to the subjacent muscles, and are not attended with retraction of the nipple. They are not disposed to soften internally, but continue to grow slowly until they have attained an enormous size when they at length burst, and a very ill-looking suppurating fungus forms upon their surface. Even in this state, however, the operation has been performed with a successful result.
>
> Swelling of the axillary glands is not a common occurrence, and when it is met with, is the consequence of simple irritation, and subsides

after the operation. The extraordinary forms which cystosarcoma phyllodes assumes, at once suggest the notion of its cancerous nature; and yet, the disease is perfectly innocent, and as far removed from carcinoma as those non-suppurating cauliflower condylomata of the penis, and of the female genitals, which have so often been mistaken for cancerous structures.

The lesion was not reported to have malignant potential until 1931, when Lee and Pack[4] reported a nonmetastatic histological malignancy in one of the 111 cases reported up to that date. In 1940 White[5] described a patient with metastases to the opposite breast, anterior mediastinum, and lung. Three years later, Cooper and Ackerman[6] reported the first case demonstrating axillary nodal metastasis. Since then, numerous other investigators have clearly established the malignant potential of this tumor.[7–10]

Cystosarcomas have subsequently shown such a variety of clinical and pathological features that, rather than constituting a single entity, they are considered a spectrum of disease including a benign form, a histologically malignant form, and a metastatic form.[11] Treves[12] has appropriately labeled them the "Dr. Jekyll and Mr. Hyde" of mammary neoplasms, sometimes as benign as the good doctor or as malignant as his vicious counterpart. The analogy is especially fitting because Treves has also postulated that this is the only breast tumor than can be transformed from a benign to a malignant process. Since Müller's description at least 62 synonyms for cystosarcoma phyllodes have been published,[13] further emphasizing the varied clinical and pathological presentations that make review difficult. Cystosarcoma is probably not the most appropriate name because of the malignant connotation of the term, but it is so firmly established in the literature that it should remain for the sake of uniformity.

Incidence

It is impossible to give an accurate estimate of incidence as such differences in histological interpretation exist. The incidence is quite low, constituting only 0.3% to 0.9% of all breast tumors in most series.[11] However, cystosarcomas account for approximately 70% of all sarcomas of the breast, with approximately 1,000 cases reported in the English literature. Treves[12] listed 93 patients with cystosarcoma phyllodes treated by the breast service of Memorial Hospital (New York) from 1950 to 1962. During these years, 3,200 fibroadenomas were observed, making the relative frequency to fibroadenomas 2.9%. The large series of Lee and Pack included only one malignant case in 111 tumors,[4] but most subsequent series show a much higher rate of malignancy—in the 25% to 30% range[7, 9]. Kessinger found only 66 cases with documented metastases in the English literature up to 1972 (approximately 16% of all patients).

Etiology

The factors influencing the development of cystosarcoma remain obscure. The gross and microscopic similarities between fibroadenoma and cystosarcoma, however, are well known. Both are tumors with connective tissue stroma growing in opposition to epithelium-lined spaces. The characteristic difference is the relative overgrowth of the connective tissue stroma in cystosarcoma phyllodes. Many pathologists have cited evidence that this tumor arises from the connective tissue of a pre-existing fibroadenoma. Of the 77 cases reported by Treves and Sunderland in 1951,[9] 21 tumors contained areas interpreted as remnants of an old intracanalicular fibroadenoma. In seven instances, the tumors had exhibited rapid growth after being present for 6 to 18 years. In six cases, fibroadenomas occurred separately from the cystosarcoma. On the other hand, 54% of the tumors in this series had been present clinically for less than 1 year, and several small tumors showed uniform cystosarcoma structure throughout. The latter two facts argue for de novo development in at least some patients.

There has been a great deal of discussion and disagreement as to the role of lactation or pregnancy in the pathogenesis of cystosarcoma.[9, 14] It is interesting, however, that patients with histologically malignant cystosarcoma have a fertility rate lower than those with benign cystosarcoma.[7] It has been shown that most cystosarcomas have progesterone receptors but lack estrogen receptors.[15] The significance of this is unclear.

Clinical Features

Cystosarcoma is limited almost exclusively to females. Although there are rare case reports of this tumor in males,[16, 17] the diagnosis has been questioned by some authors, as the male breast contains no lobules from which an adenomatous process might arise. However, prolonged administration of estrogen results in both clinical and microscopic signs of gynecomastia, including the presence of lobules similar to those in the nonlactating female breast.

Eighty to 85% of patients in the major series are Caucasians. The usual age range at the time of diagnosis is 40 to 50 years; females below age 20 years are rarely affected. However, one of the most rapidly growing tumors seen by this author was a malignant cystosarcoma in a 14-year-old girl.[18]

The presenting complaint is almost always the discovery of a painless breast mass. Often, the patient has had a small mass for years that suddenly grows rapidly. The tumors often grow to surprisingly large dimensions before the patient reaches medical attention. However, recent series generally report smaller primary tumors than those in earlier years, presumably due to earlier diagnosis. Treves[12] reported that 43% of 99 patients had tumors between 3 and 5 cm. Only 3% were greater than 20 cm. Size does not correlate well with prognosis in most series, although McDivitt et al. reported an average size of 4.6 cm for benign lesions and 6.2 cm for those histologically malignant.[7] Kessinger reported an average size of 11.8 cm in 66 cases that ultimately showed metastasis. The size range was 2 to 30 cm.[11]

Most cystosarcomas are well circumscribed, mobile, and do not involve the overlying skin or distort the nipple. However, the skin may be stretched over large tumors, producing a shiny appearance and prominence of the subcutaneous veins, as shown in Figure 9–1. The consistency of the smaller tumors is usually firm; larger tumors often contain soft areas secondary to necrosis. If pain and ulceration do occur, they are usually the result of a bulky tumor producing avascular necrosis and infection. Axillary lymph nodes are often palpable but prove to be reactive in nearly all cases.

Bilateral tumors have been reported but are rare. Interestingly, nearly all major series report a slightly greater incidence of left breast involvement.

Radiological Evaluation

The mammographic appearance of a cystosarcoma is usually indistinguishable from that of a fibroadenoma. Both form lobulated or spherical densities clearly demarcated from the surrounding breast tissue. A comparative study[19] has suggested that ultrasound might be preferable in differentiating fibroadenomas from cystosarcomas in that the presence of elongated epithelium-lined, fluid-filled cystic spaces characteristic of cystosarcoma are detected by ultrasound but not by mammography. The ultrasonographic appearance of a cyst within an otherwise solid lesion should suggest the diagnosis.

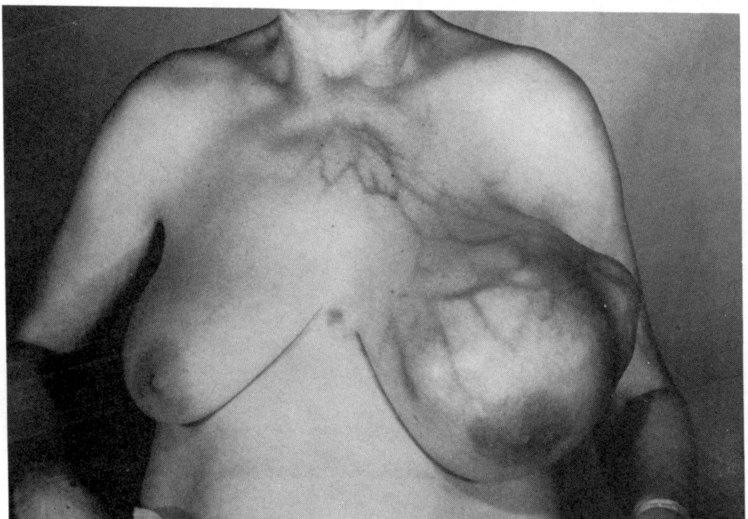

FIG 9–1.
Large, slow-growing cystosarcoma phyllodes in the breast of an elderly woman. Note the engorged subcutaneous veins. (Photograph courtesy of G. Geelhoed, M.D.)

Diagnosis

Surgical biopsy with careful histological analysis is the only reliable method of diagnosis. Clinical impressions are often inaccurate. It is vital that multiple sections be taken from all areas of the tumor for an accurate histopathological study. To rule out malignancy, the entire mass must be removed for sectioning.

Gross Pathology

There is considerable variation in the gross appearance of cystosarcoma, depending on the size of the tumor in relation to the breast size. The contour can be round, ovoid, or lobulated. The cut surface is generally bulging and pinkish gray in color. Areas of hemorrhage and necrosis are frequently evident in larger tumors. In smaller tumors, the cut surface is solid, lobulated, or granular with clefts bordered by leaflike papillary processes. Larger tumors generally have multiple cystic cavities. There is usually no gross difference between benign and malignant tumors,[9] although a "pushing" margin, as shown in Figure 9–2, usually is indicative of a better prognosis.

Microscopic Pathology

The hallmark of cystosarcoma phyllodes is stromal overgrowth and hypercellularity associated with elongated, dilated, or compressed participating ducts.[20] Cystosarcomas can be distinguished from fibroadenomas by an increase in the cellularity of the connective tissue stroma.[9] (See Figure 9–3.)

The epithelial lining of the ducts is most commonly cuboidal and generally resembles the ductal epithelium of the surrounding breast. It may show apocrine or squamous metaplasia.[7]

The classification of a given cystosarcoma as benign or malignant is based on variation in the stromal configuration[21] and not on epithelial atypia. Malignant epithelial change within cystosarcoma is possible and, indeed, there are four reported cases of microscopic foci of adenocarcinoma infiltrating the stroma of cystosarcomas.[22]

Stromal histology in malignant cystosarcomas can exhibit a number of patterns. The two most common stromal patterns seen are a spindle cell type resembling that of fibrosarcoma, and a looser, myxoid pattern similar to that of myxoliposarcoma.[7] Less common growth patterns comprise an undifferentiated type.

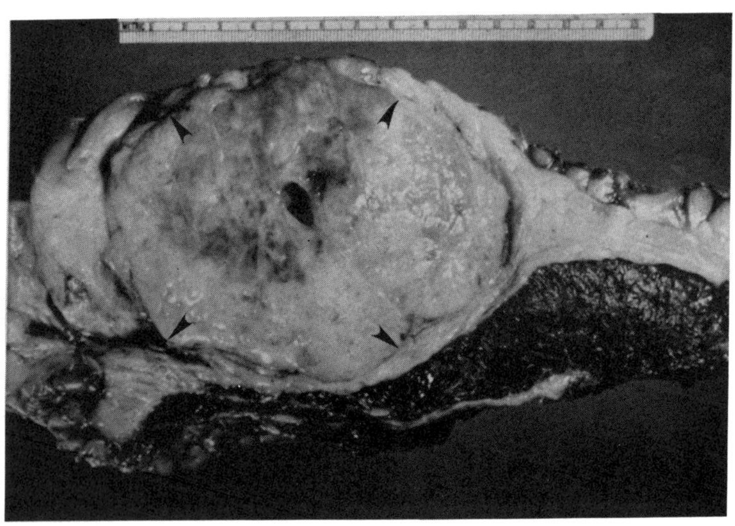

FIG 9–2.
A cross-sectional view of a large cystosarcoma phyllodes tumor occupying most of the breast but demonstrating a "pushing" margin (*arrowheads*). Involvement of the pectoralis fascia necessitated removal of the underlying muscle. (Photograph courtesy of L. V. Ackerman, M.D.)

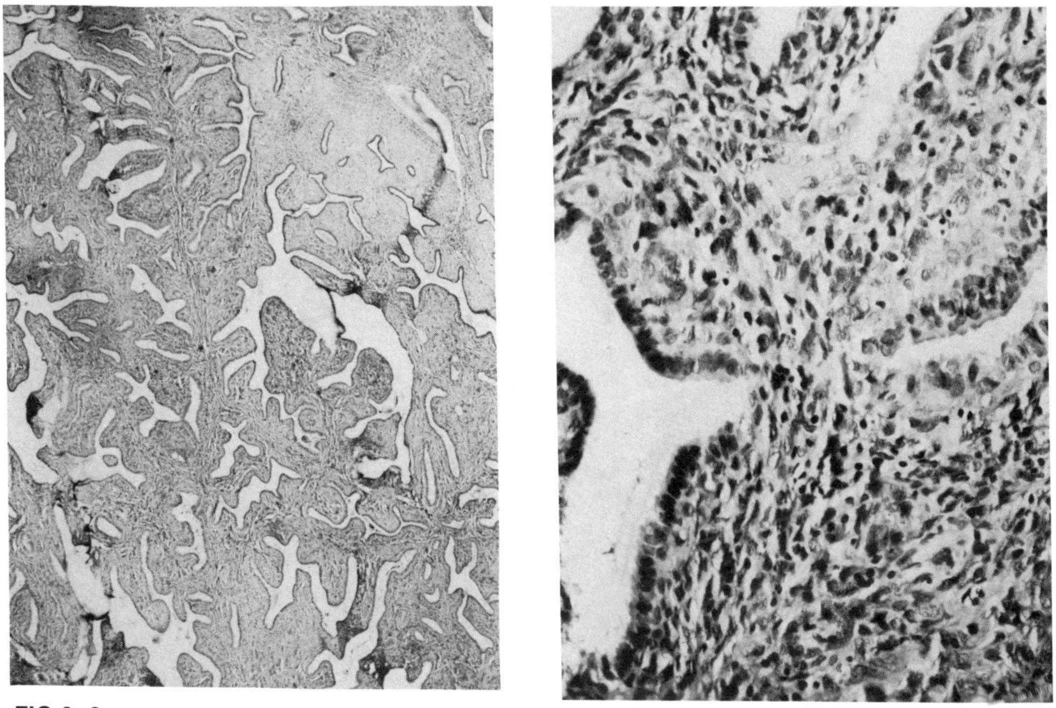

FIG 9–3.
Photomicrographs of a representative field of a primary malignant cystosarcoma phyllodes showing the typical benign ductal structures lined by normal epithelium and associated with a malignant sarcomatous stroma. (*Left*, ×35; *right*, ×350).

Although pathologists are not in agreement as to what constitutes a histologically benign or malignant cystosarcoma, some general principles apply. Malignant stroma contains increased focal cellularity, severe nuclear atypia, and atypical mitotic activity[23] (Fig 9–3). The malignant areas are often focal and easily overlooked if multiple sections are not reviewed.

The histological picture of the tumor provides a more reliable diagnosis of malignancy than the initial clinical presentation, but many tumors regarded as histologically malignant take a benign course clinically. Unfortunately, DNA histograms obtained by flow cytometry cannot yet predict malignant behavior.[24] The only proof of malignancy is invasive local recurrence or metastasis. Local recurrence is more frequently seen than metastasis. Recurrences are often more anaplastic than the primary tumor (Fig 9–4) and frequently lead to eventual metastasis and death. Metastatic lesions are always devoid of malignant epithelial elements and contain pure stromal elements.

Therapy

The treatment of cystosarcoma is surgical, but there is considerable debate as to the procedure of choice. Every major series[25–27] reports a variety of operations from local excision to radical mastectomy, with few substantial data to recommend the proper approach. Kessinger et al.[11] reported that of 65 initial surgical approaches recorded in 66 patients with subsequent metastatic disease, 31 were simple mastectomies, 18 were radical mastectomies, 11 were local excisions, and five were modified radical mastectomies. Proponents of simple mastectomy stress the "benign course" in most patients with even malignant tumors and the rarity of axillary metastases. Proponents of radical mastectomy as initial therapy point to the occasional aggressive behavior of these lesions when metastatic to regional lymph nodes.

Because no clinical or pathological criteria are reliably predictive in an individual case, this author believes that initial surgical therapy

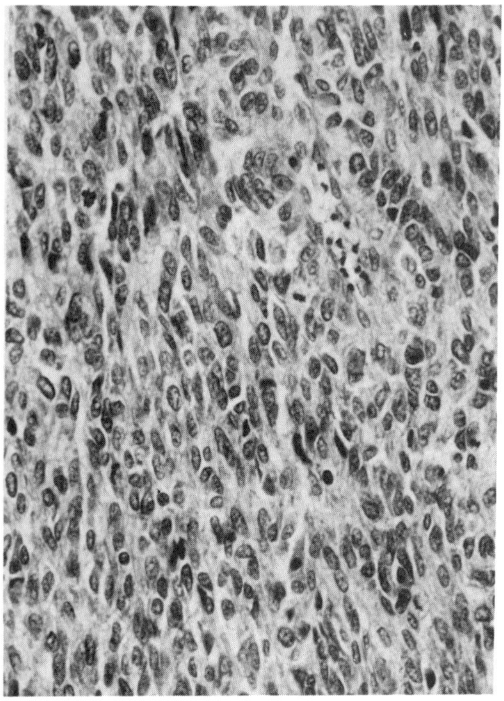

FIG 9–4.
Photomicrograph showing recurrence of the cystosarcoma phyllodes primary tumor shown in Figure 9–3. Note the absence of the epithelial components. The recurrence shows tightly packed sarcoma cells characterized by large, watery nuclei and irregular, pale-staining cytoplasm with indistinct cell membranes. Mitotic figures were numerous in this specimen. (×350.)

should be wide excision of the neoplasm. Except in small (4 cm or less), pathologically benign lesions, this usually requires a total mastectomy. If the pectoralis fascia is involved, then at least a portion of the underlying muscle should be removed. Large tumors with skin involvement often require a skin graft. If the axillary lymph nodes are clinically negative, they need not be removed unless necessary as part of an en bloc resection of a large tumor mass.

The literature is replete with reports of multiple recurrent cystosarcomas resulting from inadequate initial therapy. The histological grade often worsens with each recurrence and the risk of metastatic disease is enhanced. Ackerman[28] has defined the problem well in a recent personal communication: "Surgeons make a mistake when they don't adequately remove it; pathologists make a mistake when they don't adequately study it."

Reports of trials with chemotherapy and radiation therapy for metastatic cystosarcoma phyllodes have been very few. Our report of a response to both chemotherapy (cyclophosphamide) and irradiation in a 14-year-old girl with widely metastatic cystosarcoma[18] remains one of the few known responses to these agents. Multiple drug chemotherapy should certainly be considered in patients with nonresectible metastases in the hope of an occasional response. Endocrine therapy should be considered as well because most of the tumors contain progesterone receptors.[15]

Clinical Course

The clinical course is quite variable, depending on whether the tumor is benign or malignant, and on the stage of the disease at diagnosis. These factors are not as predictive as in other solid tumors, because benign cystosarcomas often recur if not widely excised, and patients with malignant cystosarcomas do far better on the average than patients with breast carcinoma.

Patients with benign lesions do well even after local recurrence. Recurrences are managed by excision or simple mastectomy, and the patients usually remain disease free.

Malignant recurrences are a serious matter. Although there is a divergence of opinion in the literature, most authors feel that malignant recurrences tend to be more aggressive than the original tumor. Kessinger et al.[11] reported that 51% of patients developing metastatic disease first had a malignant local recurrence.

The lungs were the most common metastatic site in the report by Kessinger, accounting for 66% of metastatic cases. The skeleton was involved in 28.3% of cases, the heart in 9.4%, and the liver in 5.6%. Metastatic lesions have been reported in virtually every organ system. Metastatic lesions are usually manifested within a few months, although they have been reported as late as 12 years after primary therapy.[9] Most patients with metastases die within 3 years of initial therapy.[11] There are no reported cures in patients with systemic metastases.

It is difficult to determine the overall prognosis for patients with malignant cystosarcomas, but at least 20% to 30% of these patients die from the disease. The obvious challenge is early detection. Norris and Taylor[8] found that all patients with lesions smaller than 4 cm were cured. As physicians and surgeons, we have the responsibility of convincing patients to allow excision of dominant breast masses.

ANGIOSARCOMA

Angiosarcoma of the breast is a malignancy that probably arises de novo within the parenchyma of the female breast.[29] It is extremely rare, with approximately 100 cases reported since its description by Schmidt in 1887.[30] The relative incidence among breast sarcomas ranges from 2.7% to 9.1%.[31, 32] In three major series[31, 33, 34] it was found to affect young women predominantly, with a median age of 34 to 49 years, but patients as old as 70 have been described.

As with cystosarcoma, the patients usually present with a rapidly enlarging, painless breast mass. Average tumor size is 4 to 5 cm, with the tumor deep within the breast in most patients. Typically the tumors are ill defined, irregular, soft, and hemorrhagic. Microscopic features are intercommunicating channels, or irregular vascular spaces lined by atypical endothelial cells confined within a thin reticulin network. A characteristic feature is the varied histological pattern, from highly cellular to bland-appearing infiltrative vascular elements that resemble benign capillary hemangiomas. Nearly 40% of cases are misdiagnosed as benign lesions at initial biopsy.[34]

Donnell and associates[33] have used the heterogeneous histological nature of the disease to define three subgroups of tumors felt to be useful as a guide to prognosis and therapy. Group I tumors show an open channel sinusoidal pattern without papillary or solid areas, with rare or absent mitotic figures and no necrotic foci. Group III tumors show the interanastomosing vascular channels, but also considerable papillary formation and solid areas with numerous mitotic figures and necrotic areas. Tumors of intermediate histopathology are classified as group II. Although most previous series of angiosarcomas of the breast had reported this disease as almost invariably fatal within 2 years, these authors found that group I and II patients rarely died, whereas 14 of 18 group III patients died of their disease. The one group I patient that died developed a local recurrence and a subsequent metastasis, both of which had the histological features of a group III lesion. Their 41% 3-year disease-free overall survival was considerably better than the 14% reported by Chen et al.[31] in their collective review. Actinomycin D, which was given to 12 of the 21 surviving patients, was credited as the probable reason for the improved survival. There is limited experience with radiation therapy in this disease.

All authors stress the necessity of a thorough excision of the primary tumor.[35, 36] At least a simple mastectomy is necessary in most cases, with modified radical or radical mastectomy reserved for large lesions encroaching on the underlying muscle or the axilla. There is only one documented case in the literature[34] of axillary nodal metastasis.

MAMMARY STROMAL SARCOMAS OF THE BREAST

Virtually all histological types of sarcoma have been described in the breast. Berg et al.[37] have suggested that all sarcomas of the breast other than hemangiosarcoma and cytosarcoma phyllodes should be classified together under the designation mammary stromal sarcomas. All are quite rare and will be mentioned only briefly.

Liposarcomas of the breast are often bulky tumors. It is quite important to distinguish this histological subtype, as they behave differently from other sarcomas of the breast, or sarcomas in general, in having a higher propensity to axillary metastasis.[29] One can make a strong argument for performing an axillary dissection for liposarcoma of the breast.

Lymphosarcomas occasionally involve the breast primarily.[38, 39] There is considerable debate regarding whether or not this is part of a generalized lymphoma that has its initial manifestation in the breast. Treatment is primarily radiotherapy and chemotherapy. The prognosis varies depending on the cell type, but 5-year cure rates as high as 64% and 49% have been reported.[38, 39]

Fibrosarcoma, leiomyosarcoma, rhabdomyosarcoma, osteogenic sarcoma, and mesenchymoma have all been reported in the breast but are exceedingly rare. There are no large series to guide us in making therapeutic decisions, but the same general principles developed for malignant cystosarcomas or angiosarcomas apply. Local tumors should be aggressively resected: this implies at least a simple mastectomy in nearly all patients. The 5-year cure rate in the series reported by Berg and colleagues[37] of 25 stromal sarcoma patients was surprisingly high at 60%. Prognosis is clearly related to stage at presentation and to the aggressiveness of the initial resective procedure. In the usual case, the stromal sarcomas are intermediate in behavior between the cystosarcomas and the highly malignant form of angiosarcomas. Adjuvant measures are not of proven benefit.

CONCLUSION

Sarcomas of the breast are a heterogeneous group of tumors with great variability of clinical behavior within each histological type. Most, however, have a better prognosis than carcinoma of the breast if the primary tumor is managed appropriately. Nearly all, including the benign form of cystosarcoma, may recur after inadequate local excision. A total mastectomy is usually required. Axillary dissection is rarely necessary as lymphatic metastases are extraordinarily rare in all histological types except liposarcoma. The proper roles for adjuvant radiotherapy and chemotherapy have not been determined.

REFERENCES

1. Hill RP, Stout AP: Sarcoma of the breast. *Arch Surg* 1942; 44:723–759.
2. Chelius M: Talsuziektasie. *Klin Ann* 1828; 4:449.
3. Müller J: *Über den feiheren Bau und die Formen der krankhafteu Geschwulste.* Berlin, G. Reimer, 1838.
4. Lee BJ, Pack CT: Giant intracanalicular fibroadenomyoxoma of the breast. The so-called cystosarcoma phyllodes mammae of Johannes Müller. *Am J Cancer* 1931; 15:2583–2609.
5. White JW: Malignant variant of cystosarcoma phyllodes. *Am J Cancer* 1940; 40:458–464.
6. Cooper WG, Ackerman LV: Cystosarcoma phyllodes with a consideration of its more malignant variant. *Surg Cynecol Obstet* 1943; 77:279–283.
7. McDivitt RW, Urban JA, Farrow JH: Cystosarcoma phyllodes. *Johns Hopkins Med J* 1967; 120:33–45.
8. Norris HJ, Taylor HB: Relationship of histologic features to behavior of cystosarcoma phyllodes: Analysis of ninety-four cases. *Cancer* 1967; 20:2090–2099.
9. Treves N, Sunderland DA: Cystosarcoma phyllodes of the breast—a malignant and a benign tumor: A study of seventy-seven cases. *Cancer* 1951; 4:1286–1332.
10. West TL, Weiland LH, Clagett OT: Cystosarcoma phyllodes. *Ann Surg* 1971; 173:520–528.
11. Kessinger A, Foley JF, Lemon HM, et al: Metastatic cystosarcoma phyllodes: A case report and review of the literature. *J Surg Oncol* 1972; 4:131–147.
12. Treves N: A study of cystosarcoma phyllodes. *Ann NY Acad Sci* 1964; 114:922–936.
13. Fiks A: Cystosarcoma phyllodes of the mammary gland—Müller's tumor. *Virchow's Arch Pathol Anat* 1981; 392:1–6.
14. Stephenson HE, Gross S, Gumport SL, et al: Cystosarcoma phyllodes of the breast. *Ann Surg* 1952; 136:856–863.
15. Rao BR, Meyer JS, Fry CG: Most cystosarcoma phyllodes and fibroadenomas have progesterone receptor but lack estrogen receptor. *Cancer* 1981; 47:2016–2021.
16. Reingold JM, Ascher GS: Cystosarcoma phyllodes in a man with gynecomastia. *Clin Pathol* 1970; 53:852–856.
17. Pantoja E, Llobeef RE, Lopez E: Gigantic cystosarcoma phyllodes in a man with gynecomastia. *Arch Surg* 1976; 111:611.
18. Hoover HC, Trestioreana A, Ketcham AS: Metastatic cystosarcoma phyllodes in an adolescent girl: An unusually malignant tumor. *Ann Surg* 1975; 181:279–282.
19. Cole-Beuglet C, Soriano R, Kurtz AB, et al: Ultrasound, x-ray mammography, and histopathology of cystosarcoma phyllodes. *Radiology* 1983; 146:481–486.
20. Oberman HA: Cystosarcoma phyllodes—a clinicopathologic study of hypercellular periductal stromal neoplasms of breast. *Cancer* 1965; 18:697–709.
21. Ward RM, Evans HL: Cystosarcoma phyllodes: A clinicopathologic study of 26 cases. *Cancer* 1986; 58:2282–2289.
22. Klausner JM, Lelcuk S, Ilia B: Breast carcinoma originating in cystosarcoma phyllodes. *Clin Oncol* 1983; 9:71–74.
23. Dyer NH, Bridger JE, Taylor RS: Cystosarcoma phyllodes. *Br J Surg* 1966; 53:450–456.
24. Layfield LJ, Hart J, Neuwirth H, et al: Relation between DNA ploidy and the clinical behavior of phyllodes tumors. *Cancer* 1989; 64:1486–1489.
25. Callery CD, Rosen PP, Kinne DW: Sarcoma of the breast: A study of 32 patients with

reappraisal of classification and therapy. *Ann Surg* 1985; 201:527–532.

26. Hart J, Layfield LJ, Trumbull WE, et al: Practical aspects in the diagnosis and management of cystosarcoma phyllodes. *Arch Surg* 1988; 123:1079–1083.
27. Chua CL, Thomas A, Ng BK: Cystosarcoma phyllodes: A review of surgical options. *Surgery* 1989; 105:141–147.
28. Ackerman LV: Personal communication, 1984.
29. Stewart FW: Tumors of the breast, in *Atlas of Tumor Pathology*, sect IX, fasc 34:75. Washington, D.C., Armed Forces Institute of Pathology, 1950.
30. Schmidt GB: Ueber das angitsarkom der mamma. *Arch Klin Chir* 1887; 26:121–127.
31. Chen KTK, Kirkeguard DO, Bocian JJ: Angiosarcoma of the breast. *Cancer* 1980; 46:368–371.
32. Steingaszuer LC, Enzinger FM, Taylor H: Hemangiosarcoma of the breast. *Cancer* 1965; 18:352–361.
33. Donnell RM, Rosen PP, Lieberman PH, et al: Angiosarcoma and other vascular tumors of the breast. Pathologic analysis as a guide to prognosis. *Am J Surg Pathol* 1981; 5:629–642.
34. Gulesserian HP, Lawton RC: Angiosarcoma of the breast. *Cancer* 1969; 24:1021–1026.
35. Hunter TB, Martin PC, Dietzen CD, et al: Angiosarcoma of the breast: Two case reports and a review of the literature. *Cancer* 1985; 56:2099–2106.
36. Rosen PP, Kimmel M, Ernsberger D: Mammary angiosarcoma: The prognostic significance of tumor differentiation. *Cancer* 1988; 62:2145–2151.
37. Berg JW, DeCosse JJ, Fracchia AA, et al: Stromal sarcomas of the breast: A unified approach to connective tissue sarcomas other than cystosarcoma phyllodes. *Cancer* 1962; 15:418–434.
38. DeCosse JJ, Berg JW, Fracchia AA, et al: Primary lymphosarcoma of the breast. *Cancer* 1962; 15:1264–1268.
39. Mambo NC, Burke JS, Butler JJ: Primary malignant lymphomas of the breast. *Cancer* 1977; 39:2033–2040.

Chapter 10

Sarcomas of the Heart and Great Vessels; Vascular Replacement

Heather N. Raaf

John H. Raaf

Although rare, soft-tissue sarcoma is the most common primary malignant tumor of the heart and great vessels. The total number of published cases of sarcomas arising in these organs is fewer than 800. In autopsy series of the general population, the incidence of any type of primary tumor of the heart and pericardium ranges between 0.0017% and 0.28%. Only 20% to 25% of such tumors are malignant.[1, 2]

SARCOMAS OF THE HEART AND PERICARDIUM

The clinical diagnosis of primary cardiac tumors is not often made pre-operatively or antemortem due to the nonspecific nature of the signs and symptoms and the low level of clinical suspicion for these rare tumors. The clinical presentation varies with anatomical location.

Tumors that spread along the pericardium and encase the heart, such as mesotheliomas and angiosarcomas, cause cardiac constriction that may result in chest pain, hypotension, tachycardia, and malaise. Diminished cardiac sounds or a friction rub may be heard. Tamponade, due to a persistent bloody pericardial effusion, eventually can cause intractable cardiac failure. Myocardial infiltration by tumor may cause refractory arrhythmias, heart block, right- or left-sided heart failure, angina, or infarction.[3] Masses within the heart may cause valvular obstruction, valvular incompetence, and congestive failure. The flow murmur of valvular insufficiency may be heard. In rare instances a pedunculated tumor may cause an audible "plop" as the tumor prolapses through a valve.

Tumor emboli from the right side of the heart to the lungs may cause dyspnea or hemoptysis, much like thrombotic pulmonary embolism. Embolization from left-sided intracavitary sarcoma may cause cerebrovascular accident or other systemic organ infarction, seizures, and peripheral metastasis. Extracardiac spread of tumor may cause signs and symptoms referable to the mediastinum, such as superior vena cava syndrome, hemoptysis from bronchial invasion, or dysphonia.[4]

The patient population, site, and gross characteristics of the various types of cardiac sarcomas vary with histological type. In adults, the most common type of cardiac sarcoma is angiosarcoma, followed by rhabdomyosarcoma (Table 10–1).

Angiosarcoma.—About 80% of cardiac angiosarcomas occur as large mural masses in the right atrium, often replacing the atrial wall and sometimes filling the entire chamber.[5] They may invade adjacent structures such as the venae cavae and the tricuspid valve. These tumors are symptomatic and rapidly fatal. A less common but nevertheless typical pattern of growth is extensive pericardial spread and encasement of the heart in continuity with a primary right atrial or ventricular component. Pericardial angiosarcoma without myocardial involvement occurs rarely (Fig 10–1). The average age of patients is 40 years (range, 10–76 years). The tumor varies in gross appearance from tan-pink, to brown, to purple and is usually hemorrhagic. The borders are poorly defined.

Kaposi's sarcoma, which is vascular in origin and often widespread in patients with acquired immunodeficiency syndrome (AIDS), was found in the heart in only three of 74 patients (4.1%) dying with this tumor in the autopsy study of Klatt and Heitz.[6] Lesions of Kaposi's sarcoma that involve the heart tend to be epicardial and asymptomatic and have no right atrial predilection. Such tumors, in the presence of typical skin lesions of Kaposi's sarcoma, may represent a subgroup of angiosarcoma with a more benign behavior. However, cases previously termed "primary Kaposi's sarcoma" of the heart, without associated skin lesions, behave clinically like angiosarcomas and should be so classified.[7]

TABLE 10–1.
Primary Malignant Tumors of the Heart and Pericardium*

Tumor Type	Percent
Angiosarcoma	31.2
Rhabdomyosarcoma	20.8
Mesothelioma	15.2
Fibrosarcoma	11.2
Extraskeletal osteosarcoma	4.0
Malignant schwannoma	3.2
Other sarcomas	2.4
Other types of primary tumor	12.0

* *Adapted from McCallister HA, Fenoglio FF: Tumors of the Cardiovascular System, in* Atlas of Tumor Pathology, *2nd series, fasc 15. Washington, D.C., Armed Forces Institute of Pathology, 1978.*

Rhabdomyosarcoma.—The second most common primary sarcoma of the heart, rhabdomyosarcoma, has been reported in all age groups. There is no predilection for a particular chamber of the heart, and in 60% of patients the tumor involves multiple sites. Pericardial invasion is common, but diffuse pericardial spread, characteristic of mesothelioma or angiosarcoma, is not found. The tumor is soft, nodular, and always has a myocardial component. Some rhabdomyosarcomas extend into a cardiac cavity to form a mass that may obstruct a valvular orifice. Invasion or partial replacement of a valve may also occur. Both juvenile (embryonal or alveolar) and adult histological types are found.

Mesothelioma.—Mesotheliomas may arise in the visceral or parietal pericardium and spread superficially to encase and constrict the heart. Unlike angiosarcomas, they do not invade the underlying myocardium. However, they may grow by direct extension to involve the pleura and mediastinum and surround the great vessels as they enter or leave the heart. They have also been reported to extend through the diaphragm and involve the peritoneum. Only rarely are they localized. The tumor tissue is firm and white, with both nodular and sheetlike growth. Mesotheliomas have been reported in all age groups. No association of pericardial mesothelioma with asbestos has been identified, despite its similarity to primary pleural mesotheliomas.

Fibrosarcoma and Malignant Fibrous Histiocytoma.—These tumors are firm and white or gray-white, with either nodular or infiltrative growth patterns. Patient ages range from 1 to 87 years. There is no propensity for a particular cardiac chamber, and over half involve multiple sites.[8] While pericardial invasion may occur, no primary fibrosarcoma of the pericardium was

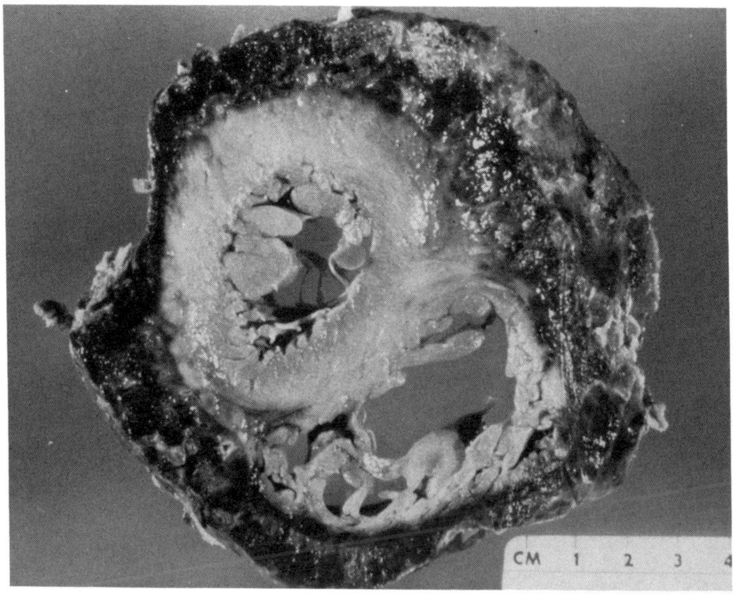

FIG 10–1.
Angiosarcoma of the heart, with pericardial encasement by hemorrhagic tumor. (Photograph courtesy of Dr. K. Marchant, Cleveland, Ohio.)

found in the largest series of cases.[1] In 50% of patients, there is an intracavitary mass causing valvular obstruction and/or invasion of a valve leaflet.

Malignant Schwannoma (Malignant Nerve Sheath Tumor).—Derived from peripheral nerve sheath, all four reported malignant cardiac schwannomas have been located at the base of the heart, on the right side, in the visceral pericardium where the vagus nerve innervates the heart.[1] In all cases the tumor invaded underlying myocardium, unlike mesothelioma. All patients were male.

Other Primary Cardiac Sarcomas.—A small number of leiomyosarcomas, liposarcomas, and one synovial sarcoma arising primarily in the heart have been reported. No primary chondrosarcomas have been reported. The majority of cardiac extraskeletal osteosarcomas arise in the left atrium, and most present as an intracavitary mass. They are otherwise grossly similar to fibrosarcomas.

Cardiac Sarcomas in Children.—Malignant cardiac tumors comprise less than 10% of all pediatric tumors, so rare that they are reported as single cases.[9] Rhabdomyosarcoma is the most commonly reported, others being fibrosarcoma and malignant schwannoma.

Metastatic Sarcoma to the Heart.—Metastases to the heart and pericardium occur 20 to 40 times more often than all primary cardiac tumors, benign or malignant. In an autopsy series of 120 adult patients who died of metastatic soft-tissue sarcoma, 25% had cardiac metastases.[10] No histological type of sarcoma is particularly likely to metastasize to the heart. The pattern of metastatic tumor growth in the mediastinum varies. Diffuse pericardial spread, similar to mesothelioma, may occur, or there may be multiple small, solid tumor nodules throughout the myocardium.

In an autopsy series of children with any type of malignant solid tumor, the incidence of metastatic tumor involving the cardiovascular system was 5.7%.[9] Some childhood tumors are more likely to spread to the heart than others. Of the sarcomas, metastasis from rhabdomyosarcoma is found most frequently, with an incidence of 11.5% in patients dying from this tumor.

Metastatic tumor to the heart may cause signs and symptoms that are overlooked or considered relatively insignificant in the context of widespread disease. When sought, however, these are often present. The usual findings are unexplained, rapid cardiac enlargement, symptoms of cardiac decompensation, congestive heart failure, and cardiac arrhythmias. Pericardial involvement by metastasis most commonly is manifested by pericardial effusion, with tamponade leading to death in some cases.

Diagnosis of Cardiac Sarcomas.—Advances in specialized diagnostic techniques have permitted accurate noninvasive assessment of cardiac pathology, improving opportunities for recognition of tumors and successful surgical intervention.

Over 75% of patients with cardiac malignancies have electrocardiographic manifestations. Patients with pericardial tumors may have tachycardia and decreased voltage. Myocardial tumors may cause arrhythmia or block. Tumor in any location may cause nonspecific ST and T wave changes.

Generalized cardiomegaly or asymmetric enlargement (e.g., right sided) may be observed on chest roentgenogram. Pulmonary congestion, edema, or pleural effusion are other frequent nonspecific findings. Occasionally there is widening of the mediastinum in the case of massive extracardiac spread of tumor, or a hilar mass with sarcoma of the pulmonary vessels. Multiple calcified densities can suggest osteosarcoma.

Echocardiography has become the method of choice for noninvasive imaging of cardiac tumors. In particular, two-dimensional echocardiography has increased the sensitivity of echocardiographic scanning, improving the rate of preoperative diagnosis of cardiac tumors and the assessment of their extent.[11] Transesophageal Doppler echocardiography may provide complementary information about the hemodynamics of intracavitary masses and possible valvular compromise caused by tumor.[12]

Computed tomography (CT) scanning is a noninvasive technique that has clearly demonstrated cardiac tumor and provided accurate information about invasion of adjacent structures. Pulmonary and hepatic metastases from a cardiac primary sarcoma may be revealed by chest and abdominal CT scans. Phillips and Williams report a case of calcified pericardial metastases from a peripheral osteosarcoma that were detected on bone scan with Tc 99m and confirmed by CT.[13]

Angiography can demonstrate intracardiac and intravascular tumors as filling defects. It is valuable for assessing coronary artery compromise or embolization by tumor and for visualization of tumor vessels. Until the advent of Doppler echocardiography, angiography was the only method available for the assessment of valvular, hence hemodynamic, function. It carries the risk of dislodging intracavitary or intravascular tumor, resulting in embolization.

Magnetic resonance imaging (MRI) has been used to visualize cardiac tumors such as rhabdomyosarcoma, and to measure response to chemotherapy.[14] In the future, MRI may provide a noninvasive method to characterize cardiac tumor tissue type.[15]

Pericardiocentesis provides fluid for cytological examination that may be positive for malignant cells, and it can also relieve tamponade. Endomyocardial biopsy to obtain tumor tissue may occasionally be diagnostic, but tissue for diagnosis is usually obtained at the time of open surgical exploration of the mediastinum.

Treatment of Cardiac Sarcomas.—Cure is seldom obtained in patients with sarcoma of the heart or pericardium, but prolongation of survival or significant palliation may be achieved. Exploratory surgery with biopsy provides tissue for histological diagnosis and determines the extent of the tumor. Total or partial excision of primary[16] or metastatic[17] cardiac sarcoma can provide hemodynamic improvement and relief of congestive heart failure, while pericardial window, pericardiectomy, or valve replacement may ameliorate symptoms. Cardiac transplantation has been successfully employed in a patient with a large unresectable fibroma of the heart[18] but is not appropriate for malignant disease. Explantation and autotransplantation of the heart may facilitate tumor resection.[19]

Complete or incomplete excision of a malignant cardiac tumor, followed by adjuvant radiation therapy and/or chemotherapy, is felt to offer optimal treatment in many cases.[3, 9] Experience with combination therapy is, however, limited by the rarity of these neoplasms. Responses of inoperable cardiac sarcoma to radiotherapy[20] and to chemotherapy[21] have been reported. Both radiation and doxorubicin are cardiotoxic.

Prognosis.—Survival data from 75 patients with primary cardiac sarcomas were studied by Burke and co-authors from the Armed Forces Institute of Pathology (Washington, DC), to determine factors affecting prognosis[22]. Mean survival was 11 months, with a median of 6 months. Histological type and presence of differentiation did not affect prognosis. Greater than ten mitoses per high-power field, or the presence of necrosis, correlated with poor prognosis. Better survival was associated with left-sided tumors and with postoperative chemotherapeutic or radiation treatment.

SARCOMAS OF THE GREAT VESSELS

The incidence of primary tumors of the great vessels is approximately 20% that of primary neoplasms of the heart and pericardium.[1] These tumors are predominantly of smooth muscle or fibroblastic origin, although some are histologically undifferentiated and reported simply as "intimal sarcomas." Fibroblastic and undifferentiated sarcomas of the great vessels are usually classified as malignant fibrous histiocytoma,[23] but electron microscopy and immunohistochemistry reveal a minority of them to be of endothelial origin.[24, 25]

Sarcomas of the great vessels cause nonspecific signs and symptoms. Patients with aortic sarcomas that obstruct the renal arteries may present with hypertension. Claudication can be seen with unilateral or bilateral loss of lower extremity pulses, or there may be abdominal or pelvic pain due to intestinal ischemia when the superior mesenteric artery is involved. Pulmonary artery sarcomas may cause exertional dyspnea, cough, hemoptysis, and chest or back pain. Regardless of the location of the tumor, there are often generalized manifestations of malignancy: fever, night sweats, weight loss, and malaise.

Aortic Sarcomas.—Approximately 30 cases have been reported. These tumors arise in the abdominal aorta more often than the thoracic aorta. The mean age of patients is 54 years.[26] Sarcomas involving the intima can form polypoid, obstructing intraluminal masses, or they may extend along the intima in a plaquelike manner resembling atherosclerosis. Such tumors often give rise to thrombo-embolic metastases, such as to the superior mesenteric artery.[27] Those arising in the media or adventitia rarely metastasize. They cause such nonspecific symptoms that a pre-operative diagnosis is seldom made.

Pulmonary Artery Sarcomas.—One hundred and ten cases have been reported.[28] The mean age of patients is about 50 years, with none younger than 20 years. The tumor appears to arise in the pulmonary trunk and may form a nodular intraluminal mass (Fig 10–2), or it may spread along the intimal surface. Retro-

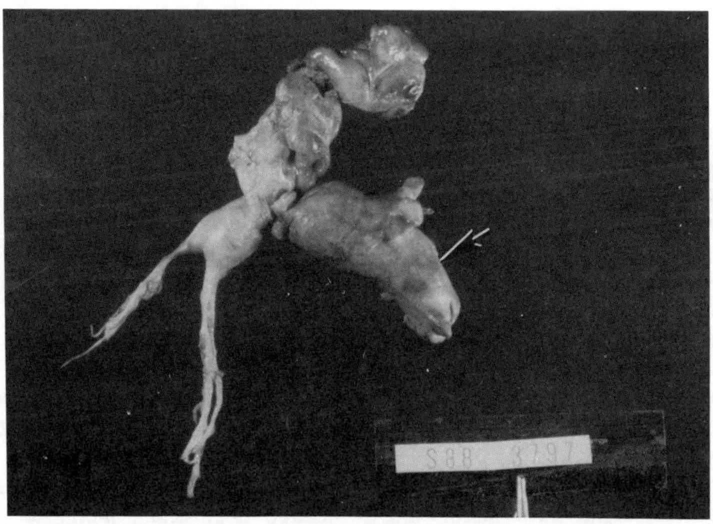

FIG 10–2.
Undifferentiated sarcoma of the pulmonary artery. Tumor growth along the main trunk (*arrow*) and right and left pulmonary arteries, and into arterial branches, grossly resembles organized thrombus. (Photograph courtesy of Dr. J. J. Berner, Cleveland, Ohio.)

grade spread can involve the pulmonary valve and right ventricle, while antegrade spread is along pulmonary artery branches into the lung. Forty percent of patients have pulmonary metastases. A sarcoma in an extremity, such as osteosarcoma of the femur,[29] may give rise to massive pulmonary tumor emboli that can occlude the main pulmonary artery.

Sarcomas of Large Veins.—These tumors comprise approximately 65% of primary neoplasms of large vessels.[1] About 85% are malignant. Of these the great majority are leiomyosarcomas, as is also true for sarcomas of muscular arteries. By contrast, malignant fibrous histiocytoma predominates in the elastic arteries (aorta and pulmonary artery). Leiomyosarcomas of the venae cavae tend to occur in adults over 60 years of age, although the age range is 24 to 83 years. Female patients outnumber male by 8:1. Leiomyosarcomas that occur in large veins other than the venae cavae have no sex predilection.

Treatment of Sarcomas of the Great Vessels.—This group of sarcomas is treated primarily by surgical excision, although a wide margin may be impossible to achieve. Long-term survival has been reported.[30] Following excision, adjuvant radiotherapy or chemotherapy[31] can be considered.

Replacement of the aorta[24, 32] or a major artery by a synthetic or autogenous graft may be required. Amputation is another option for treating tumors in the major vessels of an extremity, for example, forequarter amputation for angiosarcoma of the axillary vein.[33] Sarcomas can grow a long distance within the lumen of the inferior vena cava, extending even from the iliac vein to the heart. To remove such an intracaval and intracardiac tumor, cardiopulmonary bypass[34] or bypass with deep hypothermic circulatory arrest[35] has been successfully employed. Following cardiopulmonary bypass for removal of sarcoma from within the pulmonary artery, one must be prepared to control endobronchial reperfusion hemorrhage.[36]

VASCULAR REPLACEMENT

Soft-tissue sarcomas may grow within major blood vessels and occlude them, but more frequently they arise primarily in muscle or soft tissue and cause deviation or compression of adjacent vessels. This can lead to edema distal to the tumor, or ischemia of a limb when arterial circulation is compromised. Limb-sparing resection of a sarcoma typically spares "major structures" such as the femoral vessels (Fig 10–3) and sciatic nerve. Unresected microscopic tumor along a major structure, or even minimal visible disease, can often be sterilized by postoperative radiotherapy.

If sarcoma encases major vessels, it may not be possible to resect the tumor without sacrificing them. Examples are desmoid sarcoma surrounding the external iliac and femoral vessels in the groin (Fig 10–4), or malignant fibrous histiocytoma encasing the iliac vessels in the pelvis (Fig 10–5). In such patients the artery must be excised with the tumor and replaced.[37, 38] Sufficient collateral venous return usually exists, due to gradual compression over time by the tumor, that a partially or totally occluded vein is usually not reconstructed. Even the inferior vena cava may be sacrificed if tumor surrounds and compresses it below the renal veins (Fig 10–6). This is different from acute loss of the vena cava secondary to trauma, where reconstruction is advised.[39]

To avoid edema, a few authors have advocated simultaneous arterial and venous grafting following tumor and vessel resection in the extremity. By creating a distal arteriovenous fistula, blood flow can be increased to maintain venous graft patency, when the vein is replaced by a conduit.[40, 41]

The surgeon who intends to resect a sarcoma that is closely associated with major vessels must anticipate encasement or erosion of these structures by tumor, as illustrated by the following unusual patient.

Case Report.—In March 1989, a moderately obese 81-year-old white female developed bilateral swelling of the lower limbs after a lengthy airplane trip. The left leg edema resolved, but the right leg edema persisted. In September 1989, her physician performed a phlebogram that was considered to confirm the diagnosis of right deep venous thrombosis. She was hospitalized and treated with intravenous heparin.

While she was in the hospital, a firm mass was palpated in the medial aspect of her right thigh. This was first thought to be a hematoma related to anticoagulation, but CT scan (Fig 10–7,A) suggested a solid tumor. Magnetic resonance imaging (Fig 10–7,B) and Doppler ultrasound (Fig 10–7,C) studies of the right thigh revealed a pseudoaneurysm of the right super-

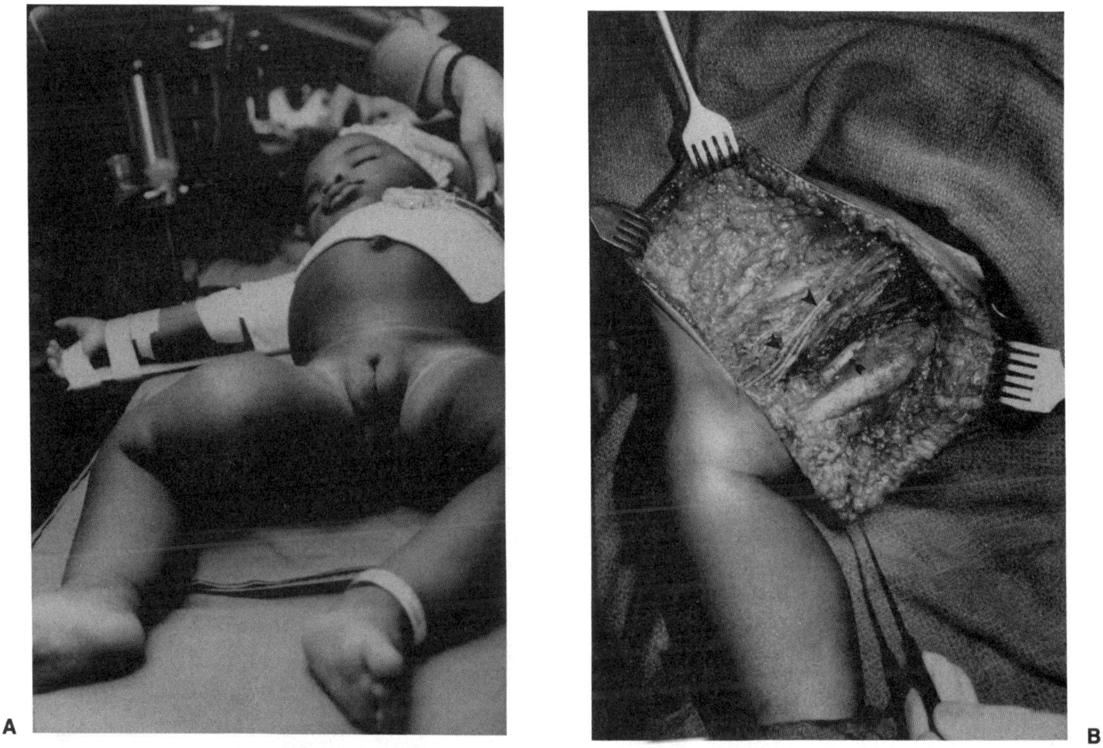

FIG 10–3.
A, fibrosarcoma in the medial right thigh of a 1-year-old child. **B,** radical resection of the adductor muscle group spared the femoral vessels (*arrowheads*). The femur (*small arrow*) is at the deepest margin of the dissection.

ficial femoral artery, within a 12-cm solid tumor. Needle biopsy showed high-grade malignant fibrous histiocytoma. There was no evidence of metastatic disease.

In November 1989, a radical limb-sparing resection was performed, including most of the adductor muscle group. The superficial femoral artery and vein, encased by tumor, were also removed (Fig 10–7,D). Pathological examination confirmed a 4-cm pseudoaneurysm of the superficial femoral artery, apparently caused by tumor erosion. A 6-mm polytetrafluoroethylene (PTFE) graft was used to reconstruct the superficial femoral artery (Fig 10–7,E). Intra-operative arteriography showed two vessel run-off into the foot, with the posterior tibial artery occluded in the midcalf. The anterior tibial and peroneal vessels were open.

Postoperatively the right foot remained viable, and the patient was able to ambulate. Two areas of necrosis developed on the edge of the posterior flap, requiring limited debridement. Dressings and antibiotics were continued for several weeks, but she was then returned to the operating room for wound re-exploration. A segment of PTFE was found to be exposed at the base of the wound, and an attempt was made to cover this with remaining hamstring muscle. Further healing of the wound occurred, and cultures remained negative, but the midsection of the PTFE graft was pushed superficially and seemed unlikely to become covered by healthy tissue (Fig 10–7,F).

Therefore, in January 1990, the above-knee PTFE femoral-popliteal bypass graft was removed. Replacement was with a right below-knee femoral PTFE graft, utilizing a lateral approach to the popliteal artery. This required excision of the fibular head. The originally placed PTFE graft was completely excised and the two ends of the superficial femoral artery suture ligated. The medial thigh wound was left open. With dressing changes, it healed rapidly by secondary intention (Fig 10–7,G). Adjuvant radiation therapy (6,000 cGy) was then delivered to the tumor bed. The patient was ambulat-

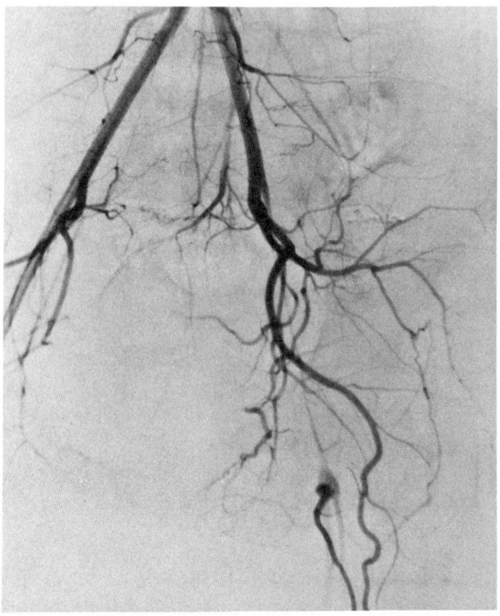
A

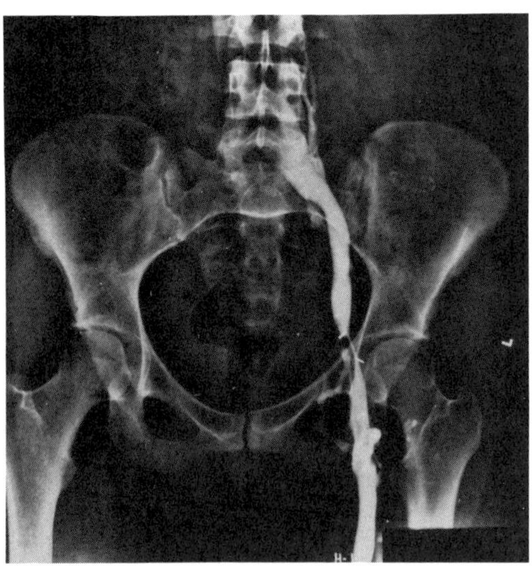
B

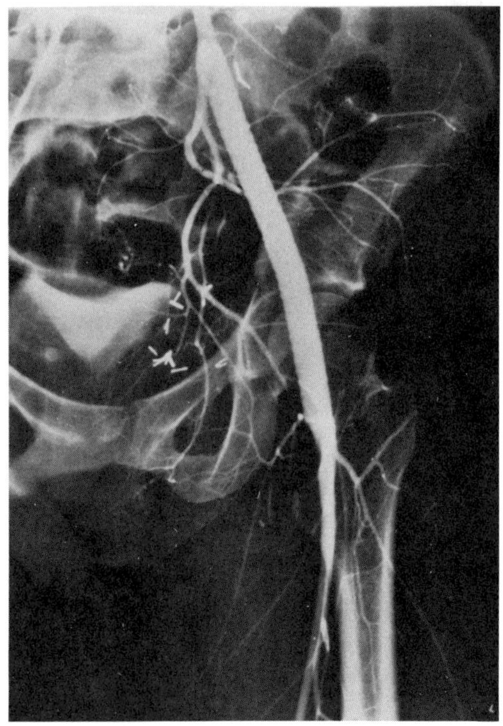
C

FIG 10–4.
A 23-year-old woman presented with left calf claudication. **A,** occlusion of, and collaterals around, the external iliac artery seen in this arteriogram was due to infiltrating desmoid fibrosarcoma of the groin and lower abdomen. **B,** venogram shows compression of the iliac vein. **C,** after resection of the tumor, the arterial supply to the leg was restored using an 8-mm dacron graft. The vein was spared, and there was no postoperative leg edema.

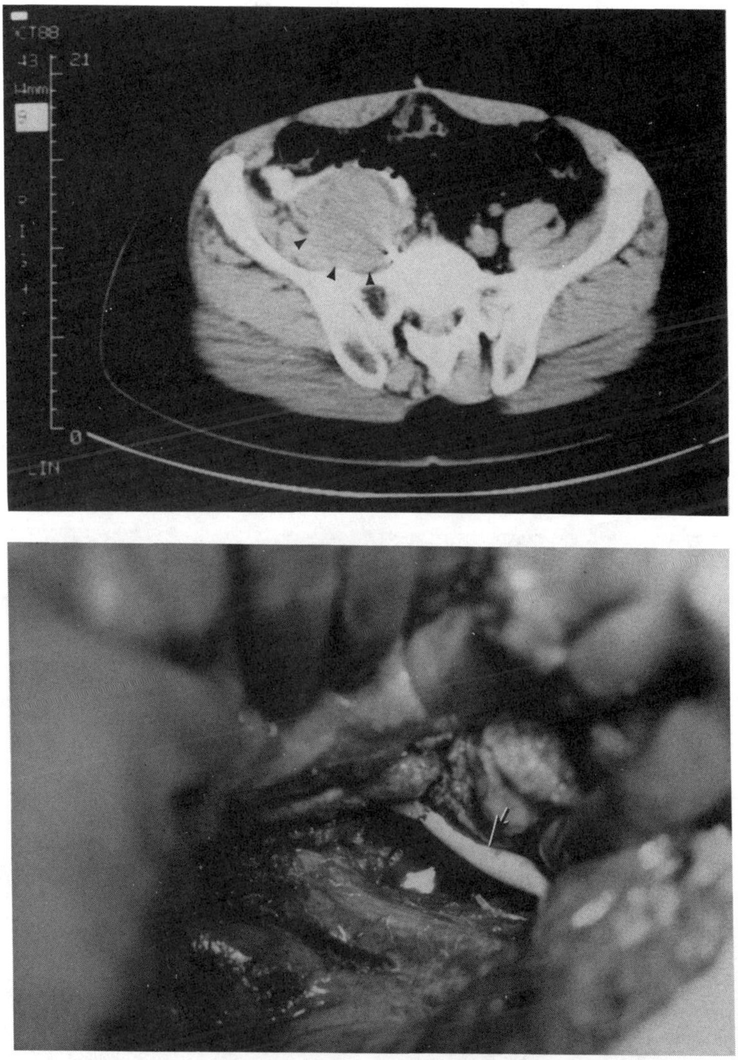

A

B

FIG 10–5.

A, recurrent malignant fibrous histiocytoma (*arrowheads*) is shown by CT scan in the right pelvis of this 57-year-old man. A loop of small bowel is seen to be adherent to the anterior surface of the tumor. **B,** during dissection, the right common iliac artery was found to be encased by tumor. It was resected and replaced by an 8-mm polytetrafluoroethylene (PTFE) graft (*arrow*). View is from right side of the patient. Postoperative radiation therapy was delivered to this area.

A

B

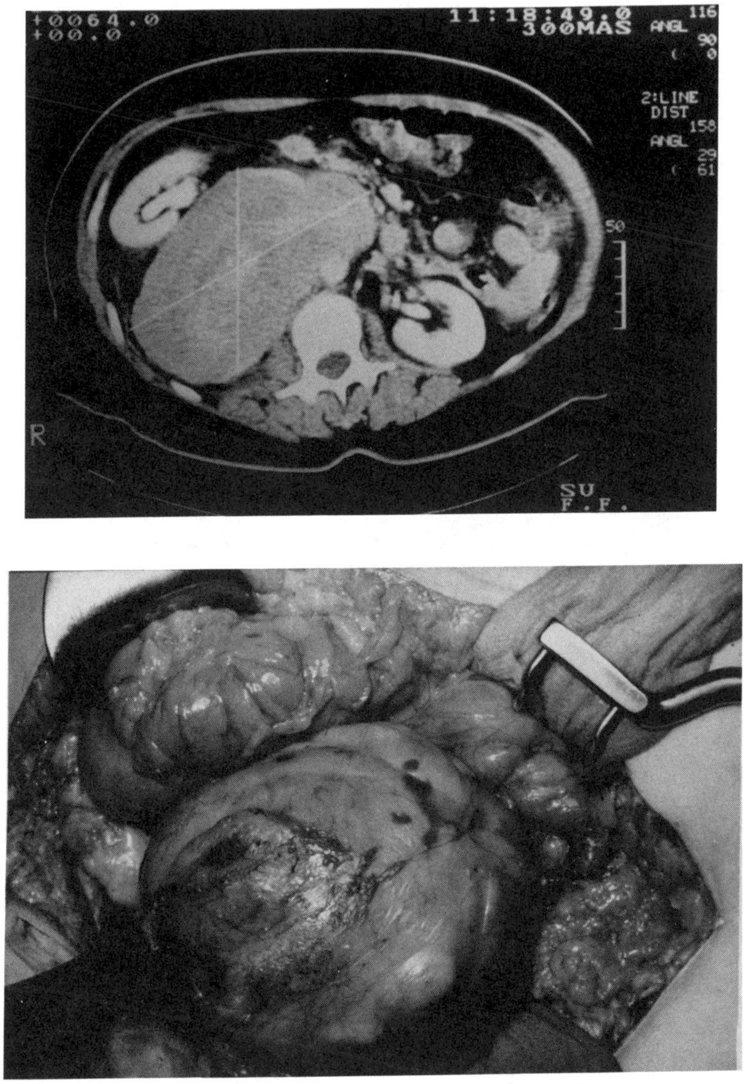

FIG 10–6.

A, liposarcoma recurred in the retroperitoneum of this 61-year-old woman. **B,** at exploration (view from patient's right side), a 24-cm-diameter tumor was dissected free of bowel and removed. A second smaller tumor was found to compress and encase the inferior vena cava (IVC) and was adherent to the aorta. The IVC was resected with this mass, from just below the renal veins to the bifurcation, and was not replaced. **C,** the tumor was dissected off the surface of the aorta (*arrow*). **D,** tumor specimen with the IVC (*arrows*) opened. Postoperatively, leg edema was minimal and quite manageable.

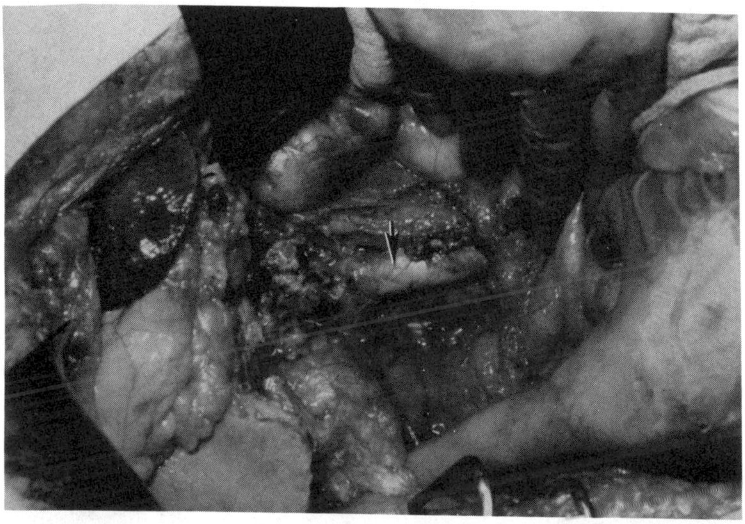

C

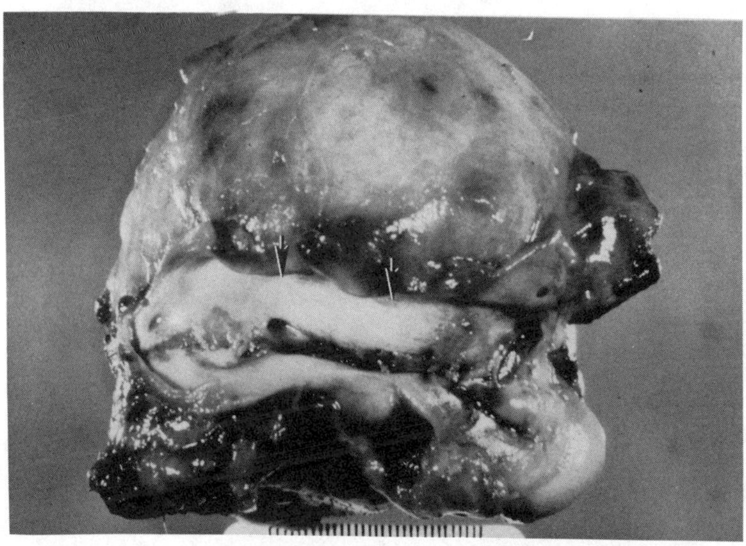

D

FIG 10–6.—*Cont.*

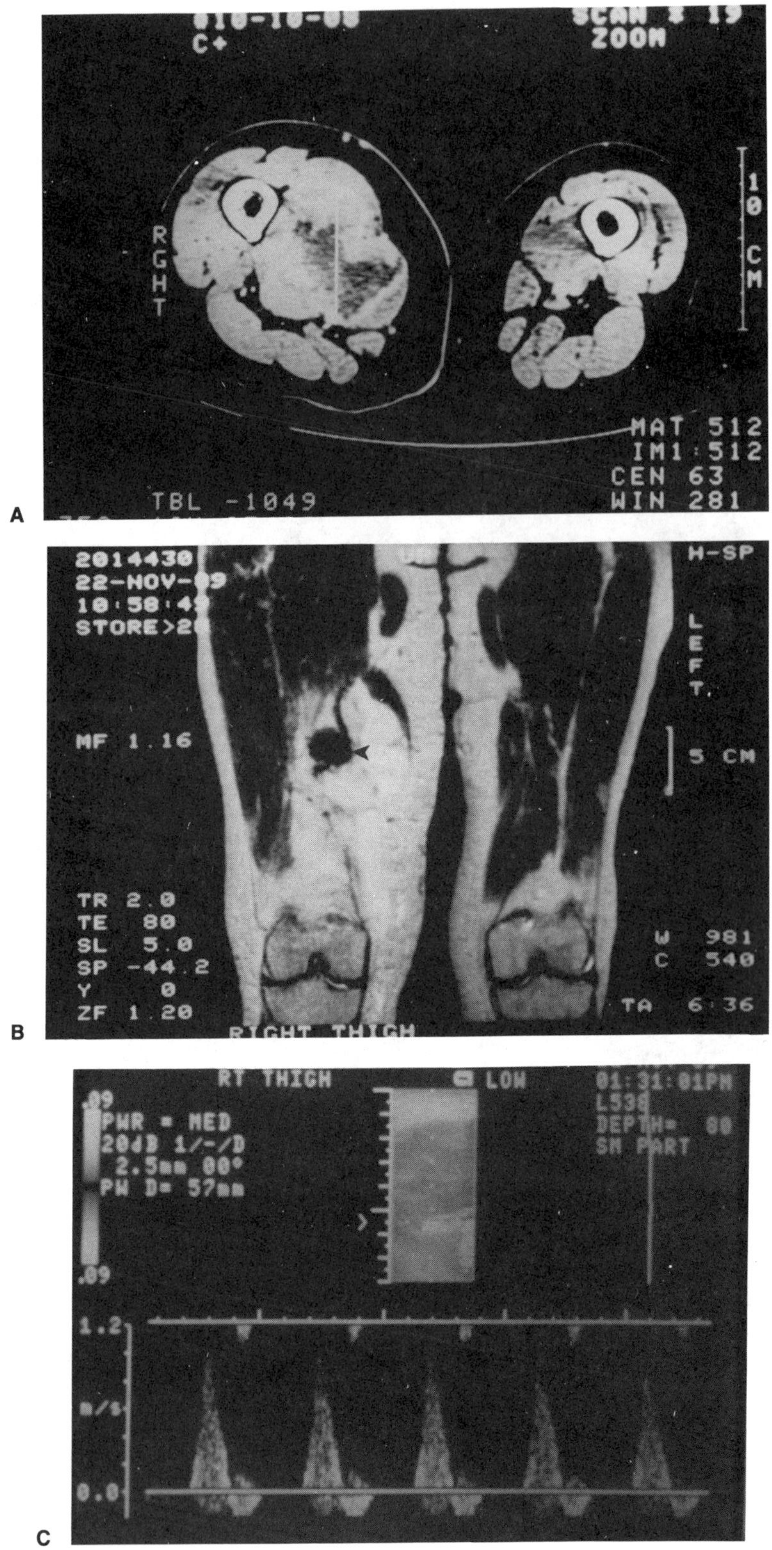

FIG 10–7.
Case report. **A,** tumor mass (malignant fibrous histiocytoma) demonstrated by CT in the medial right thigh. **B,** magnetic resonance imaging coronal view shows a pseudoaneurysm of the superficial femoral artery (*arrowhead*), with the artery entering and exiting. **C,** Doppler ultrasound of the malignant fibrous histiocytoma and aneurysm. **D,** tumor dissected free (top of photograph) except for the superficial femoral artery, which is controlled proximally and distally by vessel loops; the clamp is under the sciatic nerve. **E,** a PTFE graft was used to reconstruct the femoral artery, but the skin flaps failed to heal over it, **F. G,** after placing an extra-anatomical PTFE graft around the lateral aspect of the thigh to the popliteal artery and removal of the first graft, the wound healed. The patient ambulates without difficulty.

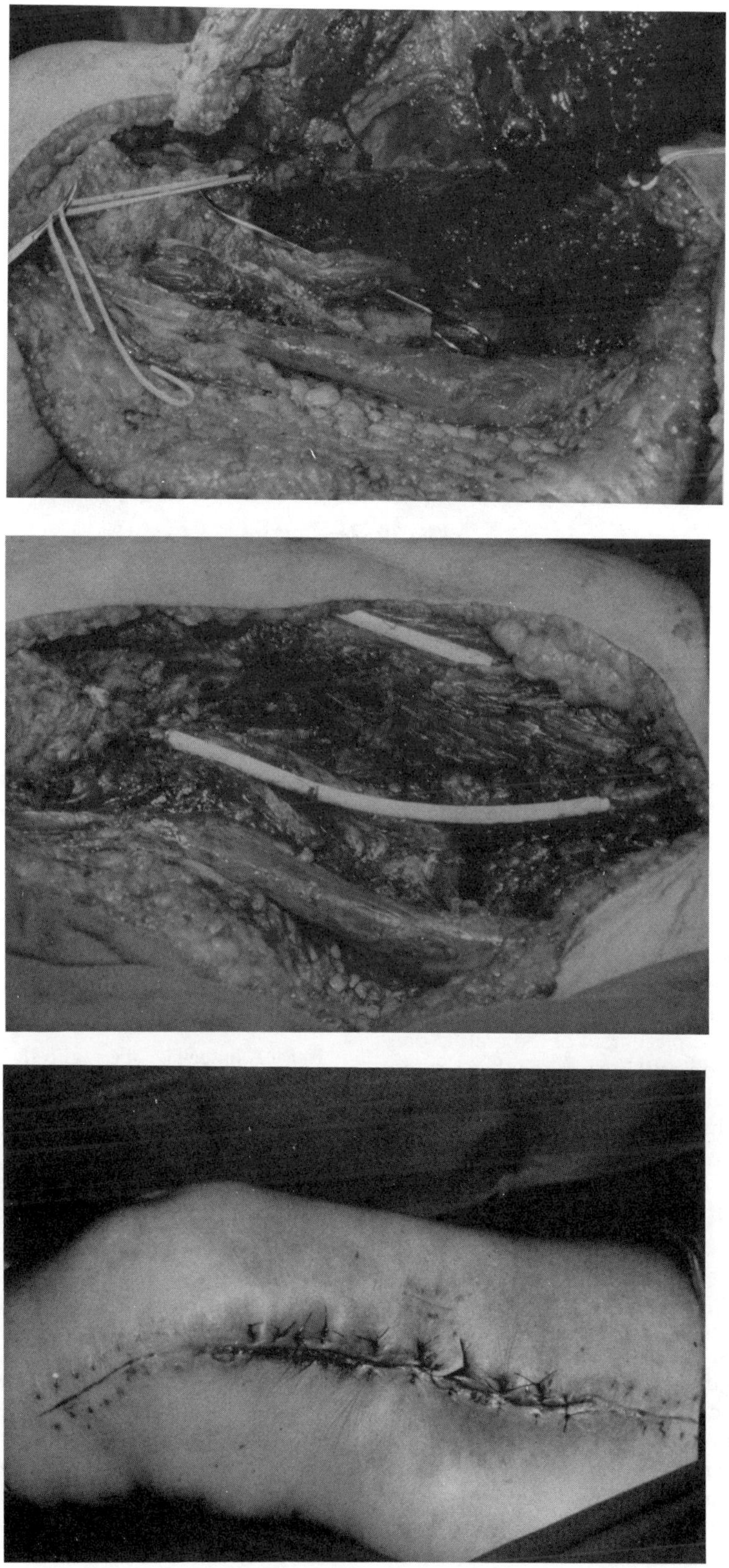

D

E

F

FIG 10–7.—*Cont.*

G 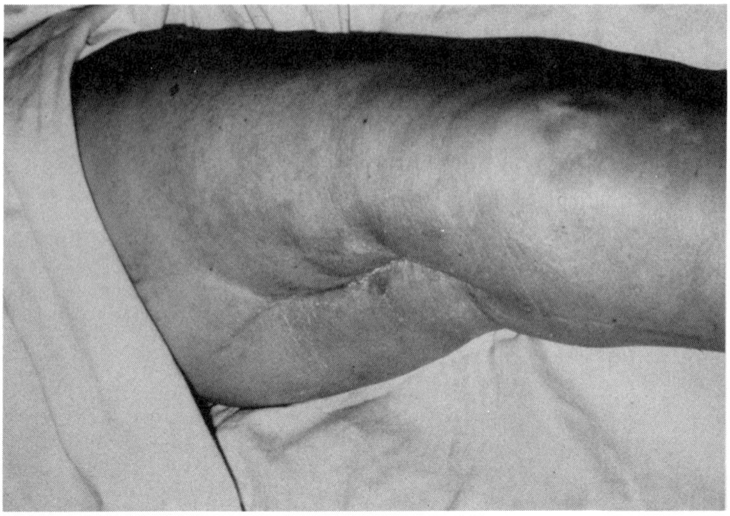

FIG 10–7.—*Cont.*

ing and without evidence of tumor in March 1992.

This patient demonstrates the challenge of resecting a malignant soft-tissue tumor that encases and erodes major vessels. In rare instances, erosion by tumor of a major artery may lead to the formation of a pseudoaneurysm. Vascular replacement may be necessary. Autogenous saphenous vein is preferred, but if the ipsilateral deep venous system is resected with the tumor, synthetic material may be required. Extra-anatomical placement of the graft is preferable to positioning it in the tumor bed because of the potential complications of persistent seroma, wound infection, or flap necrosis.

CONCLUSION

Sarcomas of the heart and great vessels are rare but interesting neoplasms. Their surgical resection is often technically challenging but may provide significant palliation or even cure. Sophisticated diagnostic techniques, including MRI and echocardiography, permit careful preoperative planning that can increase the success of complex operations. Entry of patients on multidisciplinary adjuvant trials should always be considered.

ACKNOWLEDGMENTS

The authors thank Dr. K. Marchant (Division of Laboratory Medicine, Cleveland Clinic, Cleveland, Ohio) and Dr. E. Husni (Chief of Vascular Surgery, Meridia Huron Hospital, Cleveland, Ohio) for their review of this manuscript and helpful suggestions.

REFERENCES

1. McAllister HA, Fenoglio JJ: Tumors of the cardiovascular system, in *Atlas of Tumor Pathology,* 2nd series, fasc 15. Washington, D.C., Armed Forces Institute of Pathology, 1978.
2. Dapper F, Gorlach G, Hoffmann C, et al: Primary cardiac tumors—clinical experiences and late results in 48 patients. *Thorac Cardiovasc Surg* 1988; 36:80–85.
3. Hall RJ, Cooley DA, McAllister HA Jr, et al: Neoplastic heart disease, in Hurst JW, Schlant RC (eds): *The Heart, Arteries and Veins,* ch 68. New York, McGraw-Hill, 1990, pp 1382–1403.
4. Montalescot G, Chapelon C, Drobinski G, et al: Diagnosis of primary cardiac sarcoma. Report of 4 cases and review of the literature. *Int J Cardiol* 1988; 20:209–219.

5. Janigan DT, Husain A, Robinson NA: Cardiac angiosarcomas. A review and a case report. *Cancer* 1986; 57:852–859.
6. Klatt EC, Heitz DR: Cardiac metastases. *Cancer* 1990; 65:1456–1459.
7. Glancy DL, Morales JB, Roberts WC: Angiosarcoma of the heart. *Am J Cardiol* 1968; 21:413–419.
8. McAllister HA, Hall RJ, Cooley DA. Surgical pathology of tumors and cysts of the heart and pericardium, in Waller B (ed): *Pathology of the Heart and Great Vessels,* ch 10. New York, Churchill-Livingston, 1988, pp 343–366.
9. Chan HSL, Sonley MJ, Moes CAF, et al: Primary and secondary tumors of childhood involving the heart, pericardium, and great vessels. *Cancer* 1985; 56:825–836.
10. Hallahan DE, Vogelzang NJ, Borow KM, et al: Cardiac metastases from soft-tissue sarcomas. *J Clin Oncol* 1986; 4:1662–1669.
11. Fyke FE, Seward JB, Edwards WD, et al: Primary cardiac tumors: Experience with 30 consecutive patients since the introduction of two-dimensional echocardiography. *J Am Coll Cardiol* 1985; 5:1465–1473.
12. Shapiro LM, Mulcahy D, Urban P, et al: Detection of valvar obstruction by intracardiac masses using Doppler echocardiography. *Int J Cardiol* 1988; 19:89–97.
13. Phillips GD, Williams BRJ: Osteosarcoma with pericardial metastases seen on bone scan. *Clin Nucl Med* 1987; 12:899–900.
14. Szucs RA, Rehr RB, Yanovich S, et al: Magnetic resonance imaging of cardiac rhabdomyosarcoma; quantifying the response to chemotherapy. *Cancer* 1991; 67:2066–2070.
15. Dichek DA, Holmvang G, Fallon JT, et al: Angiosarcoma of the heart: Three-year survival and follow-up by nuclear magnetic resonance imaging. *Am Heart J* 1988; 115:1323–1324.
16. Dein JR, Frist WH, Stinson EB, et al. Primary cardiac neoplasms; early and late results of surgical treatment in 42 patients. *J Thorac Cardiovasc Surg* 1987; 93:502–511.
17. Lagrange J-L, Despins P, Spielman M, et al: Cardiac metastases; case report on an isolated cardiac metastasis of a myxoid liposarcoma. *Cancer* 1986; 58:2333–2337.
18. Jamieson SW, Gaudiani VA, Reitz BA, et al: Operative treatment of an unresectable tumor of the left ventricle. *J Thorac Cardiovasc Surg* 1981; 81:797–799.
19. Cooley DA, Reardon MJ, Frazier OH, et al: Human cardiac explantation and autotransplantation: Application in a patient with a large cardiac pheochromocytoma. *Texas Heart Inst J* 1985; 12:171–176.
20. Potter R, Baumgart P, Greve H, et al: Primary angiosarcoma of the heart. *Thorac Cardiovasc Surg* 1989; 37:374–378.
21. Stevens CW, Sears-Rogan P, Bitterman P, et al: Treatment of malignant fibrous histiocytoma of the heart. *Cancer* 1992; 69:956–961.
22. Burke AP, Cowan D, Virmani R: Primary sarcomas of the heart. *Cancer* 1992; 69:387–395.
23. Fenoglio JJ Jr, Virmani R: Primary malignant tumors of the great vessels, in BF Waller (ed): *Pathology of the Heart and Great Vessels,* ch 12. New York, Churchill-Livingstone, 1988, pp 429–438.
24. Haber LM, Truong L: Immunohistochemical demonstration of the endothelial nature of aortic intimal sarcoma. *Am J Surg Pathol* 1988; 12:798–802.
25. Kanno J, Takemura T, Kasaga T: Malignant endothelioma of the aorta. *Virchow's Arch Pathol Anat [A]* 1987; 412:183–188.
26. Schipper J, van Oostayen JA, den Hollander JC, et al: Aortic tumours: Report of a case and review of the literature. *Br J Radiol* 1989; 62:35–40.
27. Higgins R, Posner MC, Moosa HH, et al: Mesenteric infarction secondary to tumor emboli from primary aortic sarcoma; guidelines for diagnosis and management. *Cancer* 1991; 68:1622–1627.
28. Nonomura A, Kurumaya H, Kono N, et al: Primary pulmonary artery sarcoma. Report of two autopsy cases studied by immunohistochemistry and electron microscopy, and review of 110 cases reported in the literature. *Acta Pathol Jpn* 1988; 38:883–896.
29. Wakasa K, Sakurai M, Uchida A, et al: Massive pulmonary tumor emboli in osteosarcoma; occult and fatal complication. *Cancer* 1990; 66:583–586.
30. Miller MM, Munnell ER, Poston A, et al: Primary angiosarcoma of the innominate vein: A case report with resection and long-term survival. *J Thorac Cardiovasc Surg* 1985; 90:148–150.
31. Weiss KS, Zidar BL, Wang S, et al: Radiation-induced leiomyosarcoma of the great vessels presenting as superior vena cava syndrome. *Cancer* 1987; 60:1238–1242.
32. Millili JJ, LaFlare RG, Nemir P Jr: Leiomyo-

sarcoma of the abdominal aorta: A case report. *Surgery* 1981; 89:631–634.

33. Alosco T, Sinning H, Harwick R, et al: Angiosarcoma of the axillary vein. *Cancer* 1989; 64:1301–1303.

34. Kaku K, Kawashima Y, Kitamura S, et al: Resection of leiomyosarcoma originating in internal iliac vein and extending into heart via inferior vena cava. *Surgery* 1981; 89:604–611.

35. Novick AC, Kaye MC, Cosgrove DM, et al: Experience with cardiopulmonary bypass and deep hypothermic circulatory arrest in the management of retroperitoneal tumors with large vena caval thrombi. *Ann Surg* 1990; 212:472–477.

36. Lyerly HK, Reves JG, Sabiston DC Jr: Management of primary sarcomas of the pulmonary artery and reperfusion intrabronchial hemorrhage. *Surg Gynecol Obstet* 1986; 163:291–301.

37. Imparato AM, Roses DF, Francis KC, et al: Major vascular reconstruction for limb salvage in patients with soft tissue and skeletal sarcomas of the extremities. *Surg Gynecol Obstet* 1978; 147:891–896.

38. Nambisan RN, Karakousis CP: Vascular reconstruction for limb salvage in soft tissue sarcomas. *Surgery* 1987; 101:668–677.

39. Dale AW, Harris J, Terry RB: Polytetrafluoroethylene reconstruction of the inferior vena cava. *Surgery* 1984; 95:625–630.

40. Fortner JG, Kin DK, Shiu MH: Limb-preserving vascular surgery for malignant tumors of the lower extremity. *Arch Surg* 1977; 112:391–394.

41. Plate G, Hollier LH, Gloviczki P, et al: Overcoming failure of venous vascular prostheses. *Surgery* 1984; 96:503–510.

Chapter 11

Gastrointestinal Leiomyosarcomas

Daniel Coit

John H. Raaf

Gastrointestinal leiomyosarcomas can occur in all parts of the alimentary canal, from esophagus to rectum. Although these tumors are unusual, Skandalakis et al.[1] collected reports of 2,525 cases of smooth muscle tumors of the alimentary tract. These tumors are biologically distinct from their epithelial counterparts in their patterns of growth, metastasis, and recurrence. Understanding these characteristics should define strategy in dealing with them. Areas of controversy in relation to these lesions include the criteria of malignancy, definition of an adequate surgical margin, and whether a complete regional lymph node dissection should be included in resection. Also, in those patients with nonresectable lesions or at high risk for recurrence or metastasis, the role of nonsurgical treatment modalities needs to be defined. Because of the relative infrequency of the lesions and lack of coordinated long-term follow-up, no definitive answers to these questions have emerged. Nevertheless, certain trends are apparent and will be reviewed here.

CRITERIA OF MALIGNANCY

Determination of malignancy in gastrointestinal smooth muscle tumors can be quite difficult. On occasion, the malignancy of a lesion is established only retrospectively, after recurrence or metastasis of what was initially thought to be an adequately resected benign leiomyoma.[2–5] Prognosis can be directly correlated with both the presence and the degree of malignant features. Finally, each tumor may be histologically heterogeneous. Ranchod and Kempson[6] have delineated guidelines for examination of multiple fields of serial sections to try to obviate this difficulty.

Among the histological criteria of malignancy there is wide agreement that the mitotic count is a reliable and reproducible indicator. Lindsay et al.,[7] in a review of gastric leiomyosarcomas, found a 58% 5-year survival in patients with fewer than five mitoses per 10 high-power fields (HPF); only 16% of those patients with over ten mitoses per 10 HPF survived 5 years.

Shiu et al.[8] included mitotic rate in a list of ten histologic criteria used to separate leiomyosarcomas into high- and low-grade categories. Included were cell shape, nuclear-to-cytoplasmic ratio, nuclear shape, chromatin pattern, vascularity, presence of necrosis, nucleolar prominence, cellularity, and stromal abundance. Using these criteria, they found an 81% 5-year survival for low-grade tumors versus a 32% 5-year survival for high-grade lesions.

Tumor size is also thought to be a reliable predictor of malignant potential. Skandalakis et al.[1] found that, in general, gastrointestinal tract leiomyosarcomas tended to be slightly larger than leiomyomas of corresponding locations (Fig. 11–1), although there is enough overlap to preclude using size alone to determine malignancy. However, once the diagnosis of sarcoma is established, size does correlate with prognosis; larger lesions have a greater tendency to metastasize than smaller ones. Shiu et al.[8] confirmed this with the finding that patients with gastric leiomyosarcoma less then 5 cm in diameter, regardless of histological grade, had a 100% 5-year survival rate following resection. Those with tumors greater than 5 cm had only a 57% 5-year survival rate. A similar correlation between size and survival was demonstrated by Chiotasso and Fazio[9] in their review of small-bowel leiomyosarcomas seen at the Cleveland Clinic (Cleveland, Ohio). Those patients with tumors greater than 9 cm had only a 14% 5-year survival rate, and all died of the disease within 7 years.

There is an unusual histological variant of the leiomyosarcoma, the malignant (epithelioid) leiomyoblastoma, which behaves similarly to the more common spindle cell leiomyosarcoma. Both lesions can be graded histologically according to the criteria outlined above. Shiu et al.[10] found that leiomyoblastomas of the small bowel behaved in an aggressive manner, while those in the stomach were more amenable to surgical cure, although the number of patients was small and the differences might have been

A

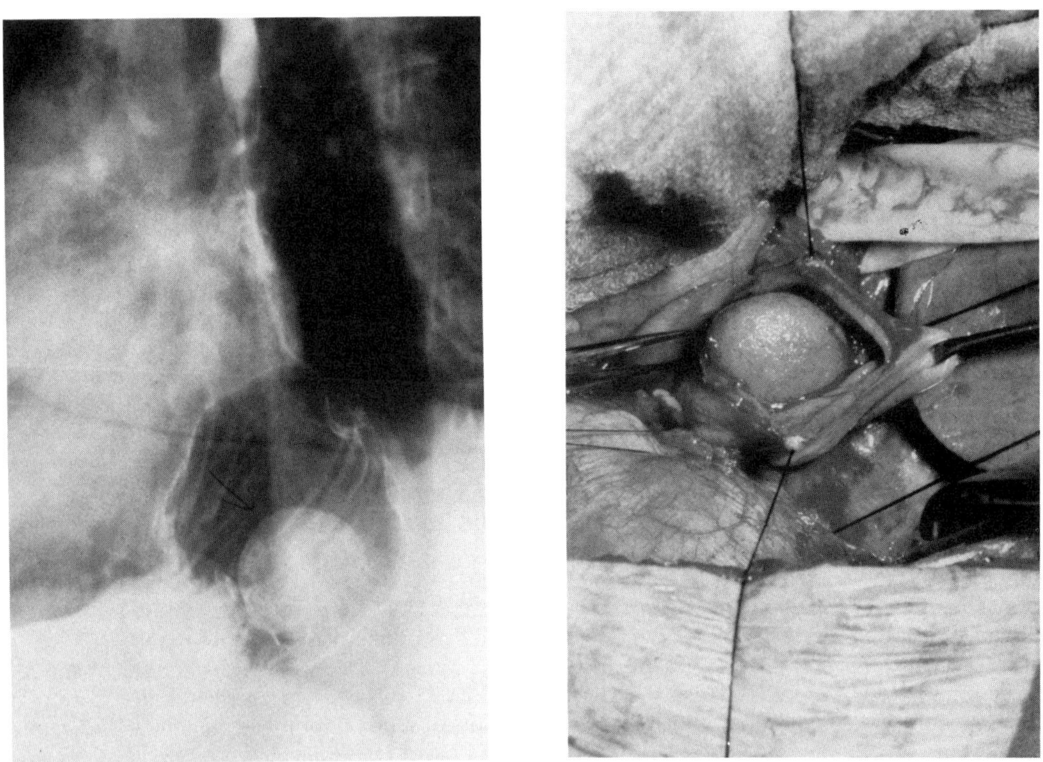

B

FIG 11–1.
A, a 2-cm submucosal tumor in the gastric wall of a hiatal hernia. The smooth, rounded contour and small size suggested the diagnosis: benign leiomyoma. **B,** the mucosa was intact over the tumor, which was removed by marginal excision, followed by repair of the hiatal hernia.

explained on the basis of the other prognostic indicators already described.

In summary, the determination of malignancy of gastrointestinal smooth muscle tumors if often made on a relative rather than absolute basis. Among histological criteria, the mitotic rate is the most widely accepted, with tumors containing more than five to ten mitoses per 10 HPF behaving more aggressively. Examination of multiple sections of tumor is essential to avoid sampling error. Any smooth muscle tumor over 5–7 cm in greatest diameter should be suspected of malignancy, regardless of histological findings. Prognosis in leiomyosarcomas greater than 7–9 cm in diameter is clearly poorer than for the smaller lesions, even if resectable. Certainly local invasion or local or distant metatases should be taken as absolute indicators of malignancy. Treatment should be governed by surgical judgment, balancing the extent of resection against the goals to be achieved.

RESECTABILITY

The treatment of choice for gastrointestinal leiomyosarcomas is surgical resection. Akwari et al.,[11] in a review of 108 patients with intestinal leiomyosarcoma at the Mayo Clinic (Rochester, Minnesota), found that 6% had unresectable disease because of invasion of adjacent organs or encasement of vital vascular pedicles. In this series, 48% of the patients were thought to have lesions resectable for cure. Overall 5- and 10-year survival rates were 50% and 35%, respectively. The remaining 46% of patients underwent palliative resections, and survival depended largely on location of the primary tumor. Five- and 10-year survival rates for small-bowel tumors were 25% and 6%, respectively. No patient survived 5 years following palliative resection of a duodenal lesion; only one patient survived 5 years following palliative resection of a colonic lesion. Chiotasso and Fazio[9] similarly found that in patients with small-bowel leiomyosarcoma with lymphatic or distant metastases, all patients died of the disease within 3 years. Thirty-seven percent of those patients underwent "palliative operation" followed by chemotherapy or radiotherapy, and all were dead within 2 years. Shiu et al.[10] found no 5-year survivors in patients with gastric leiomyosarcoma, when there was invasion of adjacent viscera at the time of initial operation.

These findings should temper enthusiasm for attempting curative radical en bloc resections of tumors that extend beyond the bowel and its mesentery. However, they should not hamper efforts at palliation, because these tumors can behave in a biologically indolent fashion once their symtomatic components have been controlled. Starr and Dockerty[12] reported a patient alive and well 19 years after resection of a 20-cm leiomyosarcoma of the distal small bowel. This same patient was alive 6 years after incidental discovery of multiple peritoneal sarcoma implants on an excised hernia sac. Kohno et al.[13] reviewed cases of resection of leiomyosarcoma metastatic to the liver (Fig 11–2 shows an obviously unresectable case, as demonstrated by computed tomography [CT] scan). Of 11 collected cases, there were four 5-year survivors, all but one of whom died of disease shortly thereafter. The single 10-year survivor underwent synchronous resection of a 14-cm jejunal tumor, three separate peritoneal implants, and an isolated right hepatic metastasis. He then required surgical re-exploration and further resection of both local recurrence and further peritoneal implants 6 and 9 years postoperatively.

Pulmonary metastases in the absence of disseminated disease are best dealt with by thoracotomy and resection. Salvage rates may be as high as 20% in properly selected patients.[14]

Local recurrences must be dealt with on an individual basis. Akwari et al.,[11] in 23 reexplorations performed on 20 patients with small-bowel tumors, found that further resection was possible on only eight occasions. In the three patients requiring a second re-exploration, nothing further could be accomplished. In the eight patients who underwent further resection, survival was not thought to be altered, except in one in which an acute small-bowel obstruction was relieved. This experience is clearly in contrast to the cases reported by Kohno et al.[13] described above. Shiu et al.[10] reported ten patients with resectable local recurrence in whom secondary procedures included pancreaticoduodenectomy in one, abdominoperineal resection in two, and pelvic exenteration in one. Survival times of 2 months to 10 years were noted, with a median survival of 25.5 months, compared with a 10.5-month median survival for those patients with initially unresectable lesions. The lone disease-free survivor at 9 years underwent total pelvic exenteration for a recurrent low-grade leiomyosarcoma invading the prostate. The approach to local recurrence must be tempered by a thorough un-

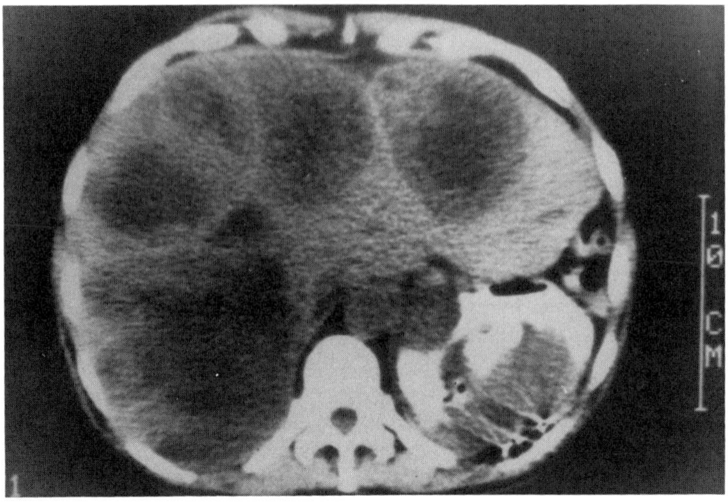

FIG 11–2.
Computed tomography scan demonstrates multiple liver metastases from a gastric leiomyosarcoma.

derstanding of the extent and morbidity of the procedure required to obtain adequate surgical margins. The outcome seems to be equally dependent on the biology of the tumor and the extent of the resection.

In summary, approximately 50% of gastrointestinal leiomyosarcomas will be resectable for cure. In the remainder, palliative resection can achieve local control of the symptomatic aspects of these tumors and can prolong median survival. Long-term prognosis in these cases is dependent on the histological grade of the tumor and the presence and extent of distant disease. Long-term survival following resection of low-grade recurrences and metastases has been reported.

NODAL METASTASES

Most investigators now acknowledge the small but finite incidence of lymph node metastases from gastrointestinal leiomyosarcomas. Lee[15] found reports of 7% to 13% in a review of series in which there were no efforts at radical resection. Lee suggested that more systematic radical resection of corresponding lymphatic drainage areas might reveal a higher incidence of occult nodal disease and might lower the rate of local and regional recurrence. A more important issue is the significance of lymph node metastases in this disease, where they often occur late in the course. Shiu at al.[10] noted that all three of their patients with intestinal leiomyosarcomas and documented nodal metastases ultimately died of their disease. The presence of lymph node metastases may predict poor long-term survival, and routine lymphadenectomy may simply be of prognostic rather than therapeutic benefit. The number of cases of nodal metastases is sufficiently small, and the reported follow-up so incomplete, that this is conjectural. Further information is required.

ESOPHAGEAL LEIOMYOSARCOMA

Esophageal leiomyosarcomas are extremely rare; only 57 cases had been reported in the world literature as of 1982.[16] They make up approximately 0.1% to 0.5% of all esophageal malignancies and about 10% of all esophageal smooth muscle tumors. The remainder are benign leiomyomas.[17, 18] There is a slight male predominance, and distribution appears to be equal throughout the length of the esophagus. These tumors present in two ways: 68% are polypoid and relatively noninvasive, and the remaining 32% are infiltrating and locally invasive,[16] which can lead to perforation (Fig. 11–3). The polypoid lesions become symtomatic relatively late, accounting for the observation of Skandalakis et al.[1] that 87% of esophageal leiomyosarcomas were greater than 5 cm in diameter. However, Franklin et al.[16] found only a 16% incidence of

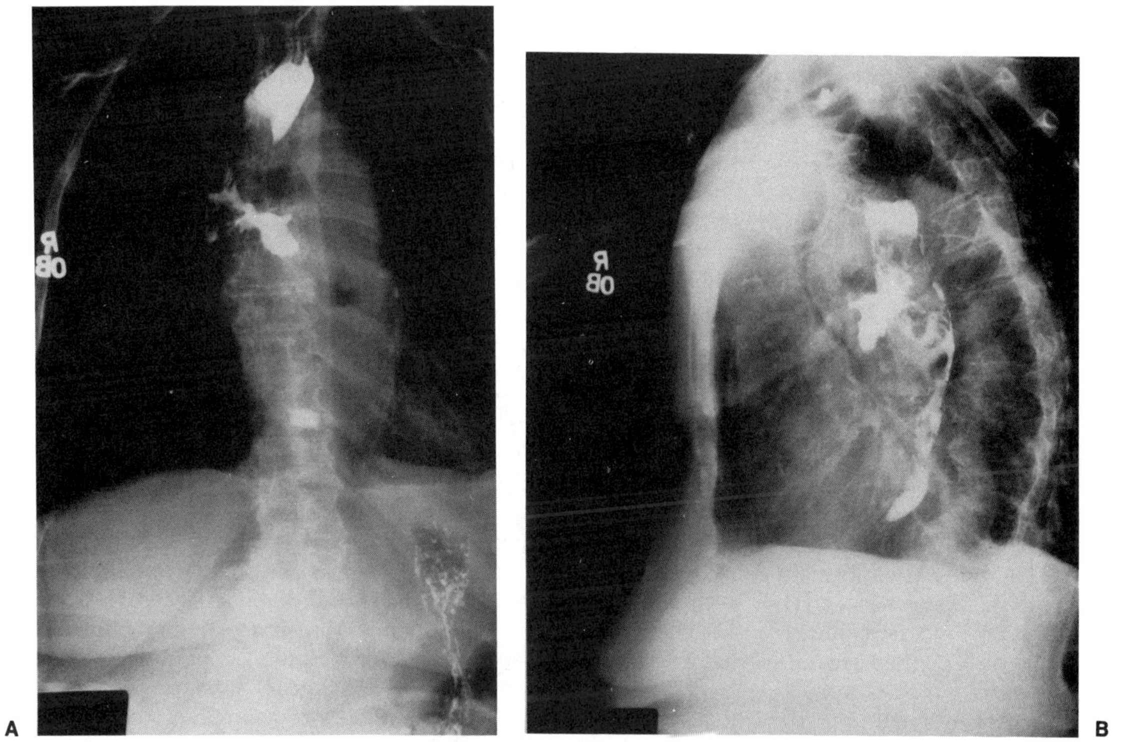

FIG 11–3.
A, an 80-year old female presented with dysphagia and weight loss (60 lb.). Upper gastrointestinal series showed a large esophageal mass. **B,** contrast extravasated from the esophageal lumen anteriorly into the body of this leiomyosarcoma.

documented metastasis, with liver, mediastinum and mediastinal nodes, and pericardium the most frequent sites.

The propensity of this tumor to remain localized suggests an aggressive surgical approach. Early surgical results were hampered by high operative mortality and incomplete follow-up. Nevertheless, Franklin et al.[16] were able to document a 26% 5-year survival rate in those patients who underwent resection, and "many others" were alive and well at 2 years. Esophagectomy is the procedure of choice for this tumor, although case reports have appeared of long-term survival following simple local excision of small, pedunculated lesions.[19]

In patients with unresectable or locally recurrent disease, transient palliative benefit has been observed in the few patients treated with radiotherapy.[16] The role of chemotherapy has yet to be defined.

Finally, it should be noted that leiomyosarcomas of the esophagus do not always occur in isolation. Approximately 10% have been noted to occur in association with a simultaneous and separate squamous cell carcinoma. Prognosis is limited by the more aggressive epithelial primary. This is distinct from the leiomyosarcoma that occurs as the mesodermal component of esophageal carcinosarcomas. These rare, usually polypoid lesions tend to remain superficial and do not invade locally or metastasize until late in their course. As such, they are thought by some to carry a prognosis similar to pure esophageal leiomyosarcomas, although this is not universally accepted.[20,21]

GASTRIC LEIOMYOSARCOMA

The stomach is the most common site of gastrointestinal leiomyosarcoma. Of all gastric smooth muscle tumors, 25% to 33% are malignant. Sarcomas make up approximately 1% to 3% of all primary gastric malignancies, of which over 90% are leiomyosarcomas. Others include neurogenic fibrosarcomas, liposarcomas, and angiosarcomas, of which only case reports can be found. The focus of this section will be on the leiomyosarcomas.[1, 2, 22]

Typically these tumors occur in patients in their sixth and seventh decades, with a roughly equal sex incidence. Symptoms tend to be nonspecific, with weight loss, epigastric fullness or mass, and upper gastrointestinal bleeding predominating. The pattern of presentation correlates with the relative endogastric or exogastric component of the individual lesions.[23] Symptomatic tumors tend to present late and are often found in the proximal two thirds of the stomach, frequently with prominent exogastric components. Diagnosis is rarely made pre-operatively. Upper gastrointestinal radiographic series are sensitive but not often specific, unless a gastric mass with a central cavity that communicates with the stomach is seen (Fig 11–4). More often an intact mucosa is found (Fig. 11–5) and endoscopic biopsy then usually fails to sample tumor tissue. [24–27]

At presentation, approximately 66% of these lesions are resectable for cure. In the remainder, resection is limited by local invasion of vital structures such as the celiac axis, peritoneal carcinomatosis, bilobar hepatic metastases, or, much less common, extra-abdominal spread.[26] Lymph node metastases at presentation are extremely rare. [2, 7, 8] Most investigators think that this finding makes extensive nodal dissection unnecessary for control of local disease. As long as an adequate surgical margin can be attained (arbitrarily defined as 4–5 cm), a resection of all gross disease is thought to be adequate. Lee[2] suggests that for lesions less than 5 cm in diameter a wedge resection is sufficient. For larger lesions a formal subtotal gastrectomy with omentectomy is advised to decrease the incidence of local recurrence. Skandalakis et al.[1] and Stavorovsky et al.[3] have documented omental metastases. Others have advocated the more aggressive total gastrectomy when dictated by the anatomy of the tumor, along with en bloc resection of adjacent viscera (liver, colon, pancreas, spleen). Even with negative surgical margins and these extensive procedures, however, survival and local recurrence rates continue to be influenced by tumor grade.[7]

Efforts have been made to discern prognostic factors in patients with gastric leiomyosarcomas, not only to aid in the selection of initial therapy but also to identify those patients at risk of failure of initial surgical control, in whom trials of adjuvant therapy might be of benefit. The two largest series to analyze these factors recently are from M. D. Anderson[7] (Houston, Texas) and Memorial Sloan-Kettering (New York).[8] Both series identify three main prognostic variables: size of the primary tumor, histological grade of the tumor, and stage of disease at presentation. as noted earlier, Shiu et al.[8] found a 57% 5-year survival rate in those patients with tumors greater than 5 cm but without adjacent organ involvement, while all patients with resected smaller tumors survived over the same period. Lindsay et al.[7] confirmed this, noting median survivals of 83 and 15.5 months in patients with tumors less than or greater than 8 cm, respectively.

Shiu's criteria for establishing histological grade have been described, and they correlate well with prognosis. The data from Lindsay's series tended to confirm this. In addition, Lindsay et al. found no differences in survival among epithelioid, pleomorphic, or spindle cell types. The most important histological variable in both of these series, as well as in prior studies, was the mitotic rate. Stage of disease at presentation was also important. Lindsay et al.[7] found that in patients with tumor confined to the stomach the median survival was 84 months; with transmural involvement this fell to 14 months. In patients with disseminated disease at presentation the median survival was only 5 months. Finally, as mentioned above, Shiu et al.[8] found no 5-year survivors among six patients undergoing extensive en bloc resection for tumor invading adjacent viscera.

Overall survival following resection for cure ranges from 35% to 50% at 5 years, substantially better than that for gastric adenocarcinoma. With none of the unfavorable prognostic indicators present (high grade, large tumor, extragastic tumor), this survival approached 100%. With one indicator present Shiu et al.[8] found 77% of patients surviving 5 years. With two present, survival was 19%.

The pattern of tumor recurrence tends to be intra-abdominal, as hepatic metastases, as peritoneal sarcomatosis, or as local perigastric recurrence. Lymphatic as well as extra-abdominal spread to lung, bone, and brain remains unusual, even in advanced stages of the disease. Radiotherapy has little to offer, either as primary or adjuvant treatment, although there are case reports of transient responses. The role of chemotherapy remains to be formally defined, but

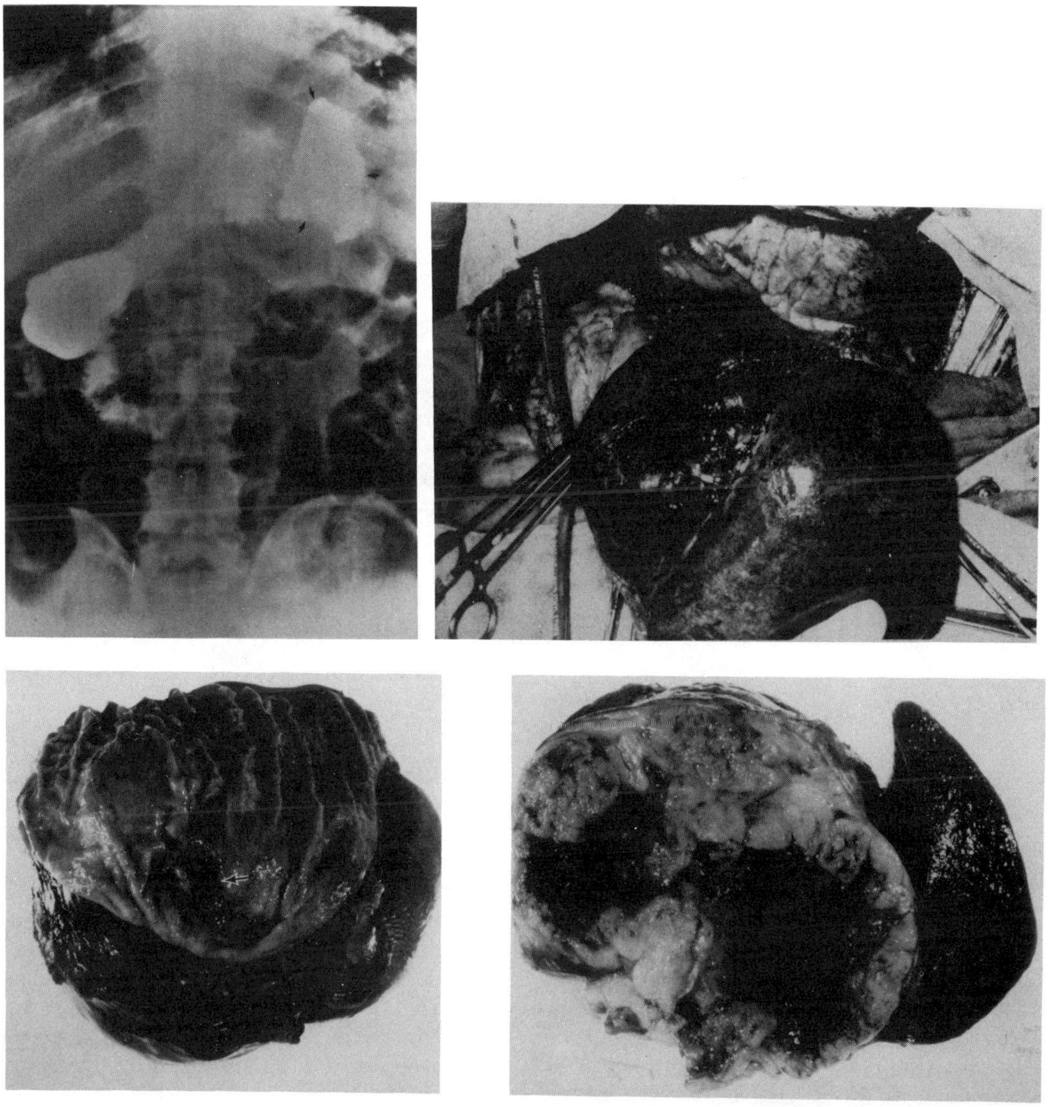

FIG 11–4.
A, a 67-year-old male presented with a 50-lb weight loss and weakness. An upper gastrointestinal series showed a gastric ulcer over a gastric mass, with extravasation of contrast into the mass (*arrows*). **B,** this gastric leiomyosarcoma was exposed through a left thoraco-abdominal incision. It arose from the gastric fundus and was attached to the spleen. **C,** the opened stomach revealed the gastric ulcer and fistula opening (*arrow*). **D,** central cavities are seen in the sectioned tumor. (From Lindsay PC, Ordonez N, Raaf JH: *J Surg Oncol* 1981; 18:399–421.)

encouraging results in the treatment of other soft tissue sarcomas may find application in the unresectable or recurrent gastric leiomyosarcomas.

Finally, and of uncertain biological significance, there appears to be an unduly high incidence of associated neoplasms prior, concurrent, or subsequent to the appearance of gastric leiomyosarcomas. Noted but not quantified by Skandalakis et al.,[1] this association was found by Shiu et al.[8] to be as high as 27% of patients with second or even third cancers. Chander et al.[28] and Carney[29] collected a series of 24 patients in whom multiple gastric epithelioid leiomyosarcomas occur as the most frequent expression of a triad that also included pulmonary chondro-

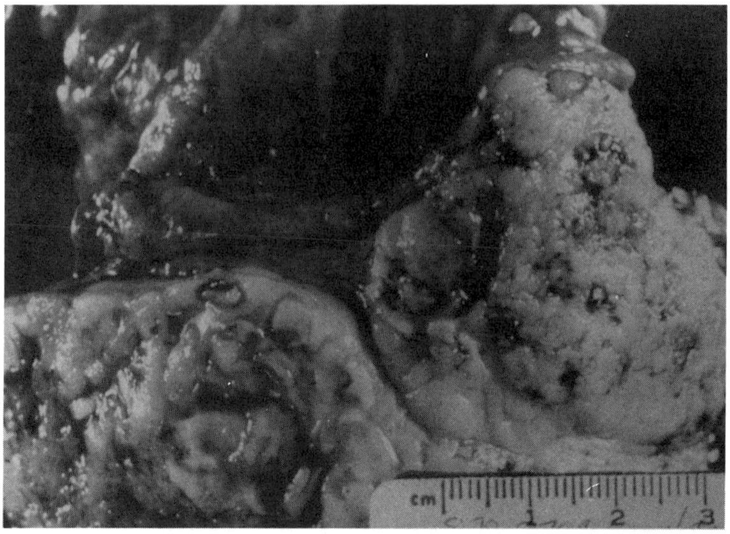

FIG 11–5.
A 66-year-old male developed left flank pain and decreased appetite. Gastroscopy suggested an extrinsic lesion along the greater curvature. Endoscopic biopsies were negative for tumor. His gastric leiomyosarcoma was found at operation to be covered by an intact gastric mucosa. (From Lindsay PC, Ordonez N, Raaf JH: *J Surg Oncol* 1981; 18:399–421.)

mas and functioning extra-adrenal paraganglioma, manifest primarily in young women.

In summary, gastric sarcomas almost exclusively are leiomyosarcomas, presenting equally in males and females in the sixth and seventh decades of life. The treatment of choice is surgical, and the goal is an adequate tumor-free margin. Extensive lymph node dissection does not seem warranted, because lymph node metastases are quite rare, even in the late stages of the disease. Assuming resectability, prognosis is determined by three variables: the size of the tumor, its histological grade, and the presence of transmural penetration or adjacent organ invasion. For resectable tumors, the 5-year survival should approach 50%. Adjuvant modalities require further formal investigation.

SMALL BOWEL LEIOMYOSARCOMA

The small bowel is the second most common site of gastrointestinal leiomyosarcoma. These tumors make up some 11% to 20% of all primary malignancies of the small intestine. There is a slight male predominance, with presentation more often in the fifth and sixth decades of life. Occult gastrointestinal bleeding is the most common presenting sign, and the diagnosis is rarely made pre-operatively. Generally vascular, these tumors are often visualized on arteriography. In various series they are found to be 50% to 80% resectable for cure. Operatively they can be separated into two distinct groups: those in the duodenum, and those distal to the ligament of Treitz.[2, 30–32]

In the former category, Barkan et al.[33] reviewed a total of 123 cases of duodenal leiomyosarcoma collected from the literature up to 1982. These represent approximately 10% of all duodenal malignancies, with 80% located in the second and third portions. Their growth pattern is such that two thirds were exoenteric, again accounting for their relatively late presentation. Jaundice is unusual.[34] Approximately 30% have metastases at the time of diagnosis. Surgery with intent to cure in the remainder almost always entails pancreaticoduodenectomy, although sleeve resections of smaller lesions in the first, third, and fourth portions of the duodenum have been reported. The role of regional node dissection in this extremely rare tumor has not been clearly defined. As the incidence of benign and malignant smooth muscle tumors has been found by Skandalakis et al.[1] to be similar, every effort should be made to establish a histological diagnosis prior to definitive surgical treatment. If malignancy is suspected or confirmed, Skandalakis recommends omentectomy as well to include any occult metastatic spread. Prognosis depends on resectability. No 5-year survivors following palliative procedures have been reported, but up to 35% of patients undergoing resection for cure survive 5 years.[34]

Distal to the ligament of Treitz, operative decisions are more straightforward. Although lymph node metastases are clearly not so common as blood-borne spread to the liver or direct peritoneal implantation, Lee [15] found the incidence of nodal metastases to be in the range of 7% to 10%. Accordingly, Lee recommends including a formal resection of the corresponding small bowel mesentery when cure is the intent. This should not have any major effect on morbidity/mortality in the case of small bowel resection and may shed further light on the natural behavior of the tumor. Deck and Silberman[30] concur with this approach. Skandalakis et al.[1] recommend inclusion of omentum in the surgical specimen for the reasons stated above. Starr and Dockerty[12] include resection of peritoneal implants and resectable hepatic metastases. The value of this, as illustrated by Kolino et al.,[13] would have to be balanced against the operative risk.

As a pathological curiosity, it should be mentioned that leiomyosarcoma is the most common malignancy in Meckel's diverticulum, as reported by Haugen et al.[35] and confirmed by Skandalakis et al.[1] and Starr and Dockerty.[12]

The prognosis of small-bowel leiomyosarcoma is determined by many factors, including size, histological grade, and stage of disease at presentation.[9, 10] Of patients suitable for resection for cure, approximately 50% will survive 5 years.[10, 30] In patients with small localized tumors, 10-year survival approaching 90% has been reported.[9] On the other hand, Shiu et al.[10] found that all three patients with intestinal leiomyosarcomas and lymphatic metastases at the time of resection ultimately died of their disease. Also notable is the continued and steady attrition seen in patients whose follow-up lasted 10 years and longer.[10, 12] While these prognostic factors should encourage efforts to develop effective adjuvant programs for patients at risk for recurrence, the surveillance of those patients clearly must be long term.

The dichotomy between the fulminance of the case that recurs early and is rapidly fatal, and the indolence of the case that recurs late with prolonged survival, highlights the broad spectrum of intestinal leiomyosarcoma. In the absence of consistently reliable and available histological criteria, this spectrum can often be seen only in retrospect. This would support a relatively aggressive surgical approach to all but the clearly terminal patient.

COLORECTAL LEIOMYOSARCOMA

Colorectal leiomyosarcoma is distinctly unusual, accounting for only 0.1% to 0.3% of all colorectal malignancies.[2] These lesions occur more frequently in the rectum, particularly the low rectum, than in the colon, where they tend to be evenly distributed. Cho and Smith [36] described a patient with multiple colonic leiomyosarcomas. Colorectal leiomyosarcomas can be divided operatively into two categories: those of the colon and upper rectum, which can be removed transabdominally, and those of the middle and lower rectum, which require abdominoperineal resection.

For lesions of the appendix, colon, and upper rectum, a standard wide resection, including corresponding mesentery, is advised. Although there are no hard data to support routine radical resection over simple sleeve resection, the small but finite incidence of 5% to 8% lymph node metastases found in various series would seem to justify this approach. Skandalakis et al.[1] recommend omental resection, because metastases have been described, although the dominant sites of metastatic disease are the liver and peritoneum.[37]

The majority of rectal leiomyosarcomas are found in the lower third, near the dentate line.[38] Surgical treatment almost always requires abdominoperineal resection.[39, 40] Diamante and Bacon[41] reported an 86% recurrence rate following local resection alone. Deyden and Wilkinson[38] confirm this, finding an 85% recurrence rate following local resection. Speculation as to the role of adjuvant radiotherapy in decreasing the rate of local recurrence has not been confirmed in prospective studies, due to the paucity of patients. Stair et al.[40] advocate consideration of adjuvant chemotherapy in patients at risk for recurrence.

Colorectal leiomyosarcomas have a poorer prognosis than their more proximal counterparts. Berkley[42] reported only a 33% 1-year survival rate for colonic lesions. Rao et al.[43] amplified this, noting a 2-year disease-free survival rate of 20% and a 5-year survival rate of only

10%. Other series are only slightly more optimistic. Diamante and Bacon[41] reported a 25% 5-year survival rate, with half of those patients ultimately succumbing to their disease. Akwari et al.[11] found that approximately half of the large bowel leiomyosarcomas were resectable, with 5-year and 10-year survivals of 60% and 20%, respectively. Only one of 13 patients undergoing palliative resection was alive at 5 years. Tang and Selamed[44] reported five patients who underwent palliative resection; all were dead of their disease within 15 months. Prognostic variables of histological grade, local invasion, and presence of metastases at original operation have been discussed. Akwari et al.[11] found size to be less predictive than did other investigators. No major differences in survival following adequate wide resection are described between colonic and rectal lesions.

There does seem to be a small subset of patients with colonic leiomyosarcoma who may have a more guardedly optimistic prognosis. Posen and Bar-Maor[45] and Ein et al.[46] described a series of pediatric patients ranging from newborn to 4 years of age. With short follow-up from 7 months to 13 years, all of those who survived operation were alive and disease free, despite the fact that two of the infants presented with perforation. Angerpointner suggested that adjuvant chemotherapy might have a role in sustaining these results.[47] Continued long-term follow-up is clearly mandated to see if this pattern persists in the younger age group.

ASSOCIATED MALIGNANCIES

An unusually high incidence of associated primary malignancies has been reported in reviews of gastrointestinal leiomyosarcomas.[8, 11, 48, 49] Shiu et al.[8] reported 11 patients with gastric leiomyosarcomas who were found to have second or even third prior, synchronous, or subsequent malignancies. Three of the four patients with synchronous second primary tumors died postoperatively, reflecting the magnitude of the surgery required to address both problems. Of the remaining seven patients, five ultimately died of the nonsarcoma malignancy. The implications are clear: follow-up in these patients must include vigilant surveillance not only for recurrent leiomyosarcoma, but also for a subsequent primary cancer that could be the determinant of survival.

As mentioned, Carney[29] collected a series of 24 patients, primarily young women, in whom multiple gastric epithelioid leiomyosarcomas occur as the most frequent expression of a triad that includes pulmonary chondromas and extra-adrenal paragangliomas. Genetic studies are needed to clarify the etiology of this syndrome. However, it does broaden the differential diagnosis of newly appearing pulmonary nodules following resection of gastric leiomyosarcoma, especially in young women.

CONCLUSION

A review of gastrointestinal leiomyosarcomas has been presented with emphasis on surgical approaches and prognostic variables. Although in general these lesions tend to have a more favorable prognosis than their epithelial counterparts in the proximal gastrointestinal tract, distally they seem to be more difficult to control. Aside from that anatomic predisposition, however, there is a much more pronounced biological spectrum of disease, ranging from the fulminance of the lesion that recurs early with rapid fatality, to the indolence of the lesion that recurs late with prolonged survival. In the absence of consistently reliable and available histological data at presentation, this spectrum can often be appreciated only in retrospect. This would support a relatively aggressive surgical approach to all but the clearly terminal patient.[50, 51]

The issue of including lymphadenectomy with resection of a primary gastrointestinal sarcoma has not been resolved. Lymphatic spread is not the major and only rarely the sole mode of metastasis. Therefore, meticulous regional lymphadenectomy beyond inclusion of corresponding mesentery would not seem indicated at this time. The primary goal of curative surgery should be the provision of adequate margins histologically free of tumor, whenever safely possible. The role of nonsurgical modalities in the treatment of these tumors has yet to be defined.

REFERENCES

1. Skandalakis JE, Gray SE, Sheperd D, et al: *Smooth Muscle Tumors of the Alimentary Tract.* Springfield, Illinois, Charles C Thomas, 1962.
2. Lee MTY: Leiomyosarcoma of the gastroin-

testinal tract: General pattern of metastasis and recurrence. *Cancer Treat Rev* 1983; 10:91–101.

3. Stavorovsky M, Morag B, Stavorovsky H, et al: Smooth muscle tumors of the alimentary tract. *J Surg Oncol* 1983; 22:109–114.
4. Starr GF: Pathologic features of smooth muscle tumors. *JAMA* 1974; 229:1219–1220.
5. Delikaris P, Golematis B, Missitzis J, et al: Smooth muscle neoplasms of the stomach. *South Med J* 1983; 76:440–442.
6. Ranchod M, Kempson RL: Smooth muscle tumors of the gastrointestinal tract and retroperitoneum; a pathologic analysis of 100 cases. *Cancer* 1977; 39:255–262.
7. Lindsay PC, Ordonez N, Raaf JH: Gastric leiomyosarcoma: Clinical and pathological review of fifty patients. *J Surg Oncol* 1981; 18:399–421.
8. Shiu MH, Farr GH, Papachristou DN: Myosarcomas of the stomach: Natural history, prognostic factors, and management. *Cancer* 1982; 48:177–187.
9. Chiotasso PJP, Fazio VW: Prognostic factors of 28 leiomyosarcomas of the small intestine. *Surg Gynecol Obstet* 1980; 155:197–202.
10. Shiu MH, Farr GH, Egeli RA: Myosarcomas of the small and large intestine: a clinicopathologic study. *J Surg Oncol* 1983; 24:67–72.
11. Akwari OE, Dozois RR, Weiland LH, et al: Leiomyosarcomas of the small and large bowel. *Cancer* 1978; 42:1375–1384.
12. Starr GF, Dockerty MB: Leiomyomas and leiomyosarcomas of the small intestine. *Cancer* 1955; 8:101–111.
13. Kohno H, Nagasue N, Araki S, et al: Ten year survival after synchronous resection of liver metastasis from intestinal leiomyosarcoma. *Cancer* 1981; 47:1421–1423.
14. DeVita VT, Hellman S, Rosenberg SA: *Cancer: Principles and Practice of Oncology*. Philadelphia, J. B. Lippincott, 1982.
15. Lee MYT: Leiomyosarcoma of the gastrointestinal tract: Should we consider metastases to regional lymph nodes? *J Surg Oncol* 1980; 15:319–321.
16. Franklin GO, Antler AS, Thelmo WL, et al: Esophageal leiomyosarcoma. *NY State J Med* 1982; 82:1100–1103.
17. Partyka EK, Sanowski RA, Kozarek RA: Endoscopic diagnosis of a giant esophageal leiomyosarcoma. *Am J Gastroenterol* 1981; 75:132–134.
18. Balthazar EJ: Gastrointestinal leiomyosarcoma—unusual sites: Esophagus, colon, and porta hepatis. *Gastrointest Radiol* 1981; 6:295–303.
19. Rainer WG, Brus R: Leiomyosarcoma of the esophagus: Review of the literature and report of three cases. *Surgery* 1965; 58:343–350.
20. Talbert JL, Cantrell JR: Clinical and pathologic characteristics of carcinosarcoma of the esophagus. *J Thorac Cardiovasc Surg* 1963; 45:1–12.
21. Miranda FJ, Kallas KN, DaCosta EA, et al: Carcinosarcoma of the esophagus. *Int Surg* 1980; 65:463–467.
22. Cathcart PM, Cathcart RS, Yarbrough DR: Tumors of gastric smooth muscle. *South Med J* 1980; 73:18–20.
23. Taylor PH: Leiomyosarcoma of the stomach. *Br J Surg* 1969; 56:187–192.
24. Burgess JN, Dockerty MB, ReMine WH: Sarcomatous lesions of the stomach. *Ann Surg* 1970; 173:758–766.
25. Nauert TC, Zornoza J, Ordonez N: Gastric leiomyosarcomas. *Am J Radiol* 1982; 139:291–297.
26. Bedekian AY, Khankhanian N, Valdivieso M: Sarcoma of the stomach: Clinicopathologic study of 43 cases. *J Surg Oncol* 1980; 13:121–127.
27. ReMine WH: Gastric sarcomas. *Am J Surg* 1979; 120:320–323.
28. Chander S, Oliverio R, Fermon C, et al: Triad of neoplasms—leiomyosarcoma, functioning extra adrenal tumors, and pulmonary chondroma. *NY State J Med* 1981; 81:392–393.
29. Carnery JA: The triad of gastric epithelioid leiomyosarcoma, pulmonary chondroma, and functioning extra-adrenal paraganglioma: A five year review. *Medicine* 1983; 62:159–169.
30. Deck KB, Silberman H: Leiomyosarcomas of the small intestine. *Cancer* 1979; 44:323–325.
31. Barclay THC, Schapira DV: Malignant tumors of the small intestine. *Cancer* 1983; 51:878–881.
32. Awrich AE, Irish CE, Vetto RM, et al: A twenty five year experience with primary malignant tumors of the small intestine. *Surg Gynecol Obstet* 1980; 151:9–14.
33. Barkan A, Wooloch Y, Dintsman M, et al: Leiomyosarcoma of the duodenum—two case reports and a literature review. *Am J Procotol Gastroenterol Col Rect Surg* 32:18–21.

34. Dodds JJ, Beahrs OH: Leiomyosarcoma of the duodenum. *AM J Surg* 1963; 105:245–249.

35. Haugen OA, Pegg, SC, Kyle J: Leiomyosarcoma of Meckel's diverticulum. *Cancer* 1970; 26:929–934.

36. Cho KC, Smith TR: Multiple leiomyosarcoma of the transverse colon: Report of a case and discussion. *Dis Col Rect* 1980; 23:118–121.

37. Meijer S, Peretz T, Gaynor JJ, et al: Primary colorectal sarcoma. A retrospective review and prognostic factor study of 50 consecutive patients. *Arch Surg* 1990; 125:1163–1168.

38. Deyden WE, Wilkinson CA: Leiomyosarcoma of the rectum. *South Med J* 1978; 71:743–745.

39. Feldtman RW, Oram-Smith JC, Teears RJ, et al: Leiomyosarcoma of the rectum: The military experience. *Dis Col Rect* 1981; 24:402–403.

40. Stair JM, Stevenson DR, Schaefer RF, et al: Leiomyosarcoma of the rectum: Report of three cases. *J. Surg Oncol* 1983; 24:180–183.

41. Diamante M, Bacon HE: Leiomyosarcoma of the rectum; report of a case. *Dis Col Rect* 1967; 10:347–351.

42. Berkley KM: Leiomyosarcoma of the large intestine, excluding the rectum. *Int Surg* 1981; 66:177–179.

43. Rao BK, Kapur MM, Roy S: Leiomyosarcoma of the colon: A case report and review of literature. *Dis Col Rect* 1980; 23:184–190.

44. Tang CK, Selamed MR: Leiomyosarcoma of the colon exclusive of the rectum. *Am J Gastroenterol* 1975; 64:376–381.

45. Posen JA, Bar-Maor JA: Leiomyosarcoma of the colon in an infant. *Cancer* 1983; 52:1458–1461.

46. Ein SH, Beck R, Allen JE: Colon sarcoma in the newborn. *J Pediatr Surg* 1979; 14:455–457.

47. Angerpointner TA, Weitz H, Haas RJ, et al: Intestinal leiomyosarcoma in childhood—case report and review of the literature. *J Pediatr Surg* 1981; 16:491–495.

48. Bedekian AY, Khankhanian N, Heilbrun LK: Primary lymphomas and sarcomas of the stomach. *South Med J* 1980; 73:21–24.

49. Berg J, McNeer G: Leiomyosarcoma of the stomach—a clinical and pathological study. *Cancer* 1960; 13:25–33.

50. Ng E-H, Pollock RE, Munsell MF, et al: Prognostic factors influencing survival in gastrointestinal leiomyosarcomas: Implications for surgical management and staging. *Ann Surg* 1992; 215:68–77.

51. Ng E-H, Pollock RE, Romsdahl MM: Prognostic implications of patterns of failure for gastrointestinal leiomyosarcomas. *Cancer* 1992; 69:1334–1341.

Chapter 12

Desmoid Fibrosarcoma; Gardner's Syndrome

Oliver J. McAnena

John M. Daly

HISTORICAL BACKGROUND

The desmoid tumor is a rare lesion arising from the musculo-aponeurotic structures of the body. Microscopically, it is a pseudo-encapsulated infiltrative growth of well-differentiated collagenous fibroblasts and fibrocytes. Its pathological diagnosis can be difficult.[1] Its management must be based on an accurate diagnosis and understanding of the natural history of this unique tumor.

The classification of desmoid tumors into benign or malignant neoplasms has been controversial ever since Macfarlane first described an anterior wall desmoid in 1832.[2] The term "desmoid" arises from the Greek work *Desmos*, which means "band or tendon." It refers to the tendon-like consistency of the tumor and was first coined by Müller in 1856.[3] Paget in 1856 described the first case of extra-abdominal desmoids.[4] Despite this and other articles,[5] the concept of desmoid tumor as a lesion confined to the anterior abdominal wall prevailed for many years.

The predilection for the musculo-aponeurotic structures of the anterior abdominal wall was first noted by Sanger in 1884.[6] Rokitansky described its microscopic appearance in 1846,[7] while Bennet subsequently described the lesion in the English literature in 1849.[8, 9] In the 19th century and earlier part of the 20th century many pathologists classified desmoid tumors as low-grade fibrosarcomas. Wilks[10] alluded to the propensity for these lesions to recur locally after their removal. In 1935, Ewing[11] classified this tumor as a low-grade fibrosarcoma. In 1948, Musgrove and McDonald[12] described the desmoid as a benign neoplasm. In a further attempt to clarify the pathology of the desmoid, Stout, in 1954, coined the term "desmoid fibromatosis."[13] This classified the desmoid under the same heading as a palmar fibromatosis (Dupuytren's contracture), implying a benign natural history for this tumor. Confusion persisted until recently, when the Soft-Tissue Task Force (1977) classified desmoids as low-grade malignant neoplasms.[14] The aggressive nature of these tumors is now well documented.[15]

The failure of pathologists to agree on the microscopic distinction between fibromatoses, desmoid tumors, and fibrosarcomas continues.[16] Differentiation of fibromatoses from well-differentiated fibrous growths such as desmoid tumors is of great clinical importance. Microscopically, this can often be difficult or even impossible. However, the location of the tumor and its history influence the surgical management more than does its microscopic appearance.

Desmoid Tumors and Gardner's Syndrome

In 1958, Smith first noted the relationship of desmoid tumors to Gardner's syndrome.[17] Eldon J. Gardner became interested in a family ("kindred 109") that had a high incidence of colon cancer. A University of Utah premedical student, Eugene Robertson, called his attention to this family during a genetics class. Gardner has since provided a unique history of this family for over 30 years.[18] In his initial presentations,[19–21] he observed the association of multiple polyposis of the colon, osteomatosis, and soft-tissue tumors of the body surface. Smith's observation in 1958[17] added the association of desmoid tumors to Gardner's syndrome. In 1962, Fader et al.[22] noted the presence of unerupted supernumerary teeth in these patients. Additional manifestations have been recognized, including mesenteric fibromatosis,[23] duodenal polyps,[24] gastric polyps,[25] periampullary carcinoma,[26] and ileal adenomas.[27] Other conditions, such as bilateral fibromatosis of the breast,[28] papillary carcinomas of the thyroid,[29, 30] and adrenal adenomas,[31] have also been reported[32, 33] as part of the syndrome. With advances in molecular biology it has become increasingly likely that these conditions reflect varying degrees of penetrance of a single gene.

Traboulsi et al.[34, 35] noted multiple pigmented ocular fundus lesions in over 90% of 16 families with Gardner's syndrome. This suggests a widespread expression of the abnormal gene in the retinal pigment epithelial cells. They also proposed that these ocular lesions were specific for Gardner's syndrome among inherited diseases with gastrointestinal polyposis.[35]

Familial polyposis coli and Gardner's syndrome differ from other genetically linked polyposis syndromes in that they involve a high risk of colonic cancer. McKusick[36] contended that polyps in Gardner's syndrome were fewer and more scattered than colonic polyps in patients with familial polyposis coli. In 1975, Sachatello and Griffen[37] developed a working classification for hereditary polypoid diseases of the gastrointestinal tract. It has become increasingly apparent that the great majority of patients with familial polyposis have extracolonic manifestations. Numerous authors have recognized that both familial polyposis coli and Gardner's syndrome follow an essentially Mendelian autosomal dominant pattern. Gardner's syndrome represents a more complete phenotypic expression of the same genotype. DeCosse et al.[38] used the term "familial polyposis coli" to describe this condition in the absence of any extracolonic manifestations, to which the classification "Gardner's syndrome" is ascribed. Reports from Japan, however, demonstrate high incidence of occult osteomas in patients with familial polyposis coli even when no other extracolonic manifestations are apparent.[39]

Genetic Studies

The introduction of chromosomal banding techniques in the 1970s[40] led to extensive investigations into the genetic basis of transmission of these associated diseases. In vitro monolayer skin culture techniques for studying affected members at increased risk in families with heritable colon cancer syndromes were used to analyze chromosomal abnormalities in these patients and distinguish them from the general population. Rasheed et al.[41] reported an ability to distinguish Gardner's syndrome and familial polyposis coli cells from those of the general population with more than 70% accuracy using such methods.

An explanation of why Gardner's syndrome presents a number of different tissue abnormalities has been proposed.[42] A single gene may manifest itself in different ways (pleiotropy). Alternatively, a close cluster of genes may rearrange at different times during embryogenesis in different individuals, so that some or all members of one generation are free of any stigmata of the syndrome. Increased tetraploidy has been identified as a marker for Gardner's syndrome and familial polyposis coli and may be helpful in identification and follow-up for probands.[43]

Molecular genetics has provided new insights into the etiology of familial polyposis. This has also advanced our understanding of the origins of colon carcinoma[44] as the genes responsible for familial polyposis play major roles in the common sporadic form of colon cancer. The current molecular evidence is consistent with the Knudson anti-oncogene model.[45] The familial polyposis gene has been mapped to chromosome 5q, and these patients frequently show allele loss on chromosome 5q.[46–48] For familial polyposis, and presumably patients with Gardner's syndrome, the first event is loss of the allele on 5q. It is possible that the polyposis gene behaves as a tumor suppressor gene, or anti-oncogene. Allele loss on 5q could occur by partial chromosome deletion, total chromosome loss, or genetic recombination. The loss of the other allele may be by point mutation. Precise localization has placed the locus for familial polyposis very close to a new marker, YN5.48 (D5S81), which represents a further step toward isolation of the genetic defect. It also provides the opportunity for preclinical diagnosis of risk status for colon cancer in families that are segregating adenomatous polyposis.[49]

The c-*myc* gene, located on human chromosome 8q24,[50] has been implicated in colon carcinogenesis. It is believed to be essential for cell proliferation either directly or by affecting other gene products that are essential for cell proliferation.[41] Elevated expression of the c-*myc* gene is a marker for carcinoma involving the familial polyposis gene; elevated *myc* expression may be an essential part of the neoplastic phenotype in such tumors.[51]

The *ras* oncogene is also putatively involved in the transition of colonic polyps to carcinoma. Ras proteins are involved in the transmission of signals generated by ligand interactions with specific cell surface receptors.[41] Current evidence supports a model in which there are two requirements for initiation of neoplastic transformation of the colonic epithelium: disruption of the cell cycle regulating pathway by an event such as deregulation of c-*myc* expression, and activation of the signal transduction pathway by an event such as *ras* point mutation.[41] The implications of these findings for patients with Gardner's syndrome are significant in terms of novel therapeutic approaches, such as methods to suppress expression of the mutated gene.

Present evidence suggests that the penetrance of Gardner's syndrome is essentially 100%. The likelihood of a "skipped generation" is minimal if the patients are fully evaluated clinically.[52] It is conceivable that in utero diagnosis may be possible in the near future. This would allow accurate genetic counseling and vigilant follow-up of affected patients.

Incidence of Desmoid Tumors

The desmoid tumor is extremely rare. Few surgeons or pathologists gain experience with more than occasional cases in their lifetime. At Memorial Sloan-Kettering Cancer Center (New York), Posner et al. identified 144 cases between 1965 and 1984.[15] Only 33 cases were reported between 1945 and 1959 from the Institute of Pathology (Lund, Sweden), an incidence of two cases per year per 1 million population.[53] From an extensive epidemiological study in Finland the incidence of desmoid tumors among the Finnish population is between 2.4 and 4.3 new cases per 1 million population per annum.[54]

Among patients with Gardner's syndrome, the incidence of desmoid tumors in the "kindred 109" originally described by Gardner is 29%.[55] McAdam and Goligher[56] reported four cases in patients with familial polyposis coli and described 89 cases in reviewing the literature. In 1962, Schiffman[57] surveyed 90 cases of Gardner's syndrome in the literature and found desmoid tumors reported in 17%. Jones and Cornell[58] reported a similar incidence. Jarvinen et al.[59] in 1982 reported an incidence of 18% desmoid tumors in 34 patients with Gardner's syndrome. Although Hayry et al.[60] noted only one case of Gardner's syndrome, they also observed 80% of 80 patients with desmoid tumors to have multiple minor bone abnormalities. This contrasted with an incidence of less than 5% in the normal control population. It is likely that desmoid tumors occur either alone or in association with Gardner's syndrome. Diagnosis of a desmoid tumor should stimulate appropriate investigations to ascertain the presence of colonic polyps or other manifestations of Gardner's syndrome.

Masson and Soule,[61] in reviewing 34 head and neck desmoids between 1915 and 1964, recorded 284 cases of desmoid tumor in all sites seen at the Mayo Clinic during that period. One hundred and twelve tumors involved the abdominal wall, 104 involved the extremities, 27 the chest wall, and seven were in miscellaneous sites.

Desmoid tumors are more common in females, with a ratio of females to males of 4–5 to 1. Reitamo[62] defined four major age categories, each demonstrating different biological properties:

1. "Juvenile" desmoid tumors: predominantly extra-abdominal and in females.

2. "Fertile": almost exclusively abdominal and in fertile females.
3. "Menopausal": predominantly abdominal and with an almost equal sex ratio.
4. "Senescent": occurring in both males and females equally and in both abdominal and extra-abdominal sites.

The frequency of intra-abdominal desmoids almost equaled the frequency of occurrence in all other sites combined, in the study reported by Reitamo.[62] Thus the abdominal wall and abdominal cavity are the commonest sites for desmoid tumors.[63–65]

The desmoid can occur at any age and at any site where musculo-aponeurotic tissues are found, even in the spinal cord and cranium.[66] A desmoid has been reported also in the parotid gland.[67] They have been mistaken for bone tumors[68] and have been found in the bladder,[69] probably by direct invasion from the posterior rectus sheath. Occasionally they have been associated with cystosarcoma phyllodes and carcinoma of the breast.[70, 71]

ETIOLOGY

Having discussed the close relationship of desmoid tumors and Gardner's syndrome, it is likely that other factors, aside from the genetic aspect, are involved.

Estrogens

Desmoid tumors have a relatively high incidence among the fertile female population.[55, 59, 60, 64] Estrogens appear to influence the growth of desmoids, particularly those involving the anterior abdominal wall. A susceptible patient is at increased risk for an abdominal wall desmoid following laparotomy.[55, 72, 73] Lipschutz and Grismali,[74] in 1944, induced infiltrative connective tissue tumors in guinea pigs following administration of estrogenic substances. Pack and Ehrlich[75] reported regression of an inoperable desmoid following X-ray castration. Svanvik et al.[76] reported a 59-year-old male who grew an abdominal wall desmoid 4 years after initiation of high-dose estradiol treatment for prostatic cancer. The tumor disappeared when estrogen therapy was interrupted. Hayry et al.[77] and Reitamo et al.[54] studied hormone receptors in four desmoid tumors and found small quantities of estrogen receptors, but not progesterone receptors, in the tumor cytosol. They also found that the growth rate of desmoid tumors roughly followed the level of endogenous estrogen in females. In males and juvenile females, growth rate was significantly slower. Fertile females with desmoid tumors had a significant predisposition to overt estrogen predominance; fewer than expected displayed progesterone predominance.

Trauma

A history of trauma has been reported in both intra- and extra-abdominal desmoids. The trauma from parturition may contribute to the increased incidence among the fertile female population.[78] There is also an increased incidence of desmoids in postoperative abdominal wounds.[79] These findings suggest that trauma is involved in the initiation of fibroblastic change in individuals susceptible to desmoid tumors. Rupture from a hematoma within the rectus sheath and subsequent abnormal growth of fibroblasts may initiate desmoid tumor formation in susceptible individuals.[80, 81]

Welch[82] noted unusual collagen fiber formations within the cytoplasm of fibroblasts from a desmoid tumor and felt they represented a pathological process in collagen fiber formation. Subsequent reports of abnormal collagen synthesis and extracellular lysis suggest that desmoid fibroblasts lack an inhibitor to prevent abnormal collagen formation.[83] These reports are compatible with the hypothesis that Gardner's syndrome/familial adenomatous polyposis and desmoid tumors comprise a spectrum of one disease.

PATHOLOGY OF DESMOID TUMORS

In general, desmoid tumors are solitary and well-defined neoplasms. They have a hard, rubbery consistency, and their cut surface exhibits a whorled grayish-white appearance. Their size at presentation varies from a few centimeters to a lesion that covers the entire abdominal wall. They possess a pseudocapsule with multiple projections into the surrounding connective tissue. Recognition of this feature is crucial to the appropriate management of these tumors.

Microscopically, it consists of well-differentiated fibroblasts and fibrocytes. The degree of cellularity is variable, but there are few or no mitoses. The cells infiltrate the surrounding muscle, and occasionally sarcolemmal giant cells are identified.

The tumor commonly compresses or even invades muscles, tendons, nerves, periosteum, bone, and lymph nodes. They do not metastasize to lymph nodes or invade skin. Thick-walled, hamartomatous vascular channels exist within the tumor.[1] More detailed pathology is outlined in Chapter 4. Desmoids have been reported to metastasize, but only rarely.[1, 15]

As a result of the disparate reports regarding pathological classification, tumor biology, and treatment alternatives, the desmoid tumor remains a poorly understood neoplasm. At Memorial Sloan-Kettering Cancer Center, the desmoid tumor is classified as a low-grade fibrosarcoma. It is considered distinct from the "aggressive fibromatoses" that tend to recur, are locally destructive, and do not metastasize.[1, 15] The distinction from fibromatosis is made less difficult if the pathologist is given an adequate biopsy specimen.

DIAGNOSIS

As desmoid tumors are so rare, the primary concern is one of recognizing their existence. Many other more common conditions present as a mass in the extremity or on the trunk. An abscess, hematoma, juxta-articular inflammatory cyst, muscle herniation, granulomatous disease, benign neoplasia such as lipomas, neurofibromas, or any other soft-tissue sarcoma ought to be considered in the differential. In general most soft-tissue masses either resolve over a couple of weeks or mandate surgical removal.

Malignant fibrosarcoma poses considerable difficulty in differentiation from a desmoid, which is a low-grade, locally invasive tumor. The natural history of desmoids distinguishes them from benign fibromatoses. Occasionally, dermatofibrosarcoma protuberans, amelanotic melanoma, Kaposi's sarcoma, or sclerosing angioma create difficulties in clinical diagnosis.

On physical examination, abdominal wall desmoid tumors are relatively easy to distinguish from intra-abdominal masses. With contraction of the rectus abdominis muscle, intra-abdominal lesions are no longer palpable and desmoids on the anterior abdominal wall are more clearly outlined. On palpation, they are hard, rubbery masses greater than 5 cm in diameter and are not fixed to the overlying skin. They are usually painless. Following resection for polyposis coli and carcinoma, presentation of a hard mass within the abdominal wound may be mistaken for a metastatic deposit. In these patients, such a presentation should alert the clinician to a desmoid tumor.

One should look for other stigmata of Gardner's syndrome if a desmoid is discovered. There may be epidermoid cysts, osteomas, dental anomalies, or gastrointestinal manifestations of the disease.[84]

RADIOLOGICAL TECHNIQUES IN DIAGNOSIS

Desmoid tumors of the extremity may display a nonspecific soft-tissue mass on plain roentgenogram or xerogram. This often interrupts the intermuscular and soft-tissue planes. With an advanced lesion, a periosteal reaction may occur.[85] On plain abdominal radiographs visceral displacement or obstruction from a large intra-abdominal desmoid may occur.[86] With contrast studies, spiculation of the mucosa and associated mural changes are seen. Ureteral displacement with obstruction may be demonstrated on intravenous urography.

The desmoid is a nonspecific echo-free mass with poor enhancement on ultrasound.[87] It is indistinguishable from rhabdomyosarcoma,[88] hematoma, abscess, or metastatic disease. Gray-scale ultrasonography may demonstrate occasional dense internal echoes within a background of low- to medium-level echoes that are indistinguishable from mesenteric adenopathy.[89]

Angiographic appearances include arterial stretching, displacement, neovascularity, and tumor staining that subsequently may not correlate with histological appearances.[90] Occasionally, the angiogram is normal.[91] There may be a positive correlation between the aggressive behavior of the tumor and the angiographic features, but this is not certain.[92]

On computed tomography (CT) it appears as a dense, soft-tissue mass. The adjacent viscera are frequently displaced. This resembles a lymphoma of the mesentery, which usually has the distinguishing feature of associated retroperitoneal lymphadenopathy.[93] Computed tomography is useful in the work-up of symptomatic Gardner's syndrome/familial polyposis patients following colon resection to detect a desmoid tumor.

SURGICAL MANAGEMENT OF DESMOID TUMORS

Failure to recognize the malignant local behavior of this tumor has led to conflicting recommendations regarding surgical management. The natural history of untreated desmoid tumors, in general, is slow, relentless growth with invasion of contiguous structures. However, a small number of patients may have regression or stabilization of their tumors.[15]

The principles of surgical management of the desmoid tumor rest on a wide margin of resection on all sides of the tumor and no evidence of tumor on microscopic examination of the margin. Resection should include the underlying fascia.[94] In a multivariate analysis of 128 patients with the desmoid tumor, Posner et al.[15] documented a significant decrease in the rate of local recurrence in patients with adequate margins of excision versus marginal or inadequate excision ($p = 0.0002$). Wide margin or compartment resection was associated with a prolonged disease-free interval compared with less extensive procedures ($p = 0.02$). Conservative resection was more likely to result in less-than-adequate margins of resection than wide margin or compartmental resection (100% vs 27%).

The primary concern in the treatment of desmoid tumors is adequate excision of the tumor to prevent local failure. Because of the finger-like projections of tumor invading contiguous structures the risk of leaving residual disease is high. Every effort must be made at the first operation to eradicate all known disease. This will not always be technically feasible due to the site of the individual tumor. The following factors are predictive of local failure[15]:

1. Age between 18 and 30 years.
2. Presentation with recurrent disease.
3. Partial or limited margin excision.
4. Tumor at or close to the microscopic margin of resection.
5. Radiation therapy not administered for gross residual disease.

An accurate diagnosis of the desmoid warrants an adequate incisional biopsy. It is imperative to adhere to the principles applied to incisional biopsy of any soft-tissue tumor. The line of incision should be in the direction of subsequent resection. Hemostasis is mandatory because a secondary hematoma may necessitate a wider resection than was originally planned. The biopsy incision is sutured securely and not used for further dissection or excision. The specimen should be sent for frozen section and analyzed by an experienced pathologist. Confirmation of the diagnosis is necessary by frozen section or permanent fixation before proceeding to formal resection.

Formal resection is performed after complete change of gown, gloves, and instruments. The biopsy incision, together with an adjacent ellipse of skin, is removed with the resection specimen.[95] Before closing the defect formed by excision of the tumor, suspicious margins should be checked microscopically. For abdominal wall lesions, if the costal margin or iliac crest are close to the tumor they should be removed en bloc to preserve at least one intact, uninvolved fascial envelope on the excised tumor specimen. This principle has been advocated for many years.[96] The difficulties with closure of what might be a large defect on the abdominal wall are not insurmountable. The abdominal wall is elastic, and large defects can often be closed primarily. Polypropylene mesh (Marlex) may be required in some cases.[97] Closed suction drains decrease accumulation of serum between mesh and overlying skin. Hemostasis is vital to prevent hematoma formation and infection. The temptation to accept tumor at a margin to allow primary wound closure must be avoided as recurrence is inevitable. Occasionally a myocutaneous flap is required to close the defect.[98, 99] Pre-operative planning and patient's understanding and consultation are vital, particularly in these difficult cases. Assistance from a plastic surgery service should be sought where appropriate (Fig 12–1).

With recurrent abdominal wall desmoids, en bloc resection of intra-abdominal viscera may be necessary. Pre-operative CT and contrast studies help to identify involved organs. Pre-operative bowel preparation should be considered in these cases.

Intra-abdominal desmoids are difficult to treat. They commonly arise between the leaves of the mesentery or retroperitoneally. Of the original Gardner "kindred 109," 55% of the total number of desmoids developed within the mesentery.[100] The application of wide en bloc resection is usually not feasible as they are often intimately related to the blood supply of a large portion of the bowel.[101] Radical resection results in the short gut syndrome. Khorsand and Karakousis[102] recommend the following approach:

A B C

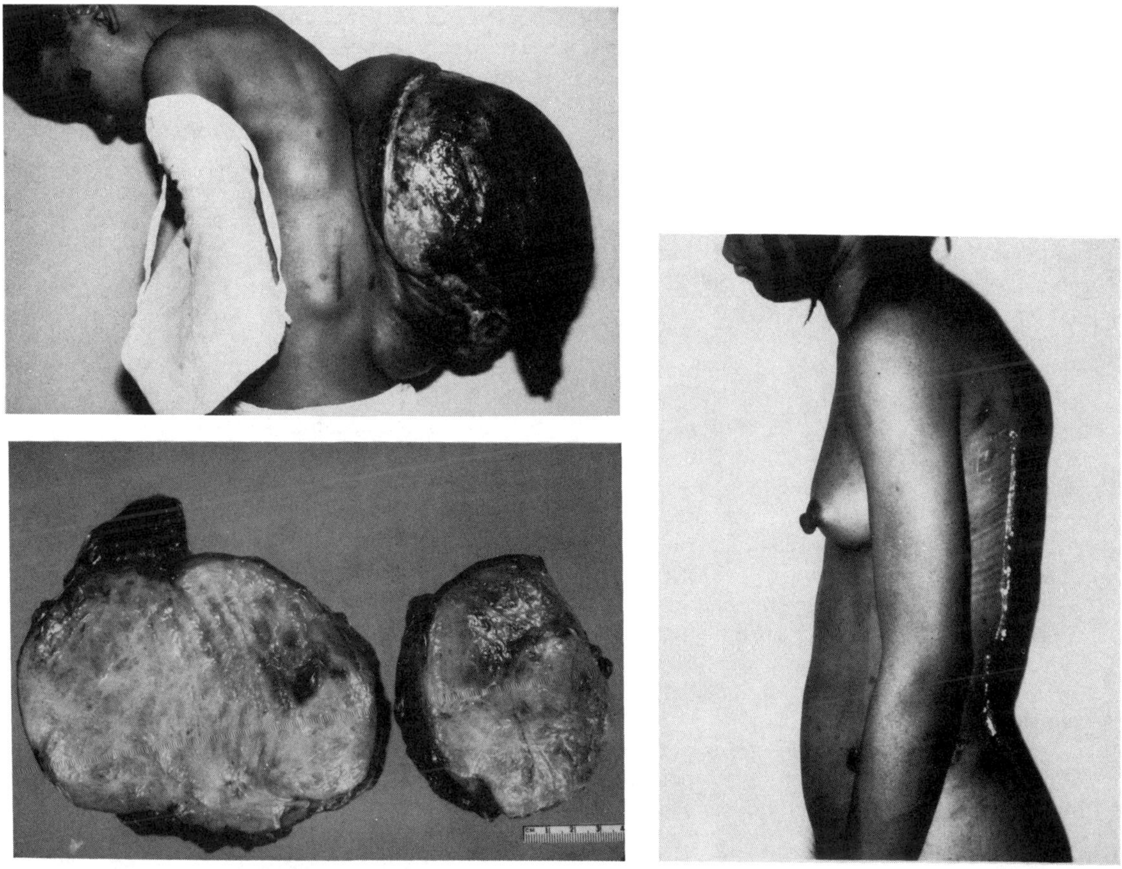

FIG 12–1.
A, a young Panamanian woman who presented with a desmoid fibrosarcoma in the soft tissue of the back, **B,** surgical specimen; **C,** primary closure of the surgical defect was possible without skin graft or myocutaneous flap. Several years later the patient developed colon cancer and died of metastatic colon carcinoma.

(1) lysis of adhesions and identification of the loops immediately proximal and distal to the tumor, (2) radial incisions in the peritoneal leaves of the mesentery proximal and distal to the tumor following visible vascular branches toward the base of the mesentery, a maneuver that leads directly to the surface of the superior mesenteric vein, which is exposed, and (3) ligation of the tributaries to the superior mesenteric vein from the involved mesentery, which are divided close to the surface of this vein. Tributaries from the distal uninvolved bowel are preserved. To the left of the vein and at a deeper plane, the superior mesenteric artery is exposed, and the branches supplying the involved portion of the mesentery are individually ligated and divided under direct vision. Thus the dissection proceeds safely, resectability is evaluated properly, and resection is completed with the maximum possible margin and the secure knowledge that the proximal and distal bowel will have an intact blood supply. Four of five patients treated in this way were alive from 2 to 8 years postoperatively. Unfortunately, complete resection is not always possible using this technique, and more radical procedures have been described.[103] These included pelvic exenteration and hemipelvectomy. The results for such procedures have been discouraging and in these cases consideration should be given to a small bowel bypass procedure for alleviation of symptoms. Adjunctive chemo- and/or radiation therapy, either by external beam or interstitial implants, may be appropriate in selected cases.

Patients who undergo colectomy for Gardner's syndrome/familial polyposis coli are at increased risk of subsequent intra-abdominal desmoids. In a review of 141 patients with familial polyposis, Sener et al.[104] found that 14 of 21 who also had desmoids developed the tumor within the abdomen following colon resection. The mean interval was 3.4 years. These patients are also at greater risk of postoperative small bowel adhesions.[104, 105]

The principles of management of desmoid tumors of the extremity are essentially the same as applied to any soft-tissue sarcoma. Limb preservation with adequate resection are the primary concerns. En bloc resection of major vessels may on occasion be required, necessitating use of autogenous or prosthetic graft material.[106] All previous incisions and biopsy paths are removed with the specimen without re-entering the paths. A wide expanse of muscular, tendinous, fascial, and aponeurotic structures contiguous with the area of known or palpable tumor is removed. The plane of surgical dissection should leave at least one fascial barrier on palpable or suspected tumor. Finally, the entire specimen is excised en bloc without at any time exposing or violating the tumor.[107]

Because of their position, desmoid tumors of the head and neck pose unique problems in management. Their presentation is similar to that of desmoid tumors in other areas of the body. They are more commonly found in the neck area than the head.[61] They may cause dyspnea or dysphagia and grow into the mediastinum with further compression of contiguous structures. Surgical management requires radical en bloc resection of the tumor with a margin of surrounding normal tissue, as far as is practicable. Masson and Soule[61] recommended radical neck dissection as the operation of choice when the tumor is first diagnosed, irrespective of its size at presentation. Desmoids at other sites such as the orbit[108] require exenteration, plastic reconstruction, and application of prosthetic materials where appropriate. As it is less likely that adequate margins of clearance can be obtained for desmoids involving the head and neck, the incidence of recurrence is expected to be higher than in other areas.

RADIATION TREATMENT OF DESMOID TUMORS

The role of radiation therapy in the management of desmoid tumors has been a subject of controversy for decades. In 1928 Ewing[109] observed that desmoid tumors responded slowly to radiation therapy. Some authors contend that there is no indication for radiation therapy, regardless of location.[63, 64] Others[56] propose that any beneficial effect from radiation therapy is secondary to its indirect effect on ovarian function, when used to treat abdominal tumors. Wara et al.[110] reported complete resolution of tumor mass in 13 of 16 patients without resorting to radical surgery. Kiel and Suit[111] recommend radiation therapy in those situations where wide-field resection without significant morbidity is not possible for gross local disease. If minimally positive margins exist after resection in a patient who may be followed carefully, frequent follow-up and prompt treatment at recurrence may be an effective alternative to immediate radiation therapy. Clearly, not all desmoids respond to radiation therapy, and most appear to need aggressive resection.[15] If at the time of initial operation it is felt that adjacent tissue planes are contaminated, postoperative radiation therapy appears to offer some benefit. Leibel et al.[112] concluded that radiation therapy may offer an excellent chance of local control in tumors that are not resectable due to their location or extension into surrounding tissues. Following resection, radiation treatment may prevent local recurrence when tumor is found at, or close to, the surgical margins, particularly when the lesion is in close proximity to bone or vital neurovascular structures.

The recommended tumor dose ranges from 40.8 to 61.2 grays (Gy). The majority of patients in Liebel's series received 50 to 55 Gy,[112] 1.6 to 1.8 Gy/fraction, five fractions per week. The radiation portals are designed to cover the tumor site with a generous margin.

CHEMOTHERAPY OF DESMOID TUMORS

There has been increasing interest in the applicability of chemotherapy in the treatment of desmoid tumors. Steroids were reported to be of some help[113] but the effect was far from dramatic. Combination chemotherapy has been used in isolated cases in children.[114, 115] This entailed a regimen of vincristine, actinomycin D, and cyclophosphamide. Such treatment regimens have been anecdotal and the exact role for combination chemotherapy at this time remains unclear.

Polynucleotides and theophylline have antitumor effects on the rate of intradermal growth of tumor cells in mice.[116] This effect is believed to be due in part to changes in AMP-mediated events in immunocompetent cells. Waddell and Gerner[117] reported diminution in size of multiple desmoid tumors in a patient following treatment with theophylline. Waddell[118] and Waddell et al.[119] subsequently reported the efficacy of indomethacin with high-dose ascorbic acid in the treatment of desmoid tumors. Conceivably, this effect results from their influence on cyclic AMP in tumor cells. Ornithine decarboxylase, inhibited by indomethacin, is critical for normal growth and the uncontrolled growth of malignancy. Another nonsteroidal drug, sulindac, has also been reported to cause regression of a desmoid tumor.[120]

Occasional reports have recommended tamoxifen in the treatment of desmoid tumors.[119, 121] The effect of estrogen blockade seems to be a restriction of RNA synthesis and alteration in transcription of genes involved in tumor growth.[122] The use of tamoxifen should be considered in selected cases although its precise role has yet to be defined.

SUMMARY

Radical tumor extirpation with resection of an adequate margin of surrounding normal tissue remains the single most important modality of treatment for desmoid tumors. Radiation therapy and various chemotherapeutic agents may be beneficial in selected cases. If there is any concern for the margins of resection, adjunctive radiation therapy should be given. Multimodal therapy should also be considered for mesenteric desmoid tumors, for which attempts at complete surgical resection are generally unsuccessful and carry a high risk of postoperative morbidity.

REFERENCES

1. Hajdu SI: *Pathology of Soft Tissue Tumors.* Philadelphia, Lea & Febiger, 1979, p 122.
2. Macfarlane J: in Robertson D (ed): *Clinical Reports of the Surgical Practice of the Glasgow Royal Infirmary.* 1832, p 63.
3. Müller J: in Berlin RG (ed):*Uber den finern bau and die Formen der Krankhaften Greschwulste.* 1838, p 80.
4. Paget J: Fibronucleated tumor of the abdomen of 14 years growth: Removal. *Lancet* 1856; 1:625.
5. Nichols RW: Desmoid tumors: a report of 31 cases. *Arch Surg* 1923; 7:277.
6. Sanger M: Uber desmoide greschwulste der bauchwand und deren operation mit resection des peritoneum parietale. *Arch Gynakol* 1884; 24:1–8.
7. Rokitansky C: *Handbuch der pathologischen anatomie.* Wein, Braumuller und Seidel, 1846, pp 1842–1846.
8. Bennet JH: *On Cancerous and Cancroid Growths.* Edinburgh, S and Knox (eds) 1849.
9. Bennet JH: Review on cancerous and cancroid growth. *Lancet* 1849; 2:429.
10. Wilks S: *Lectures on Pathological Anatomy.* London, Longman, 1859, p 467.
11. Ewing J: Fascial sarcoma and intermuscular myxoliposarcoma. *Arch Surg* 1935; 31–507.
12. Musgrove JE, McDonald JR: Extra-abdominal desmoid tumors: their differential diagnosis and treatment. *Arch Pathol* 1948; 45:513–540.
13. Stout AP: Juvenile fibromatosis. *Cancer* 1954; 7:953–958.
14. Russell WO, Cohen J, Enzinger F, et al: A clinical and pathological staging system for soft tissue sarcomas. *Cancer* 1977; 40:1562–1570.
15. Posner MC, Shiu MH, Newsome JL, et al: The desmoid tumor: Not a benign disease. *Arch Surg* 1989; 124:191–196.
16. Fine G, Hajdu SI, Morton DL, et al: Soft tissue sarcomas: Classification and treatment (a symposium). *Pathol Annu* 1982; 17:155–195.
17. Smith WG. Multiple polyposis, Gardner's syndrome and desmoid tumors. *Dis Col Rect* 1958; 1:323–332.
18. Gardner EJ, Burt RW, Friston JW: Gastrointestinal polyposis: Syndromes and genetic mechanisms. *West Med J* 1980; 132: 488–499.
19. Gardner EJ: A genetic and clinical study of intestinal polyposis, a predisposing factor for carcinoma of the colon and rectum. *Am J Hum Genet* 1951; 3:167–176.
20. Gardner EJ, Plank HP: Hereditary pattern for multiple osteomas in a family group. *Am J Hum Genet* 1952; 4:31–36.
21. Gardner EJ, Richards RC: Multiple cutaneous and subcutaneous lesions occurring simultaneously with hereditary polyposis

and osteomatosis. *Am J Hum Genet* 1953; 5:139–147.

22. Fader M, Kline SN, Spatz SS, et al: Gardner syndrome (intestinal polyposis, osteomas, sebaceous cysts) and new dental discovery. *Oral Surg* 1962; 15:153–172.
23. Simpson RD, Harrison EG, Mayo CW: Mesenteric fibromatosis in familial polyposis: A variant of Gardner's syndrome. *Cancer* 1964; 17:526–534.
24. Yao T, Iida M, Ohsato K, et al: Duodenal lesions in familial polyposis of the colon. *Gastroenterology* 1977; 73:1086–1092.
25. Hoffman DC, Goligher JC: Polyposis of the stomach and small intestine in association with familial polyposis coli. *Br J Surg* 1971; 58:126–128.
26. Jones TR, Nance FC: Periampullary malignancy in Gardner's syndrome. *Ann Surg* 1977; 185:565–571.
27. Hamilton SR, Bussey J Jr, Mendelsohn G, et al: Ileal adenomas after colectomy in nine patients with adenomatous coli/Gardner's syndrome. *Gastroenterology* 1979; 77:1252–1257.
28. Haggitt RC, Booth JL: Bilateral fibromatosis of the breast in Gardner's syndrome. *Cancer* 1970; 25:161–166.
29. Camiel MR, Mule JE, Alexander LL, et al: Association of thyroid carcinoma with Gardner's syndrome in siblings. *N Engl J Med* 1968; 278:1056–1058.
30. Keshgegian AA, Enterline HT: Gardner's syndrome with duodenal adenomas, gastric adenomyoma and thyroid papillary-follicular adenocarcinoma. *Dis Col Rect* 1978; 21:255–260.
31. Naylor EW, Gardner EJ: Adrenal adenomas in a patient with Gardner's syndrome. *Clin Genet* 1981; 20:67–73.
32. Gumpel RC, Carballo JD: A new concept of familial adenomatosis. *Ann Intern Med* 1956; 45:1045–1058.
33. McKittrick LS, Mallory TB, Talbott JH: Case records of the Massachusetts General Hospital. *N Engl J Med* 1935; 212:263–267.
34. Traboulsi EI, Krush AJ, Gardner EJ, et al: Prevalence and importance of pigmented ocular fundus lesions in Gardner's syndrome. *New Engl J Med* 1987; 316:661–667.
35. Traboulsi EI, Maumenee IH, Krush AJ, et al: Pigmented ocular fundus lesions in the inherited gastrointestinal polyposis syndromes and in hereditary nonpolyposis colorectal cancer. *Ophthalmology* 1988; 95:964–969.
36. McKusick VA: Genetic factors in intestinal polyposis. *JAMA* 1962; 182:151–157.
37. Sachatello CR, Griffen WO Jr: Hereditary polypoid diseases of the gastorintestinal tract: A working classification. *Am J Surg* 1975; 129:198–203.
38. DeCosse JJ, Adams MB, Condon RE: Familial polyposis. *Cancer* 1977; 39:267–273.
39. Doya K, Yamamoto H, Lay KM: Sclerotic masses in the mandible of a patient with familial polyposis of the colon. *J Oral Pathol* 1976; 5:305–311.
40. Borgaonkar DS: *Chromosomal Variation in Man: Catalog of Chromosomal Variants and Anomalies.* Baltimore, The Johns Hopkins University Press, 1975.
41. Rasheed S, Rhim JS, Gardner EJ: Inherited susceptibility to retrovirus induced transformation of Gardner syndrome cells. *Am J Hum Genet* 1983; 35:919–931.
42. Danes BS: In vitro studies on hereditary colon cancer. *Dis Col Rec* 1983; 26:475–478.
43. Danes BS, Boyle PD, Traganos F, et al: A standardized assay to identify colon cancer genotypes by in vitro tetraploidy in human dermal fibroblasts. *Dis Markers* 1986; 4:271–282.
44. Astrin SM, Costanzi C: The molecular genetics of colon cancer. *Semin Oncol* 1989; 16:138–147.
45. Knudson AG: Mutation and human cancer. *Adv Cancer Res* 1973; 17:317–352.
46. Bodmer WF, Bailey CJ, Bodmer J, et al: Localization for the gene for familial adenomatous polyposis on chromosome 5. *Nature Lond* 1987; 328:614–616.
47. Leppert M, Dobbs M, Scambler P, et al: The gene for familial polyposis coli maps to the long arm of chromosome 5. *Science* 1987; 238:1411–1413.
48. Okamoto M, Sasaki M, Sugio K, et al: Loss of constitutional heterozygosity in colon carcinoma from patients with familial polyposis coli. *Nature Lond* 1988; 331:273–277.
49. Nakamura Y, Lathrop M, Leppert M, et al: Localization of the genetic defect in familial adenomatous polyposis within a small region of chromosome 5. *Am J Hum Genet* 1988; 43:638–644.
50. Cole MD: The *myc* oncogene: Its role in transformation and differentiation. *Annu Rev Genet* 1986; 20:361–384.
51. Rothberg PC, Spandorfer JM, Erisman MD, et al: Evidence that c-*myc* expression defines two genetically distinct forms of

colorectal adenocarcinoma. *Br J Cancer* 1985; 52:629–632.

52. Naylor EW, Lebenthal E: Gardner's syndrome: Recent developments in research and management. *Dig Dis Sci* 1980; 25:945–949.
53. Dahn I, Jonsson N, Lundh G: Desmoid tumors: A series of 33 cases. *Acta Chir Scand* 1963; 126:305–314.
54. Reitamo JJ, Scheinin TM, Hayry P: The desmoid syndrome: New aspects in the cause, pathogenesis and treatment of the desmoid tumor. *Am J Surg* 1986; 151:230–237.
55. Naylor EW, Gardner EJ, Richards RC: Desmoid tumors and mesenteric fibromatosis and Gardner's syndrome. *Arch Surg* 1979; 114:1181–1185.
56. McAdam WAF, Goligher JC: The occurrence of desmoids in patients with familial polyposis coli. *Br J Surg* 1970; 57:618–631.
57. Schiffman MA: Familial multiple polyposis associated with soft-tissue and hard-tissue tumors. *JAMA* 1962; 179:287–300.
58. Jones EL, Cornell WP: Gardner's syndrome: Review of the Literature and report on a family. *Arch Surg* 1966; 92:287–300.
59. Jarvinen HJ, Peltokallio P, Landtman M, et al: Gardner's stigmas in patients with familial adenomatosis coli. *Br. J Surg* 1982; 69:718–721.
60. Hayry P, Reitamo JJ, Totterman S, et al: The desmoid tumor. II. Analysis of factors possibly contributing to the etiology and growth behaviour. *Am J Clin Pathol* 1982; 77:674–680.
61. Masson JK, Soule EH: Desmoid tumors of the head and neck. *Am J Surg* 1966; 112:615–622.
62. Reitamo JJ, Hayry P, Nykyri E, et al: The desmoid tumor. 1. Incidence, sex, age and anatomical distribution in the Finnish population. *Am J Clin Pathol* 1982; 77:665–673.
63. Brasfield RD, Das Gupta TK: Desmoid tumors of the abdominal wall. *Surgery* 1969; 65:241–246.
64. Kim DH, Goldsmith HS, Quan SH, et al: Intra-abdominal desmoid tumor. *Cancer* 1971; 27: 1041–1045.
65. Pearman RO, Mayo ChW: Desmoid tumors: A clinical and pathological study. *Ann Surg* 1942; 115:114–125.
66. Friede RL, Pollak A: Neurosurgical desmoid tumors: Presentation of four cases with a review of the differential diagnoses. *J Neurosurg* 1979; 50:725–732.
67. Majmudar B, Winiarski N: Desmoid tumor presenting as a parotid mass. *JAMA* 1979; 239:337–339.
68. Hardy R, Lehrer H: Desmoblastic fibroma vs. desmoid tumor of bone. *Radiology* 1967; 88:899–901.
69. Foote JW, Seemayer TA, Duignan JP, Desmoid tumor involving the bladder: case report. *J Urol* 1975; 114:147–149.
70. Abadir R: Desmoid tumor associated with cystosarcoma phyllodes of the breast. *J Surg Oncol* 1976; 8:43–48.
71. Kalisher L, Long J, Peyster RG: Extraabdominal desmoid of the axillary tail mimicking breast carcinoma. *AJR* 1976; 126:903–906.
72. Camiel MR, Solish GI: Desmoid tumor during pregnancy. *Am J Obstet Gynecol* 1982; 144:988–989.
73. Strode JE: Desmoid tumors particularly as related to their surgical removal. *Ann Surg* 1954; 139:335–340.
74. Lipschutz A, Grismali J: On the antifibromatogenic activity of synthetic progesterone in experiments with the 17-caprylic and diproprionic of G-estradiol. *Cancer Res* 1944; 4:186.
75. Pack GT, Ehrlich HE: Neoplasms of the anterior abdominal wall with special considerations of desmoid tumors: Experience with 391 cases and a collective review of the literature. *Int Abstr Surg Gynecol Obstet* 1944; 79:117–198.
76. Svanvik J, Knutsson F, Jansson R, et al: Desmoid tumor in the abdominal wall after treatment with high dose estradiol for prostatic cancer. *Acta Chir Scand* 1982; 148:301–303.
77. Hayry P, Reitamo JJ, Vihko R, et al: The desmoid tumor. III. A biochemical and genetic analysis. *Am J Clin Pathol* 1982; 77:681–685.
78. Pack GT, Ariel IM: Treatment of cancer and allied diseases, 2nd ed. VIII Hoeber Medical Division. *Tumors of the Soft Somatic Tissues and Bone.* New York, Harper and Row, 1964, pp 67–75.
79. Geschickter GF, Lewis D: Tumors of connective tissue. *Am J Cancer* 1935; 25:630–655.
80. Enzinger FM, Shiraki M: Musculoaponeurotic fibromatosis of the shoulder girdle (extra-abdominal desmoid): Analysis of thirty cases followed up for ten or more years. *Cancer* 1967; 20:1131–1140.
81. Urist MR: Trauma and neoplasm: Report

of a case of desmoid tumor following simple fracture of radius and ulna. *Am J Surg 1957; 93:682–693.*

82. Welch RA: Intracytoplasmic collagen formations in desmoid fibromatosis. *Am J Pathol* 1966; 49:515–535.
83. Allegra SR, Broderick PA: Desmoid fibroblastoma—intracytoplasmic collagenosynthesis in a peculiar fibroblastic tumor: Light and Ultrastructural study of a case. *Hum Pathol* 1973; 4:419–429.
84. Ilda M, Tsuneyoshi Y, Itoh H, et al: Natural history of duodenal lesions in Japanese patients with familial adenomatosis coli (Gardner's syndrome). *Gastroenterology* 1989; 96:1301–1306.
85. Rosen RS, Kimball W: Extra-abdominal desmoid tumor. *Radiology* 1966; 86:534–538.
86. Menuck LS: Abdominal desmoid masses in Gardner's syndrome. *Gastrointest Radiol* 1976; 1:81–84.
87. Wallace JHK: Ultrasonic diagnosis of abdominal wall desmoid tumor. *J Can Assoc Radiol* 1980; 31:120–122.
88. Goldberg B: Ultrasonic evaluation of superficial masses. *JCU* 1975; 3:91–94.
89. Baron RL, Lee JKT: Mesenteric desmoid tumors: Sonographic and computed-tomographic appearance. *Radiology* 1981; 140:777–779.
90. Miller EM, Newton TH: The angiographic appearances of extra-abdominal desmoid tumors. *Radiology* 1979; 132:305–308.
91. Yaghmai I: Angiographic features of fibromas and fibrosarcomas. *Radiology* 1977; 124:57–64.
92. Totterman S, Reitamo JJ: Desmoid tumors: An angiographic study of five cases. *Br J Radiol* 1979; 52:936–941.
93. Magid D, Fishman EK, Jones B, et al: Desmoid tumors in Gardner syndrome: Use of computed tomography. *AJR* 1984; 142:1141–1145.
94. Das Gupta TK, Brasfield RD, O'Hara J: Extra-abdominal desmoids: a clinical and pathological study. *Ann Surg* 1969; 170:109–121.
95. Shiu MH, Flanebaum L, Hajdu SI, et al: Malignant soft-tissue tumors of the abdominal wall. *Arch Surg* 1980; 115:152–155.
96. Bouffier AI: Fibrosarcoma of abdominal wall, desmoid fibroma beginning in Poupart's ligament, etc. *JAMA* 1899; 33:820–823.
97. Mungas JE, Platz CE, Block GE: Desmoid tumors of the abdominal wall. *Surg Clin N Am* 1976; 56:207–218.
98. Baffi RR, Didolkar MS, Bakamjian V: Reconstruction of sternal and abdominal wall defects in a case of desmoid tumor. *J. Thorac Cardiovasc Surg* 1977; 74:105–107.
99. Bogart JN, Rowe DS, Parsons RW: Immediate abdominal wall reconstruction with bilateral groin flaps after resection of a large desmoid tumor. *Plast Reconstr Surg* 1976; 58:716–718.
100. Richards RC, Rogers SW, Gardner EJ: Spontaneous mesenteric fibromatosis in Gardner's syndrome. *Cancer* 1981; 47:597–601.
101. Hoover JC Jr: Surgical aspects of hereditary intestinal polyposis. *Dis Col Rect* 1983; 26:409–412.
102. Khorsand J, Karakousis CP: Desmoid tumors and their management. *Am J Surg* 1985; 149:215–218.
103. Harvey JC, Quan SH, Fortner JG: Gardner's syndrome complicated by mesenteric desmoid tumors. *Surgery* 1978; 85:475–477.
104. Sener SF, Miller HH, DeCosse JJ: The spectrum of polyposis. *Surg Gynecol Obstet* 1984; 159:525–532.
105. Hunt RTN, Morgan HC, Ackerman LV: Principles in the management of extra-abdominal desmoids. *Cancer* 1960; 12:825–836.
106. Fortner JG, Kim DK, Shiu ME: Limb-preserving vascular surgery for malignant tumors of the lower extremity. *Arch Surg* 1977; 112:394.
107. Shiu ME, Hajdu SI: Management of soft tissue sarcoma of the extremity. *Semin Oncol* 1981; 8:172–179.
108. Craig RDP, Studd D: Extra-abdominal desmoid of the face involving the orbit. *Br J Surg* 1978; 65:131–134.
109. Ewing J: *Neoplastic Disease,* 2nd ed. Philadelphia, W. B. Saunders, 1928.
110. Wara WM, Phillips TL, Hill Dr, et al: Desmoid tumors—treatment and prognosis. *Radiology* 1977; 124:225–226.
111. Kiel KD, Suit HD: Radiation therapy in the treatment of aggressive fibromatoses (desmoid tumors). *Cancer* 1984; 54:2051–2055.
112. Leibel SA, Wara WM, Hill DR, et al: Desmoid tumors: Local control and patterns of relapse following radiation therapy. *Int J Radiat Oncol Biol Phys* 1982; 9:1167–1171.
113. Panos TC, Poth EJ: Desmoid tumor of the abdominal wall: Use of prednisone to pre-

vent recurrence in a child. *Surgery* 1959; 45:777–779.

114. Stein R: Chemotherapeutic response in fibromatosis of the neck. *J Pediatr* 1977; 90:482–483.

115. Hutchinson RJ, Norris DG, Schnaufer L: Chemotherapy: A successful application in abdominal fibrosis. *Pediatrics* 1979; 63:157–159.

116. Webb D, Braun W, Plescia OJ: Antitumor effects of polynucleotides and theophylline. *Cancer Res* 1972; 32:1814–1819.

117. Waddell WR, Gerner RE: Indomethacin and ascorbate inhibit desmoid tumors. *J Surg Oncol* 1980; 15:85–90.

118. Waddell WR: Treatment of intra-abdominal and abdominal wall desmoid tumors with drugs that affect the metabolism of 3′, 5′-adenosine monophosphate. *Ann Surg* 1975; 181:299–302.

119. Waddell WR, Gerner RE, Reich MP: Nonsteroid anti-inflammatory drugs and tamoxifen for desmoid tumors and carcinoma of the stomach. *J Surg Oncol* 1983; 22:197–211.

120. Belliveau P, Graham AM: Mesenteric desmoid tumors in Gardner's syndrome treated by sulindac. *Dis Col Rect* 1984; 27:53–54.

121. Kinsburner B, Ritter S, Rosenthal CJ: Tamoxifen induced remission of desmoid tumors. *Am Soc Clin Oncol* 1982; 1:180.

122. Itoh H, Ikeda S, Oohata Y, et al: Treatment of desmoid tumors in Gardner's syndrome. *Dis Col Rect* 1988; 31:459–461.

Chapter 13

Sarcomas of the Liver and Spleen*

Kamal G. Ishak

Ronald A. Malt

LIVER

Even if all reported diagnoses are considered valid, primary sarcomas of the liver are rare.[1–3] A survey from this country based on death certificates from 1966 to 1973 disclosed 205 hepatic sarcomas.[4] Of these, about 36% were angiosarcomas, 12% were leiomyosarcomas, and 7% were fibrosarcomas; the type of sarcoma was unspecified in 44%. The accuracy of the death certificate diagnosis is questionable, inasmuch as fewer than half the so-called angiosarcomas were subsequently confirmed.[4]

Because specific carcinogens such as Thorotrast (a thorium dioxide suspension) and vinyl chloride are among the known causes of angiosarcoma, etiological agents and promoting factors are likely to be demonstrable for other sarcomas, thus facilitating their prevention. The origin of sarcomas from the pseudocapsule of a pyogenic abscess[5] and the capsule of a hydatid cyst[6] suggests the promoting effects of cell proliferation in a field exposed to a potentially sarcoma-producing agent.[7, 8] Although potent chemotherapy now exists for rhabdomyosarcoma, sooner or later therapy for other sarcomas will be developed, ideally based on the inhibition of specific steps in cellular biochemistry and understanding of the etiological circumstances.

Most of the tissues of mesodermal origin composing the liver are susceptible to sarcomatous change: fibrous tissue—*fibrosarcoma;* smooth muscle—*leiomyosarcoma;* blood vessels—*Kaposi's sarcoma, epithelioid hemangioendothelioma,* and *angiosarcoma* (*malignant hemangioendothelioma*), and undifferentiated mesenchyme—*undifferentiated sarcoma.* Mixtures of several types of sarcomas are designated *malignant mesenchymomas.* Although *rhabdomyosarcomas* arise in the extrahepatic bile ducts, on occasion they can grow into the liver. Other sarcomas officially recognized by the World Health Organization,[2] such as *liposarcoma, malignant fibrous histiocytoma, lymphangiosarcoma, malignant mesothelioma,*

* The opinions or assertions contained herein are the private views of the authors and are not to be construed as official or as reflecting the views of the Army or the Department of Defense.

myxosarcoma, and *chondrosarcoma,* either have not been reported or are so rare as not to warrant discussion. A number of sarcomas (fibrosarcoma, chondrosarcoma, osteogenic sarcoma, or unclassified) have been reported to occur concurrently with primary carcinomas of the liver.[9–14] The will not be alluded to further because of their extreme rarity and the difficulty of ruling out "spindled-out" carcinomas (pseudosarcomas) in some of these reported instances. Carcinosarcomas (admixtures of carcinoma, either hepatocellular or cholangiocellular, and various sarcomatous elements)[15–20] also will not be discussed. To our knowledge, fewer than 20 primary non-Hodgkin's lymphomas of the liver have been reported,[21–24] two of which occurred in patients with acquired immune deficiency syndrome (AIDS).[22–24]

At present, resection is the best single hope for palliation or cure of hepatic sarcomas, irrespective of cell type. The value of precise histopathological classification to facilitate adjunctive therapy remains to be determined by future investigations.

Symptoms and Signs

Common to all hepatic sarcomas are symptoms related to their large bulk, or to necrosis or hypermetabolism ("tumor fever"). An erroneous diagnosis of hepatic abscess is sometimes entertained. By invading the hepatic and portal venous system, some sarcomas, for example angiosarcoma, can lead to acute portal hypertension and/or the Budd-Chiari syndrome. Some fibrosarcomas produce hypoglycemia by consuming glucose, secreting insulin or an insulin-like substance such as nonsuppressible insulin-like activity, inhibiting gluconeogenesis and lipolysis, depleting glycogen stores, or by destruction of pituitary, adrenal, or hepatic compensatory mechanisms that stimulate gluconeogensis.[25–27] All sarcomas are liable to intraperitoneal rupture and bleeding. Occasionally, the presenting symptoms and signs are related to invasion of adjacent viscera and organs or to distant metastases.

Natural History and Pathology

Fibrosarcoma.—Only about 13 cases of primary hepatic fibrosarcomas are known.[2, 5, 28–39] The age range of patients with this tumor is 30–73 years (median, 55 years). Men account for 11 of 13 (85%) of the total number of cases.

Most patients whose outcome is known die soon after diagnosis or surgery. One patient given radiotherapy lived 5 years, another 3 years, and a third patient survived for at least 1 year.

Grossly, fibrosarcomas of the liver are usually large; one of the largest weighed over 7 kg.[2] They are often well circumscribed and have a grayish-white cut surface, which may have a whorled appearance; areas of necrosis and hemorrhage (which may be cystic) are often noted (Fig. 13–1). Microscopically, these nonecapsulated tumors are composed of spindle-shaped cells arranged in interlacing bundles that may form a "herringbone" pattern (Fig. 13–2). Varying numbers of collagen fibers (arising from the tumor cells) are admixed with the sarcoma cells. The nuclei are hyperchromatic and elongated and have pointed ends; mitotic figures are present in variable numbers (Fig. 13–3).

Leiomyosarcoma.—Like leiomyomas and leiomyosarcomas of the uterus, leiomyosarcomas can be gigantic, 11.2 kg perhaps being a record.[40] There are 17 reported cases.[41, 42] These tumors occur more frequently in women, whose mean age at presentation is 52 years. The majority of patients have an upper abdominal mass, which may be continuous with the liver. About half the patients also have abdominal pain, weight loss, or both. In one patient, the diagnosis was established by peritoneoscopic biopsy.[43] The mean survival is 20 months,[41] the longest survival being 6.5 years following resection.[40]

Perhaps because they arise outside the liver and invade it, leiomyosarcomas of the ligamentum teres seem to be less aggressive than those that originate within the liver and spread through vascular channels. Of seven patients whose tumors were resected,[42] one survived for 2 years and another for 4 years.[2]

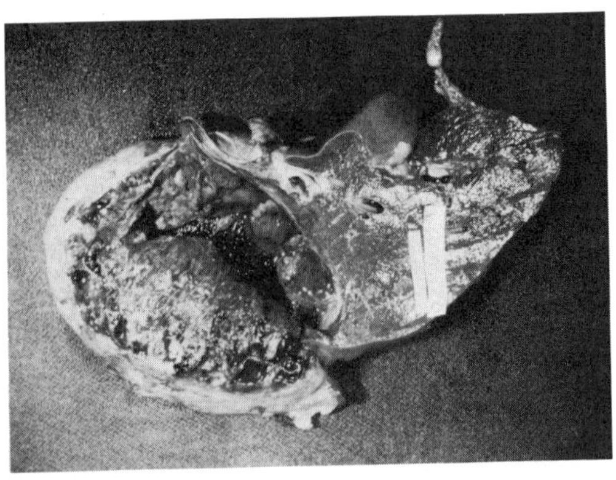

FIG 13–1.
Well-circumscribed fibrosarcoma with large area of hemorrhagic necrosis.

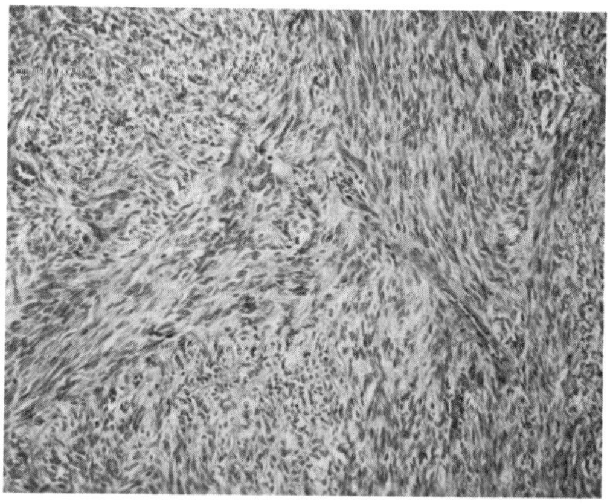

FIG 13–2.
Fibrosarcoma shows intersecting bundles of spindle-shaped cells. (Hematoxylin-eosin; ×60.)

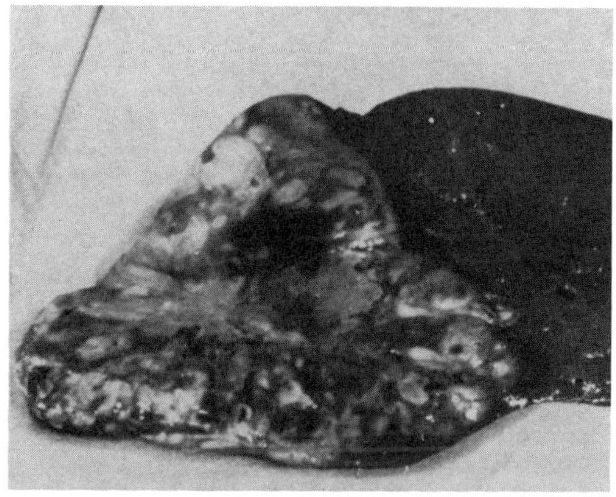

FIG 13–4.
Leiomyosarcoma is well circumscribed and has a variegated cut surface with areas of hemorrhage (dark).

The Budd-Chiari syndrome, leading to swift death, is characteristic of leiomyosarcoma arising from the hepatic veins.[44, 45] The consequences of hepatic invasion by leiomyosarcomas of the inferior vena cava, such as hematuria, proteinuria, and edema of the lower extremities, are less severe than those of chronic vena caval or renal vein obstruction from other causes.[46]

Grossly and microscopically, leiomyosarcomas of the liver resemble similar tumors in other organs and tissues. They are often well circumscribed, but nonencapsulated and moderately firm to soft in consistency (Fig. 13–4). The cut surface is pinkish-white to light tan, with yellow areas of necrosis or red-brown foci of hemorrhage. Microscopically, the leiomyosarcoma is composed of intersecting bundles of spindle cells (Fig. 13–5). The cytoplasm is eosinophilic and may exhibit longitudinal myofibrils. Desmin can be demonstrated in the cytoplasm by immunohistochemical techniques (Fig. 13–6). Nuclei, which may show palisading, are elongated and have blunt ends; they often reveal considerable variation in size and are hyperchromatic (Fig. 13–7). Mitosis are frequently observed. An ultrastructural study of one case revealed myofilaments, cystoplasmic dense bodies, and marginal dense plaques.[47]

Angiosarcoma.—Angiosarcoma is the most common hepatic sarcoma in the United States, with new cases appearing annually, and a total of over 200 worldwide.[4, 48] A nationwide survey of hepatic angiosarcoma in the United States

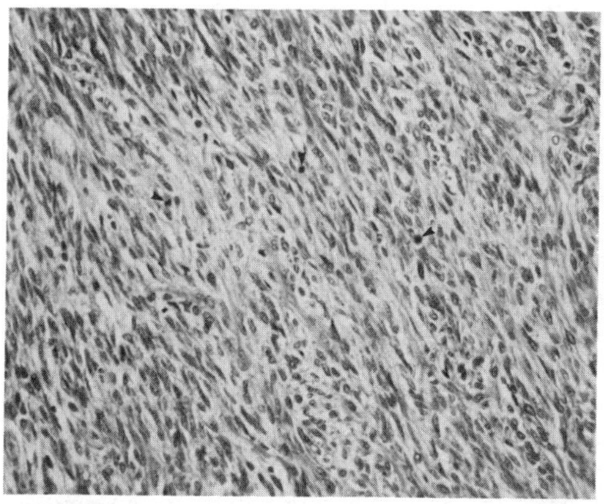

FIG 13–3.
Frequent mitoses (*arrowheads*) are noted in fibrosarcoma cells. (Hematoxylin-eosin; ×250.)

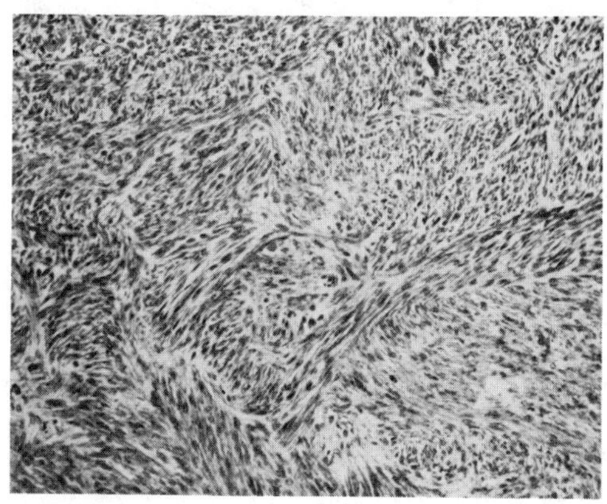

FIG 13–5.
Leiomyosarcoma is composed of intersecting bundles of elongated spindle-shaped cells. (Masson trichrome; ×160.).

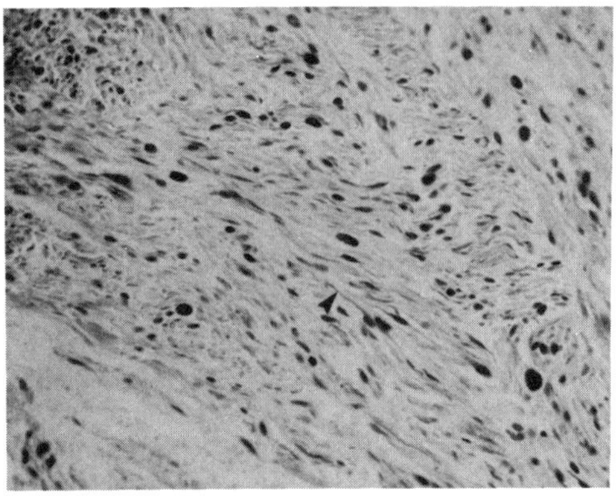

FIG 13–6.
Cytoplasm of leiomyosarcoma cells (darkly stained; *arrowhead*) contains desmin. (Peroxidase-antiperoxidase stain; ×160.)

from 1964 through 1974 identified 168 cases; only 25% of the tumors could be attributed to known causes such as Thorotrast, vinyl chloride, inorganic arsenic, and androgenic-anabolic steroids.[4] Damage by radiochemical derivatives is likely to be responsible for the effects of Thorotrast, a colloidal suspension of thorium dioxide (70% of which eventually lodges in the liver) that was being used for angiographic procedures until the mid-1950s.[49–51] The latent period after a single exposure is 12 to 30 years.[50] Thorotrast may also cause hepatocellular carcinoma and cholangiocarcinoma[51–53]; the latter is the most frequent Thorotrast-associated tumor in Japan.[53]

Exposure to vinyl chloride can lead to endothelial damage in the sinusoids, abnormalities

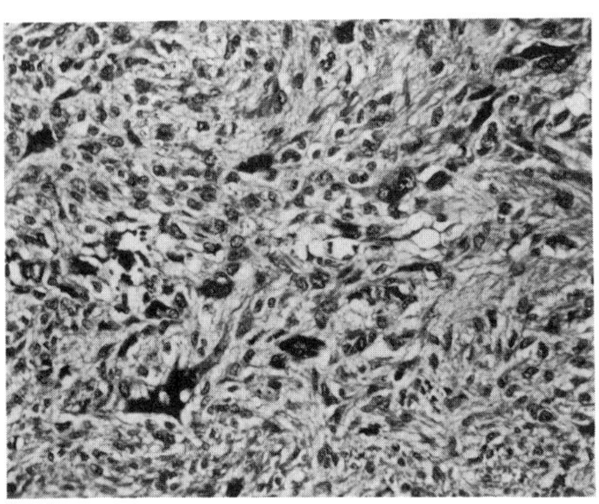

FIG 13–7.
Nuclei of leiomyosarcoma cells exhibit prominent variation in size and are darkly stained. (HE ×250). (Hematoxylin-eosin; ×250).

in DNA, focal hepatocytic hyperplasia, hepatic fibrosis, and angiosarcoma.[54–61] Even angiosarcomas (and hemangiomas) of the penis may develop,[62] and we have seen an unusual massive capillary hemangioma of the liver in an employee of a polyvinyl chloride factory. Other sources of nonindustrial exposure[59] include the use of vinyl chloride as a propellant in aerosol sprays and as an anesthetic agent. Although few new cases are being recognized, the latent period of 12 to 28 years makes it certain that more will come to light.

The carcinogenic mechanism of arsenic is unknown, even though it has long been associated with basal cell and squamous cell skin cancers. Field workers and vintners in the vineyards of the Mosel region in Germany have been at risk of hepatic angiosarcoma from exposure to arsenic-containing insecticides,[63] as were patients given Fowler's solution (potassium arsenite) for the treatment of psoriasis and other diseases.[64] In childhood, the latent period may be short,[65] however, 33 years passed before a 45-year-old man developed angiosarcoma after a 6-month medicinal exposure.[66] The latent period in Mosel vintners was 12 to 17 years.[63]

Although more frequently associated with hepatocellular carcinoma,[67–69] methyltestosterone and other anabolic steriods have manifested carcinogenicity (after a latency of about 6 years) by producing angiosarcoma in some boys thus treated for Fanconi's syndrome or aplastic anemia.[55] Oral contraceptives,[70] phenelzine[71] copper, synthetic estrogens, and hemochromatosis have also been implicated in the etiology of an angiosarcoma.[2, 4]

The peak incidence for angiosarcoma of the liver is in the sixth and seventh decades of life, and the male-to-female ratio is 3:1.[4] The modes of presentation include[2] (1) symptoms and signs of liver disease (61.8%), including hepatomegaly, abdominal pain, ascites, anorexia, nausea, occasional vomiting and jaundice—weight loss and fever occur in some patients; (2) signs and symptoms due to hemoperitoneum from rupture of the tumor (14.5%); (3) splenomegaly, with or without pancytopenia (5.5%); and (4) symptoms and signs referable to metastases to the skeleton or lungs (9.1%). Laboratory tests demonstrate anemia (sometimes a microangiopathic hemolytic anemia),[72] leukocytosis (65.6%), or leukopenia (21.9%), and thrombocytopenia (62.5%). Disseminated intravascular coagulopathy has been reported.[72, 73] Tests of liver function reveal elevation of the total serum bilirubin (greater than 10 mg/dL) in 60% of cases. Increased alkaline phosphatase activity (64%), bromsulphalein (BSP) retention (100%), and increased aminotransferase values (usually below 200 kallikrein units [KU]) have been noted in less than half the patients, and a prolonged prothrombin time (72%). Radiographically, there is displacement of various viscera, elevation of the right hemidiaphragm, and multiple defects in hepatic scans.[2, 72] Plain films of the abdomen invariably show specifically the liver, spleen, and lympth nodes because of the retained Thorotrast. Hepatic angiography can usually suggest the correct diagnosis,[59, 72] although a definitive diagnosis can be established only by liver biopsy.

Resection is usually not feasible because of the multicentric nature of the tumor. Most patients die within 3 months and almost all within a year.[2] The most frequent causes of death are hepatic failure or intra-abdominal bleeding. Spontaneous rupture of a hepatic angiosarcoma has been diagnosed by computed tomography.[74] Hepatic artery ligation and 5-fluorouracil therapy have resulted in some regression,[75] and spontaneous compression of the hepatic artery, oral 5-fluorouracil therapy, and radiotherapy have been followed by survival for at least 18 months.[76] In the experience of Dannaher et al.,[59] chemotherapy can lead to reduction in liver size or tumor size; one of seven patients who received chemotherapy lived 56 months from the time of diagnosis.

Grossly, angiosarcoma usually consists of multiple hemorrhagic foci or grayish white tissue alternating with hemorrhagic foci (Fig. 13–8). The tumor foci or nodules vary from a few millimeters to several centimeters in diameter. Both lobes are usually involved.

Microscopically, the tumor is composed of malignant endothelial cells with several or many of the following features: large, elongated cells with irregular, hyperchromatic nuclei; an eosinophilic cytoplasm; ill-defined cell borders; numerous mitoses; bizarre forms; and giant cell formation. The malignant cells either line preexisting vascular channels or form new ones (Fig. 13–9 and 13–10). Factor VIII-related antigen may be identified in tumor cells by immunohistological stains. Solid sarcomatous masses resembling fibrosarcoma may be seen (Fig. 13–11). Foci of extramedullary hematopoiesis are often present within the neoplastic vascular channels. Tumor cells rarely may display phagocytic activity. Invasion of intrahepatic portal and hepatic veins is a frequent finding (Fig. 13–12).

Thorotrast-related cases show coarsely granular, pink-brown deposits in cells of the reticuloendothelial system of the liver or lying free in the portal connective tissue (Fig. 13–13). α-Particle radiation from the thorium dioxide in Thorotrast can be demonstrated by autoradiography. The particles can easily be seen by scanning electron microscopy (Fig. 13–14) and the element thorium definitively identified by energy-dispersive X-ray microanalysis (Fig. 13–15).

Epithelioid Hemangioendothelioma.—Epithelioid hemangioendothelioma, a recently reported hepatic neoplasm,[77] can also be primary in the lung, where it has been termed "intravas-

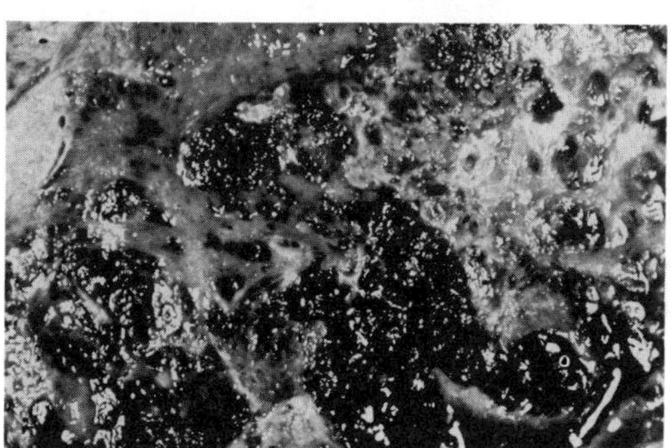

FIG 13–8.
Cut section of liver involved by angiosarcoma shows blood-filled cavitary lesions alternating with solid (white) neoplastic tissue.

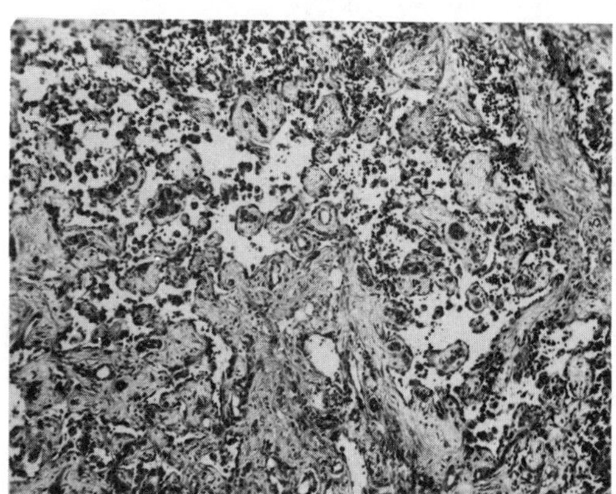

FIG 13–9.
Angiosarcoma cells line irregular vascular channels with subsequent destruction of hepatic plates. (Hematoxylin-eosin; ×90.)

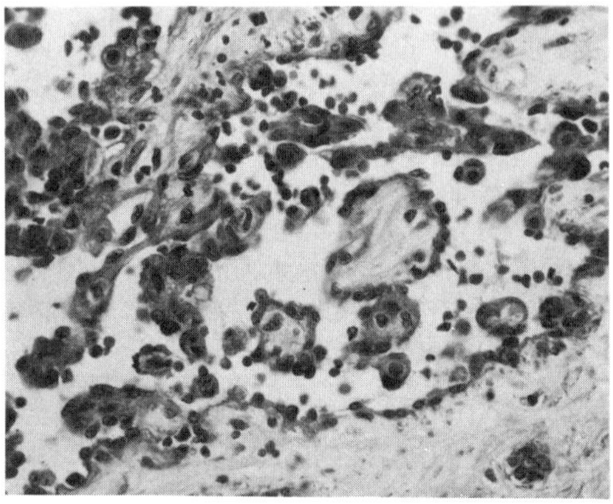

FIG 13–10.
Angiosarcoma cells line newly formed vascular channels and form tufts that project into the lumen. (Hematoxylin-eosin; ×350).

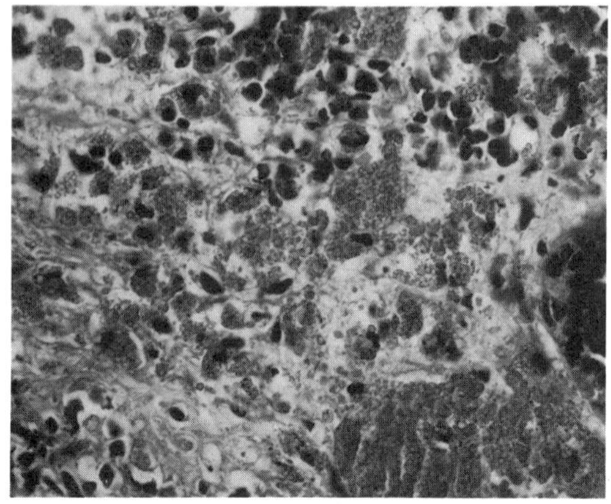

FIG 13–13.
Thorotrast particles are coarsely granular and extracellular. (Hematoxylin-eosin; ×630).

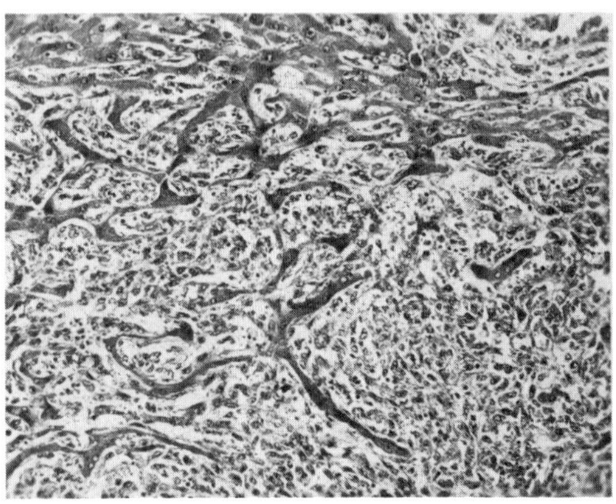

FIG 13–11.
Compact fibrosarcoma-like area in an angiosarcoma. (Hematoxylin-eosin; ×130).

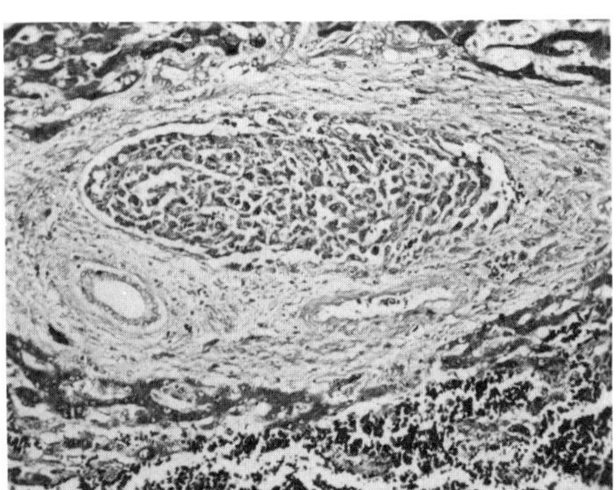

FIG 13–12.
Intrahepatic branch of portal vein is filled with angiosarcoma. (Hematoxylin-eosin; ×130).

cular bronchioloalveolar tumor,"[78] or in soft tissues.[79] It occurs more frequently in women (62.5%) than in men (37.5%). Ages of the 32 patients described in Ishak et al.[77] ranged from 19 to 86 years (average age, 50 years). The tumor was discovered incidentally in four patients. Four patients had jaundice attributable to the tumor, and one of them developed liver failure. One patient presented with an acute abdomen due to hemoperitoneum. The remaining patients had nonspecific complaints.

Nine of the 32 patients survived 5 years or more.[77] Six are alive at 5 years (two patients), two at 9 years, one at 12 years, and one at 15 years. Three patients died 7, 10, and 28 years after initial diagnosis, respectively.

Grossly, the tumors are often multiple and involve both lobes of the liver. They are gener-

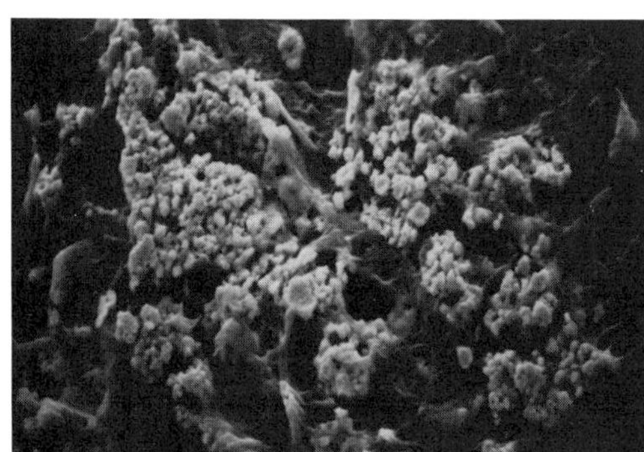

FIG 13–14.
Thorotrast particles revealed by scanning electron microscopy. (×1,250).

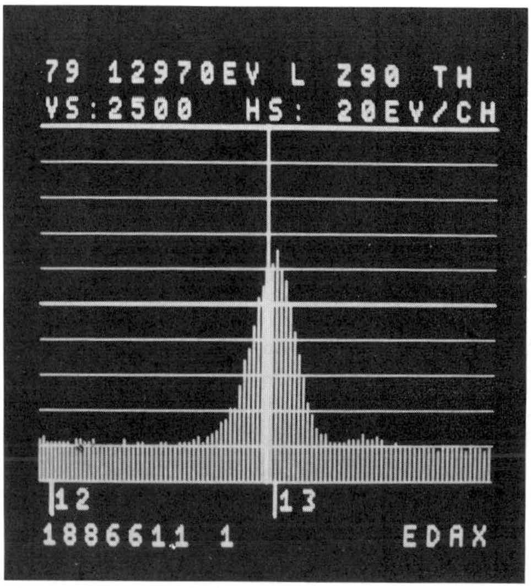

FIG 13–15.
The element thorium is positively identified in Thorotrast particles (in Fig. 13–14) by energy-dispersive X-ray microanalysis.

ally white, and firm to hard in consistency. Microscopically, the neoplastic cells infiltrate sinusoids and intrahepatic veins of all sizes. After destroying the hepatic cell plates, they form new vascular channels. Two types of tumor cells are recognized: dendritic and epithelioid (Figs. 13–16 to 13–18); they often synthesize factor VIII-related antigen (Fig. 13–19). Although the prognosis is much more favorable than for angiosarcoma, extrahepatic metastases do occur in

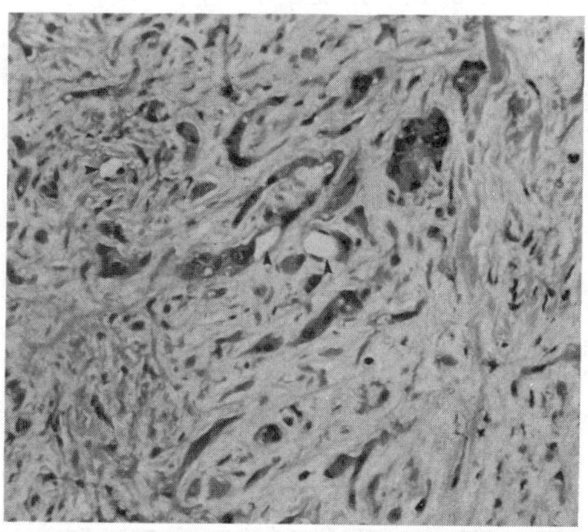

FIG 13–16.
Epitheloid hemangioendothelioma. Dendritic cells have replaced hepatic parenchyma and are forming new vessels (*arrowheads*). (Hematoxylin-eosin; ×630).

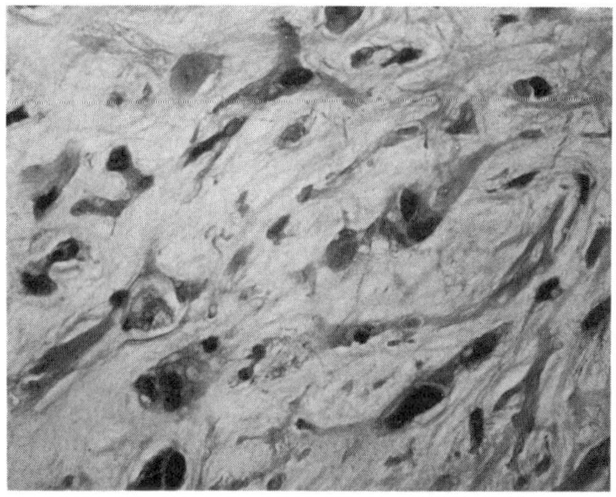

FIG 13–17.
Dendritic cells of epithelioid hemangioendothelioma have many thin processes extending into the supporting stroma. (Hematoxylin-eosin; ×250).

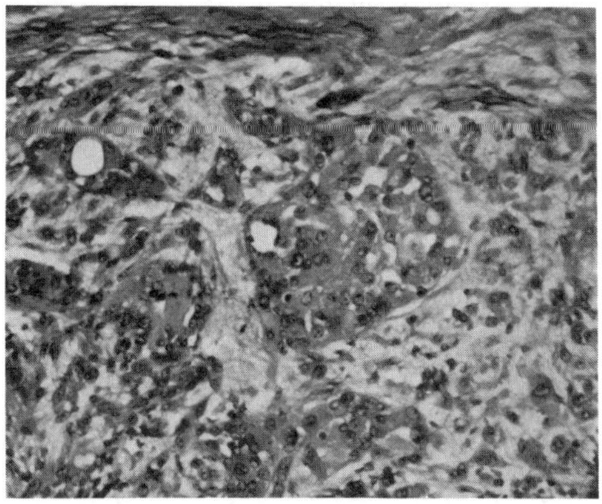

FIG 13–18.
Foci of epithelioid cells in epithelioid hemangioendothelioma. (Hematoxylin-eosin; ×250).

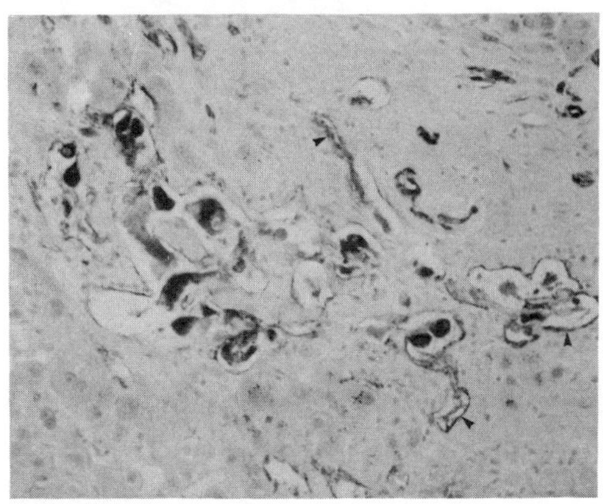

FIG 13–19.
Cells of epithelioid hemangioendothelioma demonstrate prominent factor VIII immunoreactivity (*arrowheads*). (Peroxidase-antiperoxidase stain; ×160).

28% of patients.[77] The biological behavior of the tumor may be related in part to its matrix, which may show inflammation, progressive fibrosis, and calcification.[77]

Kaposi's Sarcoma.—A number of cases of hepatic involvement with Kaposi's sarcoma have been reported in autopsy series of AIDS.[22, 24, 80] Hepatic involvement occurs in about a quarter of these cases, but does not appear to contribute to the morbidity and mortality of patients with AIDS. Functional hepatic impairment has not been documented. The lesions affect portal areas and microscopically resemble those seen in the skin and other viscera and organs (Figs. 13–20 and 13–21).

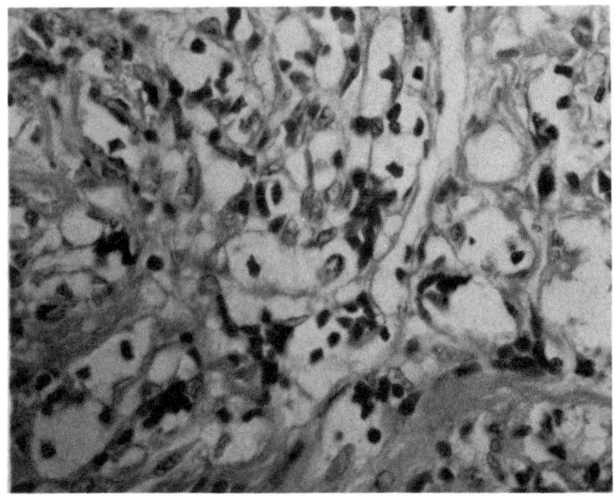

FIG 13–21.
Vessels of Kaposi's sarcoma are small. Lining cells show little pleomorphism and no mitotic activity. (Hematoxylin-eosin; ×630).

Embryonal Rhabdomyosarcoma.—Embryonal rhabdomyosarcoma (sarcoma botryoides) arises from extrahepatic bile ducts, even though they lack striated muscle. Although the victims are usually less than 5 years of age, older children and adults are also counted among them.[81–84] About 26 cases have been reported, with males and females equally affected.[84] Patients present with obstructive jaundice, often with fever and hepatomegaly. Death is usually related to the effects of local invasion by the tumor, although metastases develop in 40% of cases.[84] Early diagnosis, as accomplished in one case by transhepatic cholangiography and angiography,[85] may be the determinant of surgical excision and combination chemotherapy and the key to long-term survival.

Ideal treatment begins with resection of the bulk of the tumor even if some of it must be left behind; one patient thus treated was still alive 18 months after resection and chemotherapy.[85] In children with nonhepatic rhabdomyosarcomas, resection, even if incomplete, followed by chemotherapy and in some instances local irradiation, has resulted in high survival rates.[86, 87]

Grossly, the affected bile ducts have a thickened wall with dilatation of the biliary tract proximal to the lesion. Soft or gelatinous grapelike masses may fill the lumen. On cut section, the tumor is white or yellowish-white and glistening, with areas of hemorrhage and necrosis amidst a green liver. There may be neoplastic extension into the intrahepatic bile ducts.

Microscopically, polypoid tumor masses are covered by bile duct epithelium, which may be ulcerated (Fig. 13–22). There is a dense mass

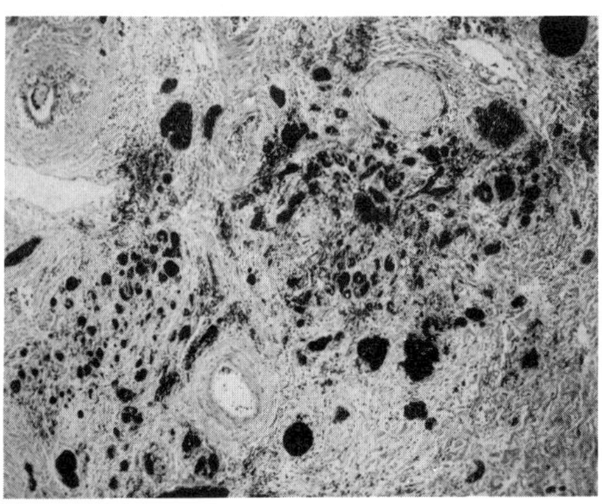

FIG 13–20.
Kaposi's sarcoma involving large portal area. Black foci represent erythrocytes in lumen of neoplastic vessels. (Hematoxylin-eosin; ×60.)

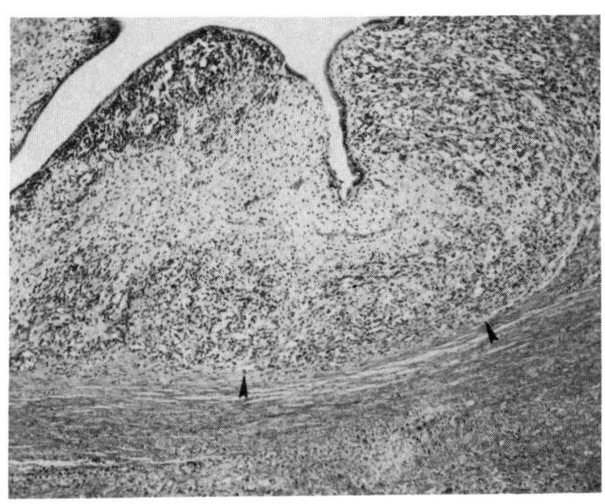

FIG 13–22.
Segment of wall of common bile duct is heavily infiltrated by cells of embryonal rhabdomyosarcoma (*arrowheads*). (Masson trichrome; ×60.)

of neoplastic cells immediately subjacent to the epithelium (cambium layer). In addition to round and spindled cells, some tumor cells may be strap shaped or racquet shaped (Fig. 13–23); cross-striations are usually identified only with difficulty. Immunohistological staining for myoglobin[83] (Fig. 13–24) and desmin may be positive. The tumor in deeper portions is more vascular and looser in texture. It is also more myxoid because of the large quantity of acid mucopolysaccharide in its matrix. Inflammatory cells, acute and chronic, and areas of necrosis and hemorrhage may be present. Ultrastructural studies reveal both thick and thin myofilaments with recognizable Z bands in some cells.[84]

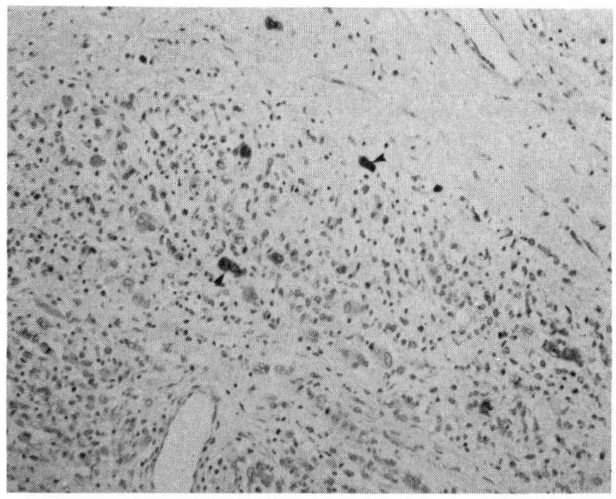

FIG 13–24.
Several cells of rhabdomyosarcoma (darkly stained) reveal myoglobin immunoreactivity (*arrowheads*). (Peroxidase-antiperoxidase stain; ×160.)

Undifferentiated Sarcoma.—Undifferentiated sarcoma has been referred to by a variety of terms, including primary sarcoma, embryonal sarcoma, malignant mesenchymoma, and fibromyxosarcoma.[88] The term *malignant mesenchyoma,* used by a number of authors,[89, 90] is justified only if the tumor shows evidence of differentiation into two or more mesenchymal elements (other than fibrosarcoma), which is rarely the case.[91–93] Although undifferentiated sarcoma is rare (some 60 cases having been reported), it is the fourth most commonly encountered pediatric tumor in the files of the Armed Forces Institute of Pathology (Washington, D.C.).[88]

Undifferentiated sarcoma occurs predominantly in the pediatric age group: the majority of patients (52%) are between ages 6 and 10.[88] Abdominal mass and pain are the usual presenting symptoms, but some patients also have fever, weight loss, and various gastrointestinal complaints. The tumor can rarely invade the inferior vena cava and grow into the right atrium, presenting clinically as a primary intracardiac tumor.[93] Hepatic scans reveal a space-occupying mass and arteriography may demonstrate a hypervascular or hypovascular mass.[88, 89] The diagnosis is generally established at exploratory laparotomy but, in at least one case, it was made by peritoneoscopy and guided biopsy.[94] The prognosis is generally very poor, with a median survival of less than 1 year following diagnosis.[88] A report of 5-year survival after excision, irradiation, and doxorubicin administration[95] holds promise of an improved prognosis after combined modality therapy in the future. A good response to palliative treatment has been reported after hepatic artery ligation and chemotherapy.[96]

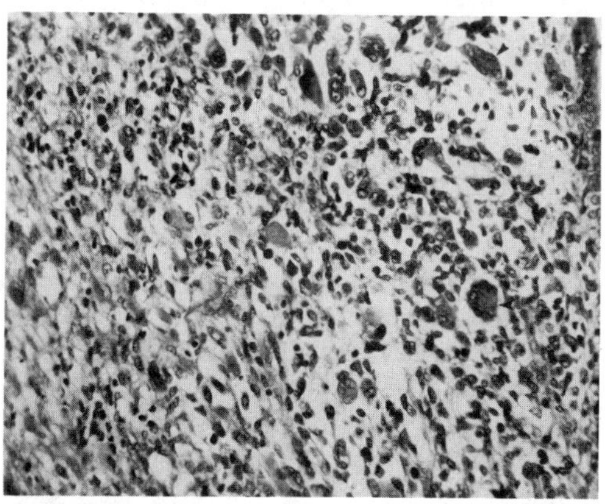

FIG 13–23.
Rhabdomyosarcoma cells are round or spindle shaped. Several tumor giant cells (*arrowheads*) are evident in the right half of the field. (Hematoxylin-eosin; ×250.)

Undifferentiated sarcoma is usually 10 to 20 cm in diameter, with an average weight of 1,310 g.[88] It is nonencapsulated and displays a variegated glistening cut surface that is yellowish-gray to tan, often with cystic areas containing necrotic debris, clotted blood, or gelatinous material (Fig. 13–25). The tumor is composed of undifferentiated sarcomatous cells, which range from spindle cells to bizzare multinucleated cells, with large hyperchromatic nuclei and atypical mitoses (Figs. 13–26 and 13–27). The stroma is fibrous and may be rich in acid mucopolysaccharides. The cytoplasm of

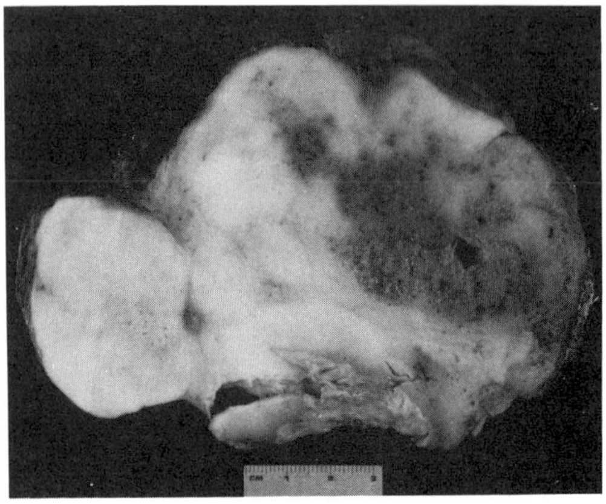

FIG 13–25.
Cut surface of undifferentiated sarcoma shows large areas of hemorrhage necrosis.

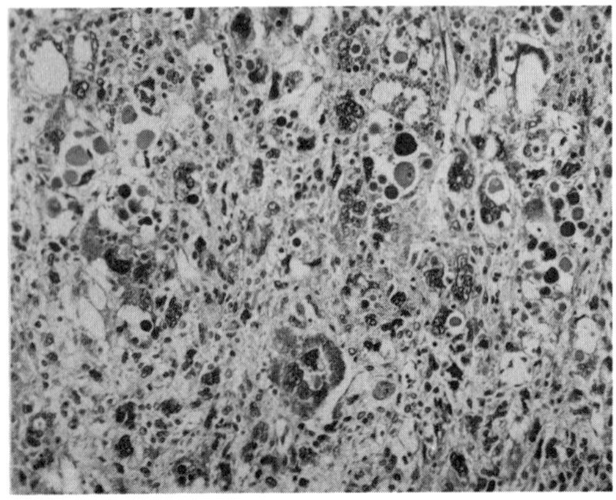

FIG 13–27.
Cells of undifferentiated sarcoma exhibit marked pleomorphism and several are multinucleated. Round globules (gray to black) are present in the cytoplasm. (Hematoxylin-eosin; ×160).

the tumor cells often contains periodic acid-Schiff stain (PAS)-positive globules that resist diastase digestion[88]; α-1-antitrypsin was identified in the globules in one case.[97] Bile ducts (sometimes dilated) are often seen at the periphery of the tumor and are thought to be entrapped ducts surviving and continuing to grow within the tumor.[88]

As is the case with most hepatic sarcomas, little is known of the induction factors in undifferentiated sarcoma, except for one intriguing report of a patient with such a tumor and birth defects, and who had been exposed prenatally to phenytoin.[98]

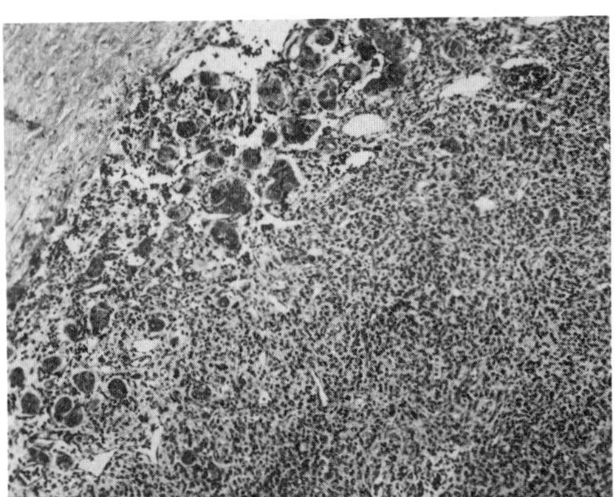

FIG 13–26.
Liver cells (upper left) are entrapped in infiltrating edge of undifferentiated sarcoma. (Hematoxylin-eosin; ×100).

Treatment

Treatment has been discussed in relation to each of the tumors covered in the previous sections. As already noted in the section of angiosarcomas, hepatic occlusion may provide palliation, and this method has been used in treating one patient with a primary undifferentiated sarcoma of the liver when used in conjunction with both intra-arterial and systemic 5-fluorouracil.[95] A better approach would seem to be resection of as much of the sarcoma as possible, followed by radiation therapy and systemic chemotherapy with a regimen as vincristine, doxorubicin, cyclophosphamide, and 5-fluorouracil, even if this program has been most extensively evaluated in carcinomas of the liver in childhood.[99]

SPLEEN

Primary sarcomas of the spleen are rare[100–105]; for all practical purposes, angiosarcoma is *the* sarcoma of the spleen. Although a number of cases of primary non-Hodgkin's lymphoma of the spleen have been reported,[100, 105, 106] it is acknowledged that differentiation of primary from secondary lymphomas is generally difficult if not impossible.[101, 102] Primary Hodgkin's disease of the spleen is also exceptionally rare.[105] Similar arguments have been advanced for splenic sarcomas other than angiosarcoma,[102] although rare cases of fibrosarcoma and malignant fibrous histiocytoma[101, 104] are on record.

Only 54 angiosarcomas of the spleen had been reported up to 1981.[103] In addition, the files of the Armed Forces Institute of Pathology up to 1981 contain 30 cases of primary angiosarcoma.[102] Other cases have since been reported.[104, 107]

The spleen can be involved by metastatic malignant vascular tumors originating in the liver, such as angiosarcoma[2] (Fig. 13–28), epithelioid hemangioendothelioma,[77] and Kaposi's sarcoma.[22, 24, 80]

Primary angiosarcoma of the spleen occurs almost equally in females and males; the mean age is 50 years.[102] Symptoms and signs include splenomegaly, abdominal pain, a microangiopathic hemolytic anemia, and, less often, a consumptive coagulopathy.[102, 107, 108] Spontaneous rupture with intraperitoneal bleeding occurs in about one third of the cases.[108] Metastases in the liver are common (80%), while metastases to other organs such as the lungs, lymph nodes, and bone occur in approximately one third of the cases.[99]

The prognosis of untreated splenic angiosarcomas is poor. Splenectomy prior to rupture is advisable; five of 19 patients treated by splenectomy survived 1 to 5 years.[108] Chemotherapy in a few cases has been of value[100]; chemotherapy and/or radiotherapy after splenectomy in four patients has resulted in survivals ranging from 10 to 24 months.[104]

The spleen affected by angiosarcoma may be three to 30 times the normal weight.[103] Microscopically, it is diffusely involved, in contrast to the more patchy lesions of hepatic angiosarcoma.[103] The histopathology is similar to that of angiosarcoma occurring in other organs and viscera and will not be further touched on. Ultrastructurally, two cell types, one resembling sinus endothelial cells of the normal spleen and the other resembling the fixed reticular cells of the red pulp, were described in one case.[103]

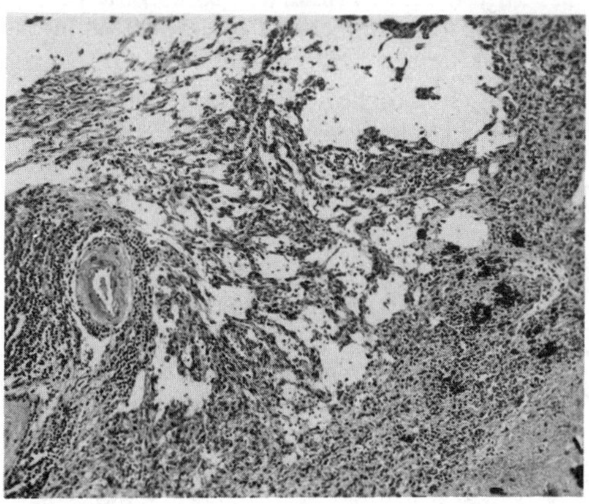

FIG 13–28.
Angiosarcoma of spleen and liver (not shown). Note black particles of Thorotrast to the right. (Hematoxylin-eosin; ×100).

Epidemiological factors of importance in angiosarcoma of the liver, such as prior exposure to Thorotrast or vinyl chloride, have not been implicated in angiosarcoma of the spleen.[103, 110]

REFERENCES

1. Edmondson HA: Tumors of the liver and intrahepatic bile ducts, in *Atlas of Tumor Pathology*, sect. 7, fasc 25. Washington, D.C., Armed Forces Institute of Pathology, 1958, pp. 139–151.
2. Ishak KG: Mesenchymal tumors of the liver, in Okuda K, Peters RL, (eds): *Hepatocellular Carcinoma.* New York, John Wiley & Sons, 1976, pp. 247–307.
3. Foster JH, Berman MM: Cystic, vascular, mesenchymal, and miscellaneous tumors. *Prob Surg* 1977; 22:179–208.
4. Falk H, Herbert J, Crowley S, et al: Epidemiology of hepatic angiosarcoma in the United States. *Environ Health Perspect* 1981; 41:107–113.
5. Goldstein, HJ: Primary sarcoma of the liver. *Int Clin* 1921; 2:73–90.
6. deVecchi: Cited by Jaffe, RH. Sarcoma and carcinoma of the liver following cirrhosis. *Arch Intern Med* 1924; 33:330–342.
7. Cayama E, Tsuda H, Sarma DSR, et al: Initiation of chemical carcinogenesis requires cell proliferation. *Nature London* 1978; 275:60–62.
8. Williamson RCN: Postoperative adaptation in the aetiology of intestinal cancer. *Mech Intest Adapt Falk Symp* 1982; 30:621–636.
9. Dominici H, Merle P: Composite tumor of liver: Carcinoma and sarcoma following cirrhosis. *Arch Med Exp Anat Pathol* 1909; 21:136–153.
10. Jaffe RH: Sarcoma and carcinoma of the liver following cirrhosis. *Arch Intern Med* 1924; 33:330–342.
11. Nagamine Y, Sorsaki K, Kaku K: Hepatic sarcoma associated with hepatoma. *Acta Pathol J* 1978; 28:645–651.
12. Shin P, Ohmi S, Sakurai M: Hepatocellular

carcinoma combined with hepatoma. *Acta Pathol J* 1981; 31:815–824.

13. Kimoto T, Ugaki M: Hepatocellular carcinoma combined with hepatic mesenchymal cell tumor and sarcoma. *Acta Pathol Jpn* 1982; 32:1131–1141.
14. Sonoda T, Toyoshima S, Enjoji M, et al: Simultaneous occurrence of primary carcinoma and chondrosarcoma in the liver: A case report and a review of the literature. *Acta Pathol Jpn* 1984; 34:919–924.
15. Millman DH, Grayzel DM: Mixed tumor of the liver. *Am J Dis Child* 1951; 81:408–420.
16. Barnett WH, Erickson EE, Halpert B: Embryonic tumor of the liver in an adult. *Cancer* 1958; 11:306–309.
17. Kerr JFR: Hepatic embryonic mixed tumor in an adult. *J Pathol Bacteriol* 1966; 92:238–240.
18. Carter R: Hepatoblastoma in the adult. *Cancer* 1969; 23:191–197.
19. Goldman RL, Friedman NB: Rhabdomyosarcohepatoma in an adult and embryonal hepatoma in a child. *Am J Clin Pathol* 1969; 51:137–143.
20. Kishimoto Y, Hijiya S, Nazasako, R: Malignant mixed tumors of the liver in adults. *Am J Gastroenterol* 1984; 79:229–235.
21. Talamo TS, Dekker A, Gurecki J, et al: Primary hepatic malignant lymphoma. *Cancer* 1980; 46:336–339.
22. Reichert CM, O'Leary TJ, Levens DL, et al: Autopsy pathology in the acquired immune deficiency syndrome. *Am J Pathol* 1983; 112:357–382.
23. Fekete F, Molas G, Tossen JC, et al: Lymphome histiocytaire primitif du foie: Etude de deux cas et revue de la litterature. *Gastroenterol Clin Biol* 1983; 7:785–791.
24. Welch K, Finkbeiner W, Alpers CE, et al: Autopsy findings in the acquired immune deficiency syndrome. *JAMA* 1984; 252:1152–1159.
25. Younus S, Soterakis J, Sossi AJ, et al: Hypoglycemia secondary to metastases to the liver: A case report and review of the literature. *Gastroenterology* 1977; 72:334–337.
26. Kahn CR: The riddle of tumor hypoglycemia revisited. *Clin Endocrinol Metab* 1980; 9:335–360.
27. Case Records of the Massachusetts General Hospital: *N Engl J Med* 1984; 310:580–7.
28. Shallow TA, Wagner FB: Primary fibrosarcoma of the liver. *Ann Surg* 1947; 125: 439–46.
29. Simpson HM, Baggenstoss AH, Stauffer MH: Primary sarcoma of the liver: a report of three cases. *South Med J* 1955; 48:1177–1182.
30. Steiner PE: Cancer of the liver and cirrhosis in Trans-Saharan Africa and the United States of America. *Cancer* 1960; 13:1085–1149.
31. Stout AP: Tumors of the soft tissues, in *Atlas of Tumor Pathology,* sect V, fasc 5. Washington, D.C., Armed Forces Institute of Pathology, 1953.
32. Snapper I, Schraft WC Jr, Ginsberg DM: Severe hypoglycemia due to fibrosarcoma of the liver. *Maandschr Kindergenees* 1964; 32:337–347.
33. Ojima A, Sugiyama T, Takeda J, et al: Six cases of rare malignant tumors of the liver. *Acta Pathol Jpn* 1964; 14:95–102.
34. Totzke HA, Hutcheson JB: Primary fibrosarcoma of the liver. *South Med J* 1965; 58:236–238.
35. Balouet G, Destombes P: A propos de quelques tumeurs mesenchymateuses hepatiques d'apparence primitive. *Ann Anat Pathol (Paris)* 1967; 12:273–286.
36. Cavallo T, Lichewitz B, Rozov T: Primary fibrosarcoma of the liver: Report of a case. *Rev Hosp Clin Fac Med Sao Paulo* 1968; 23:44–49.
37. Smith D, Rele SR: A case of primary fibrosarcoma of the liver. *Postgrad Med J* 1972; 48:62–63.
38. Walter VE, Rodner E, Lederer B: Primares fibrosarkom der leber. *Wein Klin Wochenschr* 1972; 84:8087–8010.
39. Alrenga DP: Primary fibrosarcoma of the liver: Case report and review of the literature. *Cancer* 1975; 36:446–449.
40. Fong JA, Ruebner BH: Primary leiomyosarcoma of the liver. *Hum Pathol* 1974; 5:115–119.
41. Chen KTK: Hepatic leiomyosarcoma. *J Surg Oncol* 1983; 24:325–328.
42. Callego MM, Merlo RR, Pascual BG, et al: Leiomiosarcoma hepatico primario. *Gastroenterol Hepatol* 1984; 7:77–81
43. O'Leary MR, Hill RB, Levine RA: Peritoneoscopic diagnosis of primary leiomyosarcoma of liver. *Hum Pathol* 1982; 13:76–78.
44. Koberle F, Pfleger R: Lebervenengeschwulst mit dem symptomenbild einer endophlebitis obliterans hepatica. *Wien Arch Intern Med* 1940; 34:73–85.

45. MacMahon HE, Ball HG: Leiomyosacoma of hepatic vein and the Budd-Chiari syndrome. *Gastroenterology* 1971; 61:239–243.

46. Kevorkian J, Cento DP: Leiomyosarcoma of the large arteries and veins. *Surgery* 1973; 73:390–399.

47. Bloustein PA: Hepatic leiomyosarcoma: Ultrastructural study and review of the differential diagnosis. *Hum Pathol* 1978; 9:713–716

48. Anonymous: Angiosarcoma of the liver: A growing problem? *Br Med J* 1981; 282:504–505.

49. Suckow EE, Henegar GC, Baserga R: Tumors of the liver following administration of Thorotrast. *Am J Pathol* 1961; 38:663–677.

50. Battifora HA: Thorotrast and tumors of the liver, in Okuda K, Peter RL (eds): *Hepatocellular Carcinoma.* New York, John Wiley & Sons, 1976, pp. 83–93.

51. Selinger, M, Koff, RS: Thorotrast and the liver: A reminder. *Gastroenterology* 1975; 68:799–803.

52. Rubel LR, Ishak KG: Thorotrast-associated cholangiocarcinoma: An epidemiologic and clinicopathologic study. *Cancer* 1982; 50:1408–1415.

53. Yamada S, Hosoda A, Tatero H, et al: Survey of Thorotrast-associated liver cancers in Japan. *J Natl Cancer Inst* 1983; 70:31–35.

54. Block JB: Angiosarcoma of the liver following vinyl chloride exposure. *JAMA* 1974; 229:53–54.

55. Falk H, Popper H, Thomas LB, et al: Hepatic angiosarcoma associated with androgenic-anabolic steroids. *Lancet* 1979; 11:1120–1123.

56. Blendis LM, Smith PM, Lawrie BW, et al: Portal hypertension in vinyl chloride monomer workers: A hemodynamic study. *Gastroenterology* 1978; 75:206–211.

57. Thomas LB, Popper H, Berk PD, et al: Vinyl-chloride-induced liver disease: From idiopathic portal hypertension (Banti's syndrome) to angiosarcomas. *N Eng J Med* 1975; 292:17–22

58. Schaffner F: Effect of long-term vinyl chloride exposure in mouse liver structure in Remmer H, Bolt HM, Bannasch P, et al (eds): *Primary Liver Tumors,* Falk Symp. No. 25, Baltimore, University Park Press, 1978, pp. 189–199.

59. Dannaher CL, Tamburro CH, Yam LT: Occupational carcinogenesis: The Louisville experience with vinyl chloride-associated hepatic angiosarcoma. *Am J Med* 1981; 70:279–287.

60. Tamburro CH, Makk L, Popper H: Early hepatic histologic alterations among chemical (vinylmonomer) workers. *Hepatology* 1984; 4:413–418.

61. Louagie YA, Gianello P, Kestens PJ, et al: Vinyl-chloride induced hepatic angiosarcoma. *Br J Surg* 1984; 71:322–323.

62. Ghandur-Mnaymneh L, Gonzalez MS: Angiosarcoma of the penis with hepatic angiomas in a patient with low vinyl chloride exposure. *Cancer* 1981; 47:1318–1324.

63. Roth F: The sequelae of chronic arsenic poisoning in Moselle vintners. *German Med Month* 1957; 2:172–175.

64. Lander JJ, Stanley RJ, Sumner HW, et al: Angiosarcoma of the liver associated with Fowler's solution (potassium arsenite). *Gastroenterology* 1975; 68:1582–1586.

65. Falk H, Herbert JT, Edmonds L, et al: Review of four cases of childhood hepatic angiosarcoma-elevated environmental arsenic exposure in one case. *Cancer* 1981; 47:382–391.

66. Roat JW, Wald A, Mendelow H, et al: Hepatic angiosarcoma associated with short-term arsenic ingestion. *Am J Med* 1982:933–936.

67. Johnson FL: Androgenic-anabolic steroids and hepatocellular carcinoma, in Okuda K, Peters RL (eds): *Hepatocellular Carcinoma.* New York, John Wiley & Sons, 1976, pp. 95–103.

68. Malt RA, Galdabini JJ, Jeppsson BW: Abnormal sex-steroid milieu in young adults with hepatocellular carcinoma. *World J Surg* 1983; 7:247–253.

69. Hendersen BE, Preston-Martin S, Edmondson HA, et al: Hepatocellular carcinoma and oral contraceptives. *Br J Cancer* 1983; 48:437–440.

70. Monroe PS, Riddell RH, Siegler M, et al: Hepatic angiosarcoma: Possible relationships to long-term oral contraceptive ingestion. *JAMA* 1981; 64–65.

71. Daneshmend TK, Scott GL, Bradfield JWB: Angiosarcoma of liver associated with phenelzine. *Br Med J* 1979; 1:1679.

72. Locker GY, Doroshow JH, Zwelling LA, et al: The clinical features of hepatic angiosarcoma: A report of four cases and a review of the English literature. *Medicine* 1979; 58:48–64.

73. Truell JE, Peck SD, Reiquam CW: Heman-

giosarcoma of the liver complicated by disseminated intravascular coagulation: A case report. *Gastroenterology* 1973; 65:936–942.

74. Mahoney B, Jeffrey B, Federle MP: Spontaneous rupture of hepatic and splenic angiosarcoma demonstrated by CT. *Am J Radiol* 1982; 138:965–966.
75. Nagasue N, Ogawa Y, Inokuchi K: Hemangiosarcoma of liver and spleen treated by hepatic artery ligation, intraportal infusion, chemotherapy, and splenectomy. *Cancer* 1976; 38:1386–1390.
76. Langley JR, Rosato FE, El-Mahdi A: Primary malignant hemangioendothelioma of the liver: Survival following non-operative treatment. *J Surg Oncol* 1978; 10:533–541.
77. Ishak KG, Sesterhenn IA, Goodman ZD, et al: Epithelioid hemangioendothelioma of the liver: A clinicopathologic and follow-up study of 32 cases. *Hum Pathol* 1984; 15:839–852.
78. Dail DH, Leibow AA, Gymelich JT, et al: Intravascular, bronchiolar, and alveolar tumor of lung (IVBAT): An analysis of twenty cases of a peculiar sclerosing endothelial tumor. *Cancer* 1983; 51:452–464.
79. Weiss SW, Enzinger FM: Epithelioid hemangioendothelioma: A vascular tumor often mistaken for a carcinoma. *Cancer* 1982; 50:970–981.
80. Guarda LA, Luna MA, Smith IL, et al: Acquired immune deficiency syndrome: Postmortem findings. *Am J Clin Pathol* 1984; 81:549–557.
81. Davis GL, Kissane JM, Ishak KG: Embryonal rhabdomyosarcoma (sarcoma botryoides) of the biliary tree. *Cancer* 1969; 24:333–342.
82. Mori H, Matsubara N, Fuji M, et al: Alphafetoprotein producing rhabdomyosarcoma of the adult liver. *Acta Pathol. Jpn* 1979; 29:485–491.
83. Brooks JJ: Immunochemistry of soft tissue tumors: Myoglobin as a tumor marker for rhabdmyosarcoma. *Cancer* 1982; 50:1757–1763.
84. Lack EE, Perez-Atayde AR, Schuster SR: Botryoid rhabdomyosarcoma of the biliary tract: Report of five cases with ultrastructural observations and literature review. *Am J Surg Pathol* 1981; 5:643–652.
85. Cannon PM, Legge DA, O'Donnell B: The use of percutaneous transhepatic cholangiography in a case of embryonal rhabdomyosarcoma. *Br J Radiol* 1979; 52:326–327.
86. Raney RB, Ragab AH, Ruymann FB, et al: Soft tissue sarcoma of the trunk in childhood: Results of the intergroup rhabdomyosarcoma study. *Cancer* 1982; 49:2612–2616.
87. Grosfeld JL, Weber TR, Weetman RM, et al: Rhabdomyosarcoma in childhood: Analysis of survival in 98 cases. *J Ped Surg* 1983; 18:141–146.
88. Stocker JT, Ishak KG: Undifferentiated (embryonal) sarcoma of the liver: Report of 31 cases. *Cancer* 1978; 42:336–348.
89. Stanley RJ, Dehner LP, Hesker AE: Primary malignant mesenchymal tumors (mesenchymoma) of the liver in childhood. *Cancer* 1973; 32:973–984.
90. Cozzutto C, DeBernardi B, Comelli A, et al: Malignant mesenchymoma of the liver in children: A clinicopathologic and ultrastructural study. *Hum Pathol* 1981; 12:481–485.
91. Sumiyoshi A, Nicho Y: Primary osteogenic sarcoma of the liver: Report of an autopsy case. *Acta Pathol Jpn* 1971; 21:305–312.
92. Lagacé R, Delage C, Robert J: Le mesenchymome primitif du foie: Etude ultrastructurale. *Ann Anat Pathol* 1974; 19:275–286.
93. Gallivan MVE, Lack EE, Chun B, et al: Undifferentiated ("embryonal") sarcoma of the liver: Ultrastructure of a case presenting as a primary intracardiac tumor. *Pediatr Pathol* 1983; 1:291–300.
94. Esposito R, Pollavini G, deLalla F: A case of primary undifferentiated sarcoma of the liver diagnosed by peritoneoscopy and guided biopsy. *Endoscopy* 1976; 8:108–110.
95. Smithson WA, Telander RL, Carney JA: Mesenchymoma of the liver in childhood: Five-year survival after combined modality treatment. *J Pediatr Surg* 1982; 17:70–72.
96. Tanner AR, Bolton PM, Powell LW: Primary sarcoma of the liver: Report of a case with excellent response to hepatic artery ligation and infusion chemotherapy. *Gastroenterology* 1978; 74:121–123.
97. Abramowsky CR, Cebelin M, Choudhury A, et al: Undifferentiated (embryonal) sarcoma of the liver with alpha-1-antitrypsin deposits: Immunohistochemical and ultrastructural studies. *Cancer* 1980; 45:3108–3113.
98. Blattner WA, Henson DE, Young RC, et al: Malignant mesenchymoma and birth defects: Prenatal exposure to phenytoin. *JAMA* 1977; 238:334–335.

99. Evans AE, Land VJ, Newton WA, et al: Combination chemotherapy (vincristine, adriamycin, cyclophosphamide, and 5-fluorouracil) in the treatment of children with malignant hepatoma. *Cancer* 1982; 50:821–826.
100. Gupta PP, Coombes B, Brasfield RD: Primary malignant neoplasms of the spleen *Surg Gynecol Obstet* 1965; 120:947–960.
101. Rappaport H: Tumors of the hematopoietic system, in *Atlas of Tumor Pathology* sect III, fasc 8. Washington, D.C., Armed Forces Institute of Pathology, 1966.
102. Garvin DF, King FM: Cysts and nonlymphomatous tumors of the spleen. *Pathol Annu* 1981; 16:61–80.
103. Silverman ML, Federman M, O'Hare CJ: Malignant hemangioendothelioma of the spleen: A case report with ultrastructural observations. *Arch Pathol Lab Med* 1981; 105:300–304.
104. Wick MR, Smith SL, Scheithauer BW, et al: Primary nonlymphoreticular malignant neoplasms of the spleen *Am J Surg Pathol* 1982; 6:229–242.
105. Kraemer BB, Osborne BM, Butler JJ: Primary splenic presentation of malignant lymphoma and related disorders: A study of 49 cases. *Cancer* 1984; 54:1606–1619.
106. Burke JS: Surgical pathology of the spleen: An approach to the differential diagnosis of splenic lymphomas and leukemia. I. Diseases of the white pulp. *Am J Surg Pathol* 1981; 5:551–563. II. Diseases of the red pulp. *Am J Surg Pathol* 1981; 5:681–694.
107. Hermann GG, Fogh J, Graem N, et al: Primary hemangiosarcoma of the spleen with angioscintigraphic demonstration of metastases. *Cancer* 1984; 53:1682–1685.
108. Autry JR, Weitzner S: Hemangiosarcoma of spleen with spontaneous rupture. *Cancer* 1975; 35:534–539.
109. Aranha GV, Gold J, Grage TB: Hemangiosarcoma of the spleen: Report of a case and review of previously reported cases. *J Surg Oncol* 1976; 8:481–487.
110. Chen KTK, Bolles JC, Gilbert EF: Angiosarcoma of the spleen: A report of two cases and review of the literature. *Arch Pathol Lab Med* 1979; 103:122–124.

BIBLIOGRAPHY

Aldabagh SM, Shibata CS, Taxy JB: Rhabdomyosarcoma of the common bile duct in an adult. *Arch Pathol Lab Med* 1986; 110:547–550.

Caccamo D, Pervez NK, Marchevsky A: Primary lymphoma of the liver in the acquired immunodeficiency syndrome. *Arch Pathol Lab Med* 1986; 110:553–555.

DeMent SH, Mann RB, Staal SP, et al: Primary lymphomas of the liver. Report of six cases and review of the literature. *Am J Clin Pathol* 1987; 88:255–263.

Dich NH, Goodman ZD, Klein MA: Hepatic involvement in Hodgkin's disease. Clues to histologic diagnosis. *Cancer* 1989; 64:2121–2126.

Forbes A, Portmann B, Johnson P, et al: Hepatic sarcomas in adults: A review of 25 cases. *Gut* 1987; 28:668–674.

Hasan FA, Jeffers LJ, Welsh SW, et al: Hepatic involvement as the primary manifestation of Kaposi's sarcoma in the acquired immune deficiency syndrome. *Am J Gastroenterol* 1989; 84:1449–1451.

Inoue J, Nomura M, Nakagawa S: A case of primary hepatic lymphoma with cirrhosis of the liver. *Acta Hepatol Jpn* 1987; 28:794–800.

Ishak KG: Malignant mesenchymal tumors of the liver, in Okuda K, Ishak KG (eds): *Neoplasms of the Liver.* Tokyo, Springer-Verlag, 1987, pp 159–176.

Ito Y, Kojiro M, Nakashima T, More T: Pathomorphologic characteristics of 102 cases of Thorotrast-related hepatocellular carcinoma, cholangiocarcinoma, and hepatic angiosarcoma. *Cancer* 1988; 62:1153–1162.

Jaffe ES: Malignant lymphomas: Pathology of hepatic involvement. *Semin Liver Dis* 1987; 7:257–268.

Lisker-Melman M, Pittaluga S, Pluda M, et al: Primary lymphoma of the liver in a patient with acquired immune deficiency syndrome and chronic hepatitis B. *Am J Gastroenterol* 1989; 84:1445–1448.

Maki HS, Hubert BC, Sajjad SM, et al: Primary hepatic leiomyosarcoma. *Arch Surg* 1987; 122:1193–1196.

Ryan J, Straus DJ, Lange C, et al: Primary lymphoma of the liver. *Cancer* 1988; 61:370–375.

Ruymann FB, Raney RB Jr, Crist WM, et al: Rhabdomyosarcoma of the biliary tree in childhood. A report from the Intergroup Rhabdomyosarcoma Study. *Cancer* 1985; 56:575–581.

Steiner M, Bostrum B, Leonard AS, et al: Undifferentiated (embryonal) sarcoma of the liver. A clinicopathologic study of a survivor treated with combined technique therapy. *Cancer* 1989; 64:1318–1322.

Taylor RW, Sylwestrowicz T, Kossakowska AE, et al: Leiomyosarcoma of the inferior vena cava presenting as Budd-Chiari syndrome. *Liver* 1987; 7:201–205.

Thomaszewski M-M, Kuenster JT, Hartman K: Leiomyosarcoma of ligamentum teres of liver: Case report. *Ped Pathol* 1986; 5:147–156.

Chapter 14

Retroperitoneal and Abdominal Wall Sarcomas

William C. Wood
Joel Tepper

Soft-tissue sarcomas of the retroperitoneum account for only 10% to 15% of the 4,500 new sarcomas seen annually in the United States. The rarity of these tumors, the variety of their histological diagnoses and grades, and their various locations and stages defeat all attempts to make statistically valid generalizations.[1, 2]

CLINICAL FEATURES

The distensibility of the retroperitoneum permits tumors to attain considerable size before attracting notice. Early symptoms are so vague that nearly 25% of these patients have evident metastases at presentation.[2–4] The most common complaint is pain in the abdomen or back. An abdominal mass is palpable in 75% of these patients.[2] Retroperitoneal tumors grown large produce symptoms and findings related to the organs they compress or invade. These typically include obstructive symptoms of the gastrointestinal or urinary tracts, venous obstructions from occlusion or compression of the inferior vena cava or iliac veins, or compression of nerves to the lower extremity.

DIAGNOSTIC STUDIES

The evaluation of patients with a clinical diagnosis of retroperitoneal sarcoma requires definition of the extent of the mass and involvement of adjacent organs. Ultrasonography and computed tomography have largely replaced contrast studies and angiography as the primary means of imaging of these tumors. Although ultrasonograms are commonly obtained when an asymptomatic retroperitoneal or abdominal mass is discovered, or in the evaluation of abdominal pain of uncertain etiology, computed tomography can delineate more accurately the dimensions of the tumor. It can define involvement or displacement of adjacent blood vessels and organs to allow the planning of biopsy approaches, radiation therapy fields, and surgical resection. Although angiographic studies are helpful in certain locations where tumors appear to encase or displace major blood vessels, their general use is no longer required.

Although such large lesions are easily visualized radiographically, primary diagnosis by needle biopsy is discouraged because the diagnosis of soft-tissue sarcoma requires sufficient tissue for grading as well as examination of histological pattern over several microscopic fields. Its use in primary diagnosis has also been associated with seeding of the needle tract on multiple occasions.[5] Consequently, incisional biopsy is preferred. During the biopsy, every effort must be made to minimize the danger of tumor spillage or local implantation. Retroperitoneal sarcomas are exquisitely capable of seeding and implantation.[3] At the time of open biopsy, the anatomical dimensions of the tumor should be marked by clips.

Excision of retroperitoneal sarcomas for biopsy will commonly compromise the opportunity for later definitive resection. This is particularly true when the attempt is made to bluntly excise an "encapsulated" tumor. Such an enucleation allows the large sheet of compressed tumor cells forming this false capsule to be disseminated throughout the raw surfaces created by the surgery.

Staging retroperitoneal sarcomas should include computed tomography (CT) or plain tomography of the lungs.[6–8] Extent of disease can be evaluated by the same CT scan used to examine the retroperitoneal tumor itself. Intravenous urography is helpful in demonstrating the position of the ureters and the persence of bilateral renal function, as nephrectomy may be required in up to 25% of complete resections of retroperitoneal sarcoma.[2] Myelograms are required to evaluate intraspinal extension in neurogenic tumors arising near the vertebrae.

HISTOLOGICAL CLASSIFICATION

Liposarcomas remain the most common retroperitoneal soft-tissue sarcoma, accounting for 28% to 40% of the total.[1, 9, 10] Although fatty tissue tumors elsewhere in the body are generally benign, those found in the retroperitoneum are more commonly malignant. These, with leiomyosarcomas, fibrosarcomas, and neurogenic sarcomas, account for the majority of retroperitoneal sarcomas. Malignant fibrous histiocytomas is described with increasing frequency in more recently reported series.[3, 11] As is true with sarcomas arising in other locations, the grade of sarcoma correlates strongly with prognosis.[2, 12]

The pattern of spread is primarily by direct invasion. Although low-grade tumors may displace adjacent organs before invading them, high-grade tumors tend to invade adjacent organs and tissue planes directly. As is true of sarcomas in other locations, high-grade tumors are much more prone to metastasis than are low-grade tumors. Unlike extremity sarcomas, which exhibit a known propensity for pulmonary metastasis, retroperitoneal sarcomas produce a different pattern of distant metastasis. Although pulmonary metastases occur (26% to 50% of all distant metastases), the greater access to the portal venous system commonly produces hepatic metastases (27% to 63% of distant metastases).[2, 3, 13]

TREATMENT

Surgery remains the mainstay of treatment for resectable sarcomas.[14] As might be anticipated, completely resected sarcomas with radiation of the tumor bed have a more favorable outcome than incompletely resected tumors treated by radiation.[2, 11, 15] Although the significance of this finding is blunted by the fact that tumors of low grade are more likely to be resectable than high-grade ones, soft-tissue sarcomas at all sites are best completely resected. The operative plan is complete resection of the sarcoma and adjacent organs or tissues involved by the tumor insofar as that is feasible. This often involves the use of a thoraco-abdominal incision. These are particularly challenging operations because each must be uniquely designed to meet the location and growth pattern of the specific tumor.

It has been appreciated for several decades that soft-tissue sarcomas extend microscopically well beyond their apparent borders; hence the importance of extensive resection, or resection and aggressive radiation treatment of the periphery, to avoid almost certain local recurrence. Unfortunately, large sarcomas of the retroperitoneal space do not lend themselves to resection with generous margins.

By analogy to sarcomas at other sites,[16] irradiation might be expected to sterilize subclinical deposits of tumor in the environs and, coupled with complete resection of the primary tumor mass, achieve local control. The presence of overlying bowel, liver, kidney, and ureter limit the dose of radiation. Radiation can be given either per-operatively or postoperatively. Preoperative irradiation can shrink the tumor mass and facilitate surgical resection, and decreases the possibility of tumor seeding at surgery.[11, 16] Postoperative irradiation has been used successfully in some series.[1, 2, 17] The use of interstitial radiation sources and, more recently, intra-operative irradiation boosts to achieve doses in the range of 60–65 Gy have been associated with good local control.[11] The therapeutic effectiveness and toxicity of intra-operative radio therapy compared to standard external beam irradiation are under investigation.[18] The small numbers involved, and the extreme variability of the tumors treated, preclude meaningful comparisons of differing treatment techniques.

Although the addition of irradiation as an adjunct to complete resection of retroperitoneal sarcoma has not been proved beneficial in randomized trials, the existing data suggest a clear benefit from its use. Cody et al,[2] analyzed the results in 158 patients treated at the Memorial Sloan-Kettering Cancer Center (New York, New York) between 1951 and 1977. A 5-year disease-free interval was obtained in only 17% of patients (4 of 23) treated with complete excision alone compared with 33% (5 of 15) of patients treated with complete excision plus postoperative irradiation.[2] Local recurrence was observed in 77% of patients who had complete resections. In a series from the Massachusetts General Hospital Cancer Center (Boston, Massachusetts) the actuarial 5-year survival and local control were both 54% (10 of 17) after resection plus high-dose radiation therapy. Among 37 patients treated at the National Cancer Institute with complete resection of gross tumor, actuarial continuous disease-free survival at 5 years was 38%. Of 47 patients seen at the Massey Cancer Center, 18 had complete tumor excision: the 5-year disease-free survival was 50% and the overall survival 70% at 5 years. There was no clear advantage to adjuvant irradiation in this series.[15]

Adjuvant chemotherapy with presently available agents has not demonstrated benefit in retroperitoneal sarcoma. A randomized study from the National Cancer Institutes showed no advantage in the use of adjuvant doxorubicin and Cytoxan (cyclophosphamide) after resection and irradiation.[1]

The importance of achieving local control of the tumor by a combination of as radical a resection as feasible with irradiation of tissues remaining at risk cannot be overemphasized. Although retroperitoneal sarcomas metastasize to lungs and liver, the majority of patients who die of this disease die of local recurrence. Local recurrence more than doubles the probability of death from retroperitoneal sarcoma.[19]

The use of irradiation, with or without chemotherapy, for unresectable or imcompletely resected retroperitoneal sarcoma is associated with a few long-term survivors. Particularly with low-grade tumors, however, such survival is possible and worth pursuing. Such low-grade tumors may not respond rapidly, but slowly shrink over a period of years.[20] Significant palliation can be achieved by judicious use of irradiation with or without surgery directed toward the symptomatic lesions.[17, 21]

When retroperitoneal sarcoma recurs, it can sometimes be resected one or more times (Fig 14–1). This is particularly true of low-grade sarcomas and of liposarcoma especially.[22] Periodic

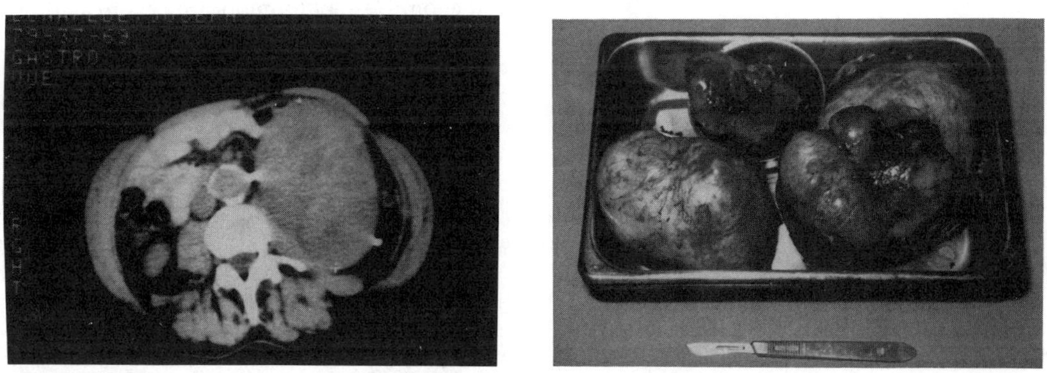

A B

FIG 14–1.

A, computed tomography scan showing recurrent left retroperitoneal liposarcoma in a 55-year-old man. **B,** exploration of the abdomen was performed through a generous midline incision. The colon and small bowel were dissected away from the tumor and two large tumor masses resected. The invaded, nonfunctioning left kidney was also removed.

CT scan, usually at 4- to 6-month intervals for the first 2 years, is invaluable in detecting early recurrence in the retroperitoneum.

There are certain special presentations of retroperitoneal sarcoma that deserve mention, and are described in the following sections.

LEIOMYOSARCOMA OF THE INFERIOR VENA CAVA

Leiomyosarcoma of the inferior vena cava is rare, occurring almost exclusively in women of middle age or older. Symptoms are vague and the diagnosis is rarely made early. These tumors most commonly involve the proximal inferior vena cava, producing Budd-Chiari syndrome by obstruction of the hepatic veins with tumor or associated thrombosis and can be demonstrated by inferior vena cavography. An enlarged, tender liver with ascites and jaundice and edema of the extremities may suggest the diagnosis. Tumors at this level of the inferior vena cava do not lend themselves to resection. Tumors at or below the level of the renal veins are usually seen in conjunction with peripheral edema and may be resected with particular care to avoid embolization.[23] The suprarenal, infrahepatic vena cava many be resected and the left kidney will usually function satisfactorily because of its collateral venous tributaries. Consequently, a right nephrectomy should usually be performed at resection of the tumor.[24, 25]

MESENTERIC SOFT-TISSUE SARCOMA

Mesenteric soft-tissue sarcomas can be resected when peripheral in the mesentery. Those that are central and encase the superior mesenteric artery and its branches are unresectable. Irradiation of such sarcomas has occasionally been associated with prolonged survival.

RETRORECTAL SARCOMA

The most common tumor arising in the retrorectal space is the chordoma. Tumors of the retrorectal space are usually bulky when discovered. Pain is the most constant symptom—often present for months or years before the mass is appreciated. It is readily palpated on rectal examination but may destroy the sacrum and present as a posterior mass as well. A chordoma arising anterior to the sacrum may extend to fill the pelvis, producing obstruction of the rectum and urinary tracts. These tumors invariably destroy the sacrum and usually encase the lower sacral nerve roots. An abdominosacral approach is helpful in resecting these tumors.[26] The sacrum must be resected at a vertebra above the radiological extent of tumor. Whenever possible, preservation of at least one S2 nerve root may allow some retention of urinary and fecal continence. However, it is important to resect these nerve roots if involved by tumor. Because local failure is the most common type of tumor recurrence, it is important that the first resection be aggressive. Once the tumor has recurred it is virtually ineradicable. High-dose irradiation given pre-operatively may minimize the chance of seeding the tumor into the wound, as these are very implantable tumors.

SOFT-TISSUE SARCOMA OF THE ABDOMINAL WALL

Sarcomas of the abdominal wall are uncommon tumors that present problems in the reconstruction of the abdominal wall. Relatively benign, slowly growing, desmoid tumors were originally described on the abdominal wall, although subsequent series have not demonstrated a particular predilection for this site.[9, 27] These low-grade fibrosarcomas occur more commonly in females, especially those of child-bearing age. Case reports describe childhood desmoid tumors regressing spontaneously at the onset of puberty, but this is an uncommon phenomenon. Desmoid tumors are best treated by resection with an adequate margin. There are reports of incomplete resection with no recurrence over many years of follow-up, but the tumor is not always so cooperative. Positive margins should be followed by prompt resection. Local recurrence may be controlled by radiation therapy. On the anterior abdominal wall, electron beam techniques or tangential fields are used to avoid high-dose radiation to the abdominal viscera. Irradiation of such recurrent desmoid tumors may lead to gradual regression, often over a period of more than a year.[20, 28]

Higher grade, more aggressive sarcomas of the soft tissues of the abdominal wall require resection to even wide margins. The use of Marlex mesh (Bard Vascular Systems Division, C. R. Bard Inc., Billerica, MA) to restore continuity of the supporting fascial planes of the abdominal wall, together with primary coverage with myocutaneous flaps, has made aggressive surgical resection relatively uncomplicated. It is important to resect adjacent skeleton and adherent viscera to extirpate these tumors totally.[29, 30]

CASE HISTORY

A 58-year-old white male was hospitalized in the October 1976, with a 3-month history of fatigue and fevers. Intravenous urography and ultrasonic examination demonstrated a mass dorsal to and distorting the left kidney. At laparotomy on October 7, 1976, an inflamed mass was seen posterior to the left kidney. The tumor was completely resected to grossly clear margins. Pathological examination demonstrated an inflammatory malignant fibrous histiocytoma, high grade. The patient received postoperative irradiation to 44 Gy via external beam techniques. A 2,500-rad boost was accomplished via interstitial iridium 192. After completion of radiation therapy, chemotherapy was administered with a combination of doxorubicin, Cytoxan, and DTIC (dacarbazine). He has had no evidence of local recurrence or distant metastases seven and a half years after the initial surgical resection.

SUMMARY

The expansile nature of the retroperitoneal space allows these rare tumors to reach considerable size before attracting diagnostic attention. They are best visualized radiographically by computed tomography. Complete surgical resection is desirable whenever feasible. The addition of radiation therapy, either pre-operatively or postoperatively, appears beneficial. Adjuvant chemotherapy does not.

REFERENCES

1. Glenn J, Sindelar WF, Kinsella T, et al: Results of multi-modality therapy of resectable soft-tissue sarcomas of the retroperitoneum. *Ann Surg* 1985; 97:316–324.
2. Cody HS III, Turnbull AD, Fortner JA, et al: The continuing challenge of retroperitoneal sarcomas. *Cancer* 1981; 27:2147–2152.
3. Storm FK, Eilber FR, Mirra J, et al: Retroperitoneal sarcomas: A reappraisal of treatment. *J Surg Oncol* 1981; 17:1–7.
4. Braasch JW, Mon AB: Primary retroperitoneal tumors. *Surg Clin Am* 1967; 47:663–678.
5. Hindai H, Sakuramoto T, Miura T, et al: Needle tract seeding following puncture of retroperitoneal liposarcoma. *Eur Urol* 1983; 9:368–369.
6. Lindell MM, Wallace S, DeSantos LA, et al: Diagnostic techniques for the evaluation of the soft tissue sarcoma. *Semin Oncol* 1981; 8:160–171.
7. Neifeld JP, Walsh JW, Lawrence W Jr, et al: Computed tomography in the management of soft tissue tumors. *Surg Gynecol Obstet* 1982; 155:535–540.
8. Kreel L, Bydder GM: Evaluation of retroperitonal sarcoma with computed tomography. *Comput Tomogr* 1981; 5:111–116.
9. Hajdu SI: *Pathology of Soft Tissue Tumors*. Philadelphia, Lea & Febiger, 1979, pp 122–135.
10. Benamark S, Hafstrom L, Jonsson PE, et al: Retroperitoneal sarcoma treated by surgery. *J Surg Oncol* 1980; 14:307–314.
11. Tepper JE, Suit HD, Wood WC, et al: Radiation therapy of retroperitoneal soft tissue sarcomas. *Int J Radiat Oncol Biol Phys* 1984; 10:825–830.
12. Russell W, Cohen G, Enzinger F, et al: A clinical and pathological staging system for soft tissue sarcomas. *Cancer* 1977; 40:1562–1570.
13. Kinne DW, Chu FCH, Huvos AG, et al: Treatment of primary and retroperitoneal liposarcoma. *Cancer* 1973; 31:53–64.
14. Adam YG, Oland J, Halevy A, et al: Primary retroperitoneal soft tissue sarcomas. *J Surg Oncol* 1984; 25:8–11.
15. McGrath PC, Neifeld JP, Lawrence W Jr, et al: Improved survival following complete excision of retroperitoneal sarcomas. *Ann Surg* 1984; 200:200–204.
16. Wood WC, Suit HD, Mankin HJ, Cohen AM, et al: Radiation and conservative surgery in the treatment of soft tissue sarcoma. *Am J Surg* 1984; 147:537–541.
17. Moore SV, Aldrete JS: Primary retroperitoneal sarcomas. The role of surgical treatment. *Am J Surg* 1981; 142:358–361.
18. Kinsella TJ, Sindelar WF, Lack E, et al: Preliminary results of a randomized study of adjuvant radiation therapy in resectable adult retroperitoneal soft tissue sarcomas. *J Clin Oncol* 1988; 6:18–25.

19. Canton J, McNeer GP, Chu FC, et al: The problem of local recurrence after treatment of soft tissue sarcoma. *Ann Surg* 1968; 168:47–53.
20. Suit HD, Russell WO: Radiation therapy of soft tissue sarcomas. *Cancer* 1975; 37:759–764.
21. Fortner JG, Martin S, Hajdu S, et al: Primary sarcoma of the retroperitoneum. *Semin Oncol* 1981; 8:180–184.
22. Binder SC, Katz B, Sheridan B: Retroperitoneal liposarcoma. *Ann Surg* 1978; 187:257–261.
23. Arbeit JM, Flye MW, Mundinger GH, et al: Latent pulmonary embolus from a retroperitoneal sarcoma. *Cancer* 1980; 46:1492–1498.
24. Bailey RV, Stribling J, Weitzner S, et al: Leiomyosarcoma of the inferior vena cave. *Ann Surg* 1976; 184:169–173.
25. Brewster DC, Athanasoulis CA, Darling RC: Leiomyosarcoma of the inferior vena cava. *Arch Surg* 1976; 11:1081–1085.
26. Localio SA, Eng K, Ranson JHC: Abdominosacral approach for retrorectal tumors. *Ann Surg* 1980; 191:555–560.
27. Pearman RO, Mayo CW: Desmoid tumors. *Ann Surg* 1942; 115:114–125.
28. Rosenberg SA, Suit HD, Baker LH, et al: Sarcomas of the soft tissue and bone, in De vita VT, Hellman S, Rosenberg SA (eds): *Cancer: Principles and Practice of Oncology.* Philadelphia, J. B. Lippincott, 1982, pp 1036–1093.
29. Karakousis CP: Exposure and reconstruction in the lower portion of the retroperitoneum and abdominal wall. *Arch Surg* 1982; 117:840–844.
30. Shiu MH, Flancbaum L, Hajdu SI, et al: Malignant soft tissue tumors of the anterior abdominal wall. *Arch Surg* 1980; 115: 152–155.

Chapter 15

Sarcomas of the Female Genital Tract

Arlan F. Fuller, Jr.

Donald Patterson

David S. Shimm

INTRODUCTION

Sarcomas arising in the female genital tract constitute less than 1% of gynecological malignancies. The clinical course and prognosis of these tumors vary widely, from extensive local growth and invasion in some, to widespread early metastases in others. A detailed review of this diverse behavior may provide both a source of guidance to the practicing physician and a framework for better understanding of pathogenesis and interrelationships.

To provide a resource for practical management by the clinician, we have categorized these lesions, reviewed the important distinguishing pathological characteristics, and provided the clinicopathological correlations that may assist in the diagnosis, treatment, and follow-up of these uncommon lesions. To delineate perspective, we have critically reviewed the end results of treatment to assess sites of treatment failure, and suggest directions for improved therapy.

CLASSIFICATION

The upper female genital tract (fallopian tubes, uterus, cervix, and upper vagina) has a common derivation from the Müllerian ducts. These ducts, in turn, are paired structures resulting from the invagination of the coelomic epithelium of the genital ridge; this same primitive epithelium covers the peritoneal surfaces of the ovaries and, as the so-called "germinal" epithelium, represents the origin of the common epithelial tumors of the ovary.[1]

The embryonic mesenchyme surrounding the ducts also participates in the development of the genital tract. As the ducts differentiate into the epithelial components, so too does the mesenchyme arise from its subcoelomic site of origin and develop into the muscle and supporting stroma of the fallopian tube, uterine myometrium, endometrium, and cervical stroma.

Just as the epithelial components appear to recapitulate the epithelial derivatives of their embryonic tissue of origin, so may the mesenchymal components of each organ follow a similar path in neoplastic transformation. Thus, one encounters the mixed müllerian tumor, unique to the female genital tract, arising in the ovary, fallopian tube, cervix, or uterus. Because of the prevalence of this lesion among genital sarcomas and its unique nature, the classification of these upper genital tract tumors into those of müllerian mesenchymal origin contrasts with those pure soft-tissue sarcomas originating in the vulva and vagina (Table 15–1).

Further substantiation of this pathogenesis comes from the recognition that primary endometrial stromal sarcomas may originate in other müllerian tissues, particularly in the myometrium[2] and cervix.[3] The origin of gynecological sarcomas from the müllerian derivatives of the "subcoelomic mesenchyme"[4] further serves to explain the etiology of leiomyomatosis peritonealis disseminata (LPD), a rare benign disease occurring in premenopausal women and characterized by multiple subperitoneal nodules of well-differentiated smooth muscle on peritoneal surfaces in the pelvis and abdomen. Some of these nodules contain foci of müllerian epithelial tissue, such as endometrial glands and stroma.[5]

SARCOMAS OF THE LOWER GENITAL TRACT

Vulvar Sarcoma

Primary sarcoma of the vulva is a rare malignancy comprising no more than 1% to 3% of all vulvar cancer. The exact incidence is difficult to determine because the histology may be confused with melanoma, undifferentiated carcinoma, necrobiotic granuloma,[6] and even squamous carcinoma with spindle cell transformation.[7]

In contrast to squamous cell carcinoma of the vulva, which has a peak incidence in the seventh and eighth decade of life, sarcoma of the vulva occurs in a younger age group with a peak incidence at 30 to 50 years.[8] The majority of sarcomas are confined to the labia majora (50% to 60%) and the labia minora (25%). These lesions generally present as a mass in the vulva beneath the surface epithelium, often associated with local discomfort. Confusion with a benign Bartholin's gland lesion often delays the diagnosis of sarcoma. Several studies have suggested a 1-year delay in diagnosis in 30% to 35% of patients.[9, 10] Successful treatment requires early diagnosis by biopsy of any persistant subepithelial mass.

The clinical behavior of the vulvar sarcomas varies widely with histology. Rhabdomyosarcoma is associated with rapid growth and early metastasis to regional nodes as well as distant sites. Leiomyosarcoma and malignant fibrous histiocytoma may grow slowly with extensive local invasion; recurrences predominate at local sites following primary therapy, with distant metastasis occurring late in the disease.

The general approach to management is either wide local excision or radical vulvectomy.

TABLE 15–1.
Classification of Genital Tract Sarcomas

Sarcoma	Characteristics
Müllerian	Arising in the uterus, ovary, fallopian tube, and cervix
Pure homologous	All tissue of müllerian origin
Pure heterologous	Tissue of extra müllerian origin
Mixed müllerian tumors	Containing a malignant epithelial component as well; these may be homologous (carcinosarcoma) or heterologous
Nonmüllerian	Arising in the lower female genital tract with the general pathological characteristics and clinical behavior of the common soft-tissue sarcomas

The extent of the procedure is determined by the location of the tumor, the extent of disease, both locally and regionally, as well as by the histological type of tumor (the distinction between these two procedures for any large tumor is only semantic). Dermatofibroma requires only wide local excision and rarely metastasizes. Leiomyosarcoma requires at least wide local excision; if local recurrence develops, then more extensive local excision, even radical vulvectomy and bilateral groin lymphadenectomy, is necessary. Primary radical vulvectomy and bilateral groin lymphadenectomy have also been suggested.[11]

Epithelioid sarcoma of the vulva differs markedly in its clinical behavior from extragenital lesions of similar histology. The tumor frequently recurs locally after wide local excision and is usually followed by distant metastasis, particularly to the lungs. This behavior suggests potential benefit from a more extensive local excision or radical vulvectomy as well as benefit from adjuvant therapy. No data are presently available for adjuvant chemotherapy, although a brief response to doxorubicin has been noted in one case.[12] Malignant fibrous histiocytoma is prone to local recurrence and there may be a role for postoperative local radiation therapy in this disease. Endometrial stromal sarcoma needs aggressive radical surgery and lymph node dissection and may benefit from resection of late solitary distant metastasis. Kaposi's sarcoma should be treated with radiation or chemotherapy following surgical biopsy.[13]

Common surgical complications of radical vulvar surgery include wound infection, necrosis, and separation, as well as late effects of leg edema and introital stenosis. Traditionally, vulvar tissue has been thought to tolerate radiation poorly. However, reports of excellent responses of advanced vulvar carcinoma to external radiation therapy indicate that although local reactions may be severe, they are short lived and may justify treatment, particularly if the perineum can be kept dry. Radiation therapy in the past has generally been reserved for surgical failures and for treatment of pelvic nodes in patients with groin node metastasis.

In contrast to the tumors of the surface epithelium of the vulva, where an adequate deep margin can be obtained by radical surgery, the sarcomatous lesions arising in the deep vulvar tissues and margins are compromised in all but the smallest of low-grade lesions. In light of the propensity for local recurrence in many of these tumors, there is a role for adjuvant radiation therapy, particularly if wide local excision is performed. In the extragenital soft-tissue sarcomas, this approach has led to local control and survival rates comparable to ablative radical surgery.[14, 15]

Studies of the role for chemotherapy have been anecdotal to date. They have included single-agent therapy such as methotrexate and multiple-agent therapy such as actinomycin D, Cytoxan (cyclophosphamide), and DTIC (dacarbazine) with limited success. A greater role for adjuvant therapy will require development and clinical trials of more effective chemotherapeutic agents.

Vaginal Sarcoma

In the adult, primary sarcoma of the vagina represents a distinctly rare entity: a small proportion of the cancers arising in a site bearing less than 2% of all gynecological malignancies. The majority of these tumors originate in the smooth muscle wall of the vagina and range from benign leiomyomas or cellular myomas with a distinct pseudocapsule to fully developed, infiltrative lesions with marked cellular atypism and a high mitotic index.

The clinical presentation is that of a subepithelial mass, identified either in an asymptomatic patient on routine examination, or in evaluating complaints of pain, particularly with coitus. The tumor may be within the vaginal wall itself, or paravaginal in location. The majority of the 60 smooth muscle tumors reviewed by Tavassoli and Norris[16] from the files of the Armed Forces Institute of Pathology (AFIP) (Washington, DC) were either benign or locally aggressive neoplasms, with recurrences in only five cases. They concluded that the five tumors with recurrences all were 3 cm or more in size and demonstrated the presence of five or more mitoses per ten high-power fields on microscopic examination. The one patient with an infiltrating tumor margin developed pulmonary metastases. Five such leiomyosarcomas were reported from the Swedish Cancer Registry; four patients with high-grade lesions were dead within 36 months, whereas one patient with a low-grade lesion was alive at 10 years after wide local excision.[17]

These lesions require careful clinical assessment. If the lesion is small with well-defined borders, excisional biopsy will provide both diagnosis and sufficient therapy for most lesions. With cellular atypia or a high mitotic index, additional therapy will be required because of the risk of both local recurrence and distant metastasis. If the lesion is large with diffuse margins, or if it is situated anteriorly (as were three of the five Swedish cases noted), or lateral to the vaginal wall, needle biopsy prior to definitive therapy may be warranted. We have approached the low-grade paravaginal sarcomas from an extraperitoneal route following diagnosis by needle biopsy. Typically the report will be "smooth muscle tumor" with rare or absent mitoses. The differential diagnosis in recent cases has included lymphoma or granulocytic sarcoma. Should the lesion be large and involve the upper third of the vagina and cervix, then hysterectomy will be required with retroperitoneal dissection of the ureter and bladder on the affected side.

The large, low-grade lesions have been treated with postoperative pelvic radiation therapy. Choice of treatment for the rarer, high-grade sarcomas is presently unclear, because of the uniformly fatal results with local recurrence as well as distant metastases. It should probably include adjuvant chemotherapy as well as postoperative radiotherapy.

Primary lymphoma of the vagina is another rare cancer that must be distinguished from the smooth muscle tumors arising in this site, because both may present as an asymptomatic paravaginal mass. We have treated several patients with primary lymphoma involving either the cervix[18] or vagina with a combination of surgical resection and pre- or postoperative radiotherapy. The role of surgery beyond diagnosis appears limited; two patients with disease confined to the anterior vagina, bladder, and retropubic space, not amenable to nonradical surgical excision, were treated with primary radiation therapy and have remained free of disease beyond a 5-year interval.

Embryonal rhabdomyosarcoma of the vagina (sarcoma botryoides) is commonly recognized as a disease of infancy, with more than 50% of cases occurring in the first 2 years of life.[19] Its treatment is discussed elsewhere in this book (Chapter 17), and involves the use of combination chemotherapy with conservative, nonmutilating surgery and radiation therapy for patients with uncertain surgical margins. Survival is related to the initial extent of disease and to the adequacy of resection; survival exceeds 80% in completely resected, localized disease. It should be noted as well that this disease may occur in adults, involving the vagina, cervix, or uterus, with a poorer prognosis than in childhood.[20] Thirteen adult patients with genitourinary rhabdomyosarcoma had a 38% 5-year survival following surgery and radiation and there was a marked tendency to distant metastases (lung, bone, liver, and lymph nodes).

SARCOMAS OF THE UPPER GENITAL TRACT

Malignant lesions of the upper genital tract (cervix, uterus, fallopian tube, and ovary) share common histological characteristics and presumably a common origin in the same primordial müllerian stem cell. The explanation for simultaneous neoplasia of both mesenchymal and epithelial elements in the mixed müllerian tumors of these organs remains unclear, but represents an inescapable fact. Tumors initially presenting as poorly differentiated carcinoma and recurring as sarcoma (especially in the ovary) are usually found to have small foci of sarcomatous elements on retrospective review of the initial specimen. Selection of cells resistant to therapy may lead to subsequent proliferation of the resistant clone and overgrowth with persistence or recurrence as a sarcoma. No evidence exists at present for conversion of these two cell types.

Cervical Sarcomas

Cervical sarcoma is a rare primary malignant neoplasm with a generally poor prognosis, usually presenting as a polypoid mass during the late reproductive and the perimenopausal years. Ulceration of the mass and vaginal bleeding may accompany progression of disease. The exact incidence of this tumor is uncertain; reports suggest an incidence of 0.2% to 0.5% of all cervical cancers.[21–23] Tumors should be considered to arise in the cervix *only* in the absence of involvement of the corpus uteri.[3] The majority of these tumors are of müllerian origin and represent the pure homologous tumor (Table 15–1). In the adult, leiomyosarcomas and endometrial stromal sarcomas predominate, with rare cases of mixed tumors, either adenosarcoma or mixed müllerian tumors.

Cervical leiomyosarcomas may be associated with pre-existing cervical leiomyomas. These smooth muscle sarcomas are described histologically as consisting of neoplastic, spindle-shaped muscle cells with large hyperchromatic nuclei. Mitotic activity may be evaluated by the criteria of Norris and Taylor[24] for uterine sarcomas. The presence of ten or more mitoses per ten high-power fields (HPF) indicates a poorer prognosis and differentiates high-grade from low-grade lesions.

The typical patient is in her fifth decade and presents with complaints of vaginal bleeding; a polypoid cervical lesion or diffuse cervical enlargement is evident. Initial treatment is similar to that for cervical carcinoma of corresponding extent. Local disease is treated with either radical hysterectomy or radiation therapy; combined modality therapy involves planned post-radiation total hysterectomy for bulky uterine disease or postoperative radiation therapy when extensive invasion is present in the surgical specimen. The therapeutic value of pelvic node dissection is unclear, but it should be performed with primary radical hysterectomy to assess the extent of disease. The frequency of nodal metastases is uncertain, but in light of their prevalence with similar tumors of the uterine body,[25] lymphadenectomy should be undertaken. Although reports are few, cervical leiomyosarcomas appear to have a very poor prognosis, regardless of treatment, because of a high risk of distant dissemination, even when local control can be achieved.

Cervical stromal sarcomas arise from müllerian tissue in the cervix and may, therefore, resemble the corresponding uterine sarcoma. Abel and Ramirez[3] have reported the results of treatment in 12 cases; patients typically presented with vaginal bleeding and a polypoid, occasionally ulcerated cervical mass. Surgery was the primary mode of therapy in seven patients; two others received a combination of radiation therapy with either surgery or chemotherapy, and one was treated with chemotherapy alone. Two patients were not treated, because of the extent of their metastatic disease. Seven of the 12 died within 2 years of diagnosis; most survivors had low-grade primaries. In our own experience, the only high-grade lesion associated with long-term survival was one in which the tumor arose in a polyp and was not invasive of its base.

Cervical adenosarcoma is a low-grade form of mixed müllerian tumor containing benign neoplastic glands associated with a sarcomatous stroma. The histological appearance of the stroma is characteristic of endometrial stromal sarcoma; when invasion is present, it is circumscribed. Patients are usually postmenopausal and present with abnormal bleeding. Total abdominal hysterectomy yields low recurrence rates. Two patients in their teenage years were treated conservatively in a report from the AFIP and did not develop recurrence after either subtotal excision of the cervix or wide local excision of polypoid cervical lesions.[26] Our own experience with a third patient treated by cone biopsy alone has been successful to date; the teenage nulligravida is still free of recurrence after 3 years of very close observation.

Mixed müllerian tumors contain malignant epithelial and connective tissue elements. The epithelial component may be either squamous or glandular carcinoma. The sarcomatous component may be either homologous, containing elements of only uterine derivation, or heterologous, containing neoplasms of cartilaginous, bony, or striated muscle origin. Both components arise from the pluripotential müllerian cells in the cervix. The tumors have a very poor prognosis, like their uterine counterparts, regardless of histological subtype. Sixty-six percent of the patients described by Rotmench et al.[27] died with local and disseminated disease within 15 months of diagnosis.

Uterine Sarcomas

Uterine sarcomas represent approximately 4% of all uterine malignancies and are associated with a poor prognosis because of their propensity for widespread dissemination within the abdomen and hematogenous metastases as well as local pelvic recurrence. According to the classification described by Kempson and Bari,[28] uterine sarcomas can also be classified into three major groups, the mixed müllerian tumors (MMT) and two forms of pure homologous sarcoma: leiomyosarcomas (LMS), and endometrial stromal sarcomas (ESS). These represent approximately 50%, 25%, and 15%, respectively, of uterine sarcomas, with the balance being sarcomas of other histological types. These groups will be discussed in general as one entity, because most major clinical reports include all three subtypes. Where specific differences occur, they will be described.

The typical patient is a woman in the seventh or eighth decade of life, although the average age at diagnosis of leiomyosarcoma is approximately 10 years younger. Symptoms are nonspecific, including vaginal discharge or bleeding, pelvic pain, an abdominal mass, or ascites. There is no clear-cut relation between parity or hormonal exposure in those tumors, with the exception of a solitary report of a risk ratio of 1.5 (95% confidence interval, 1.3 to 1.8) for women who were never married.[29] Some series have implicated prior exposure to ionizing radiation as an etiological factor in mixed müllerian tumors.[30]

Although the diagnosis of endometrial stromal sarcoma or mixed müllerian tumor can be readily made by diagnostic endometrial curettage, the identification of a uterine mass as leiomyosarcoma is considerably more difficult, as it is usually not contiguous with the endometrial cavity. Occasionally the diagnosis of leiomyosarcoma may be made pre-operatively on the basis of circumstantial evidence, that is, a rapidly enlarging "fibroid," but this event is rare. The incidence of leiomyosarcoma was reported by Meigs[31] over 50 years ago as 0.6% of all fibroids. This number is abnormally high for the general population at risk, because only a small number of women ever came to surgery for their symptomatic leiomyomas. Nonetheless, similar figures continue to be quoted in leading texts, raising undue apprehension and leading to a lower threshold for hysterectomy. Wallach et al.[32] have estimated that as many as 30% of women in their late 30s and 40s may have leiomyomata. Given the prevalence of leiomyomas in the population at risk, the incidence of leiomyosarcoma is no more than 0.01%, and probably an order of magnitude less. With the use of diagnostic ultrasound, which can both quantitate changes in size and detect central necrosis, and with repetitive pelvic examinations, it is possible to improve the precision of diagnosis. Leibsohn and colleagues[33] also emphasized the importance of age and menopause; of 1,429 women who came to hysterectomy for presumed leiomyomas, 10 had leiomyosarcomas. Seven of the ten patients had symptoms of abnormal uterine bleeding. From the fourth to the seventh decade of age, the incidence rose from 0.2% to 0.9% to 1.4% to 1.9%, respectively.

Although uterine sarcomas are not included within the International Federation of Obstetrics and Gynecology (FIGO) staging system for endometrial carcinomas, a number of authors have adopted the FIGO staging system to describe their patients. The stage at diagnosis in a number of series, including all histologies, is shown in Table 15–2.[34–39] For all 349 patients included in these series, only 53% presented with disease confined to the uterine corpus. Leiomyosarcomas typically present with a lower stage than do the other uterine sarcomas; for patients described in Table 15–2, 71/115 (62%) presented with stage I disease.

TABLE 15–2.
Distribution of Clinical Stage in Patients with Uterine Sarcoma

Author	Stage (%) I	II	III	IV	Total Patients
Badib et al[35]	56	11	19	14	147
Salazar et al[36, 37]	56	16	17	11	73
Mantravadi et al[38]	56	10	21	13	52
Tanga and Delgado[39]	41	18	18	22	49
Shimm et al[34]	46	11	36	7	28
Average	53	14	19	14	349

Clinical stage at presentation is the most important prognostic factor in determining survival. Once the tumor has spread beyond the uterine corpus, the chance for cure is small, as shown in Table 15–3. For leiomyosarcoma, the most powerful prognostic feature is the origin of the tumor. Van Dinh and Woodruff[40] reviewed 43 cases and found similar 5-year survivals for sarcomas arising in submucous (80%), intramural (88%), and subserous fibroids

TABLE 15–3.
Survival by Clinical Stage in Uterine Sarcoma

Author	Stage I	II	III	IV
Badib et al[35]	50/82 (61%)	4/17 (24%)	1/27 (4%)	0/18
Mantravadi et al[38]	17/29 (59%)	2/5 (40%)	0/11	0/7
Salazar et al[36, 37]	64%		20%	
Shimm et al[34]	32%		15%	

TABLE 15–4.
Association of Survival with Mitotic Counts in Thirty Patients with Leiomyosarcoma*

Number of Mitoses per HPF†	Five-Year Survival (%)	Number of Mitoses per Ten HPF	Five-Year Survival (%)
2–3 (11)††	100	1–4 (9)	100
4–5 (13)	69	5–9 (16)	75
6–7 (3)	33	>10 (5)	20
8–9 (5)	33		

* *From Van Dinh T, Woodruff JD: Leiomyosarcoma of the uterus.* Am J Obstet Gynecol *1982; 144:817–823. Used by permission.*
† *Number of mitoses in the most anaplastic high-power field (HPF).*
†† *The number in parentheses is the total number of patients.*

(100%), while those developing de novo in the myometrial wall had a 25% 5-year survival. The physical separation of the malignancy from the myometrium by the myoma may serve to explain this difference. This has been suggested by the observation that most patients with leiomyosarcoma in larger (6 to 10 cm) myomas had the best survival.[40] A low mitotic count was an additional favorable prognostic feature (Table 15–4).

The prognosis of the mixed müllerian tumor does not vary according to its histological constituents, regardless of the presence of homologous or heterologous elements.[41] The Johns Hopkins group also noted a 76% 2-year survival with invasion of less than one half of the myometrial thickness compared with a 17% survival if more than one half of the wall was involved. They also noted that all of the latter group had evidence of spread of disese beyond the uterus. The Gynecologic Oncology Group[42] studied nodal metastases in patients with disease apparently limited to the uterus. Ten of 28 patients had histologically positive pelvic nodes and 4 of these 10 had para-aortic nodal metastases as well. All patients with nodal metastases had evidence of myometrial invasion beyond the inner third of the uterine wall. The report by Chen[25] (previously cited) also demonstrated a high rate of nodal metastasis. Nine of 20 patients were found to have pelvic nodal metastases (3) or both pelvic and para-aortic metastases. All nine patients with nodal metastases died of the disease.[25]

Endometrial stromal tumors are commonly subdivided into three groups: (1) the endometrial stromal nodule, a benign neoplasm with well-demarcated, noninfiltrating margins, (2) endolymphatic stromal myosis, the invasive form with evidence of some mitotic activity (generally two to ten mitoses per 10 HPF) and a relatively good prognosis, and (3) endometrial stromal sarcoma, a highly anaplastic tumor (more than ten mitoses per HPF and near-uniform fatality.[43] The term "endolymphatic stromal myosis" may actually be a misnomer, as three-dimensional reconstruction of the tumor and immunohistochemical studies disclosed that two such tumors were growing in the intravascular space.[44] The benign and low-grade malignant forms may be referred to as endometrial "stromatosis." Terminology may vary; in a series of patients from the M. D. Anderson Hospital (Houston, TX), Evans[45] subdivided endometrial sarcomas into endometrial stromal sarcomas and poorly differentiated endometrial sarcomas. The endometrial stromal sarcomas, with low mitotic counts and good survival, correspond to the traditional endolymphatic stromal myosis. The poorly differentiated endometrial stromal sarcomas generally behave in a manner similar to that of the traditional endometrial stromal sarcoma. Age and menopause heavily influenced survival, because all patients younger than 50 years of age had well-differentiated, low-grade lesions, whereas all the patients with poorly differentiated, high-grade lesions were over 50 years of age. The low-grade lesions are diploid when analyzed by flow cytometry[46] and bear progesterone receptors.[47]

Uterine adenosarcoma is a variant of the mixed müllerian tumor with benign glands admixed with a sarcomatous stroma, most commonly endometrial stromal sarcoma. All patients described by Clement and Scully[48] were women in their seventh to ninth decades who presented with postmenopausal bleeding and were found to have bulky polypoid tumors. Only one patient had a deeply invasive malignancy; this was the only tumor to metastasize, although indolent local recurrences developed in the vagina in three of the remaining nine patients. A study from the AFIP confirmed this tendency to late local recurrence: 10 of 25 patients experienced local recurrence, with a median disease-free interval of 5 years. They also identified deep myometrial invasion as the only adverse prognostic factor.[49] The propensity for local recurrence suggests a role for postoperative intracavitary brachytherapy.

A benign variant of the uterine smooth muscle tumor, leiomyomatosis peritonealis disseminata, bears the gross clinical characteristics of metastatic carcinoma, with tumor nodules studding the peritoneal surfaces, yet a benign histological appearance. This condition was identified in pregnancy in 7 of 12 patients reviewed by Williams and Pavlick[50] and in 1 patient the concurrent presence of a granulosa cell tumor of the ovary was reported. They concluded that the genesis of this tumor from the subcoelomic mesenchyme was the response to persistent estrogen secretion. This conclusion was supported by the subsequent experimental development of this disease in guinea pigs with constant estrogen administration.[51] Therapy for this condition, usually identified incidentally at cesarian section, is conservative, with spontaneous regression common, and oophorectomy a last resort. There have been only two reports of malignancy arising within the field of leiomyomatosis peritonealis disseminate; both patients had highly malignant lesions and short survival following diagnosis. We have seen one woman with a low-grade lesion whose tumor could be completely excised following pre-operative hypogastric embolization with autologous thrombus and in continuity resection of the descending and rectosigmoid colon.[52] The use of pre-operative embolization for large pelvic sarcomas permits control of the deep hypogastric vessels prior to mobilization of these bulky tumors and, along with deliberate hypotensive anesthesia, minimizes operative blood loss.[53]

Intravenous leiomyomatosis (IL) and benign metastasizing leiomyomata (BML) represent two other uncommon forms of benign smooth muscle tumor that mimic malignancy. The clinical picture may include pulmonary metastases on chest radiograph or a tumor mass within veins of the myometrium or pelvic side wall. It is clear that myometrial vessels do respond to estrogens with proliferation during the follicular phase of the menstrual cycle and this condition may represent a further benign proliferation of those responsive vessels that originate in the endomyometrium. Banner et al.[54] have reported complete remissions in these diseases after oophorectomy. Our experience has been with occasional local recurrence of IL requiring resection and postoperative pelvic radiation therapy and pulmonary metastases with both IL and BML. Although some solitary lesions have responded to progestins, wedge resection of the involved lung is often necessary for long-term control.

As the peak age of incidence of leiomyosarcoma is considerably younger than that of other uterine sarcomas, many patients will be premenopausal and a number of these will have had myomectomy as initial treatment of this malignancy. Since premenopausal patients have a better prognosis than their postmenopausal counterparts, serious consideration must be given to uterine preservation rather than hysterectomy in selected patients who wish to preserve childbearing.[55] Van Dinh and Woodruff[40] reviewed the outcome of nine patients in whom the diagnosis was made after myomectomy. Three of the nine underwent hysterectomy as part of their primary treatment; six others, ages 22 to 33 elected "conservative" therapy and five of the six survived free of disease. One patient had a recurrence in the uterus and abdomen and was alive with metastases six years after initial myomectomy.

The difference in prognosis for leiomyosarcoma between pre- and postmenopausal women also merits further investigation. Lantta et al.[56] reported the presence of high levels of estrogen and progesterone receptors in leiomyosarcomas. One could hypothesize that concurrent bilateral oophorectomy in the premenopausal patient might have a significant therapeutic effect on occult metastases. Examination of resected specimens for steroid receptors may clarify this further and correlate with subsequent response to exogenous progestin treatment.

Radiation therapy has been employed as a primary means of therapy for this disease in patients with advanced disease or poor medical condition. As expected, results have been poor. External beam therapy or intracavitary irradiation has been employed in an adjuvant setting by a number of investigators. Although whole abdominal irradiation has been reported in an anecdotal fashion, most experience has involved pelvic irradiation. Although a few series have demonstrated a slight survival advantage following pelvic irradiation, most have not, in keeping with the frequent extrapelvic spread of these tumors. On the other hand, where pelvic control has been evaluated, most series have shown improvement with pelvic irradiation, as shown in Table 15–5.[35–38, 57–60] Reported techniques of irradiation have varied, including pre-operative and postoperative external pelvic irradiation, as well as pre-operative intracavitary irradiation, but no technique appears to yield noticeably better or poorer results. In our series of patients, most treated with postoperative external pelvic irradiation,[34] multivariate analysis showed that pelvic control varied with the dose delivered to the pelvis. On that basis, when pelvic irradiation is used to improve local control, we recommend giving radiation to the tolerance of pelvic structures, regardless of technique: approximately 50 Gy pre-operative external pelvic radiation, 45 Gy postoperative external pelvic radiation, or 9,000 to 10,000 mg-hr pre-operatively using tandem, ovoids and Simon capsules.

In a disease such as uterine sarcoma which can recur locally, spread over peritoneal surfaces, or disseminate through the blood stream, there is an obvious need for effective chemotherapy. However, clinical experience with chemotherapy for advanced disease has been disappointing. The M. D. Anderson Hospital has published the results of a study of 74 patients with advanced uterine sarcomas treated with a combination of cyclophosphamide, vincristine, and actinomycin D.[61] Thirteen percent were complete responders, with a median duration of 16 months, whereas 16% were partial responders, with a median duration of 5.5 months. Other studies employing combinations including doxorubicin have reported more partial responders, but no more complete responders, and no increase in remission durability. The M. D. Anderson group also reported their results with adjuvant chemotherapy in early uterine sarcomas, which were no better than their results in an untreated historical control group.[62] Studies with more intensive therapy in the adjuvant setting for high-risk stage I uterine sarcomas have more promise: Piver et al.[63] reported a 36% estimated 5-year survival rate with surgery alone vs. 63% for surgery plus doxorubicin. In another study with adjuvant cyclophosphamide, vincristine, doxorubicin, and dacarbazine, Piver reported an 89% 5-year survival rate. Peters et al.[64] studied the effects of adjuvant high-dose cisplatin and doxorubicin (100 mg and 45–60 mg/m^2, respectively) on patients with stromal sarcomas and mixed mesodermal tumors of the uterus. The excellent re-

TABLE 15–5.
Effect of Pelvic Radiation on Outcome in Pelvic Sarcoma

Author*	Histology†	Local Control (S)‡	Local Control (S + X)	Survival	Survival (S + X)
DiSaia et al[57]	MMT	2/5	19/24	2/5	14/24
Badib et al[35]	LMS	16/26	10/12	15/32	11/26
	MMT	3/11	1/9	5/14	6/18
	ESS	4/9	4/6	6/10	7/10
Mantravadi et al[38]	LMS	15/18	9/9	12/18	4/9
	MMT			2/8	5/10
		8/13	10/14		
	ESS			1/4	1/2
Salazar et al[36, 37]	All	12/33	7/31		
Vongtama et al[58]	All	40%	54%	26/61	23/31
Saksela et al[59]	LMS	2/4	9/19		
	MMT	0/2	6/8		
	ESS	3/4	6/14		
Perez et al[60]	All	3/9	8/13		

* *Disaia et al: Stage I, 2-year absolute survival, 2-year absolute local control; Badib et al: All stages, 5-year absolute survival, ultimate local control; Mantravadi et al: All stages, 5-year absolute survival, ultimate local control; Salazar et al: All stages, ultimate local control; Vongtama et al: Stages I and II, 5-year actuarial survival, ultimate local control; Saksela et al: All stages, 5-year absolute survival; Perez et al: Stages I and II, 3-year absolute survival.*
† *MMT = mixed müllerian tumor; LMS = leiomyosarcoma; ESS = endometrial stromal sarcoma.*
‡ *S = Surgery; X = Radiation therapy.*

sults with high-risk patients, if confirmed, support a role for adjuvant therapy in stage I uterine sarcoma.

Sarcoma of the Fallopian Tube

Müllerian tumors containing both glandular and stromal elements represent a rare primary neoplasm of the fallopian tube. Fewer than 50 patients have been reported in the literature to date.[65, 66] These tumors are found predominantly in postmenopausal women (median age, 58 years). Symptoms can include vaginal bleeding, abdominal swelling, and abdominal pain, but, like the ovarian neoplasms, minimal symptoms are generally present in the early stages of the disease. A hydrosalpinx may result from a slow-growing intraluminal polypoid mass. Tumor histology is identical to its counterpart in the uterus and ovary and includes mixed müllerian tumor (homologous and heterologous), carcinosarcoma, and leiomyosarcoma.[67] This is consistent with the multipotentiality of the mesoderm of the müllerian system. The malignant potential is expressed by local infiltration, peritoneal implants, metastasis to lymph nodes, ovaries, contralateral tube, and distant viscera. In the very rare case of tumor confined to the tube with a smooth outer surface, there may be a favorable outcome.[68] The disease generally presents in an advanced stage with metastases[69]; early lesions may be incidental findings.

The prognosis is grim and relates to the diagnosis of the disease in advanced stages. The mean survival is 7 to 8 months.[70] The treatment is primarily surgery, followed by radiation and/or chemotherapy.[71] Chemotherapy has included vincristine, actinomycin D, and cyclophosphamide,[72] Adriamycin (doxorubicin) and DTIC,[72] cyclophosphamide and 5-fluorouracil,[71] and cisplatin and cyclophosphamide.[69] The results from our unit with cisplatin and cyclophosphamide and cisplatin and doxorubicin have been encouraging.

Ovarian Sarcoma

Ovarian sarcomas may be derived from three sources of connective tissue in the pelvis: (1) the totipotential müllerian cell and associated subcoelomic mesenchyme, (2) the mesenchymal tissue of the ovarian stroma itself, and (3) the mesenchymal component of an adult teratoma.[73]

Regardless of the tissue of origin, early detection is rare, and the patient usually presents with abdominal bloating and cramps similar to the symptoms of advanced ovarian carcinoma. Surgical resection remains the mainstay of treatment in concert with precise operative staging of the extent of disease. Surgery alone has provided mixed success, being particularly useful in the low-grade endometrial stromal sarcomas; these alone appear to have a favorable outcome.

The teratoid sarcoma may arise either de novo from undifferentiated embryonic sarcoma, or from a benign cystic (adult) teratoma. It is a disease of young women; only one of the first ten patients reported was over 25 years old. The tumor usually contains undifferentiated elements and has a poor prognosis despite the fact that it is frequently confined to a single ovary.

The sarcoma of ovarian stromal (mesenchymal) origin also occurs predominantly in young women. The histological appearance of the tumor reflects its origin; in Woodruff's series, there was an equal distribution of the predominant subtypes: stromal (spindle cell) sarcoma and fibrosarcoma/leiomyosarcoma.

The mixed mesodermal tumors are extremely aggressive, presenting at advanced stages following rapid growth. The major prognostic factor is the stage at diagnosis, particularly the presence of spread beyond the ovary. The optimal treatment remains unclear, as responses have generally been anecdotal. Morrow et al.[74] reported the results of treatment of 30 patients with mixed müllerian tumors of the ovary. These patients were treated with vincristine, actinomycin D, and cyclophosphamide (VAC); 22 patients received the drug only, the other 8 were treated with whole abdominal irradiation and a pelvic boost. Two of the eight patients receiving the combination were surviving at 32 and 54 months, whereas none of the chemotherapy-only group survived. The use of platinum-based chemotherapy has shown more promise, with a high initial response rate, but limited improvement in overall survival.[75]

CHEMOTHERAPY IN THE TREATMENT OF ADVANCED GYNECOLOGICAL SARCOMAS

In general, the role of chemotherapy in the treatment of advanced gynecological sarcomas is still limited by its relative inefficacy. The need for treatment of disease beyond the pelvis is readily apparent in the poor survival of most patients with high-grade lesions. Barker[76] has stated that the rarity of gynecological sarcomas allows for limited controlled trials of adequate chemotherapy. The müllerian tumors of the uterus may respond more frequently than the other gynecological sarcomas, because of the early stage of disease at diagnosis. Lele et al.[77] reported 35 cases of mixed müllerian tumors of the ovary with a 12% primary response to vincristine, Cytoxan, Adriamycin, and DTIC as a first-line drug combination. They report a 7% response using vincristine, actinomycin D, and Cytoxan as a second-line drug combination. DTIC and cisplatin was used as third-line combination with few partial responses. They concluded there was no clear-cut difference in the effectiveness of the various combinations. There were no significant long-term remissions following any of the systemic chemotherapeutic regimens.

Buchsbaum et al.[78] reported on the use of adjuvant chemotherapy in early stage leiomyosarcomas (stages I and II). Ten patients were treated with vincristine, actinomycin D, and Cytoxan. There were no concurrent controls. With 3- to 7-year follow-up, five patients were free of disease, two patients died of intercurrent disease free of tumor, and one patient was alive with tumor.[78] Piver and Lurain[79] reported no benefit in this setting from Adriamycin.

Six patients with leiomyosarcomas were treated by Azizi et al.[80] with DTIC, Adriamycin, and vincristine; three had a complete response, with a mean disease-free interval of 15.6 months.

Omura et al.[81] reported on patients with advanced uterine sarcomas (stages III and IV) using Adriamycin and Adriamycin plus DTIC. Sixteen percent responded to single-agent chemotherapy (13 of 80) compared to 24% in the combination group (16 of 66). The disease-free interval was 10 months, but there was no increase in survival. Patients with leiomyosarcomas seemed to have a longer survival. The addition of DTIC was associated with more hematological and gastrointestinal toxicity. Further treatment with vincristine, actinomycin D, and Cytoxan after either combination yielded no apparent benefit.[81] Other chemotherapeutic agents have included cisplatin,[82] methotrexate,[83] and 5-FU.[84]

CONCLUSION

Sarcomas of the female genital tract comprise a heterogeneous group of uncommon tumors with diverse behavior. In the lower genital tract, the histological type of the tumor best predicts prognosis, whether indolent local recurrence or virulent distant metastasis. In the upper genital tract, the derivatives of the subcoelomic mesenchyme predominate and the clinical behavior appears, in part, to be related to such local factors as the tissue of origin and locally invasive behavior. A notable exception is the ovarian sarcoma, in which a uniformly poor prognosis is evident. Future progress must depend on a means of early diagnosis and the development of effective chemotherapy for both advanced disease as well as the adjuvant setting.

REFERENCES

1. Donahoe PK, Fuller AF Jr, Scully RE, et al: Mullerian inhibiting substance inhibits growth of a human ovarian cancer in nude mice. *Ann Surg* 1981; 194:472–480.
2. Norris HJ, Taylor HB: Mesenchymal tumors of the uterus. I. A clinical and pathologic study of 53 endometrial stromal tumors. *Cancer* 1966; 19:755–766.
3. Abel MR, Ramirez JA: Sarcomas and carcinosarcomas of the uterine cervix. *Cancer* 1973; 31:1176–1192.
4. Ober WB, Black MB: Neoplasms of the subcoelomic mesenchyme. *Arch Pathol* 1955; 59:698–705.
5. Kaplan C, Benirschke K, Johnson KC: Leiomyomatosis peritonealis disseminata with endometrium. *Obstet Gynecol* 1980; 55:119–122.
6. Gallup DG, Abell MR, Morley, GW: Epithelioid sarcoma of the vulva. *Obstet Gynecol* 1976; 48:14s–17s.
7. Steeper TA, Piscioli F, Rosai J: Squamous cell carcinoma with sarcoma-like stroma of the female genital tract. *Cancer* 1983; 52:890–898.
8. DiSaia PJ, Rutledge F, Smith JP: Sarcoma of the vulva. *Obstet Gynecol* 1971; 38:180–184.
9. Davos I, Abell MR: Soft tissue sarcomas of the vulva. *Gynecol Oncol* 1976; 4:70–86.
10. Morley GW: Cancer of the vulva: A review. *Cancer* 1981; 48:597–601.

11. Malkasian GD: Gynecologic Sarcomas. [In] Cancer Medicine, Holland JF, Frei E, (eds), Lea and Febiger, Philadelphia 1973, pp. 1753–1756.
12. Ulbright TM, Brokaw SA, Stehman FB, et al: Epithelioid sarcoma of the vulva: Evidence suggesting a more aggressive behavior than extra-genital epithelioid sarcoma. *Cancer* 1983; 52:1462–1469.
13. Hall DJ, Burns JC, Goplerud, DR: Kaposi's sarcoma of the vulva: A case report and brief review. *Obstet Gynecol* 1979; 54:478–483.
14. Rosenberg SA, Tepper J, Glaststein E, et al: The treatment of soft tissue sarcomas of the extremities. Prospective randomized evaluations of limb sparing surgery plus radiation therapy compared with amputation and the role of adjuvant chemotherapy. *Ann Surg* 1982; 196:305–315.
15. Suit H, Mankin H, Wood W, et al: Treatment of the patient with stage M0 soft tissue sarcoma. *J Clin Oncol* 1988; 6:854–862.
16. Tavassoli FA, Norris HJ: Smooth muscle tumors of the vagina. *Obstet Gynecol* 1979; 53:689–693.
17. Rastogi BL, Bergman B, Angervall L: Primary leiomyosarcoma of the vagina: A study of five cases. *Gynecol Oncol* 1984; 18:77–86.
18. Muntz HG, Ferry JA, Flynn D, et al: Stage IE primary malignant lymphoma of the uterine cervix. *Cancer,* in press.
19. Hilgers RD: Pelvic exenteration for vaginal embryonal rhabdomyosarcoma. *Obstet Gynecol* 1975; 45:175–180.
20. Lloyd RV, Hajdu SI, Knapper WH: Embryonal rhabdomyosarcoma in adults. *Cancer* 1983; 51:557–565.
21. Crawford E, Tucker F: Sarcomas of the uterus. *Am J Obstet Gynecol* 1959; 77:286–291.
22. Chang H, Melin J, Vellois F, et al: Leiomyosarcomas of the uterus. *Obstet Gynecol* 1957; 9:212–218.
23. *Surveillance, Epidemiology, and Results; Incidence and Mortality Data 1973–1977.* National Cancer Institute Monograph 57, Bethesda, MD.
24. Norris H, Taylor H: Mesenchymal tumors of the uterus. III. A clinical and pathologic study of 31 carcinosarcomas. *Cancer* 1966; 49:1459–1465.
25. Chen SS: Propensity of retroperitoneal lymph node metastasis in patients with stage I sarcoma of the uterus. *Gynecol Oncol* 1989; 32:215–217.
26. Zaloudek C, Norris HJ: Adenofibroma and adenosarcoma of the uterus. *Cancer* 1981; 48:354–366.
27. Rotmench J, Rosenshein NB, Woodruff JD: Cervical sarcoma: A review. *Obstet Gynecol Surv* 1983; 38:456–460.
28. Kempson R, Bari W: Uterine sarcomas: Classification, diagnosis, and prognosis. *Hum Pathol* 1970; 1:331–349.
29. Schwartz SM, Weiss NS: Martial status and incidence of sarcomas of the uterus. *Cancer Res* 1990; 50:1886–1889.
30. Meredith RF, Eisert DR, Kaka Z, et al: An excess of uterine sarcomas after pelvic irradiation. *Cancer* 1986; 58:2003–2007.
31. Meigs, JV: *Tumors of the Female Pelvis.* New York, Macmillan, 1934, pp 147–157.
32. Wallach EE, Hammond CB, Goldfarb AF, et al: Symposium: Problems linked to uterine myomas. *Contemp OB/GYN* 1983; November.
33. Leibsohn S, d'Ablaing G, Mishell DR Jr, et al: Leiomyosarcoma in a series of hysterectomies performed for presumed uterine leiomyomas. *Am J Obstet Gynecol* 1990; 162:968–976.
34. Shimm D, Bell D, Fuller AF Jr, et al: Sarcomas of the uterine corpus: Prognostic factors and treatment. *Radiother Oncol* 1984; 2:201–207.
35. Badib A, Vongtama V, Kurohoar S, et al: Radiotherapy in the treatment of sarcomas of the corpus uteri. *Cancer* 1969; 24:724–729.
36. Salazar O, Bonfiglio T, Patten S, et al: Uterine sarcomas: Natural history, treatment, and prognosis. *Cancer* 1978; 42:1152–1160.
37. Salazar O, Bonfiglio T, Patten S, et al: Uterine sarcomas: Analysis of failures with special emphasis on the use of adjuvant radiation therapy. *Cancer* 1978; 42:1161–1170.
38. Mantravadi R, Bardawil W, Lochman D, et al: Uterine sarcomas: An analysis of 69 patients. *Int J Radiat Oncol Biol Phys* 1981; 7:917–922.
39. Tanga R, Delgado G: Uterine sarcoma. *Intern Surg* 1982; 67:339–344.
40. Van Dinh T, Woodruff JD: Leiomyosarcoma of the uterus. *Am J Obstet Gynecol* 1982; 144:817–823.
41. Lotocki R, Rosenshein NB, Grumbine F, et al: Mixed mullerian tumors of the uterus: Clinical and pathologic correlations. *Int J Gynaecol Obstet* 1982; 20:237–243.
42. DiSaia PJ, Morrow CP, Boronow R, et al:

Endometrial sarcoma: Lymphatic spread pattern. *Am J Obstet Gynecol* 1978; 130:104–105.

43. Yoonessi M, Hart WR: Endometrial stromal sarcomas. *Cancer* 1977; 40:898–906.
44. Suzuki M, Aizawa S, Ushigome S: Endometrial stromal sarcoma of low grade malignancy. Immunohistochemical and three-dimensional reconstruction study with special emphasis on the inadequate terminology of endolymphatic stromal myosis. *Acta Pathol Jpn* 1989; 39:260–265.
45. Evans HL: Endometrial stromal sarcoma and poorly differentiated endometrial sarcoma. *Cancer* 1982; 50:2170–2182.
46. el Naggar AK, Abdul-Karim FW, Silva EG, et al: Uterine stromal neoplasms: A clinicopathologic and DNA flow cytometric correlation. *Hum Pathol* 1991; 22:897–903.
47. Sabini G, Chumas JC, Mann WJ: Steroid hormone receptors in endometrial stromal sarcomas. A biochemical and immunohistochemical study. *Am J Clin Pathol* 1992; 97:381–386.
48. Clement PB, Scully RE: Mullerian adenosarcoma of the uterus. *Cancer* 1974; 34.1138–1149.
49. Zaloudek CJ, Norris HJ: Adenofibroma and adenosarcoma of the uterus: A clinicopathologic study of 35 cases. *Cancer* 1981; 48:354–366.
50. Williams LJ, Pavlick FJ: Leiomyomatosis peritonealis disseminata. *Cancer* 1980; 45:1726–1733.
51. Fujii S, Nakashima N, Okamura H, et al: Progesterone-induced smooth muscle-like cells in the subperitoneal nodules produced by estrogen—experimental approach to leiomyomatosis peritonealis disseminata. *Am J Obstet Gynecol* 1981; 139:164–172.
52. Fuller AF Jr: Malignant leiomyomatosis peritonealis disseminata; complete surgical resection of a low grade recurrence, submitted for publication.
53. Falkenberry SS, Muntz HG, Fuller AF Jr: Successful surgical resection of an extrauterine pelvic hemangiopericytoma following preoperative angiographic embolization, submitted for publication.
54. Banner AS, Carrington CB, Emory WB, et al: Efficacy of oophorectomy in lumphangioleiomyomatosis and benign metastasizing leiomyoma. *N Engl J Med* 1981; 305:204–209.
55. Fuller AF Jr: Myomectomy with unexpected leiomyosarcoma, in Nichols DH (ed): *Clinical Problems, Injuries and Complications of Gynecologic Surgery*, ed 5. Baltimore, Williams & Wilkins, 1988.
56. Lantta M, Karkkainen J, Wahlstrom T, et al: Estradiol and progesterone receptors in gynecologic sarcomas. *Acta Obstet Gynecol Scand* 1984; 63:505–508.
57. DiSaia P, Castro J, Rutledge F: Mixed mesodermal sarcoma of the uterus. *Am J Rorentgenol* 1973; 117:632–636.
58. Vongtama V, Karlen J, Piver S, et al: Treatment results and prognostic factors in stage I and II sarcomas of the corpus uteri. *Am J Roentgenol* 1976; 126:139–147.
59. Saksela E, Lampinen V, Procope B-J: Malignant mesenchymal tumors of the uterine corpus. *Am J Obstet Gynecol* 1974; 120:452–460.
60. Perez C, Askin F, Baglan R, et al: Effects of irradiation on mixed mullerian tumors of the uterus. *Cancer* 1979; 43:1274–1284.
61. Hannigan E, Freedman R, Elder K, et al: Treatment of advanced uterine sarcoma with vincristine, actinomycin D, and cyclophosphamide. *Gynecol Oncol* 1983; 15:224–229.
62. Hannigan E, Freedman R, Rutledge F: Adjuvant chemotherapy in early uterine sarcoma. *Gynecol Oncol* 1983; 15:56–64.
63. Piver MS, Lele SB, Marchetti DL, et al: Effect of adjuvant chemotherapy on time to recurrence and survival of stage I uterine sarcoma. *J Surg Oncol* 1988; 38:233–239.
64. Peters WA, Rivkin SE, Smith MR, et al: Cisplatin and Adriamycin combination chemotherapy for uterine stromal sarcomas and mixed mesodermal tumors. *Gynecol Oncol* 1989; 34:323–327.
65. Deppe G, et al: Combination chemotherapy for mixed mullerian tumors of the fallopian tube. *Cancer* 1984; 54:1517–1520.
66. Muntz HG, Rutgers JL, Tarraza HM, et al: Carcinosarcomas and mixed mullerian tumors of the fallopian tube. *Gynecol Oncol* 1989; 34:109–115.
67. Jacoby AF, Thor A, Muntz HG, et al: Case report: Primary sarcoma of the fallopian tube, submitted for publication.
68. Wu JP, Tanner WS, Fardal P: Malignant mixed mullerian tumors of the uterine tube. *Obstet Gynecol* 1973; 41:707–712.
69. Jain V: Mixed mullerian tumors of the fallopian tube. *Md State Med J* 1977; 26:43–45.
70. Acosta AA, Kaplan AL, Kaufman RH:

Mixed mullerian tumor of the oviduct. *Obstet Gynecol* 1974; 44:84–90.

71. Disaia PJ, Creasman W: *Clinical Gynecologic Oncology*. St. Louis, C. V. Mosby, 1981, pp 351–356.
72. Hanjani P, Peterson RO, Bonnell SA: Malignant mixed mullerian tumors of the fallopian tube. *Gynecol Oncol* 1980; 9:381–393.
73. Azoury RS, Woodruff JD: Primary ovarian sarcomas. *Obstet Gynecol* 1971; 37:920–941.
74. Morrow C, d'Ablang G, Brady L: A clinical and pathological study of 30 cases of malignant mixed mullerian epithelial and mesenchymal ovarian tumors: A Gynecologic Oncology Group study. *Gynecol Oncol* 1984; 18:278–292.
75. Anderson WA, Young DE, et al: Platinum-based combination chemotherapy for malignant mixed mesodermal tumors of the ovary. *Gynecol Oncol* 1989; 32:319–322.
76. Barker GH. *Chemotherapy of Gynaecological Malignancy*. Castle House Publishing, 1983, pp 129–133.
77. Lele SB, Piver MS, Barlow JJ: Chemotherapy in the management of mixed mesodermal tumors of the ovary. *Gynecol Oncol* 1980; 10:298–302.
78. Buchsbaum HJ, Lifshitz S, Blythe, JG: Prophylactic chemotherapy for stage I and II uterine sarcomas. *Gynecol Oncol* 1979; 8:346–348.
79. Piver MS, Lurain JR: Uterine sarcoma: Clinical features and management, in Coppleson M (ed): *Gynecologic Oncology*, Churchill Livingstone, 1981, pp 615–616.
80. Azizi F, et al: Remission of uterine leiomyosarcomas treated with vincristine, Adriamycin and dimethyl triazeno-imidazole carboxamide. *Am J Obstet Gynecol* 1979; 133:379–381.
81. Omura GA, et al: A randomized study of Adriamycin with and without dimethyl triazenoimidazole carboxamide in advanced uterine sarcomas. *Cancer* 1983; 52:626–632.
82. Karakousis CP, Holtermann OA, Holyoke ED: Cis-dichlorodiammineplatinum (II) in metastatic soft tissue sarcomas. *Cancer Treat Rep* 1979; 63:2071–2075.
83. Karakousis CP, Rao U, Carlson M: High-dose methotrexate as secondary chemotherapy in metastatic soft-tissue sarcomas. *Cancer* 1980; 46:1345–1348.
84. Malkasian GD, Mussey T, Decker DG, et al: Chemotherapy of gynecologic sarcomas. *Cancer Chemother Rep* 1967; 51:507–516.

Chapter 16

Sarcomas of the Kidney, Urinary Bladder, Prostate, Spermatic Cord, Paratestis, and Testis in Adults

Taiji Tsukamoto

Michael M. Lieber

This chapter is a study of genitourinary sarcomas in adults. Sarcomas of the kidney, urinary bladder, prostate, spermatic cord, testis, and paratestis will be reviewed. Sarcomas of the female genital tract are covered in Chapter 15, and rhabdomyosarcomas of the urogenital tract in children age 15 years and under are described in Chapter 17. Standard urogenital sarcomas in adults will be reviewed first; the extremely rare carcinosarcomas of the adult urogenital system will be discussed separately at the end of this chapter.

Sarcomas of the genitourinary system in adults (excluding those of the female reproductive tract) are quite rare: from the 1930s to the present, only 511 cases have appeared in the English literature (Table 16–1). Thus, true sarcomas of the genitourinary tract in adults appear to be two to four orders of magnitude less common than carcinomas of the same organs.

The most common genitourinary sarcomas in adults are those of the spermatic cord, testis, and paratestis, with 212 cases described. Renal sarcomas are the next most common, followed by sarcomas of the urinary bladder and prostate (Table 16–1).

Because genitourinary sarcomas in adults are so rare, we have systematically reviewed the English literature over the last 45 years in an attempt to provide reasonable guidelines for the management of these tumors.

TABLE 16–1.
Urogenital Sarcomas in Adults (511 Cases)

Sarcoma Type	Kidney* (1950–1984)	Bladder (1954–1984)	Prostate (1938–1984)	Spermatic Cord, Testis, Paratestis (1950–1984)
Sarcoma of fibrous tissue	16 (13.0%)	3 (3.8%)	6 (6.2%)	35 (16.5%)
Sarcoma of adipose tissue	18 (14.6%)	1 (1.3%)	1 (1.0%)	47 (22.2%)
Sarcoma of muscle	53 (43.1%)	64 (81.0%)	75 (77.4%)	120 (56.6%)
Sarcoma of vessels	12 (9.8%)			
Sarcoma of peripheral nerve	1 (0.8%)			
Extraskeletal bone sarcoma	8 (6.5%)	7 (8.9%)	1 (1.0%)	
Miscellaneous	15 (12.2%)	4 (5.1%)	14 (14.4%)	10 (4.7%)
Total	123	79	97	212

** Including 10 cases with renal pelvic sarcoma.*

SARCOMAS OF THE KIDNEY IN ADULTS

The sarcomas of the kidney are uncommon, with only 123 such tumors being reported in the urologic literature since 1950.[1-66] Approximately 1% of primary renal tumors are true sarcomas.[25, 67] Sarcomatoid renal cell carcinoma appears to be more common than true sarcomas,[68, 69] but several histological types of sarcomas do arise in the kidney (Table 16–2). The most common renal sarcoma in adults is leiomyosarcoma, accounting for approximately 40% of reported cases. Liposarcomas are the next most common tumor, making up 15% of cases. Most other histological types of sarcoma are also reported in the kidney in smaller percentages.

In 75 cases, the most common symptoms and signs of renal sarcoma in adults were pain (57%), a palpable renal mass (56%), and hematuria (28%) (Table 16–3). Thus, hematuria, the most common symptom for renal cell carcinoma, is much less common for renal sarcomas.

TABLE 16–2.
Sarcoma of the Kidney in Adults

Sarcoma Type	Total Number	Number by Subtype
Sarcoma of fibrous tissue	16	
Fibrosarcoma		9 (7.3%)
Malignant fibrous histiocytoma		7 (5.7%)
Sarcoma of adipose tissue	18	
Liposarcoma		18 (14.6%)
Sarcoma of muscle	53	
Leiomyosarcoma		47 (38.2%)
Rhabdomyosarcoma		6 (4.9%)
Sarcoma of vessel	12	
Hemangiopericytoma		11 (9.0%)
Angiomyoliposarcoma		1 (0.8%)
Sarcoma of peripheral nerve	1	
Malignant schwanoma		1 (0.8%)
Extraskeletal bone sarcoma	8	
Osteogenic sarcoma		8 (6.5%)
Miscellaneous	15	
Malignant mesenchymoma		2 (1.6%)
Mixed sarcoma		6 (4.9%)
Round cell sarcoma		1 (0.8%)
Spindle cell sarcoma		4 (3.3%)
Undifferentiated sarcoma		2 (1.6%)
Total	123	(100%)

TABLE 16–3.
Major Symptoms and Signs in Sarcoma of the Kidney (75 Cases)

Symptom/Sign	Number of Occurrences
Pain	43 (57%)
Mass	42 (56%)
Hematuria	21 (28%)
Tenderness	14 (19%)
Gastrointestinal	
Vomiting	8 (11%)
Nausea	6 (9%)
Diarrhea	2 (3%)
General nonspecific	
Weight loss	22 (29%)
Fever	12 (16%)
Anorexia	8 (11%)

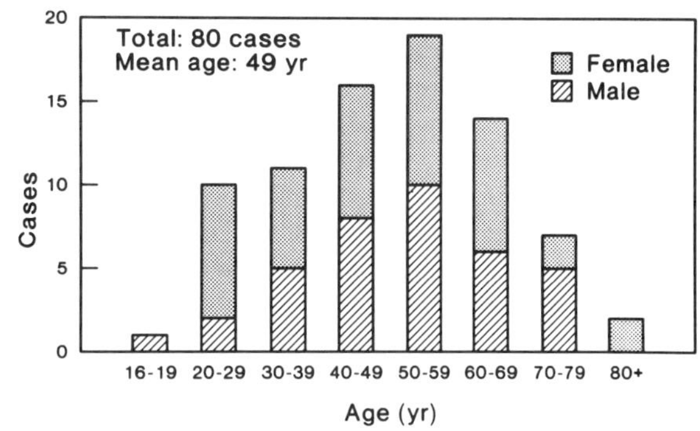

FIG 16–1.
Age and sex distribution in sarcoma of kidney. Total number of cases, 80; mean age, 49 years.

The high prevalence of a palpable renal mass and flank pain suggests the advanced local stage of renal sarcomas at the time such patients first present for diagnosis. Age and sex distribution in 80 cases of renal sarcoma is presented in Figure 16–1. Approximately equal numbers of males and females were seen (male, 38 cases; female, 42 cases), and age distribution for all renal sarcomas is typical of that seen in renal cell carcinoma, with a peak incidence in the fifth decade (median age, 51 years). All of the different histological subgroups of renal sarcoma basically show the same male-to-female ratio and age distribution, except for hemangiopericytoma and angiomyoliposarcoma, which show a younger age distribution and female predominance, but the total number of patients is small.

Diagnosis and Staging

Renal sarcomas typically present as a large, mass lesion of the kidney indistinguishable by standard radiological imaging techniques from the much more common renal cell carcinoma. As noted above, tumors are usually quite large at the time of diagnosis. Renal sarcomas are usually solid lesions and generally indistinguishable from a renal cell carcinoma on excretory urography, ultrasound examination of the kidney, and by computed tomography (CT). The hypervascularity and neovascularity seen on angiography in the majority of renal cell carcinomas is usually not seen with a renal sarcoma. Angiographic findings in 20 patients have been reported. Of these, seven showed hypervascularity and 13 showed hypovascularity. Four of the seven patients with hypervascular tumors had leiomyosarcomas. All fibrosarcomas and liposarcomas were hypovascular. Preoperative diagnosis of renal sarcomas by radiological imaging techniques and their differentiation from renal cell carcinoma is not normally possible. Rather, the typical case of renal sarcoma is approached as if it were renal cell carcinoma; its true nature becomes apparent only after radical nephrectomy.

Typically, then, the pre-operative management of a patient with renal sarcoma consists of imaging techniques to assess the extent of tumor involvement of renal cell carcinoma. Current evaluation would include and excretory urogram, a chest X-ray, CT of the abdomen and chest to detect metastatic disease, and ultrasound examination of the inferior vena cava and renal vein to look for a tumor thrombus. Depending on the physician's choice, a radionuclide bone scan would be indicated to search for osseous metastasis for renal sarcoma, and a CT of the head would be indicated in the presence of any neurological symptoms. Standard preoperative hematological and biochemical tests should be carried out, but the hypercalcemias and hepatic dysfunction syndrome seen with renal cell carcinoma have not been reported with renal sarcomas. Although rare, hemangiopericytomas are sometimes associated with hypoglycemia: nine such cases have been reported, three of which were renal.[19, 25, 59]

Treatment

The treatment selected for a renal sarcoma in general will be that indicated for a similar stage of renal cell carcinoma, because a preoperative tissue diagnosis is unlikely. In the absence of evidence of metastatic disease by pre-operative evaluation, radical nephrectomy would be the treatment of choice. Standard radical nephrectomy with wide local excision of the kidney and tumor within Gerota's fascia is the most appropriate treatment for both renal cell carcinoma and renal sarcoma. At present, there is no reason to recommend a formal retroperitoneal lymph node dissection for either renal cell carcinoma or renal sarcoma.[70] For patients who present with obvious metastatic disease, usually in the chest or other sites, but with a renal primary tumor visualized radiologically, a tissue diagnosis must be made at some site. A sarcoma of the kidney is more likely to be responsive to radiotherapy or cytotoxic chemotherapy than a renal cell carcinoma, so a tissue diagnosis is particularly important. Unresectable tumors causing local symptoms such as pain or bleeding can be treated by renal artery embolization, as in the case of renal cell carcinoma, although this has rarely been done or reported for renal sarcomas.[59, 61] The initial treatment regimen for patients with a sarcoma of the kidney in 71 cases is described in Table 16–4.

Because soft-tissue sarcomas may be responsive to radiotherapy[71] (in contrast to renal cell carcinomas), postoperative radiotherapy of the renal fossa can be considered depending on histological type seen. Leiomyosarcoma, the most common renal sarcoma, has such a poor prognosis that this tumor type as well as osteosarcoma of the kidney should be aggressively treated with postoperative radiotherapy to the renal bed, as well as with postoperative adjuvant chemotherapy via an Adriamycin (doxorubicin)-based combination chemotherapy regimen.[72] In addition to the use of Adriamycin as an adjuvant or therapeutic chemotherapy, the combination of cyclophosphamide, vincristine, and actinomycin D with or without DTIC (dacarbazine) has been reported to be effective for urogenital sarcomas.[57] Adjuvant chemotherapy seems to be more important than radiotherapy, because blood-borne metastases occur more frequently than regional (lymph node) metastases.

Prognosis

Death for most patients with sarcomas of the kidney results from the tumor. Survival curves for renal sarcomas in adults are presented in Figure 16–2. Hemangiopericytomas and angiomyoliposarcomas, quite rare tumors,

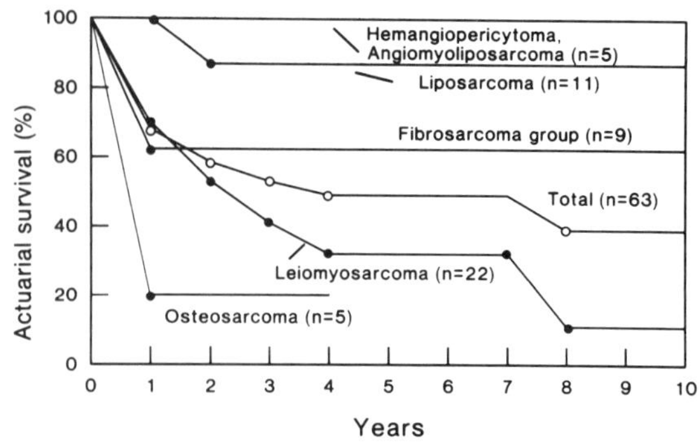

FIG 16–2.
Ten-year survival rate in sarcoma of the kidney. Three patients died of postoperative complications and were excluded from assessment of the survival rate. Total number includes patients with miscellaneous sarcomas whose survival rates are not shown separately in this figure. The fibrosarcoma group comprises fibrosarcoma and malignant fibrous histiocytoma.

have a favorable prognosis, with just two deaths from tumor seen in this group. Renal liposarcomas and tumors of the fibrosarcoma group (fibrosarcoma, malignant fibrous histiocytoma), usually of relatively low grade and limited metastatic potential, also have a fair prognosis. These histological types justify aggressive attempts at total local excision. Leiomyosarcomas, the most common renal sarcoma, have a much poorer prognosis than other histological types. At 5 years, survival is approximately 30%, and at 10 years only 10%. Osteosarcomas of the kidney have an even poorer prognosis, with 62% of patients dead from metastatic disease within 1 year. Once again, for these latter histological types, aggressive postoperative local radiotherapy and aggressive systemic adjuvant chemotherapy seem appropriate. Overall, the prognosis in renal sarcomas and renal cell carcinoma is much the same; the average 5-year survival rate is about 45%.[73]

SARCOMAS OF THE URINARY BLADDER IN ADULTS

Whereas rhabdomyosarcoma of the bladder is a common pediatric malignancy, sarcomas of the urinary bladder in adults are quite rare, with only 79 such cases being reported in the English literature since 1954[26, 57, 74–107] (Tables 16–1 and 16–5). Because carcinomas of the bladder (particularly transitional cell carcinoma of the blad-

TABLE 16–4.

Initial Treatment Regimen for Sarcoma of Kidney (71 Cases)

Treatment	Fibrosarcoma Group	Liposarcoma	Leiomyosarcoma	Rhabdomyosarcoma	Hemangiopericytoma Group	Osteogenic Sarcoma	Miscellaneous	Total
Radical nephrectomy group	5	1	5	1	3	2	3	20
Radical nephrectomy	(4)	(1)	(4)*		(1)	(1)	(2)	(13)
+ Retroperitoneal lymph node dissection	(1)							(1)
+ Radiotherapy			(1)		(1)			(2)
+ Chemotherapy				(1)				(1)
+ Radiotherapy							(1)†	(1)
+ Embolization					(1)			(1)
+ Embolization					(1)			(1)
Nephrectomy Group	6	10	21	1	3	4	2	47
Nephrectomy	(5)	(8)	(15)*,†	(1)	(2)	(4)	(1)	(36)
+ Radiotherapy	(1)	(2)	(1)		(1)			(5)
+ Chemotherapy			(3)				(1)	(4)
+ Radiotherapy			(1)					(1)
+ Adrenalectomy			(1)					(1)
Tumor excision		1						1
Nonsurgical group	1	1	1			1		3
Chemotherapy			(1)			(1)		(2)
+ Radiotherapy	(1)							(1)

** Including one patient case who received radial nephrourecterectomy and two who had nephrourecterectomy.*
† Including one patient who had vena caval resection.

TABLE 16–5.
Sarcoma of the Bladder in Adults

Sarcoma Type	Total Number	Number by Subtype
Sarcoma of fibrous tissue	3	
Fibrosarcoma		3 (3.8%)
Sarcoma of adipose tissue	1	
Myxoid liposarcoma		1 (1.3%)
Sarcoma of muscle	64	
Leiomyosarcoma		36 (46.4%)
Rhabdomyosarcoma		25 (30.8%)
Myosarcoma		1 (1.3%)
Leiomyosarcoma + rhabdomyosarcoma		2 (2.5%)
Extraskeletal bone sarcoma	7	
Osteogenic sarcoma		7 (8.8%)
Miscellaneous	4	
Mixed sarcoma		1 (1.3%)
Spindle cell sarcoma		1 (1.3%)
Undifferentiated sarcoma		2 (2.5%)
Total	79	(100%)

der and its relatives) are among the most common urinary tract tumors in adults, with about 50,000 new cases a year being reported in the United States alone, the relative scarcity of sarcomas of the urinary bladder is readily apparent. The incidence of bladder sarcoma is often estimated to be 0.4% to 1.4% of all primary bladder tumors, but is probably even lower.[87, 88, 108]

Nearly all sarcomas of the urinary bladder are sarcomas of muscle, with nearly half being leiomyosarcomas and one third rhabdomyosarcomas. The remaining histological types of sarcomas make up just a small fraction of tumor types observed. Carcinosarcoma is also common in this organ and will be discussed later. Age and sex distribution for patients with sarcoma of the urinary bladder is presented in Figure 16–3. Bladder sarcomas are most common in the fifth and sixth decades, and the male-to-female distribution is 1:0.57 (male, 42 cases; female, 24 cases). The median age of adult patients with sarcomas of the bladder was 59 years.

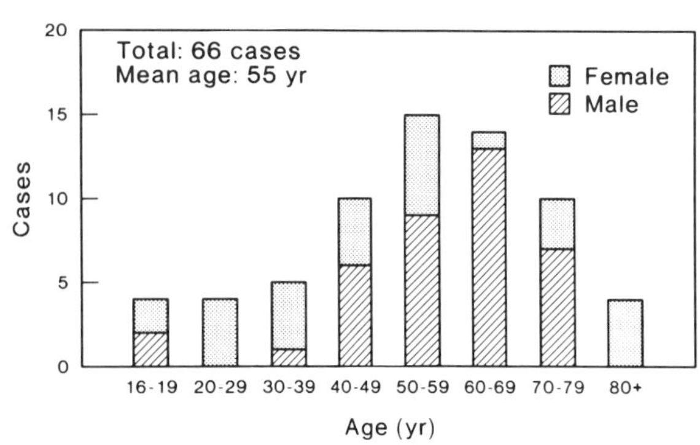

FIG 16–3.
Age and sex distribution for sarcoma of the bladder. Total number of cases, 66; mean age, 55 years.

Hematuria was the most common presenting symptom of patients with sarcoma of the bladder and was seen in approximately 80% of patients. Bladder irritation was also common (Table 16–6).

Diagnosis and Staging

The presence of gross hematuria usually prompts urological referral and then cystoscopy. Diagnosis of sarcoma of the urinary bladder is thus commonly made after cytoscopic biopsy. Sarcomas cannot be readily differentiated from sessile invasive transitional cell carcinoma or squamous cell carcinoma of the bladder by cystoscopic appearance. However, these tu-

TABLE 16–6.
Major Symptoms in Sarcoma of the Bladder (43 Cases)

Symptom	Number
Gross hematuria	33 (77%)
(Painless)	(16) (37%)
Frequency	15 (35%)
Dysuria	10 (32%)
Urgency	6 (14%)
Lower abdominal pain or suprapubic pain	5 (12%)

mors usually have a different appearance from the typical low-grade papillary transitional cell carcinomas that make up the bulk of bladder tumors. Bladder sarcomas usually present as a sessile ulcerative mass involving the bladder wall. No particular location within the bladder is typical of a sarcoma. In the present series of cases in which information was reported, three cases were seen in the bladder neck, nine in the trigone, 12 on the posterior wall, ten on the lateral wall, nine in the dome or anterior wall, two diffusively, and one in a diverticulum. In males, differentiation between a sarcoma of the prostate and sarcoma of the bladder, when the region of the bladder neck is involved, can be quite difficult.[92]

Endoscopic biopsy of the tumor mass by the cold-cup biopsy instrument or by hot loop resection will generally yield a valid tissue diagnosis. Bimanual examination under anesthesia performed at the same time as the cytoscopic biopsy should give some indication about the anatomical extent of the tumor and the possibilities for open surgical resection. Sarcomas of the bladder normally arise in the muscular wall of the bladder (rather than in the epithelium) and cannot normally be treated successfully by endoscopic resection. Rather, formal open surgery is currently indicated for patients with sarcomas of the bladder.

Standard radiological imaging techniques for staging sarcomas of the bladder are similar to those used for patients with invasive transitional cell carcinoma of the bladder. Patients with the diagnosis of sarcoma of the urinary bladder made by cystoscopic biopsy should have a chest radiograph and a CT of the abdomen and pelvis to delineate any metastatic disease post-operatively. Excretory urography to show upper tract anatomy should also be done.

Treatment

For patients with no evidence of metastatic disease, wide local surgical excision is indicated. Because vesicle sarcoma is not a field-change disease like transitional cell carcinoma, every attempt should be made, depending on the histology, size, and location of the tumor, to perform a partial cystectomy in order to save a functional bladder.[92] A wide local excision, taking the overlying perivesical fat and reimplanting the ureter if necessary, is the operation of choice. If the tumor involves the bladder neck and trigone, a formal radical cystectomy may be indicated. We would also recommend a unilateral or bilateral pelvic *lymph node dissection* in this setting because pelvic nodal metastases, if present, would indicate the need for systemic adjuvant cytotoxic chemotherapy.

Because leiomyosarcomas and rhabdomyosarcomas are often radiation sensitive, radiotherapy along with surgery can be used in the treatment of patients with sarcoma of the bladder (Table 16–7). We recommend postoperative radiotherapy in the tumor bed after the bladder is healed for patients with relatively low-grade leiomyosarcomas in which local tumor recurrence is apt to be the most common problem. For patients with high-grade leiomyosarcomas, rhabdomyosarcomas and other more anaplastic tumors, and for those patients with positive pelvic lymph nodes, we recommend aggressive adjuvant combination cytotoxic chemotherapy including Adriamycin.[72] Combination chemotherapy with cyclophosphamide, vincristine, and actinomycin D with or without DTIC has been tried; these combinations are effective in some patients, but its efficacy in sarcomas of the urinary bladder has yet to be established.[57]

Prognosis

Survival for patients with sarcomas of the urinary bladder is presented in Figure 16–4. Overall, the prognosis is not particularly poor, with the overall group of patients showing 50% survival after 5 years, and those with leiomyosarcomas showing a 5- and 10-year survival of 62% and 54%, respectively. Rhabdomyosarcomas of the bladder have a much poorer prognosis than leiomyosarcomas. To re-emphasize, leiomyosarcomas, usually of low or intermediate grade, are the most common sarcomas found in the urinary bladder. Because these tumors are locally aggressive but do not often metastasize early, aggressive local measures including surgery and radiotherapy should be used initially.

SARCOMA OF THE PROSTATE IN ADULTS

Prostate sarcoma is rare, with only 97 cases reported in the English urological literature from 1938 to 1984.[26, 57, 84, 92, 99, 109–150] Once again, this incidence is much lower than in adenocarcinoma of the prostate, now one of the most common malignancies in the adult male. The incidence of sarcoma of the prostate has been estimated to be 0.1% to 0.3% of malignant prostate tumors, but this may be high.[136, 138, 141] The

TABLE 16–7.
Initial Treatment Regimen for Sarcoma of the Bladder (58 Cases)

Treatment	Fibrosarcoma Group	Leiomyosarcoma	Rhabdomyosarcoma	Osteogenic Sarcoma	Miscellaneous	Total
Radical surgery group		9	10		2	21
Pelvic exenteration			(1)			(1)
Radical cystectomy		(6)	(4)		(2)	(12)
Total cystectomy		(3)	(4)			(7)
+ Radiotherapy			(1)			(1)
Conservative surgery group	1	18	3	2	3	27
Partial cystectomy		(8)	(1)	(1)	(1)	(11)
+ Pelvic lymph node dissection		(1)			(1)	(2)
Transurethral resection	(1)	(1)			(1)	(3)
+ Radiotherapy		(4)				(4)
+ Suprapubic excision		(1)				(1)
Suprapubic excision		(2)	(1)	(1)		(4)
+ Fulguration			(1)			(1)
Cryosurgery + chemotherapy		(1)				(1)
Surgical excision group*		3				3
+ Chemotherapy		(2)				(2)
+ Radiotherapy		(1)				(1)
Nonsurgical group	1	1	4		1	7
Radiotherapy		(1)	(3)			(4)
+ Chemotherapy	(1)		(1)		(1)	(3)

* *No further information available.*

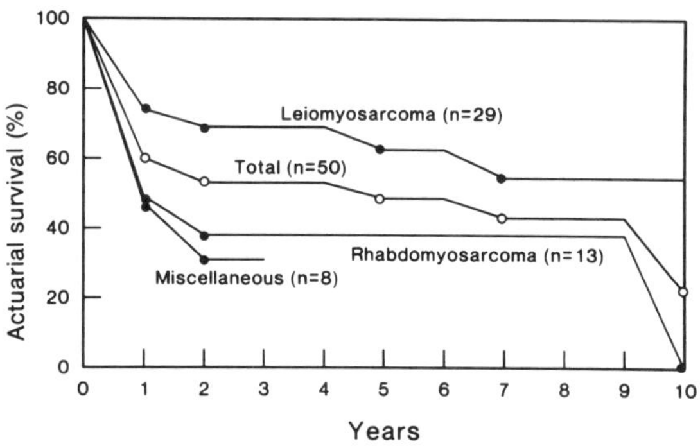

FIG 16–4.
Ten-year survival rate for sarcoma of the baldder. Six patients died of postoperative complications and were excluded from survival rate assessment.

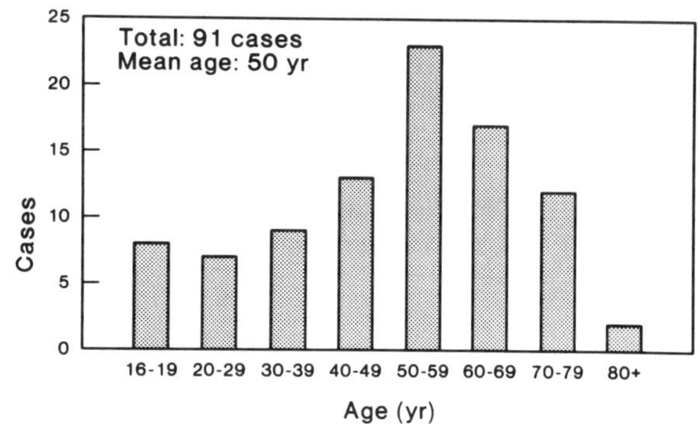

FIG 16–5.
Age distribution for sarcoma of the prostate. Total, 91 cases; mean age, 50 years.

histological types of sarcoma seen in the adult prostate are presented in Table 16–8. The spectrum of tumor types reported is quite similar to that seen for sarcoma of the urinary bladder. Leiomyosarcoma is by far the most common tumor type, occurring in slightly more than 50% of patients, and rhabdomyosarcoma, the next most common tumor type, is seen in about 20%. The other types of sarcomas are vanishingly rare. The age distribution of patients with sarcoma of the prostate is illustrated in Figure 16–5. The median age is 54 years. Of considerable interest and importance is the fact that leiomyosarcoma, the most common tumor, is seen in an older group of patients, the majority over the fifth decade of life (median age, 55 years). Rhabdomyosarcoma is much more common in younger patients (few patients with rhabdomyosarcoma of the prostate are seen over age 60).

Diagnosis

Most patients with sarcomas of the prostate present with symptoms related to prostatic obstruction (Table 16–9). Thus, in 74 cases in which the information was available, 85% of patients reported symptoms of urinary obstruction. In about 15% of patients, the main symptoms related to obstruction of the rectum. Typi-

TABLE 16–8.
Sarcoma of the Prostate in Adults

Sarcoma Type	Total Number	Number by Subtype
Sarcoma of fibrous tissue	6	
Fibrosarcoma		5 (5.2%)
Myxofibrosarcoma		1 (1.0%)
Sarcoma of adipose tissue	1	
Myxoid liposarcoma		1 (1.0%)
Sarcoma of muscle	75	
Leiomyosarcoma		52 (53.6%)
Rhabdomyosarcoma		18 (18.6%)
Myosarcoma		5 (5.2%)
Extraskeletal bone sarcoma	1	
Osteogenic sarcoma		1 (1.0%)
Miscellaneous	14	
Myosarcoma		1 (1.0%)
Spindle cell sarcoma		8 (8.2%)
Undifferentiated sarcoma		2 (2.1%)
Sarcoma (unknown origin)		3 (3.1%)
Total	97	(100%)

TABLE 16–9.
Major Symptoms and Characteristics of the Prostate on Palpation in Sarcoma of Prostate

Symptoms/Characteristics	Number of Cases	Percent of Total
Symptoms	74	
Related to prostatic obstruction		
(+)		85
(−)		15
Related to rectal obstruction		
(+)		16
(−)		84
Characteristics on palpation		
Surface	29	
Smooth		62
Globular		7
Irregular		31
Consistency	36	
Soft or boggy		25
Elastic or tense		19
Firm or hard		56

cal adenocarcinoma of the prostate is usually quite hard and nodular, but on rectal prostatic examination sarcomas are often found to be smooth and globular and soft/elastic in contrast to the usual findings with prostatic carcinoma (Table 16–9).

Diagnosis is usually made by needle biopsy of the prostate. The "True-cut"® or Vim-Silverman biopsy needle introduced through the perineum or rectally usually provides adequate tissue cores for diagnosis. Extensive diagnostic sampling of the prostate may be necessary to make a conclusive diagnosis of a low- or intermediate-grade leiomyosarcoma by this method, because smooth muscle cells are usually found in the prostate stroma and capsule under normal circumstances. With adequate tissue sampling, differentiating leiomyosarcoma or rhabdomyosarcoma of the prostate from adenocarcinoma should be fairly straightforward.

Staging a prostatic sarcoma would normally include a careful bimanual examination under anesthesia to check for local resectability, cystoscopy to check for involvement of the bladder base, CT of the abdomen and pelvis, and a chest X-ray to detect pulmonary metastases.

Treatment

In the absence of evidence of metastatic disease, aggressive local surgical excision should be used to treat prostatic sarcomas. Occasionally a small, low-grade leiomyosarcoma may be confined within the prostate capsule and can be treated by radical prostatectomy. However, prostate sarcomas are usually quite large at the time of diagnosis so that surgical excision of the prostate, bladder, and seminal vesicles (radical cystoprostatectomy) would normally be the local extirpative procedure of choice. For particularly large tumors that involve the rectum as well, a total pelvic exenteration may be indicated. We would normally perform bilateral pelvic lymphadenectomy at the same time as radical cystectomy/prostatectomy for the staging information it yields. Patients with relatively low-grade leiomyosarcomas and with positive resection margins would normally receive postoperative radiotherapy to the pelvis to lower the risk of local recurrence. Patients with high-grade leiomyosarcomas or rhabdomyosarcomas, and those with positive lymph nodes, should generally receive adjuvant cytotoxic chemotherapy because these patients commonly die of disseminated disease. Once again, some combination chemotherapy regimen based on Adriamycin seems most advisable, although there are no "hard" data to support such adjuvant treatment programs for prostate sarcomas at present.[72, 151] Pelvic radiation therapy should also be used if local resection margins are small, or if tumor is left behind or is not resectable. Indeed, many initial treatment regimens for sarcoma of the prostate have been reported in the literature, but no strong support for any one treatment can be gleaned from this experience (Table 16–10).

TABLE 16–10.
Initial Treatment Regimen for Sarcoma of the Prostate (77 Cases)

Treatment	Fibrosarcoma Group	Leiomyosarcoma	Rhabdomyosarcoma	Miscellaneous	Total
Radical surgery group		9		3	12
Translumbar amputation				(1)	(1)
Pelvic exenteration		(2)			(2)
Radical (or total) cystectomy		(1)		(1)	(2)
Radical (or total) prostatectomy		(3)			(3)
+ Radiotherapy		(3)		(1)	(4)
Conservative surgery group	4	27	9	7	47
Prostatectomy	(2)	(14)	(5)	(2)	(23)
+ Radiotherapy		(4)	(1)	(3)	(8)
+ Chemotherapy	(1)				(1)
Transurethral resection		(2)	(2)	(1)	(5)
+ Radiotherapy	(1)	(2)	(1)	(1)	(5)
+ Chemotherapy		(2)			(2)
Excision		(2)			(2)
+ Radiotherapy		(1)			(1)
Nonsurgical group	3	6	3	6	18
Radiotherapy	(2)	(3)	(2)	(5)	(12)
+ Chemotherapy	(1)	(1)	(1)		(3)
Chemotherapy		(2)		(1)	(3)

Prognosis

Patients with sarcomas of the prostate do less well than those with sarcomas of the urinary bladder. In general, this is because prostate sarcomas reach a much larger size before causing symptoms, whereas sarcomas of the bladder cause hematuria at a smaller size and earlier stage. Leiomyosarcomas of the prostate have a better prognosis than rhabdomyosarcomas, with 44 cases of leimyosarcoma showing a 5-year survival rate of 38% in contrast to a 15% 5-year survival rate for rhabdomyosarcoma (Fig 16–6).

Because the survival experience for high-grade leiomyosarcomas of the prostate and particularly for rhabdomyosarcomas of the prostate is so poor, aggressive local therapy and aggressive cytotoxic adjuvant chemotherapy is indicated for young patients who present with this disease.

For patients who have evidence of metastatic disease at the time of initial presentation, which is fairly common with rhabdomyosarcoma and high-grade leiomyosarcoma, palliative treatment should include external beam radiotherapy to the prostate, and combination cytotoxic chemotherapy. Because rhabdomyosarcomas and high-grade leiomyosarcomas locally grow so rapidly, palliative urinary and fecal diversion may be necessary in such patients.

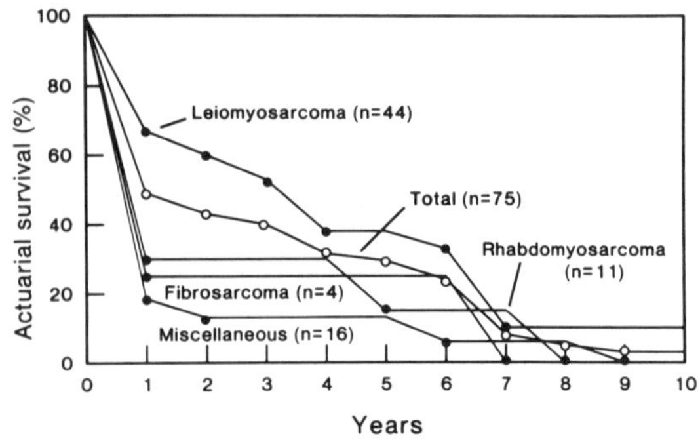

FIG 16–6.
Ten-year survival rate for sarcoma of the prostate. Five patients died of postoperative complications and were excluded from survival rate assessment.

SARCOMAS OF THE SPERMATIC CORD, TESTIS, AND PARATESTIS IN ADULTS

Sarcomas of the spermatic cord, testis, and paratestis in adults are the most common adult male genitourinary tract sarcomas. From 1950 through 1984, 212 cases of sarcoma of the spermatic cord, testis, and paratestis were reported in adults[26, 57, 152–240] (Table 16–11). Sarcomas of muscle origin made up more than half of these tumors, with rhabdomyosarcomas seen in

TABLE 16–11.
Sarcoma of Spermatic Cord, Testis, and Paratestis in Adults

Sarcoma Type	Total Number	Number by Subtype
Sarcoma of fibrous tissue	35	
Fibrosarcoma		25 (11.8%)
Myxofibrosarcoma		2 (0.9%)
Malignant fibrous histiocytoma		8 (3.8%)
Sarcoma of adipose tissue	47	
Liposarcoma		39 (18.4%)
Myxoliposarcoma		4 (1.9%)
Fibroblastic liposarcoma		2 (0.9%)
Lipoblastic liposarcoma		1 (0.5%)
Lipofibromyosarcoma		1 (0.5%)
Sarcoma of muscle	120	
Leiomyosarcoma		52 (24.5%)
Rhabdomyosarcoma		64 (30.2%)
Myosarcoma		4 (1.9%)
Miscellaneous	10	
Spindle cell sarcoma		3 (1.4%)
Mixed sarcoma		4 (1.9%)
Undifferentiated sarcoma		3 (1.4%)
Total	212	(100%)

30% of cases and leiomyosarcomas in 25%. The next most common histological type was liposarcoma of the spermatic cord, which accounted for 18% of tumors reported. Fibrosarcomas made up 12% of tumor types. The age distribution for sarcomas of the spermatic cord, testis, and paratestis is presented in Figure 16–7. Almost all of the large number of patients under age 30 had rhabdomyosarcomas. Leiomyosarcomas, liposarcomas, and fibrosarcomas were most common in the fifth and sixth decades; rhabdomyosarcomas occurred only rarely after age 30.

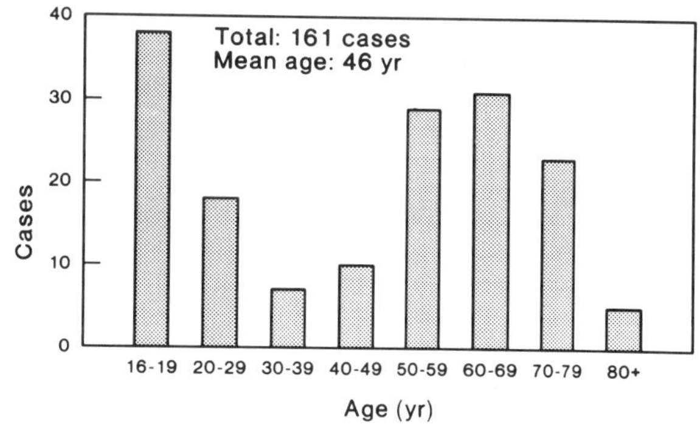

FIG 16–7.
Age distribution for sarcoma of the spermatic cord, testis, and paratestis. Total number of cases, 161; mean age, 46 years.

Sarcomas of the spermatic cord, testis, and paratestis nearly always present as firm, painless, palpable mass lesions in these areas. Table 16–12 presents an analysis of the anatomical location of these sarcomas. Although fibrosarcomas were seen in equal numbers on the right and left side, rhabdomyosarcomas, leiomyosarcomas, and liposarcomas were most common on the right side of the scrotum. Fibrosarcomas generally occurred in the spermatic cord with an equal number in the intrascrotal region and inguinal canal. Most liposarcomas also involved the spermatic cord or paratestis in the intrascrotal region, with about one third being found in the inguinal canal. The majority of leiomyosarcomas involved the spermatic cord in the intrascrotal or inguinal region, but a substantial number arose in the epididymis (25%). Nearly all rhabdomyosarcomas were found within the scrotum and arose from the spermatic cord, testis, epididymis, tunica vaginalis, or in the paratestis area.

Diagnosis

If a hard mass is palpated in the paratesticular area or in the spermatic cord, either within the scrotum or in the inguinal canal, sarcoma should be suspected. Germ cell tumors of the testis, however, usually form a hard mass in the substance of the testis (within the tunica albuginea), whereas a sarcoma is felt as a hard mass outside the tunica albuginea. If the malignant mass in the scrotum is quite large, preoperative differentiation between a primary germ cell testicular tumor and a sarcoma in this region may be impossible. Because most lesions in the scrotum are benign, and include such common findings as spermatoceles and cysts of various kinds, the current availability of high-resolution testicular ultrasonography for delineating the solid or cystic character of intrascrotal pathology is particularly important. Any abnormal lesion in the scrotum, external to the tunica albuginea, that is not cystic and that appears solid should be explored. Although adenomatoid tumors of the epididymis and paratestis are the most common solid lesions in an extratesticular location within the scrotum, their diagnosis cannot be made with confidence preoperatively, and require inguinal surgical exploration.

Treatment

As for most other urogenital sarcomas, a large number of treatment methods have been used for patients with sarcomas of the spermatic cord, testis, and paratestis (Table 16–13). No definitive conclusion about treatment can be made from this varied experience. Nevertheless, we recommend that patients with a suspicious lesion of the spermatic cord, testis, or paratestis be formally explored through an inguinal incision for a formal operative biopsy and potential radical orchiectomy including the spermatic cord. Transcrotal biopsy and excision of tumor is not recommended. If at the time of inguinal exploration of the spermatic cord, testis, or paratestis a sarcoma is diagnosed, then radical orchiectomy with high ligation of the cord at the internal ring should be performed. Additional therapy would depend on the histological type of tumor seen.

Liposarcomas of the spermatic cord are a special group. These tumors rarely metastasize and/or cause death (Fig 16–8). Thus, liposarcomas of the spermatic cord need be treated only by aggressive local excision.[240] In patients with rhabdomyosarcomas, leiomyosarcomas, or fi-

TABLE 16–12.
Location of Spermatic Cord, Testicular, and Paratesticular Sarcoma

	Side			Intrascrotal Region					Inguinal Region	
Sarcoma Type	Right	Left	Unknown	Spermatic Cord	Testis	Epididymis	Vaginalis	Paratestis	Spermatic Cord	Total Cases
Fibrosarcoma group	12 (46%)	13 (50%)	1 (4%)	10 (38%)		5 (19%)		1 (4%)	10 (38%)	26
Liposarcoma	16 (55%)	13 (45%)		15 (52%)				4 (14%)	10 (34%)	29
Leiomyosarcoma	24 (67%)	10 (28%)	2 (5%)	15* (42%)		9 (25%)	2 (5%)	1 (3%)	9 (25%)	36
Rhabdomyosarcoma	29 (51%)	21 (37%)	7 (12%)	21 (37%)	6 (11%)	7 (12%)	5 (9%)	14 (25%)	4 (6%)	57
Miscellaneous	1 (50%)		1 (50%)	2 (100%)						2
Total	82 (55%)	57 (37%)	11 (8%)	63 (42%)	6 (4%)	21 (14%)	7 (5%)	20 (14%)	33 (22%)	150

** Testicular or paratesticular sarcoma found simultaneously in two patients.*

TABLE 16–13.
Initial Treatment Regimen for Sarcoma of Spermatic Cord, Testis, and Paratestis (157 Cases)

Treatment	Fibrosarcoma Group	Liposarcoma	Leiomyosarcoma	Rhabdomyosarcoma	Miscellaneous	Total
Radical surgery group	15	24	25	40	4	108*
Radical orchiectomy	(12)	(23)	(19)	(16)	(3)	(73)
+ Retroperitoneal lymph node dissection			(1)	(1)		(2)
+ Inguinal lymph node dissection			(1)			(1)
+ Chemotherapy				(10)		(10)
+ Radiotherapy				(2)		(2)
+ Chemotherapy + radiotherapy				(3)		(3)
+ Inguinal lymph node dissection			(1)	(1)		(2)
+ Radiotherapy	(2)	(1)	(2)	(2)	(1)	(8)
+ Chemotherapy	(1)		(1)	(1)		(3)
+ Chemotherapy + radiotherapy				(3)		(3)
+ Immunotherapy				(1)		(1)
Nonradical surgery group	9	5	13	19	1	47*
Orchiectomy	(7)	(2)	(8)	(8)	(1)	(26)
+ Retroperitoneal lymph node dissection				(1)		(1)
Radiotherapy + chemotherapy				(1)		(1)
+ Inguinal lymph node dissection				(1)		(1)
+ Radiotherapy			(1)	(2)		(3)
+ Chemotherapy				(1)		(1)
+ Radiotherapy				(1)		(1)
Excision	(2)	(3)	(4)	(4)		(13)
Nonsurgical group				2		2
Chemotherapy				(1)		(1)
+ Radiotherapy				(1)		(1)

** Hemiscrotectomy or wide scrotal excision was also performed in 13 patients*

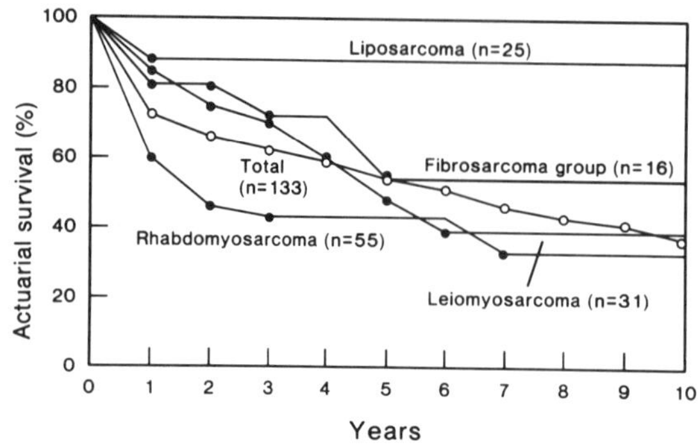

FIG 16–8.
Ten-year survival rate for sarcoma of spermatic cord, testis, and paratestis. One patient died of postoperative complications and was excluded from the assessment of survival rate. Total number of patients includes six patients with miscellaneous sarcomas whose survival rates are not shown separately in this figure. The fibrosarcoma group comprises fibrosarcoma, myxofibrosarcoma, and malignant fibrous histiocytoma.

brosarcomas in this anatomical group, the retroperitoneal lymph nodes must be staged by CT and lymphangiography after radical orchiectomy is performed. In the presence of *obvious metastatically involved retroperitoneal lymph nodes,* we recommend aggressive cytotoxic chemotherapy. Patients with rhabdomyosarcoma of the spermatic cord, testis, and paratestis have the poorest prognosis in this group (Fig 16–8). If large metastatic nodes are detected by CT of the abdomen, then aggressive chemotherapy should be given. If the lymph nodes appear normal, we recommend a formal retroperitoneal lymph node dissection.

In this review, we discovered 17 patients with rhabdomyosarcoma of the spermatic cord in which retroperitoneal lymph node dissection had been performed. Of these, eight patients (47%) had metastases to the retroperitoneal nodes. Moreover, in a total group of 33 patients with rhabdomyosarcoma of the spermatic cord, 16 of 33 patients (48%) had retroperitoneal lymph node metastases at the time of initial presentation, or such metastases became apparent during their subsequent clinical course. Patients with positive lymph nodes (even microscopically) should receive aggressive combination cytotoxic chemotherapy based on Adriamycin.[59, 72] Because most patients with paratesticular rhabdomyosarcoma are young men under age 30, an aggressive surgical approach and adjuvant chemotherapy seem indicated, much as in the treatment of patients with germ cell testicular tumors.[219]

CARCINOSARCOMA OF THE KIDNEY, BLADDER, AND PROSTATE

Fifty-one cases of carcinosarcoma of the kidney, bladder, and prostate have been reported in the English urological literature over the last 50 years[26, 79, 95, 241–268] (Table 16–14). The majority of these tumors were in the urinary bladder. Many different sarcomatous components have been found in carcinosarcomas of the kidney, bladder, and prostate (Table 16–15). In general, the carcinoma component in carcinosarcoma of the urinary bladder is transitional cell carcinoma. Carcinosarcoma of the kidney is found in roughly equal numbers in both males and females, whereas carcinosarcoma of the bladder is much more common in males (23 males, seven females). The age distribution for carcinosarcoma of the kidney, bladder, and prostate is presented in Figure 16–9. Carcinosarcoma of the kidney, bladder and prostate is seen in elderly patients with a mean age of 67 years; many patients are in the eighth decade of life. The diagnosis of carcinosarcoma in these anatomical sites is unusual, unsuspected, and normally made by the diagnostic methods described previously. Because sarcomatoid renal cell cancer makes up about 3% of renal carcinomas, carcinosarcomas of the kidney, which do not have a transitional cell carcinoma component, most likely should be reclassified in the former category.[68, 69] Such sarcomatoid renal cell carcinomas have a particularly poor prognosis.[69] Many different initial treatment regimens have been used for patients with carcinosarcoma of the kidney, bladder, and prostate (Table 16–16), but so few cases have been seen that no definite recommendations can be drawn. Because the prognosis for patients with carcinosarcoma of

TABLE 16–14.
Urogenital Carcinosarcoma in Adults

Type	Number of Cases
Kidney (1950–1984)	12
Bladder (1954–1984)	32
Prostate (1938–1984)	7
Total	51

TABLE 16–15.
Sarcomatous and Epithelial Components in Carcinosarcoma of Kidney, Bladder, and Prostate (40 Cases)

Component	Location: Kidney* (12 Cases)	Bladder (22 Cases)	Prostate (6 Cases)	Total (40 Cases)
Sarcomatous				
Fibrosarcoma	3 (25%)	2 (9%)		5 (13%)
Malignant fibrous histiocytoma		1 (5%)		1 (3%)
Leiomyosarcoma		3 (14%)	1 (17%)	4 (10%)
Rhabdomyosarcoma	3 (25%)	3 (14%)	1 (17%)	7 (18%)
Myosarcoma		1 (14%)		1 (3%)
Osteogenic sarcoma	5 (42%)	7 (32%)	3 (50%)	15 (38%)
Chondrosarcoma	2 (17%)	8 (36%)	3 (50%)	13 (35%)
Spindle cell sarcoma	1 (8%)	4 (18%)		5 (13%)
Sarcoma	1 (8%)			1 (3%)
Undifferentiated sarcoma		3 (14%)		3 (8%)
Epithelial				
Adenocarcinoma	8	6	4	
Transitional cell carcinoma	4	15		
Squamous cell carcinoma		7	1	
Undifferentiated carcinoma		1	1	

** Including four patients with carcinosarcoma in renal pelvis.*

the kidney, bladder, and prostate is poor (Fig 16–10), we recommend an aggressive treatment plan for these patients, modified by their chronological and physiological age. Patients with carcinosarcoma of the kidney or sarcomatoid renal cell carcinoma should be treated with radical nephrectomy and adjuvant chemotherapy. Almost all of these patients will die of metastatic disease within 2 years. Patients with carcinosarcoma of the bladder and prostate without evidence of metastatic disease should be treated by radical cystectomy-prostatectomy and bilateral pelvic lymphadenectomy. The exact role for pre-operative or postoperative radiotherapy for these patients has yet to be defined, and we would recommend it at present. Patients with positive lymph nodes should receive some cytotoxic adjuvant chemotherapy treatment, *which should be chosen according to the histological findings of the metastatic lesion (i.e., either carcinoma or sarcoma, or both)*, For the elderly patient, or those with poor physiological age, one should probably attempt local control via external beam radiotherapy alone.

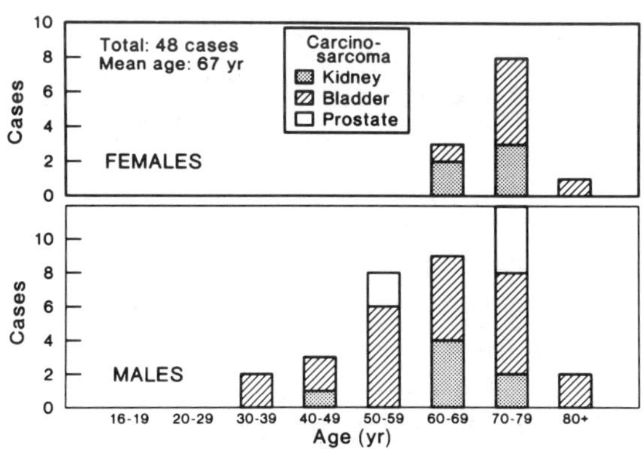

FIG 16–9.
Age and sex distribution for carcinosarcoma of kidney, bladder, and prostate. Total number of cases, 48; mean age, 67 years.

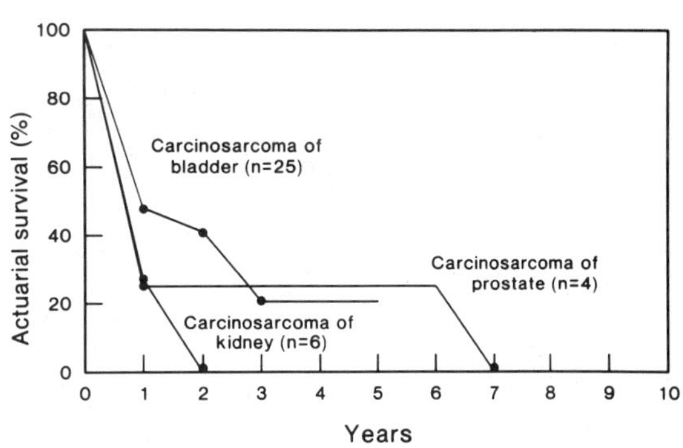

FIG 16–10.
Survival rate for carcinosarcoma of kidney, bladder, and prostate. Two patients died of postoperative complications and were excluded from survival rate assessment in carcinosarcoma of the bladder.

TABLE 16–16.
Initial Treatment Regimen for Carcinosarcoma of Urogenital Tract (41 Cases)

Location and Treatment	Number of Cases	Location and Treatment	Number of Cases
Kidney	10	Bladder	27
Radical nephrectomy group	2	Radical surgery group	11
Radical nephrectomy	(1)*	Radical cystectomy	(1)
+ Radiotherapy	(1)*	+ Radiotherapy	(2)
		Total cystectomy	(5)
Nephrectomy group	8		
		+ Radiotherapy	(1)
Nephrectomy	(6)†		
		+ Chemotherapy	(1)
Partial nephrectomy	(2)	+ Radiotherapy + chemotherapy	(1)
Prostate	4	Conservative surgery group	15
Radical surgery group	2	Partial cystectomy	(8)
Pelvic exenteration	(1)	+ Pelvic lymph node dissection	(1)
Radical cystectomy + radiotherapy	(1)		
		+ Radiotherapy	(2)
Conservative surgery group	2	Transurethral resection	(2)
TUR	(2)	+ Radiotherapy	(1)
		Suprapubic excision	(1)
		Nonsurgical group	1
		Radiotherapy	(1)

** All patients had radical nephroureterectomy.*
† Including two patients who had nephroureterectomy.

CONCLUSIONS

Sarcomas of the kidney, bladder, prostate, spermatic cord, testis, and paratestis in adults are so uncommon that no one urological oncologist, radiotherapist, or medical oncologist will have had much experience with this kind of cancer. Nevertheless, gathering the reported experience in the literature with these tumors allows the formulation of some general guidelines about their natural history and treatment. First, each histological type of sarcoma in these anatomical sites has a different natural history, so the treatment of sarcomas in these organs must be modulated accordingly. For example, patients with liposarcomas of the kidney or liposarcomas of the spermatic cord have a good prognosis when treated by aggressive local surgery alone. Those with rhabdomyosarcomas or carcinosarcomas in these same organs do poorly, and aggressive surgery, radiotherapy, and chemotherapy give the best chance at long-term control. Patients with intermediate types of tumors such as low- and intermediate-grade leiomyosarcomas deserve our best individualized approach to obtain a good chance of cure, while avoiding radical exenterative surgery if feasible anatomically. Because some histological types of sarcoma are sensitive to chemotherapeutic agents, we hope that additional active compounds will be identified and combined in potentially curative combinations. Thus, we can realistically hope for the day when adult patients with sarcomas of the bladder and prostate can be treated by biopsy and combination chemotherapy without exenterative surgery, as are children with rhabdomyosarcomas of the genitourinary tract.[269]

REFERENCES

1. Petkovic S: Myomatous tumors of the kidney. *Urol Cutan* 1951; 55:730–734.
2. Brady L: Liposarcoma of the kidney. *Urol Cutan* 1981; 55:741–744.
3. Edelman L: Liposarcoma of the kidney. *J Mt Sinai Hosp* 1951; 17:659–670.
4. Kretschmer HL: Leiomyosarcoma of the kidney. *J Urol* 1952; 68:36–38.

5. Bruce J, McNaught GHD: Leiomyosarcoma of the kidney. *Br J Urol* 1953; 25:114–115.
6. Ruff TE: Fibrosarcoma of the adult kidney: Case Report. *J Urol* 1953; 69:474–479.
7. Lazurus JA, Friedmann F: Leiomyosarcoma of the kidney. *Am J Surg* 1954; 87:251–258.
8. Higbee DR, Atkins DM: Leiomyosarcoma in a double kidney. *J Urol* 1954; 71:166–170.
9. Black HR, Heinemann S: Hemangiopericytoma: Report of a case involving the kidney. *J Urol* 1955; 74:42–46.
10. Frehling S: Leiomyosarcoma of the kidney: Report of a case, with review of the literature. *Arch Surg* 1956; 73:346–352.
11. Hudson HC: Osteogenic sarcoma involving the left kidney. *J Urol* 1956; 75:21–24.
12. Williams JP, Savage PT: Liposarcoma of kidney. *Br J Surg* 1958–1959; 46:225–231.
13. Berk LE, Ering AL, McManus RG: Hemangiopericytoma involving a kidney. *N Engl J Med* 1962; 263:1185–1187.
14. MacDermont EN, Kennedy JD: Liposarcoma of the kidney. *Br J Urol* 1960; 32:282–284.
15. Lee HC, Kay S: Hemangiopericytoma: Report of a case involving the kidney with an 11-year follow-up. *Ann Surg* 1962; 156:125–128.
16. Gupta JC, Nagrath C, Chagwat AC: A leiomyosarcoma of the kidney. *Indian J Pathol Bacteriol* 1963; 6:66–70.
17. Naib ZM, Young JD, Philippidjis PJ: Exfoliative cytology of a primary fibrosarcoma of the kidney. *J Urol* 1963; 90:386–390.
18. Sankaran V: Fibrosarcoma of the kidney. *J Indian Med Assoc* 1964; 43:81–83.
19. Simon R, Greene RC: Perirenal hemangiopericytoma: A case associated with hypoglycemia. *JAMA* 1964; 189:181–182.
20. Fein RL, Hamm FC: Malignant schwannoma of the renal pelvis: A review of the literature and a case report. *J Urol* 1965; 94:356–361.
21. Soto PJ Jr, Rader ES, Martin JM, et al: Osteogenic sarcoma of the kidney: Report of a case. *J Urol* 1965; 94:532–535.
22. Addison NV: Smooth muscle tumors of the kidney. *Br J Urol* 1966; 38:382–387.
23. Bazaz-Malik G, Gupta DN: Leiomyosarcoma of the kidney; Report of a case and review of the literature. *J Urol* 1966; 95: 754-8.
24. Seabury JC Jr: Renal rhabdomyosarcoma. *JAMA* 1967; 201:1043–1044.
25. Farrow GM, Harrison EG Jr, Utz DC, et al: Sarcomas and sarcomatoid and mixed malignant tumors of the kidney in adults. Part I. *Cancer* 1968; 22:545–550.
26. Tripathi VNP, Dick VS: Primary sarcoma of urogenital system in adults. *J Urol* 1969; 101:898–904.
27. Islam MU, Talibi MA, Boyd PF: Leiomyosarcoma of the kidney. *JAMA* 1970; 212:2266–2267.
28. Johnson LA, Ancona VC, Johnson T, et al: Primary osteogenic sarcoma of the kidney. *J Urol* 1970; 104:528–531.
29. Dalinka MK, Fiveash AE, Aston JK: Metastatic extraosseous osteosarcoma to the liver. *J Nucl Med* 1971; 12:754–755.
30. Das P, Gupta CK, Gupta SC: Fibrosarcoma of the kidney. *Indian J Med Sci* 1971; 25:877–878.
31. Jenkins JD, Anderson CK, Williams RE: Renal sarcoma. *Br J Urol* 1971; 43:263–267.
32. Gupta OP, Dube MK: Rare primary renal sarcoma. *Br J Urol* 1971; 43:546–551.
33. Zitter FMH, Wieche DR, McAndrews JF: Renal leiomyosarcoma: A case report with angiographic findings. *J Urol* 1971; 105:726–778.
34. Colabawealla BN: Renal hamartoma, angiomyoliposarcoma: A case report. *Br J Urol* 1972; 44:112–116.
35. Loomis RC: Primary leiomyosarcoma of the kidney: Report of a case and review of the literature. *J Urol* 1972; 107:557–560.
36. Newman LB, Anderson EE, Bucy JG: Small round cell sarcoma of the renal pelvis: A case report. *J Urol* 1972; 108:227–229.
37. Lien WM: Liposarcoma of the kidney. *Postgrad Med J* 1973; 49:600–603.
38. Rifai GM: Renal and perirenal hemangiopericytoma. *Urology* 1973; 1:148–150.
39. Rios JT: Renal liposarcoma with hypertension. *Urology* 1973; 1:246–248.
40. Tolia BM, Hajdu SI, Whitmore WF Jr: Leiomyosarcoma of the renal pelvis. *J Urol* 1973; 109:974–976.
41. Busuttil A, More IAR: Two malignant soft tissue tumors of the kidney: An ultrastructural appraisal. *J Urol* 1974; 112:24–29.
42. Helmbrecht LJ, Cosgrove MD: Triple therapy for leiomyosarcoma of the kidney. *J Urol* 1974; 112:581–584.

43. Niceta P, Lavengood RW Jr, Fernandes M, et al: Leiomyosarcoma of the kidney. *Urology* 1974; 3:270–277.
44. Gallagher JC, Winslow DJ, Grossman A: Coexistent chondrosarcoma and transitional-cell carcinoma in kidney. *Urology* 1974; 3:473–477.
45. Bennington JL, Beckwith JB: Tumors of the kidney, renal pelvis, and ureter, In *Atlas of Tumor Pathology*, fasc 12. Washington, D.C., Armed Forces Institute of Pathology, 1975, pp 229–231.
46. Chambers A, Carson R: Primary osteogenic sarcoma of the kidney. *Br J Urol* 1975; 48:316–317.
47. Cano JY, D'Altorio RA: Renal liposacoma: Case report. *J Urol* 1976; 115:747–749.
48. Granmayeh M, Wallace S, Barret AF: Sarcoma of the Kidney: Angiographic features. *AJR* 1977; 129:107–112.
49. Kotecha NM: Embryonal rhabdomyosarcoma of the kidney. *J Urol* 1977; 118:325–326.
50. Axelrod R, Naideck HJ, Myers J, et al: Primary osteosarcoma of the kidney. *Cancer* 1978; 41:724–727.
51. Osamura RY, Watanabe K, Yoneyama K, et al: Malignant fibrous histiocytoma of the renal capsule: Light and electron microscopic study of a rare tumor. *Virchows Arch* [Pathol Anat] 1978; 380:327–334.
52. Thomas ML: Angiographic features of a primary leiomyosarcoma of the kidney. *Aust Radiol* 1978; 22:155–157.
53. Chen KTK: Fibroxanthosarcoma of kidney. *Urology* 1979; 13:439–440.
54. Beccia DJ, Elkort RJ, Krane RJ: Adjuvant chemotherapy in renal leiomyosarcoma. *Urology* 1979; 13:652–654.
55. Biggers R, Stewart J: Primary renal osteosarcoma. *Urology* 1979; 13:674–676.
56. Meier WL, Willscher MK, Novicki DE, et al: Evaluation of perihilar and central renal masses using the chiba needle. *J Urol* 1979; 121:414–416.
57. Sinkovics JG, Plager C, von Eschenbach A, et al: Sarcoma of the genitourinary tract: Case histories, in Johnson DE, Samuels ML (eds): *Cancer of the Genitourinary Tract*. New York, Raven Press, 1979, pp 281–299.
58. Raghavaiah NV, Mayer RF, Hagitt R, et al: Malignant fibrous histiocytoma of the kidney. *J Urol* 1980; 123:951–953.
59. Asam SL, Bedard YC, Buckspan MB, et al: Spontaneous hypoglycemia associated with hemangiopericytoma of the kidney. *J Urol* 1981; 125:864–867.
60. MacEachern NH, Anderson KR, Wright WL: Fibroxanthosarcoma of the kidney: Report of a case. *J Urol* 1981; 126:684–685.
61. Bollack C, Cinqualbre J, Warter A, et al: Primary osteosarcoma of the kidney. *Br J Urol* 1982; 54:435–436.
62. Guice SL III, Beckmann EN, Kantrow CM, et al: Clinicopathological conference: Sudden anuria and renal failure in an elderly man. *J Urol* 1982; 127:289–293.
63. Mead JH, Herrera GA, Kaufman MF, et al: Case report of a primary cystic sarcoma of the kidney demonstrating fibrohistiocytic, osteoid and cartilaginous component (malignant mesenchymoma). *Cancer* 1982; 50:2211–2214.
64. Singh EO, Barrett DM, Adams VI: Synchronously occurring malignant fibrous histiocytoma of the kidney with contralateral renal cell carcinoma. *J Urol* 1982; 128:586–588.
65. Brenner R: Primary renal leiomyosarcoma: Report of two cases. *J Am Osteopathol Assoc* 1983; 82:558–561.
66. Reed HM, Poppiti R, Siviva M: Malignant mesenchymoma of kidney and inferior vena cava. *Urology* 1983; 22:297–299.
67. Bennington JL, Beckwith JB: Tumors of the kidney, renal pelvis, and ureter, in *Atlas of Tumor Pathology*, fasc 12. Washington, D.C., Armed Forces Institute of Pathology, 1975, pp 25–29.
68. Farrow GM, Harrison EG Jr, Utz DC: Sarcomas and sarcomatoid and mixed malignant tumors of kidney in adults. Part III. *Cancer* 1968; 22:556–563.
69. Tomera KM, Farrow GM, Lieber MM: Sarcomatoid renal carcinoma. *J Urol* 1983; 130:657–659.
70. Lieber MM: Management of renal cell carcinoma, in Skinner DG (ed): *Urologic Cancer*. New York, Grune & Stratton, 1983, pp 425–434.
71. Lindberg RD, Martin RG, Romsdahl MM, et al: Conservative surgery and radiation therapy for soft tissue sarcoma, in M. D. Anderson Hospital and Tumor Institute (ed): *Management of Primary Bone and Soft Tissue Tumors*. Chicago, Year Book Medical Publishers, 1977, pp 289–298.
72. Rosenberg SA, Suit HD, Baker LH, et al: Sarcoma of the soft tissue and bone, in De Vita VT Jr, Hellman S, Rosenberg SA (eds): *Cancer, Principles and Practice of Oncology*.

Philadelphia, J.B. Lippincott, 1982, pp 1063–1067.

73. Lieber MM: Renal adenocracinoma in young adults: Survival and variable affecting prognosis. *J Urol* 1981; 125:164–168.
74. Ober WB, Edgcomb JH: Sarcoma botryoides in the female urogenital tract. *Cancer* 1954; 7:45–91.
75. Sadler RN, Shelley HS, McCarty JE; Leiomyosarcoma of the urinary bladder; Report of a case. *J Urol* 1954; 72:211–216.
76. McCrea LE, Post EA: Sarcoma of the bladder. *Urol Surv* 1955; 5:307–356.
77. Silbar JD, Silbar SJ: Leiomyosarcoma of bladder: Three case reports and a review of literature. *J Urol* 1955; 73:103–111.
78. Nourse MH: Primary ostenogenic sarcoma of the bladder. *J Urol* 1957; 77:634–638.
79. Pang LSC: Bony and cartilaginous tumors of the urinary bladder. *J Pathol Bacteriol* 1958; 76:357–377.
80. Parker P, Smith PL, Rathmell TK: Sarcoma botryoides of the bladder: Successful therapy by cystectomy. *J Urol* 1959; 82:494–496.
81. Bacon RJ: Rhabdomyosarcoma of the urinary bladder. *J Int Coll Surg* 1961; 35:732–734.
82. Hellstrom HR, Fisher ER: Embryonal rhabdomyosarcoma of the bladder in the aged. *J Urol* 1961; 86:336–339.
83. Bohne AW, Urwiller RD, Pintos TG: Leiomyosarcoma of the urinary bladder with review of the literature. *Henry Ford Hosp Med Bull* 1962; 10:445–448.
84. Batsakis JG: Urogenital rhabdomyosarcoma: Histogenesis and classification. *J Urol* 1963; 90:180–186.
85. Jones CB Jr, Oberman HA: Rhabdomyosarcoma of the bladder: Occurrence in childhood and in advanced age. *J Urol* 1964; 91:354–356.
86. Uehling D, Firable WJ: Myosarcoma of the bladder: Report of two cases. *J Urol* 1964; 91:354–356.
87. Brown H: Leiomyosarcoma of the bladder: Follow-up report of two cases with 4 and 10 year's survival. *J Urol* 1965; 94:247–251.
88. Evans AT, Bell TE: Rhabdomyosarcoma of the bladder in adult patients: Report of three cases. *J Urol* 1965; 94:573–575.
89. Kikuchi K, Nakamura K, Nakajima F, et al: An autopsy case of primary osteogenic sarcoma of the urinary bladder. *Acta Pathol Jpn* 1965; 15:287–293.
90. Joshi DP, Wessely Z, Seery WH, et al: Rhabdomyosarcoma of the bladder in an adult: Case report and review of literature. *J Urol* 1966; 96:214–217.
91. Reeves JF Jr, Powell EB, Powell NB: Leiomyosarcoma of the bladder: Case report with autopsy. *J Urol* 1967; 97:486–489.
92. Mackenzie AR, Whitmore WF Jr, Melamed MR: Myosarcomas of the urinary bladder and prostate. *Cancer* 1967; 22:833–844.
93. Mackenzie AR, Sharma TC, Whitmore WF Jr, et al: Non-extirpative treatment of myosarcomas of the bladder and prostate. *Cancer* 1971; 28:329–334.
94. Chitiyo ME: Primary osteogenic sarcoma of the urinary bladder. *J Pathol* 1973; 111:53–56.
95. Ostroff, EB, Alperstein JB, Young JD Jr: Neoplasm in vesical diverticula: Report of 4 patients, including a 21 year old. *J Urol* 1973; 110:65–69.
96. Tara HL, Mentus NL: Leiomyosarcoma of urinary bladder. *Urology* 1973; 2:460–462.
97. Haworth J: Sarcoma of the bladder in an adult. *Practitioner* 1976; 217:268–269.
98. Krumerman MS, Katatikan V: Rhbdomyosarcoma of the urinary bladder with intraepithelial spread in an adult. *Arach Pathol Lab Med* 1976; 100:395–397.
99. Narayana AS, Loenig S, Weimar GW, et al: Sarcoma of the bladder and prostate. *J Urol* 1978; 119:72–76.
100. Keenan RA, Buchanan JD: Fibrosarcoma of bladder exhibiting endocrine characteristics of phaechromocytoma. *J R Soc Med* 1979; 72:618–620.
101. Wilson TM, Fauver HE, Weigel JW: Leiomyosarcoma of urinary bladder. *Urology* 1979; 8:565–567.
102. Papacharalambous AN, Pavlakis AJ; Leiomyosarcoma of the bladder. *Br J Urol* 1979; 51:321.
103. Alabaster AM, Jordan WP Jr, Soloway MS, et al: Leiomyosarcoma of the bladder and subsequent urethral recurrence. *J Urol* 1981; 125:583–585.
104. Punekar SV, Sane SY, Patel B, et al: Embryonal rhabdomyosarcoma of urinary bladder in an adult. *J Postgrad Med* 1982; 28:174–176.
105. Patterson DE, Barrett DM: Leiomyosarcoma of urinary bladder. *Urology* 1983; 21:367–369.
106. Rowland RG, Eble JN: Bladder leiomyosarcoma and pelvic fibroblastic tumor follow-

ing cyclophosphamide therapy. *J Urol* 1983; 130:334–346.

107. Rosi P, Selli C, Carini M, et al: Myxoid liposarcoma of the bladder. *J Urol* 1983; 130:560–561.
108. Flint LD, Dick VS: Myosarcoma of the urinary bladder: Preliminary report of favorable cases. *Lahey Clin Bull* 1950; 6:181–186.
109. Hess E: Sarcoma of prostate and adjacent retrovesical structures. *J Urol* 1938; 40:629–640.
110. Fein MJ: Spindle cell sarcoma of the prostate. *Am J Clin Pathol* 1939; 9:564–571.
111. Stirling WC, Ash JE: Sarcoma of the prostate. *J Urol* 1939; 41:515–533.
112. Counseller VS, Bedard RE: Sarcoma of the prostate gland. *J Urol* 1940; 43; 836–843.
113. Stevens AR, Barringer BS: Sarcoma of the prostate. *J Urol* 1940; 44:83–108.
114. Taylor HE: Sarcoma of the prostate (with report of a case of rhabdomyosarcoma). *Can Med Assoc J* 1940; 42:120–122.
115. Prince CL, Vest SA: Leiomyosarcoma of the prostate. *J Urol* 1941; 46:1129–1143.
116. Melicow MM, Pelton TH, Fish GW: Sarcoma of the prostate gland; review of literature; table classification; report of four cases. *J Urol* 1943; 49:675–707.
117. Miller S, Barshay E: Sarcoma of the prostate gland. *Med Bull Vet Admin* 1944; 20:417–421.
118. Rapport AE, Nixon CE, Colonel L: Sarcoma of prostate: A report of one case of rhabdomyosarcoma of the prostate. *Am J Clin Pathol* 1945; 15:456–466.
119. Seng M, Siminovitch M: Sarcoma of the prostate. *Can Med Assoc J* 1947; 56:425–427.
120. Kawaichi GK, Cooper P: Leiomyosarcoma of the prostate: A case report. *Urol Cutan Rev* 1950; 54:399–401.
121. Ostry H: Leiomyosarcoma of the prostate. *J Urol* 1950; 63:162–164.
122. Riba LW, Wheelock MC: Leiomyosarcoma of prostate. *J Urol* 1950; 63:162–164.
123. Barone AM, Joelson JJ: Leiomyosarcoma of the prostate: Report of a case. *J Urol* 1950; 63:533–538.
124. Pack GT, Eberhart WF: Rhabdomyosarcoma of skeletal muscle. *Surgery* 1952; 32:1023–1064.
125. Derian GH: Spindle cell sarcoma of prostatic gland: Case report. *J Urol* 1953; 69:544–546.
126. Smith GG: Three unusual cases of prostatic malignancy: Adenocarcinoma with mucus cells; malignant lymphoma; leiomyosarcoma. *J Urol* 1953; 70:267–274.
127. Scardino PC, Prince CL: Prostatic sarcoma: Survival following radical perineal prostatectomy. *J Urol* 1954; 72:729–730.
128. Graves RS, Coleman MW: Sarcoma of the prostate: An unusual survival. *J Urol* 1954; 72:731–734.
129. Bell R, Stinson RF Jr: Leiomyosarcoma of prostate. *J Urol* 1955; 73: 716–717.
130. Rattner WH: The rare prostatic neoplasms. *Am Practitioner* 1959; 10:1533–1535.
131. Fitzpatrick TJ, Stump G: Leiomyosarcoma of the prostate: Case report and review of the literature. *J Urol* 1960; 83:80–83.
132. Goldfarb M, Bertcher RW: Primary osteochondrosarcoma of the prostate gland: A case report. *J Urol* 1960; 84:402–405.
133. Murphy G, Bradley J: Primary sarcoma of the prostate. *J Urol* 1961; 85:973–976.
134. Siegel J: Sarcoma of the prostate: a report of four cases and a review of current therapy. *J Urol* 1963; 89:78–83.
135. Torres LF, Estrada JY, Esquivel EL Jr: Sarcoma of the prostate gland: Report of four cases. *J Urol* 1966; 96:380–384.
136. Mackenzie AR, Miller TR, Randall HT: Translumbar amputation for advanced leiomyosarcoma of the prostate. *J Urol* 1967; 97:133–136.
137. Stenron U, Holby LE: A case of circumscribed myosarcoma of the prostate. *Cancer* 1969; 24:803–806.
138. Christofferen J: Leiomyosarcoma of the prostate. *Acta Chir Scand [Suppl]* 1973; 433:75–84.
139. Peterson LJ, Paulson DF: Rhabdomyosarcoma in adult prostate. *Urology* 1974; 3:689–692.
140. Chatterjee AC: Leiomyosarcoma of the prostate. *Br J Urol* 1975; 47:577.
141. Schmidt JD, Welch MT Jr: Sarcoma of the prostate. *Cancer* 1976; 37:1908–1912.
142. King DG, Finney RP: Embryonal rhabdomyosarcoma of the prostate. *J Urol* 1977; 117:88–90.
143. Cea PC, Ward NJ: Sarcoma of the prostate 13 years after suprapubic prostatectomy. *J Urol* 1977; 117:129–130.
144. Stallwood G, Davidson JW: Leiomyosarcoma of the rectum and prostate. *Can J Surg* 1977; 20:446–449.
145. Vereecken RL, Lauweryns J, Drochmans

A, et al: Leiomyosarcoma of prostate; A case report. *Eur Urol* 1977; 3:370–372.

146. Guha T: Leiomyosarcoma of the prostate: a case report. *Clin Oncol* 1979; 5:261–265.
147. Witherow R, Molland E, Oliver T, et al: Leiomyosarcoma of prostate and superficial soft tissue. *Urology* 1980; 15:513–515.
148. Dupree WB, Fisher C: Rhabdomyosarcoma of prostate in adult. Long-term survival and problem of histologic diagnosis. *Urology* 1982; 19:802.
149. Shehata WM, Kerr AA, Boss HH, et al: Leiomyosarcoma of the prostate apparently cured by surgery and radical irradiation: Report of case. *Int J Radiat Oncol Biol Phys* 1982; 8:1814–1815.
150. Carmel M, Masse SR, Lehous JG: Leiomyosarcoma of prostate. *Urology* 1983; 22:190–193.
151. Rosenberg SA, Tepper J, Glatstein E, et al: Prospective randomized evaluation of adjuvant chemotherapy in adults with soft tissue sarcomas of the extremities. *Cancer* 1983; 52:424–434.
152. Fitzpatrick RJ, Orr LM, Glanton JB: Tumor of the spermatic cord: Review of literature and report of two cases. *JAMA* 1952; 148:259–261.
153. Hansen JL, Enos WE, Park OK, et al: Rhabdomyosarcoma of spermatic cord. *U.S. Armed Forces Med J* 1952; 3:621–626.
154. Herbut PA: *Urological Pathology.* Philadelphia, Lea & Febiger, 1952, pp 1029–1030.
155. Schottenfeld LE, Grayzel DM, Trattler AJ: Sarcoma of the testis. *Am J Surg* 1952; 83:589–594.
156. Sherwin B, Bergman H: Primary malignant neoplasms of the spermatic cord and epididymis: 2 case reports. *J Urol* 1952; 67:208–215.
157. Wessel HN: Leiomyosarcoma of the spermatic cord. *J Urol* 1953; 69:823–829.
158. Eason TJ, Solitau HK: Sarcoma of the epididymis. *Br J Surg* 1953–1954; 41:331–332.
159. Bevan PG: Malignant leiomyoma of spermatic cord. *Br J Surg* 1954; 42:101–102.
160. Jessen C, Storm O: Fibrosarcoma of the epididymis: Report of a case. *Acta Chir Scand* 1955; 110:246–249.
161. Cannon EM, Altheide JP, Allen HC: Malignant tumors of the spermatic cord and testicular tunica. *South Med J* 1956; 49:17–24.
162. Powell HDW: Fibrosarcoma of the spermatic cord. *Br J Urol* 1956; 28:194–197.
163. Cruse K: Leiomyosarcoma of the spermatic cord: Report of a case and review of literature. *Arch Srug* 1958; 76:151–154.
164. Enterline HT, Horn RC Jr: Alveolar rhabdomyosarcoma: A distinctive tumor type. *Am J Clin Pathol* 1958; 29:356–366.
165. Kohler FP, Murphy JJ: Rhabdomyosarcoma of the male genital tract. *J Urol* 1959; 82:500–503.
166. Statler EJ, Heidner FC II, Wear JB: Primary sarcoma of the spermatic cord and epididymis. *J Urol* 1959; 82:148–154.
167. Pearlman CK, Mackey JF Jr: Intrascrotal rhabdomyosarcoma: Case report. *J Urol* 1960; 83:303–304.
168. Dreyfuss, W, Goodsitt E: Tumors of spermatic cord. *J Urol* 1960; 84:658–665.
169. Fagundes LA, Hampe O: Leiomyosarcoma of the spermatic cord. *J Urol* 1961; 85:835–837.
170. Walker WF, Cameron HM: Rhabdomyosarcoma of the epididymis. *Br J Surg* 1961; 49:319–321.
171. Bhansali SK: Rhabdomyosarcoma of the spermatic cord. *Br J Surg* 1962; 50:883–884.
172. Wagner M, Teresi JL: Primary fibroleiomyosarcoma of spermatic cord. *Wis Med J* 1963; 62:342–347.
173. Miller Al Jr, Sharp L: Unusual intrascrotal tumors. *J Urol* 1964; 91:273–279.
174. Samellas W: Malignant neoplasms of spermatic cord. *NY State J Med* 1964; 64:1213–1215.
175. Arean VM, Kreager JA: Paratesticular rhabdomyosarcoma. *Am J Clin Pathol* 1965; 43:418–427.
176. Graf RA: Malignant tumors of the spermatic cord: A brief review and presentation of lipofibromyxosarcoma of spermatic cord. *J Urol* 1965; 93:74–76.
177. Ravich L, Lerman PH, Drabkin JW, et al: Pure testicular rhabdomyosarcoma. *J Urol* 1965; 94:596–599.
178. Ashby BS, MacGillivray JB: Paratesticular lipoma. *Br J Surg* 1966; 53:828–830.
179. Kyle VN: Leiomyosarcoma of the spermatic cord: A review of the literature and report of an additional case. *J Urol* 1966; 96:795–800.
180. Fox TA, Collier RL: Rhabdomyosarcoma of the spermatic cord. *Am Surg* 1967; 33:483–489.
181. Lundbald RR, Mellinger GT, Gleason DF: Spermatic cord malignancies. *J Urol* 1967; 98:393–396.

182. Abell MR, Holitz F: Testicular and paratesticular neoplasms in patients 60 years of age and older. *Cancer* 1968; 21:852–870.
183. Alexander F: Intrascrotal sarcomas. *Br J Cancer* 1968; 22:486–497.
184. Housfield KF, Guira AC: Liposarcoma of the spermatic cord: Case report. *Ohio State Med J* 1968; 64:1036–1037.
185. Sharma MP: Leiomyosarcoma of the spermatic cord. *Br J Urol* 1968; 40:464–467.
186. Tanimura H, Fukuta M: Rhabdomyosarcoma of the spermatic cord. *Cancer* 1968; 22:1215–1220.
187. Arlen M. Grabstold H, Whitmore WF Jr: Malignant tumors of the spermatic cord. *Cancer* 1969; 23:525–532.
188. Williams G, Banerjee R: Paratesticular tumors. *Br J Urol* 1969; 41:332–339.
189. Yadau SB, Patil PN, Karkhanis PB: Primary tumor of the spermatic cord, epididymis and rete testis. *J Postgrad Med* 1969; 15:49–52.
190. Young TW: Malignant tumors of spermatic cord. *Br J Surg* 1969; 56:260–262.
191. Rosas-Uribe A, Cuna MA, Guinn GA: Paratesticular rhabdomyosarcoma. *Am J Surg* 1970; 120:787–791.
192. Tanaka T, Harada M, Hara M, et al: Three cases of rhabdomyosarcoma originiated from relatively unusual sites. *Acta Pathol Jpn* 1970; 20:103–110.
193. Datta NS, Singh SM, Bapna BC: Liposarcoma of the spermatic cord: Report of a case and review of the literature. *J Urol* 1971; 106:888–889.
194. Rushworth GF: Leiomyosarcoma of epididymis. *Proc R Soc Med* 1971; 64:999.
195. Cole AT, Straus FH, Gill WB: Malignant fibrous histiocytoma: An unusual inguinal sarcoma. *J Urol* 1972; 107:1005.
196. Jenkins DG: Subbuswamy: Leiomyosarcoma of the spermatic cord. *Br J Surg* 1972; 59:408–410.
197. Malek RS, Utz DC, Farrow GM: Malignant tumors of the spermatic cord. *Cancer* 1972; 29:1108–1113.
198. Sinclair-Smith, CC: Paratesticular rhabdomyosarcoma. *South Afr J Surg* 1972; 10:56–57.
199. D'Abrera VS, Burfitt-Williams W: A giant scrotal liposarcoma. *Med J Aust* 1973; 2:854–856.
200. Mostofi FK, Price EB Jr: Tumor of the male genital system, in *Atlas of Tumor Pathology*, 2nd series, fasc 8. Washington, D.C., Armed Forces Institute of Pathology, 1973, pp 166–167.
201. Remzi D: Tumors of the tunica vaginalis. *South Med J* 1973; 66:841–842.
202. Weitzner S: Leiomyosarcoma of spermatic cord and retroperitoneal lymph node dissection. *Am Surg* 1973; 39:352–354.
203. Dimacopoulos DG: Paratesticular liposarcoma. *Br J Urol* 1974; 46:347.
204. Mackenzie I, Roberts H: Liposarcoma of paratesticular origin: A case report. *Br J Urol* 1974; 46:467–470.
205. Farah RN, Bohne AW: Malignant fibrous histiocytoma of spermatic cord. *Urology* 1974; 3:782–783.
206. Somani IK, Sharma HSD, Arora MM: Primary fibrosarcoma of the epididymis. *Ind J Med Sci* 1974; 19:72–74.
207. Skeel DA, Drinker JR, Witherington R: Rhabdomyosarcoma of the spermatic cord: Report of 3 cases with review of the literature. *J Urol* 1975; 13:279–284.
208. McCormack M: Bilateral fibrosarcoma of the epididymis. *J Clin Pathol* 1975; 28:576–579.
209. Jungling MJ, Culp DA: Case report of embryonal rhabdomyosarcoma of the testis with an 8-year survival. *J Urol* 1975; 114:313–315.
210. Davides KC, King LM. Paat F: Primary leiomyosarcoma of the epididymis. *J Urol* 1975; 114:642–644.
211. de Luise VP, Draper JW, Gray FG Jr: Smooth muscle tumors of the testicular adnexa. *J Urol* 1976; 115:685–688.
212. Bissada NK, Finkenbeiner AE, Redman JF: Paratesticular sarcoma: Review of remanagement. *J Urol* 1976; 116:198–200.
213. Zegel HG, Goldsmith HS: Rhabdomyosarcoma of the spermatic cord. *Clin Oncol* 1976; 2:261–266.
214. Beall ME, Young IS: Spermatic cord rhabdomyosarcoma: Case report. *J Urol* 1977; 117:807.
215. Malek RS, Kelalis PP: Paratesticular rhabdomyosarcoma in childhood. *J Urol* 1977; 118:450–453.
216. Curnes JH, Pratt CB, Hustu O: Five-year survival after disseminated paratesticular rhabdomyosarcoma. *J Urol* 1977; 118:662–665.
217. Dikranian HA: Rhabdomyosarcoma of spermatic cord. *Urology* 1977; 9:329–331.
218. Senoh K, Osada Y, Kawachi J: Spermatic cord liposarcoma. *Br J Urol* 1978; 50:429.

219. Sogani RC, Grabstald H, Whitmore WF Jr: Spermatic cord sarcoma in adults. *J Urol* 1978; 120:301–305.

220. Johnson DE, Harris JD, Ayala AG: Liposarcoma of spermatic cord. *Urology* 1978; 11:190–192.

221. Bellinger MF, Gibbons MD, Koontz WW Jr. et al: Paratesticular liposarcoma. *Urology* 1978; 11:285–288.

222. Dias R, Fernandes M, Gaetz HP: Malignant fibrous histiocytoma of spermatic cord. *Urology* 1978; 12:365–367.

223. Banik S, Guha PK: Paratesticular rhabdomyosarcomas and leiomyosarcomas: A clinicopathological review. *J Urol* 1979; 121:823–862.

224. Gould L, Klein K, Patel M: Ultrasound evaluation of a spermatic cord myxoliosarcoma. *J Med Soc N J* 1979; 76:203–205.

225. Olney LE, Narayana A, Loening S, et al: Intrascrotal rhabdomyosarcoma. *Urology* 1979; 14:113–125.

226. Turetz F, Smulewicz JJ, Hecht H: Liposarcoma of the spermatic cord: Report of a case and pitfalls in sonographic differential diagnosis. *Mt Sinai J Med* 1979; 46:199–200.

227. Sane SY, Nimbkar SA, Bapat RD: Leiomyosarcoma of hydrocele sac. *J Postgrad Med* 1980; 26:145–146.

228. Williamson JC, Johnson JD, Lamm DL, et al: Malignant fibrous histiocytoma of the spermatic cord. *J Urol* 1980; 123:785–788.

229. Farrell MA, Donnelly BJ: Malignant smooth muscle tumors of the epididymis. *J Urol* 1980; 124:151–153.

230. Reyes CV: Spermatic cord liposarcoma. *Urology* 1980; 15:416–417.

231. Hoekstra JH, Wobbes T, Brouwers TM, et al: Embryonal rhabdomyosarcoma of spermatic cord. *Urology* 1980; 16:360–363.

232. Blitzer PH, Dosoretz DE, Proppe KH, et al: Treatment of malignant tumors of the spermatic cord: A study of 10 cases and a review of the literature. *J Urol* 1981; 126:611–614.

233. Buckley RM: Leiomyosarcoma of the spermatic cord. *Br J Urol* 981; 53:193.

234. Treadwell T, Treadwell MA, Owen M, et al: Giant liposarcoma of the spermatic cord. *South Med J* 1981; 74:753–755.

235. Trippitelli A, Rosi P. Selli C, et al: Rhabdomyosarcoma of spermatic cord in adult. *Urology* 1982; 19:533–535.

236. Sago AL, Novicki DE: Rhabdomyosarcoma of spermatic cord. *Urology* 1982; 19:606–608.

237. Riehle RA Jr, Venkatachalam H: Electron microscopy in diagnosis of adult paratesticular rhabdomyosarcoma. *Urology* 1982; 19:658–661.

238. Smailowitz Z. Koneti J, Sober I, et al: Management fibrous histiocytoma of the spermatic cord. *J Urol* 1983; 130:150–151.

239. Puts JG, Boerema JJ, van Hielst UJGM: Leiomyosarcoma of spermatic cord. *Urology* 1984; 23:189–193.

240. Vorstman B, Block NL, Politano VA: The management of spermatic liposarcoma. *J Urol* 1984; 131:66–69.

241. Fauci PA Jr, Therhag HG, Davis JE: Carcinosarcoma of the renal pelvis. *J Urol* 1961; 85:897–902.

242. Fisher ER, Davis ER: Carcinosarcoma of the kidney. *J Urol* 1962; 87:109–118.

243. Hou LT, Willis RA: Renal carcino-sarcoma, true and false. *J Pathol Bacterial* 1963; 85:139–144.

244. Newman D, Vellios F: Adult carcinosarcoma (adult Wilms' tumor) of the kidney. *Am J Clin Pathol* 1964; 42:45–54.

245. Elliott JT, Pontius EE, McCallum DC: Carcinosarcoma of kidney. *Urology* 1973; 1:151–153.

246. Ridolfi RL, Eggelston JC: Carcinosarcoma of the renal pelvis. *J Urol* 1978; 119:569–572.

247. Dent EB: Carcinosarcoma ("collision tumor") of the urinary bladder. *J Urol* 1955; 74:104–108.

248. Powers JF, Hawn CVZ, Carter RD: Osteogenic sarcoma and transitional cell carcinoma occurring simultaneously in the bladder. *J Urol* 1956; 76:263–269.

249. Thompson IM, Coppridge AJ: Bladder sarcoma. *J Urol* 1959; 82:329–332.

250. Brinton JA, Ito Y, Olsen BS: Carcinosarcoma of the urinary bladder: A case report and review of literature. *Cancer* 1970; 25:1183–1186.

251. Delides GS: Bone and cartilage in malignant tumors of the urinary bladder *Br J Urol* 1972; 44:571–581.

252. Holtz F, Fox JE, Abell MR: Carcinosarcoma of the urinary bladder. *Cancer* 1972; 29:294–304.

253. Shive AV, Kherdekar KKS: Carcinosarcoma of the urinary bladder: A case report and review of literature. *Ind J Med Sci* 1973; 27:932–934.

254. McCarthy LJ, Whale WM, Moosey NA: Carcinosarcoma of the urinary bladder: A case report. *J Indiana State Med Assoc* 1975; 68:722–724.

255. Patterson TH, Dale GA: Carcinosarcoma of the bladder: Case report and review of the literature. *J Urol* 1976; 115:753–755.

256. Johansen SE, Stenwig AE, Tveter KJ: Carcinosarcoma of the urinary bladder in an adult male. *Scand J Urol Nephrol* 1979; 13:117–122.

257. Schoborg TW, Saffos RO, Rodriguez AP, et al: Carcinosarcoma of the bladder. *J Urol* 1980; 124:724–727.

258. Babaian RJ, Johnson DE, Manning J, et al: Mixed mesodermal tumors of urinary bladder: Prognosis and management. *Urology* 1980; 15:261–264.

259. Uyama T, Moriwaki S: Carcinosarcoma of urinary bladder. *Urology* 1981; 18:191–194.

260. Guirguis AB, Milam J, Richardson DH: Carcinosarcoma. *Urology* 1983; 22:553–555.

261. Smith JA Jr, Herr HW, Middleton RG: Bladder carcinosarcoma: Histologic variation in metastatic lesions. *J Urol* 1983; 129:829–831.

262. Kusaba Y, Yushita Y, Suzu H, et al: Carcinosarcoma of the bladder. *J Urol* 1984; 131:118–119.

263. Meeter UL, Richards JN: Osteogenic sarcoma of the prostate. *J Urol* 1960; 84:654–657.

264. Hamlin WB, Lund PK: Carcinosarcoma of the prostate: a case report. *J Urol* 1967; 97:518–522.

265. Haddad JR, Reyes EC: Carcinosarcoma of prostate with matastasis of both elements: Case reprot. *J Urol* 1970; 103:80–83.

266. Martin SA, Fowler M, Catalona WJ, et al: Carcinosarcoma of the prostate: Report of a case with ultrastructural observations. *J Urol* 1979; 122:709–711.

267. Krastanova LJ, Addonizio JC: Carcinosarcoma of prostate. *Urology* 1981; 18:85–88.

268. Quay SC, Proppe KH: Carcinosarcoma of the prostate: Case report and review of the literature. *J Urol* 1981; 125:436–438.

269. Hays DM: Pelvic rhabdomyosarcoma in childhood. *Cancer* 1980; 45:1810–1814.

Chapter 17

Genitourinary Rhabdomyosarcoma in Childhood

Stephen A. Kramer

Neoplasms of the urinary tract are rare in children and predominantly mesothelial in origin. Rhabdomyosarcoma is the most common soft-tissue sarcoma of childhood. This neoplasm accounts for 10% to 15% of all solid tumors in children, and from 15% to 20% of these tumors arise from the genitourinary tract.[1] The estimated annual incidence for rhabdomyosarcoma of the urogenital tract is 0.5 to 0.7 case per million children younger than 15 years. Boys are affected more often than girls, in a ratio of 3:1.

PATHOLOGY

Rhabdomyosarcomas arise from undifferentiated mesenchyme, which undergoes various degrees of differentiation into myxomatous tissue, fibrous tissue, or striated muscle.[2] These tumors are highly malignant and have a propensity for early invasion of local structures. Lymphatic metastatic lesions and hematogenous dissemination to the lungs and liver have been noted in up to 30% of patients at autopsy.[2]

Rhabdomyosarcomas have been traditionally divided into four histological types: pleomorphic, alveolar, embryonal, and botryoid.[3] A proposal by the Intergroup Rhabdomyosarcoma Study (IRS) III differentiates cytohistological subtypes into "unfavorable" and "favorable" categories.[4] Proposed unfavorable histological types include (1) anaplastic rhabdomyosarcoma (markedly enlarged and bizarre mitotic figures with nuclear hyperchromatism and nuclear pleomorphism), (2) monomorphous round cell rhabdomyosarcoma (marked uniformity in size and cytological characteristics of the total tumor cell population), and (3) alveolar tumors. All other rhabdomyosarcomas are included in the favorable category, regardless of cellular constituents or tissue organization.

BLADDER RHABDOMYOSARCOMA

Bladder lesions occur twice as often in boys as in girls, and most patients are younger than 5 years at the first presentation. Rhabdomyosarcoma of the bladder usually originates in the submucosa and superficial layers of the trigone. The tumor extends into the membranous urethra in the male and throughout the entire length of the female urethra. Extension of tumor into the prostate, vulva, and vagina occurs before lymphatic or hematogenous metastatic lesions develop. This tendency for expansive growth explains why local recurrence is a more frequent cause of treatment failure than either regional or distant metastasis.

Tumor of the bladder tends to occur in a distinctive botryoid form and may reach massive size before producing symptoms (Fig. 17–1). Bladder outlet obstructive symptoms are common at presentation, and occasionally children have acute urinary retention or passage of tissue fragments through the urethra. Gross hematuria, infrequent in occurrence, results from disruption of the overlying bladder mucosa.

The tumor is often palpable as a suprapubic mass and may be mistaken for a distended bladder. The excretory urogram reveals ureteropyelocaliectasis in more than 50% of patients, and the cystogram shows the characteristic negative filling defects within the bladder (Fig. 17–2).[5] Definitive diagnosis is made at endoscopic evaluation, when the typical polypoid, whitish growth can be removed for histological examination.

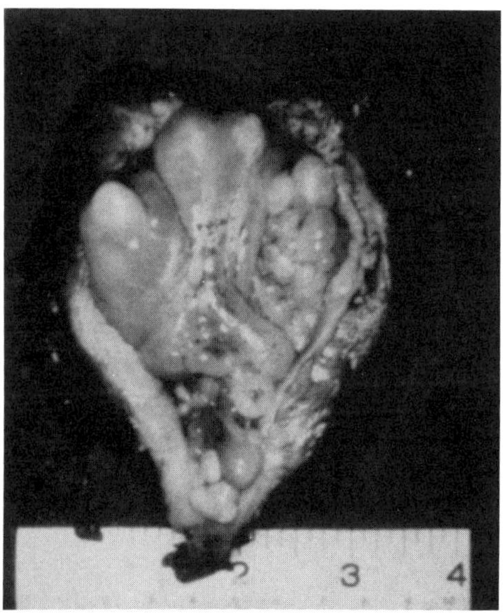

FIG 17–1.
Rhabdomyosarcoma of the bladder in a girl with urinary retention: gross appearance of tumor after radical cystectomy. Lobules of tumor are prolapsed into the uretha. (From Tank ES, Kelalis PP: Lower urinary tract, in Kelalis PP, King LR, Belman AB (eds): *Clinical Pediatric Urology*, vol 2. Philadelphia, W. B. Saunders, 1976, pp. 928–936. Used by permission.)

PROSTATIC RHABDOMYOSARCOMA

The median age of patients with prostatic lesions is 3.5 years. Prostatic rhabdomyosarcoma tends to be solid rather than botryoid. Continuous spread into the bladder often makes it difficult to distinguish histologically whether this tumor originates primarily in the prostate or in the bladder. The tumor infiltrates the bladder neck and posterior portion of the urethra and causes bladder outlet obstruction. Infiltration of the rectum by tumor may produce constipation as a presenting syndrome.

Lymphatic metastases occur much more frequently with this tumor than with bladder rhabdomyosarcoma. Twenty percent of patients with prostatic rhabdomyosarcomas have lymphogenous metastases, and up to 40% have hematogenous dissemination.[6]

The tumor is easily palpable on rectal examination, and a distended bladder from outlet obstruction is usually palpable suprapublically. Excretory urography demonstrates elevation of the bladder base, and voiding cystourethrography shows distortion of the prostatic urethra (Fig. 17–3). Diagnosis is established by transurethral biopsy (if possible) or by perineal biopsy.

VAGINAL AND UTERINE RHABDOMYOSARCOMA

Rhabdomyosarcoma of the vagina and uterus usually appears when the patient is between 6 and 18 months of age. This tumor usually occurs on the anterior vaginal wall adjacent to the cervix,[7] but it may arise from the distal portion of the vagina or from the labia.[8] Often the tumor extends through the vesicovaginal septum into the bladder and urethra (Fig. 17–4).[9] Interestingly, the rectovaginal septum acts as a barrier to posterior spread of tumor, so that the rectal wall is infrequently involved.

Patients may present with a prolapsing mass, vaginal discharge, or bleeding. Distant metastases are uncommon at initial presentation. Diagnosis is established by cystoscopy, vaginoscopy, and biopsy.

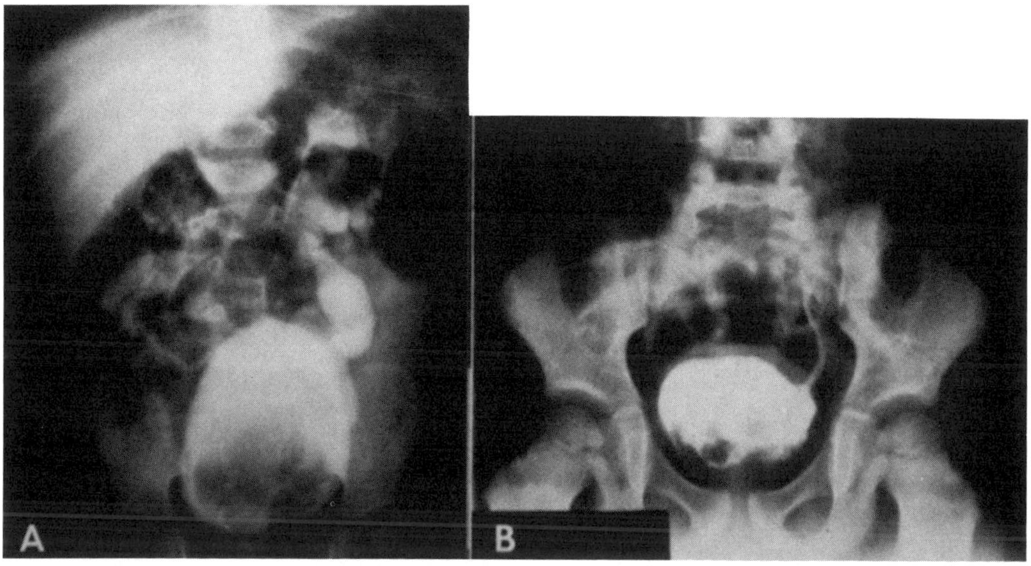

FIG 17–2.
Excretory urograms. **A,** intravesical rhabdomyosarcoma of bladder with bilateral ureteral obstruction. **B,** characteristic lobulated filling defects on excretory cystogram from patient with botyroid sarcoma of bladder. (From Tank ES, Kelalis PP: Lower urinary tract, in Kelalis PP, King LR, Belman AB (eds): *Clinical Pediatric Urology,* vol. 2. Philadelphia, W. B. Saunders, 1976, pp. 928–936. Used by permission.)

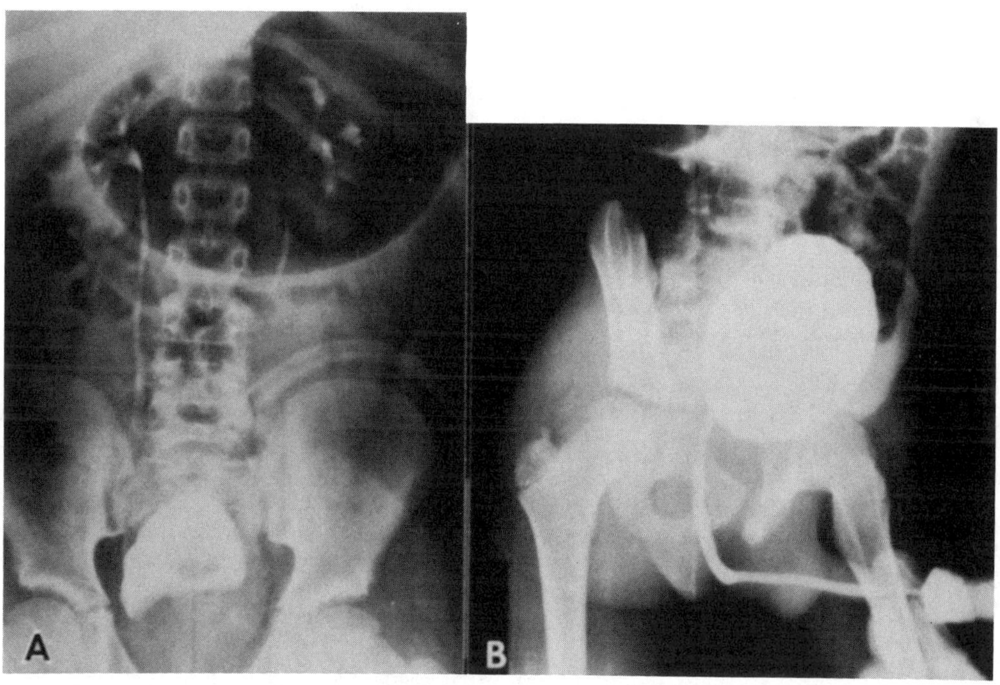

FIG 17–3.
Rhabdomyosarcoma of prostate. **A,** excretory urogram shows elevation of bladder by huge prostatic mass. **B,** retrograde urethrogram shows elongation and distortion of prostatic uretha by solid variety of tumor. (From Tank ES, Kelalis PP: Lower urinary tract, in Kelalis PP, King LR, Belman AB (eds): *Clinical Pediatric Urology,* vol. 2. Philadelphia, W. B. Saunders, 1976, pp. 928–936. Used by permission.)

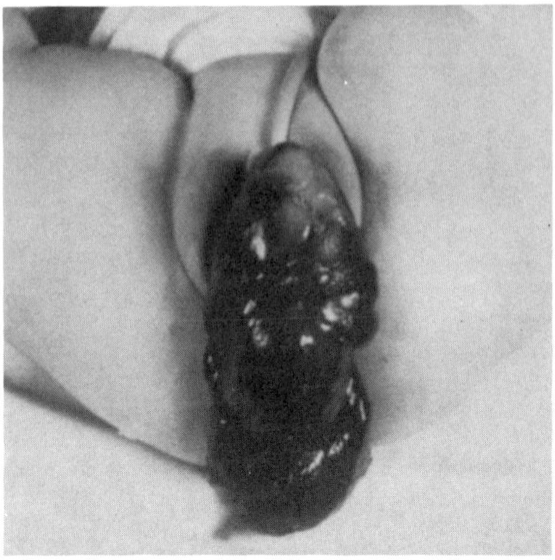

FIG 17–4.
Large vaginal rhabdomyosarcoma in 3-month-old child. (From Fleming ID, Etcubanas E, Patterson R, et al: *Ann Surg* 1984; 199:509–514. Used by permission.)

STAGING AND PROGNOSIS

Clinical staging is based on local extent of tumor, presence or absence of metastatic disease, and microscopically verified completeness of surgical removal (Box 17–1). Computed tomography, ultrasonography, and magnetic resonance imaging are used routinely to determine size and anatomical extent of disease. The most favorable prognostic indicators of survival are clinical staging, histological findings, and the site of the primary tumor.

BOX 17–1.
Staging of Rhabdomyosarcoma*

Group I
- Localized disease, completely resected
  - Tumor confined to the muscle or organ of origin
  - Infiltration outside this structure without involvement of regional nodes

Group II
- Grossly resected tumor with "microscopic residual disease"
- Regional disease, completely resected, in which nodes may be involved or tumor extends into adjacent organ
- Regional disease with involved nodes grossly resected but with evidence of "microscopic residual disease"

Group III
- Incomplete resection or biopsy with gross residual disease

Group IV
- Distant metastatic disease present at onset

*Modified from Hays DM, Raney RB Jr, Lawrence W Jr, et al: *Cancer* 1982; 50:1472.

THERAPY

Before the advent of multiagent chemotherapy, rhabdomyosarcoma of the prostate or bladder was treated by radical cystectomy or pelvic exenteration.[10] Rhabdomyosarcoma of the vagina and uterus was managed by radical hysterectomy and excision of the vaginal cuff. Local excision or segmental resection uniformly resulted in pelvic recurrence and subsequent tumor dissemination.[6, 7, 11–16] Furthermore, chemotherapy alone or a combination of chemotherapy and radiation therapy has not controlled genitourinary rhabdomyosarcoma.[17]

Combined therapy, including extirpative surgery, local radiation therapy, and 2-year multiagent chemotherapy, has produced survival rates of greater than 90% in patients with localized disease.[15, 18–21] These excellent survival rates were reproduced by IRS I.[7] Vincristine, actinomycin D, and cyclophosphamide (VAC) are the most effective chemotherapeutic agents, and combination chemotherapy has been superior to single-agent treatment.[6, 13, 22]

Although some groups continue to advocate pelvic exenteration as an integral part of treatment for genitourinary rhabdomyosarcoma,[23] concerns about impotency and sterility and problems associated with urinary or bowel diversions have raised questions about the use of radical surgery in these children.

In 1975, Rivard et al.[24] proposed biopsy of tumor alone followed by aggressive chemotherapy and radiation therapy. Their series included nine children with pelvic rhabdomyosarcoma who were given intensive chemotherapy or radiation therapy, or both, pre-operatively. Five patients survived, each of whom was managed successfully with excision of residual tumor only. No patients were subjected to anterior exenteration. All four deaths occurred in patients with stage IV disease.

In 1979, Ortega[25] updated the Los Angeles Children's Hospital experience to include a group of 13 children treated initially with cytoreductive triple-agent chemotherapy. Eight children were alive and well without evidence of disease from 2 to 8 years after diagnosis. Only one patient had required anterior pelvic exenteration.

Disenchantment with pelvic exenteration and the documented effectiveness of primary intensive multiagent chemotherapy have brought about significant changes in the treatment of pelvic rhabdomyosarcoma.[5, 18, 20] IRS II was established to evaluate the impact of limited surgery and limited radiation therapy in children with genitourinary rhabdomyosarcoma. In the current approach to children with pelvic rhabdomyosarcoma, the diagnosis is confirmed by biopsy, and multi-agent chemotherapy with pulse VAC (vincristine, 2 mg/m^2 for 1 day [maximum daily dose, 2 mg]; actinomycin D, 0.015 mg/kg/day for 5 days [maximum daily dose, 0.5 mg]; and cyclophosphamide, 10 mg/kg/day for 3 days) is repeated twice, 4 weeks apart (Fig. 17–5).[18] Clinical evaluation is undertaken at the end of 8 weeks, and if the tumor has shrunk at least 50%, chemotherapy is continued to 16 weeks. Then, exploratory laparotomy is performed, and residual tumor is excised. With this approach, it is often possible to perform radical prostatectomy for prostatic tumors or partial cystectomy for bladder tumors. Radiation therapy is added postoperatively if there is evidence of microscopic or gross residual disease.

If there is evidence of progressive disease at any time after 2 weeks or no response at 8 weeks, the patient is treated with irradiation. Triple-agent chemotherapy, in which doxorubicin (Adriamycin) may be alternated with actinomycin D, is continued for 2 years irrespective of the surgical findings.

Recent data from IRS II concern the effects of primary chemotherapy in 79 patients with localized sarcoma of the prostate, bladder, or vagina.[26] Thirty-six patients had prostatic tumors, 29 had bladder tumors, and 14 had vaginal tumors. The relapse-free survival rates at 2 years were 16 of 29 (55%) for prostate, 14 of 25 (56%) for bladder, and 4 of 9 (44%) for vagina. The actuarial survival rate at 2 years was 34 of 63 (54%). Twenty of 34 patients retained their bladder (59%). These results are certainly not as impressive as those of IRS I, in which the overall 2-year relapse-free survival rate was 21 of 27 (78%) (Table 17–1). The IRS I bladder salvage rate was 16 of 21 (76%). The overall actuarial survival rate at 3 years in IRS 1 was 17 of 23 (74%), compared with 26 of 44 (59%) in IRS II.

It appears that although immediate cystectomy is not necessary at the time of diagnosis, radiation therapy is usually necessary for patients with prostatic and bladder tumors, and partial vaginectomy is often necessary for those with vaginal tumors. Unfortunately, primary

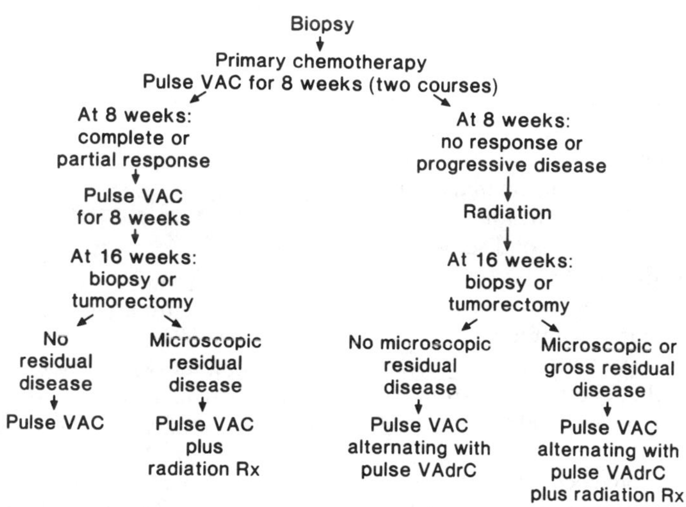

FIG 17–5.
Current therapeutic recommendations for pelvic rhabdomyosarcoma (bladder, prostate, vagina, uterus). VAC-vincristine, actinomycin D, and cyclophosphamide; VAdrC-vincristine, doxorubicin (Adriamycin), and cyclophosphamide. (From Kramer SA: *Urol Clin Am* 1985; 12:31–42. Used by permission.)

TABLE 17–1.
Bladder or Prostate Rhabdomyosarcoma: Relapse-Free Survival at 2 Years*

	Patients			
	IRS I†		IRS II†	
	Number	Percent	Number	Percent
Alive with no evidence of disease	21	78	34	54
With intact bladder or after partial cystectomy	(16)		(20)	
After anterior exenteration or total cystectomy	(5)		(14)	
Dead	6	22	29	46
Total	27		63	

* *Kramer SA, Kelalis PP: Pediatric urologic oncology, in Gillenwater JY, Grahack JT, Howards SS, et al (eds): Adult and Pediatric Urology, vol 2. Chicago, Year Book Medical Publishers, 1987, pp 2001–2042.*
† *IRS = Intergroup Rhabdomyosarcoma Study.*

chemotherapy as given in this study appeared relatively ineffective in producing relapse-free survival at 2 years. Currently, IRS III is adding radiation therapy sooner and a more aggressive chemotherapy regimen.

PARATESTICULAR RHABDOMYOSARCOMA

Paratesticular rhabdomyosarcoma is the most frequent spermatic cord tumor of childhood.[27] This neoplasm usually is a unilateral painless, firm, and nontender mass in the scrotum, lying superior to the testis. The tumor may originate in the testis itself,[28] the epididymis,[29] or the testicular tunics.[30] The tumor tends to grow rapidly and has a predilection for early lymphogenous metastatic spread.

In 1977, Malek and Kelalis[31] reviewed the Mayo Clinic experience in ten children with paratesticular rhabdomyosarcomas. Three patients with noninfiltrative tumors treated by radical orchiectomy and adjunctive irradiation were alive and well without evidence of disease from 8 to 44 years after diagnosis. Retroperitoneal nodel metastases developed in all seven patients with cord-infiltrating tumors. Interestingly, two of the seven patients were salvaged with early retroperitoneal lymphadenectomy followed by postoperative irradiation and multi-agent cyclic chemotherapy.

Radical inguinal orchiectomy at the level of the internal inguinal ring remains the first method of therapy. Resection of scrotal skin is indicated in patients who have had transcrotal biopsy or who have fixation of the scrotal skin by tumor. The incidence of nodal involvement disclosed by lymph node dissection ranges from 40% to 50%; thus, all patients with paratesticular rhabdomyosarcomas should undergo retroperitoneal lymphadenectomy.[32] Patients with groups I and II disease are treated with retroperitoneal lymphadenectomy and postoperative chemotherapy with VAC for 2 years. Patients with group III (gross retroperitoneal disease) or group IV disease (distant metastasis) are treated initially with cytoreductive chemotherapy and then by retroperitoneal node dissection and postoperative radiation therapy.

In a review of patients with paratesticular rhabdomyosarcoma between 1960 and 1974, Raney et al.[32] reported that 44 of 74 patients (60%) were alive without evidence of disease 2 years after diagnosis. Current figures from IRS I indicate that 16 of 18 patients (89%) were alive without evidence of disease at a median of 2 years after treatment.[32]

REFERENCES

1. Fleischmann J, Perinetti EP, Catalona WJ: Embryonal rhabdomyosarcoma of the genitourinary organs. *J Urol* 1981; 126:389–392.
2. Mostofi FK, Morse WH: Polypoid rhabdomyosarcoma (sarcoma botryoides) of bladder in children. *J Urol* 1952; 67:681–687
3. Horn RC Jr, Enterline HT: Rhabdomyosarcoma: A clinicopathological study and classification of 39 cases. *Cancer* 1958; 11:181–199.
4. Children's Cancer Study Group: Protocol CCG-212: Intergroup Rhabdomyosarcoma Study-III. Unpublished.

5. Hays DM, Raney RB Jr, Lawrence W Jr, et al: Primary chemotherapy in the treatment of children with bladder-prostate tumors in the Intergroup Rhabdomyosarcoma Study (IRS-II). *J Pediatr Surg* 1982; 17:8'2–819.
6. Tefft M, Jaffe N: Sarcoma of the bladder and prostate in children: Rationale for the role of radiation therapy based on a review of the literature and a report of fourteen additional patients. *Cancer* 1973; 32:1161–1177.
7. Hays DM: Pelvic rhabdomyosarcomas in childhood: Diagnosis and concepts of management reviewed. *Cancer* 1980; 45:1810–1814.
8. Talerman A: Sarcoma botryoides presenting as a polyp on the labium majus. *Cancer* 1973; 32:994–999.
9. Hilgers RD, Malkasian GD Jr, Soule EH: Embryonal rhabdomyosarcoma (botryoid type) of the vagina: A clinicopathologic review. *Am J Obstet Gynecol* 1970; 107:484–502.
10. Grosfeld JL, Smith JP, Clatworthy HW Jr: Pelvic rhadbomyosarcoma in infants and children. *J Urol* 1972; 107:673–675.
11. Ghazali S: Embryonic rhabdomyosarcoma of the urogenital tract. *Br J Surg* 1973; 60:124–128.
12. Hays DM, Raney RB Jr, Lawrence W Jr, et al: Rhabdomyosarcoma of female urogenital tract. *J Pediatr Surg* 1981; 16:828–834.
13. Ray R, Grabstald H, Exelby PR, et al: Bladder tumors in children. *Urology* 1973; 2:426–435.
14. Williams DI, Schistad G: Lower urinary tract tumours in children. *Br J Urol* 1964; 36:51–65.
15. Clatworthy HW Jr, Braren V, Smith JP: Surgery of bladder and prostatic neoplasms in children. *Cancer* 1973; 32:1157–1160.
16. Timmons JR Jr, Burgert EO JR, Soule EH, et al: Embryonal rhabdomyosarcoma of the bladder and prostate in childhood. *J Urol* 1975; 113:694–697.
17. Scholtmeijer RJ, Tromp CG, Hazebroek FWJ: Embryonal rhabdomyosarcoma of the urogenital tract in childhood. *Eur Urol* 1983; 9:69–74.
18. Maurer HM: The Intergroup Rhabdomyosarcoma Study II: Objectives and study design. *J Pediatr Surg* 1980; 15:371–372.
19. Ehrlich FE, Haas JE, Kiesewetter WB: Rhabdomyosarcoma in infants and children: Factors affecting long-term survival. *J Pediatr Surg* 1971; 6:571–576.
20. Ghavimi F, Exelby PR, D'Angio GJ, et al: Combination therapy of urogenital embryonal rhabdomyosarcoma in children. *Cancer* 1973; 32:1178–1185.
21. Hays DM, Raney RB Jr, Lawrence W Jr, et al: Bladder and prostatic tumors in the Intergroup Rhabdomyosarcoma Study (IRS-I): Results of therapy. *Cancer* 1982; 50:1472–1482.
22. Pratt CB, James DH Jr, Holton CP, et al: Combined therapy including vincristine (NSC-67574) for malignant solid tumors in children. *Cancer Chemother Rep* 1968; 52:489–495.
23. McDougal WS, Persky L: Rhabdomyosarcoma of the bladder and prostate in children. *J Urol* 1980; 124: 882–885.
24. Rivard G, Ortega J, Hittle R, et al: Intensive chemotherapy as primary treatment for rhabdomyosarcoma of the pelvis. *Cancer* 1975; 36:1593–1597.
25. Ortega JA: A therapeutic approach to childhood pelvic rhabdomyosarcoma without pelvic exenteration. *J Pediatr* 1979; 94:205–209.
26. Ramey B, Hays D, Nauer H, et al: Primary chemotherapy ± radiation therapy (RT) and/or surgery for children with localized sarcoma of the prostate, bladder, or vagina: Preliminary results of the Intergroup Rhabdomyosarcoma Study (IRS)-II [abstract]; in Hammond D (chairman): Children's Cancer Study Group: Study Committee Reports, Seattle, April 24–27, 1985.
27. Young JL Jr, Miller RW: Incidence of malignant tumors in U.S. children. *J Pediatr* 1975; 86:254–258.
28. Jungling MJ, Culp DA: Case report of embryonal rhabdomyosarcoma of the testis with an 8-year survival. *J Urol* 1975; 114:313–315.
29. Walker WF, Cameron H McD: Rhabdomyosarcoma of the epididymis. *Br J Surg* 1961; 49:319–321.
30. Areán VM, Kreager JA: Paratesticular rhabdomyosarcoma. *Am J Clin Pathol* 1965; 43:418–427.
31. Malek RS, Kelalis PP: Paratesticular rhabdomyosarcoma in childhood. *J Urol* 1977; 118:450–453.
32. Raney RB Jr, Hays DM, Lawrence W Jr, et al: Paratesticular rhabdomyosarcoma in childhood. *Cancer* 1978; 42:729–736.

Chapter 18

Sarcomas of the Lower Extremity

Richard E. Wilson*

In the treatment of soft-tissue sarcomas, the relationship of surgery to irradiation and chemotherapy has become better defined in the past decade. Each of these modalities has progressed in dramatic fashion. Better equipment, deeper knowledge of radiobiology, new drugs and drug combinations, and a better understanding of pharmacokinetics have led to a more cooperative effort on the part of physicians using these forms of treatment. The surgeon has come to recognize a practical and extremely useful staging[1] system, the difference between low- and high-grade sarcomas has become apparent, and the value of aggressive resection of malignant tumors and surrounding normal tissues in an anatomical relationship has been appreciated. With these new concepts and greater collaborative enterprise, the end results of sarcoma therapy as well as rehabilitation efforts have improved.

Nowhere is this more true than in the management of sarcomas of the lower extremity. For purposes of this chapter, the lower extremity will include the buttock, posteriorly, and all tissue below the inguinal ligament, anteriorly. Because sarcomas of the soft tissues are more often found on the extremity than on the trunk in adults, and more frequently on the lower extremity than the upper, the lower extremity is, therefore, the most common site for these cancers. Fortunately, more lower extremity sarcomas, as well as upper extremity lesions, are located in the proximal portion of the limb. Thus, there is a real opportunity for limb preservation, while at the same time performing an adequate resection of the malignant process. The concept of limb salvage has sparked an entire array of new technical approaches in the treatment of thigh and buttock sarcomas,[2] which have stimulated the interest of surgical oncologists and increased the potential role of radiation therapy, the place of chemotherapy in lower extremity sarcomas is not nearly as clear, but the question is under thorough investigation by appropriate cooperative studies.[3–5]

It is essential that the surgeon resecting such extremity sarcomas be thoroughly familiar with the anatomy and musculoskeletal physiology in order to achieve the most satisfactory results. The use of magnetic resonance (MR), computed tomography (CT), and angiography has helped the surgeon to become more aware of the anatomical relationships. These sarcomas behave in a reproducible fashion as they grow. Low-grade sarcomas virtually never metastasize, but have a high propensity to recur locally if inadequately resected. They grow more steadily with a "pushing" border. Both low- and

* Deceased.

high-grade sarcomas have only a pseudocapsule, consisting of the tumor border interface with normal tissue. However, the border is easier to see and encompass when the tumor is of lower grade. Still, the surgeon must not be deceived by an apparently easily defined tumor border and accede to the temptation to "shell out" the mass.

High-grade sarcomas have a less well-defined border and show streaming of cells (microscopically) and frequent extension of tumor (grossly) into adjacent tissues. Thus, for high-grade sarcomas, the resection must be wider; adjunct radiotherapy is necessary for local and regional control. Fortunately, the lymph nodes are rarely involved and can usually be preserved. This permits better lymphatic drainage and less leg swelling, despite extensive surgery.

Lower extremity sarcomas of the thigh and calf generally grow in a longitudinal fashion, extending upward within the sheath of a given muscle. Extension to adjacent muscles occurs only as the tumor enlarges. Blood vessels and nerves are often pushed aside, until large tumors emerge. These tumors rarely extend from one compartment to another, but when they do, they can usually be identified by a combination of physical examination and CT or MR. The surgeon can take advantage of this behavior in planning the operative procedure. On the other hand, tumors around the ankle, knee, and pelvis do not generally behave in such a favorable manner. They are more likely to involve vital structures and to require a major amputation for curative resection. Tumors of the buttock are common and, again, often stay confined to one muscle area. They are frequently in the large subcutaneous fat pad overlying the gluteal musculature. Depending on the size and location of these sarcomas in the buttock region, a resection can be achieved with an excellent functional result.

In the course of this chapter, the following aspects of treatment of lower extremity sarcomas will be presented: methods of diagnosis, pre-operative treatment planning, types of tumor excision, concepts of surgical therapy, the roles of chemotherapy and irradiation, the interaction of the surgeon and the pathologist, and anticipated results of treatment. Special categories to be discussed will include patients with local recurrence and those presenting with an untreated primary sarcoma and synchronous distant metastases (stage IVB).

METHODS OF DIAGNOSIS

A wide variety of histological types of soft-tissue sarcomas can occur in the lower extremities, as in any other area of the body. These include malignant fibrous histiocytoma, fibrosarcoma, rhabdomyosarcoma, leiomyosarcoma, synovial sarcoma, liposarcoma, hemangiopericytoma, angiosarcoma, neurofibrosarcoma, and extraskeletal osteogenic or chondrosarcoma. In addition, aggressive fibromatosis can be seen in the plantar fascia and in the proximal thigh. We have learned that histological grade is more important than cell type of origin, as far as treatment and prognosis are concerned. Frequently, pathological decision as to cell type changes, depending on which pathologist reviews the tissues. However, the use of electron microscopy has increased the sophistication of these decisions. Certain of these sarcomas behave in a more reproducible manner: synovial sarcoma often occurs near the knee and ankle joint, liposarcoma in the buttock, and chondrosarcoma adjacent to the pelvic bones. Also, synovial sarcoma may have lymph node metastases in adults.

The key to diagnosis and treatment is early biopsy! Many of these tumors occur in young, active patients who are constantly subjected to minor trauma. Often these sarcomas are misdiagnosed as hematomas, cysts, or even benign solid lesions. In the case of high-grade sarcomas, the growth rate can be exceedingly rapid, yet the tumor can be generally asymptomatic, even in a weight-bearing extremity. Any new lesion of the extremity, particularly one that is enlarging, should be considered as a possible sarcoma. No radiograph, ultrasound, MR, CT, or radionuclide scan can definitively confirm this diagnosis. Fortunately, lesions on the extremity can be found earlier than those in the pelvis and retroperitoneum; this may be one of the reasons for their better prognosis. Biopsy of many sarcomas of the extremity can be performed with local anesthesia, often as an outpatient procedure.

Excisional biopsy of a potential sarcoma should not be attempted because the final resection is more accurately performed with the original mass in place and its relationships to surrounding structures undisturbed. Cytological needle aspiration and core needle biopsy, although often useful, are not always successful. In addition, the pathologist requires adequate tissue to define the grade. Thus, the preferred technique is open incisional biopsy under local anesthesia. The biopsy must be planned so that the incision and tract can be completely excised at the time of definitive surgery. When located between joints, it must be longitudinal. Around or near joints, it is best curved in a horizontal manner or S-shaped, whereas on the buttock it can be oblique. It is often necessary to enter the muscle bundles to obtain an adequate specimen; an interrupted suture closure of muscle poses no problems. Frozen section should be obtained to be certain that the pathologist has adequate tissue, because necrosis can often occur in some of the high-grade lesions. The pathologist can frequently make a "suggestive" diagnosis from frozen section, but these tumors are hard to distinguish from poorly differentiated carcinomas and some lymphomas without permanent sections. Also, the pathologist cannot accurately stage the tumor on frozen section alone.

The delay required for final pathological review permits the surgeon to perform noninvasive staging and plan therapeutic strategy. Sometimes the pathological diagnosis is difficult to determine, and consultation with other pathologists will be required before a final decision can be made. Because strategies differ for different cellular grades, this delay is necessary for definition of stage.

PRE-OPERATIVE TREATMENT PLANNING

Extensive tumor cell heterogeneity can occur within every one of these sarcomas.[6] Thus, low-grade and high-grade tumors can coexist in the same mass. All of the tumor must be removed before the grade is finally determined. The biological behavior of each sarcoma is generally determined by the highest component grade. Thus, a small segment of high-grade sarcoma within a large low-grade liposarcoma, for example, can be responsible for eventual pulmonary metastases. As a result, all lesions should be evaluated for pulmonary metastases regardless of the biopsy-defined stage. The angioinvasive nature of these tumors makes pulmonary metastases the most likely site for occult disease. Approximately 10% of such lesions will be missed on the standard chest radiograph, (postero-anterior, and lateral). Although full lung tomography has been a major contribution to the management of these patients, CT of the lung and mediastinum is more sensitive and accurate.

Of equal importance is the evaluation of the extent of regional disease. This is most true for the lower extremity, particularly the proximal area and the buttock where options exist as to the extent of resection. In lesions about the knee and ankle, and for many in the calf or foot, there is a limited amount of normal tissue available in the region around a sarcoma, which makes wide tumor excision and wound closure more difficult. In the region of the thigh and buttock, however, there is almost always adequate skin and subcutaneous tissue available to permit primary wound closure after even the most extensive type of sarcoma resection. It is therefore necessary to define as accurately as possible the full extent of the malignant process so that the proper operative approach can be selected and adequate tumor margins maintained during the surgical procedure.

Computed tomography and, increasingly, MR have proved to be the best tools for this type of evaluation. Although physical examination provides important information to the surgeon in evaluating the mobility of the tumor, its freedom from bone involvement, the proximal extension of disease, and the character of the overlying skin, CT and MR provide more specific information. Decisions can be made as to which muscle or groups of muscles are involved, the full proximal and distal extent of the tumor within the muscles, whether or not the periosteum has been invaded, the presence of absence of necrosis within the tumor mass, and the status of fibrous septae dividing the high compartments. One can evaluate the patency of the femoral artery and vein and whether these and other vessels have been displaced by the tumor. In this author's experience, CT and MR have replaced the need for ultrasound or xeroradiography to study the mass and arteriography to evaluate its vasculature. Only the use of intra-arterial infusion chemotherapy prior to resection necessitates pre-operative arteriography. The vascular anatomy is so easily defined at operation that the surgeon does not routinely require identification of feeding vessels to the tumor mass pre-operatively.

Lymph node involvement is rare with primary tumors. Usually, palpation is the best way to identify nodes with suspected metastases. Lymphangiography is rarely indicated unless one wishes to evaluate the iliac, hypogastric, or peri-aortic nodes.

Bone scans are generally not as useful as CT for evaluating local bone involvement. On occasion, however they can be helpful in determining destruction of a bone adjacent to a primary sarcoma and may also be used to rule out occult bone lesions in patients with chondrosarcomas. Because simple radiographs will often adequately demonstrate whether bones are involved with soft-tissue sarcomas, these should be ordered first.

TYPES OF TUMOR EXCISION

By its very name, excision implies removal of the tumor. The types of excision used are defined by the kind of margin obtained around the primary tumor mass.

Local Excision.—Local excision makes no attempt to obtain wide margins around the tumor, but does depend on total excision with histologically "free" margins. No resection should be contemplated that accomplishes less than that. Under no circumstances should a tumor be "shelled out" from the surrounding tissues. There is never a true capsule about any sarcoma, regardless of grade, and a rim of normal tissue must always be excised. Obviously, the anatomical relationships of the tumor determine the extent of normal tissue that can be removed around the sarcoma. For example, despite a wide muscle margin, the tumor may extend to the periosteum of the femur, and only the thin periosteal layer can be seen to cover the border of the specimen at that point. This is not a rare situation.

Wide Excision.—Wide excision is best typified by the muscle group or compartmental resection. It is necessary to assess the extent of the tumor, both pre-operatively and intraoperatively, and then remove all muscle tissue within the compartment that lies adjacent to the tumor mass. When there is uncertainty as to the involvement of any specific muscle or muscle component, it is essential that that muscle be removed as part of the specimen (Fig 18–1). Ideally, the entire operative procedure should avoid any contact with the tumor. When the primary tumor is still intact, it is relatively easy to determine those structures that must be removed to provide a wide excision.

Re-excision after previous inadequate resection is an entirely different situation. Under those circumstances, the operating surgeon attempts to convert an initially inadequate operation to a wide and satisfactory resection by, once again, purposely avoiding contact with the previous operative site.

In all circumstances, a wide resection is arbitrarily meant to include a margin of at least 2 cm around all identifiable tumor. Some surgeons further classify the extent of resection with the term *radical resection,* which is generally defined as a minimal margin of 4 cm about all the tumor. However, that definition is problematic because, for small tumors, such an extended margin is possible; for larger tumors, however, it is rarely possible to maintain such a wide margin in all directions. Obviously, the closest margin to the tumor is the only one that counts! Usually, the close margins will be near a major nerve, vessel, or bone, and that will be the limiting structure.

Amputation.—Resection by amputation of the extremity at a point appropriately proximal to the sarcoma was considered the treatment of choice until the majority of surgical oncologists began to use limb salvage techniques. A major impetus to limp-sparing procedures came with the use of bone prosthetic devices for osteogenic sarcoma.[7] In these patients, the soft tissue could generally remain intact with replacement of the diseased bone. The reverse is true, obviously, for soft-tissue sarcomas, permitting sparing of bone, vessels, and nerves to maintain limb function despite large muscle group excision. There are, however, some patients who will still require amputation for lower extremity sarcomas. Tumors of the foot and ankle region, if high grade, are often best treated by amputation (Fig 18–2). These are difficult locations in which to direct adequate irradiation and still have a good functioning extremity. Unless extensive or recurrent, sarcomas of the lower leg above the knee can usually be treated without amputation. Again, wide resection of recurrent tumor more often requires amputation, because closure, even with microvascular techniques for pedicle grafting, may be a serious problem. The other tumor locations for which amputation must be considered are those lying at the inguinal ligament, in the buttock, or high in the medial compartment. When primary tumor resection is carried out for sarcomas in these locations, adequate excisional margins may be possible, but if

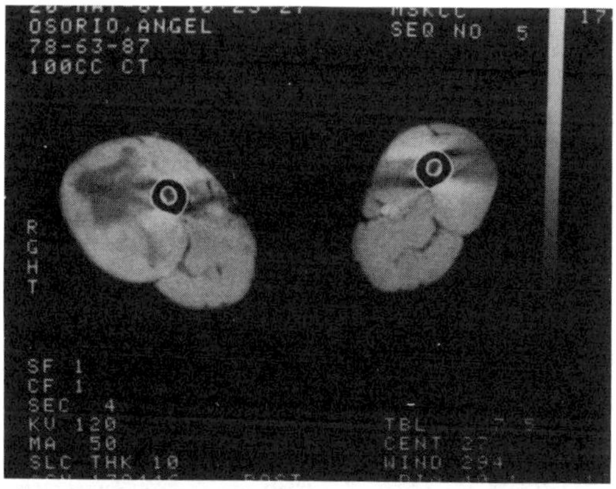

A

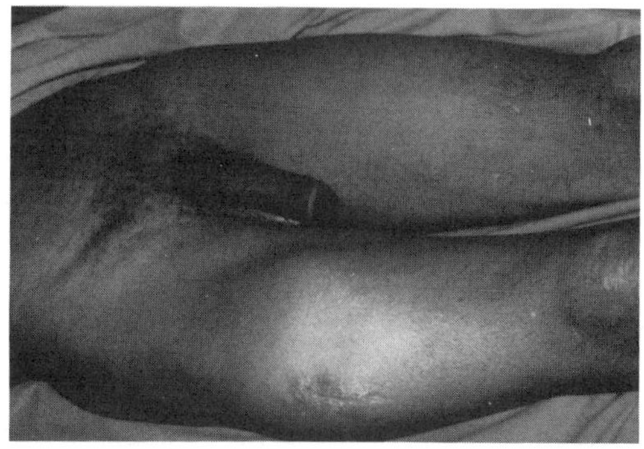

B

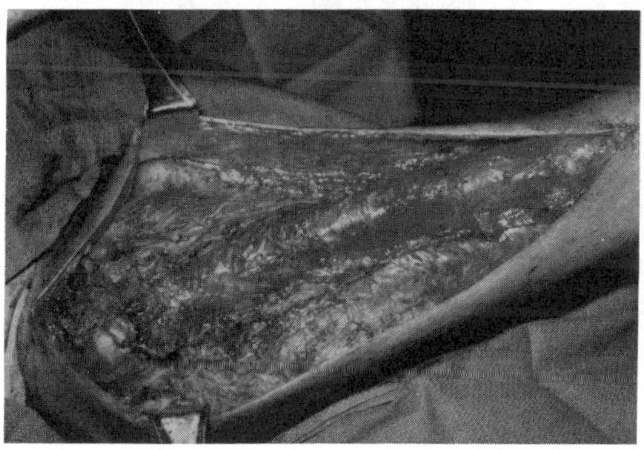

C

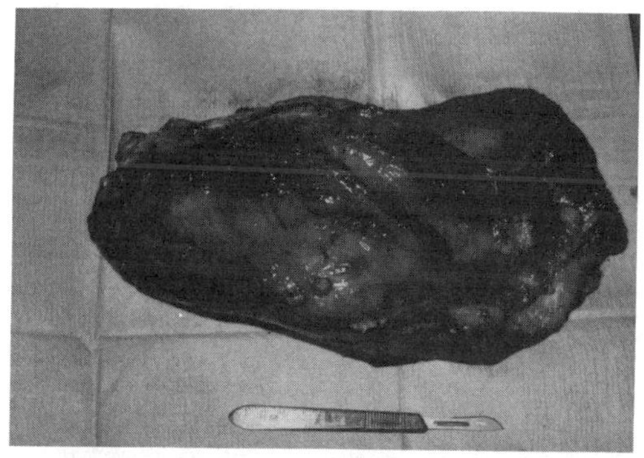

D

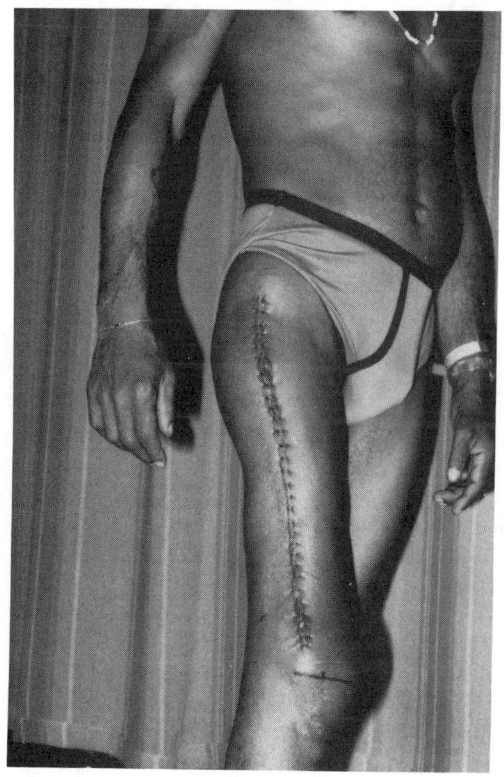

E

FIG 18–1.
Presentation of a painless mass in the anterolateral aspect of the right thigh was shown by CT to fill the vastus lateralis muscle. **A,** Appropriate biopsy was performed through a short longitudinal incision directly over the mass and showed a high-grade spindle cell sarcoma. **B,** Wide en bloc resection was performed, **C,** leaving a cuff of normal muscle around all aspects of the tumor. **D,** Despite removal of almost all the quadriceps muscle, the patient was able to ambulate 1 week later without support, **E.**

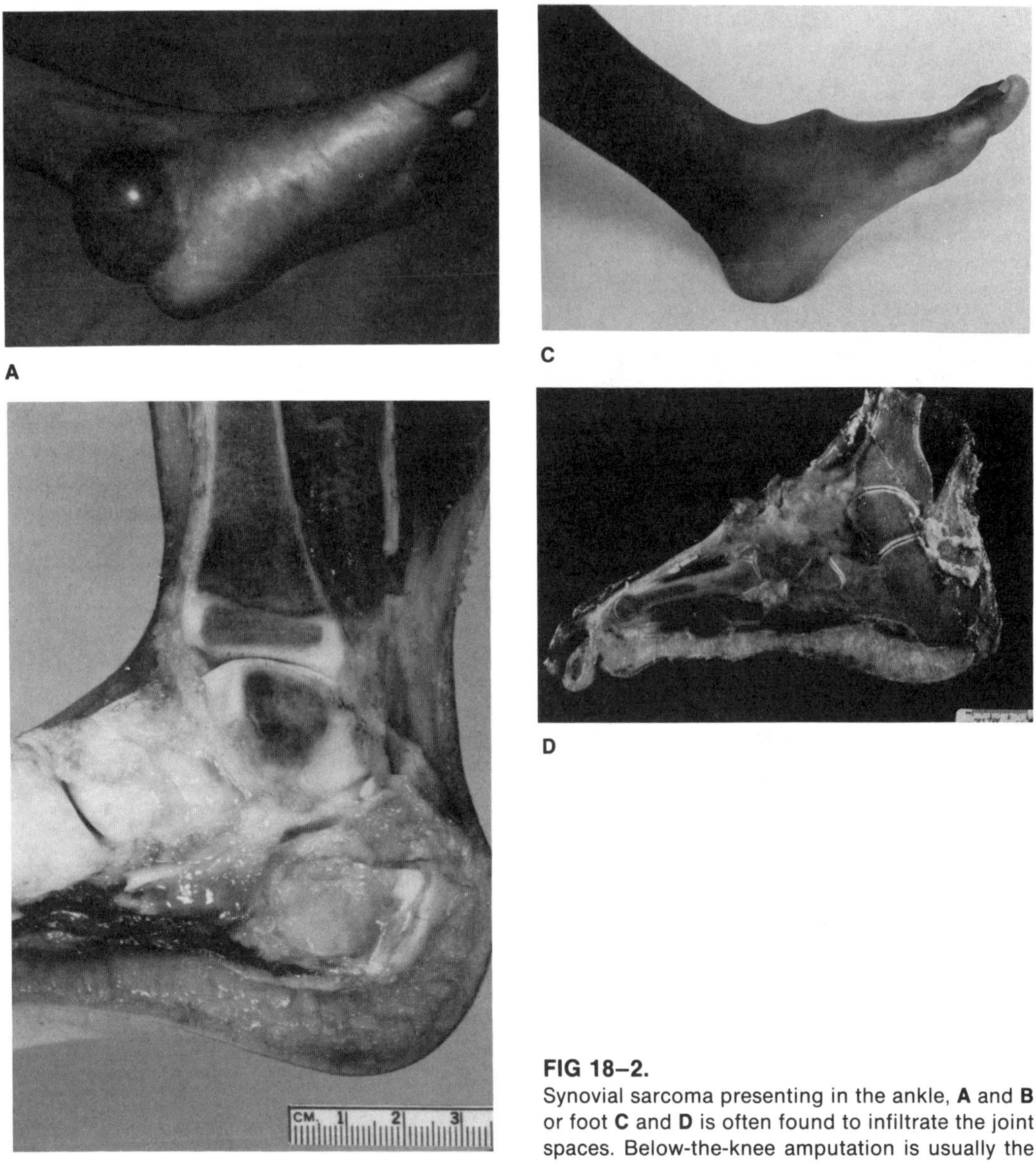

FIG 18–2.
Synovial sarcoma presenting in the ankle, **A** and **B** or foot **C** and **D** is often found to infiltrate the joint spaces. Below-the-knee amputation is usually the best approach.

one is treating recurrence in these sites then amputation is almost a certainty. Hip disarticulation is to be selected over hemipelvectomy, if the lesion is high in the thigh. This permits use of an ischial weight-bearing prosthesis and provides for a better functional result.

Hemipelvectomy may be required for tumors involving bone or periosteum of the pelvis, for those growing through the sciatic or obturator foramina, for tumors arising from the bone surface (such as chondrosarcomas), or for those involving the common femoral or iliac arteries. If the lesion is high on the buttock (within the gluteal musculature or arising from the iliac crest area), it is possible to resect the iliac wing with the specimen, preserving a strut of inferior iliac bone and the acetabulum. The patient thus suffers minimal loss of function. Hemipelvectomy can be performed with retention of the lower extremity, provided the iliac and femoral vessels, as well as the sciatic nerve, can be spared.[8] Fibrosis will occur to provide sufficient stability of the femur so that the patient can eventually bear weight on this extremity. Hemipelvectomy with total limb amputation, however, must remain in the surgeon's armament. This operation should be selected in the appropriate circumstance to achieve curative resection. It is now used less often for primary sarcomas, but is much more frequent for recurrent high-grade sarcoma of the proximal thigh or hip region. Patients can function extremely well after this procedure, most without a prosthesis.

CONCEPTS OF SURGICAL THERAPY

The general concept of surgical therapy for lower extremity sarcomas involves curative resection of the cancer with the least morbidity and loss of function. The operative approach must be based on a careful analysis of the anatomical relations of the primary tumor and a thorough staging of the patient for distant metastases. As already stated, small incisional biopsies are preferred to provide accurate information about the grade and type of tumor before the surgeon embarks on a resection with curative intent.

All biopsy site incisions should be included with the resected specimen. The skin and the biopsy tract should be left in place over the tumor, with an ellipse of skin left around the scar. The key to adequate surgical resection is the development of large skin flaps. The flaps use the dissection plane between the deep fascia and the subcutaneous fat, once adequate margins are obtained around the tumor itself. This is particularly true if the tumor arises in or involves subcutaneous tissue. In that situation, the dissection proceeds obliquely through normal subcutaneous tissue until the fascial plane is reached. I prefer S-shaped incisions, either longitudinal or oblique, that extend far beyond the area of the tumor. They permit the best exposure of large anatomical areas and still provide the most satisfactory and cosmetic wound closure. Meticulous hemostasis is important because large surface areas are exposed after resection, and hematoma formation interferes with skin flap healing and often leads to sepsis.

Low-grade sarcomas require local excision, but because they do not tend to infiltrate as extensively as high-grade tumors can, wide excision is generally not necessary. If the margins are not histologically "clean," the tumor will recur locally. Devereux et al.[9] showed that adding chemotherapy or radiation therapy to the resection of low-grade sarcomas did not compensate for histologically "dirty margins." Intraoperative frozen sections should be taken, both of the border of the resected specimen and of the residual tissue bed, to determine margin status. Low-grade sarcomas rarely involve major nerves, arteries, or veins.

High-grade sarcomas of the lower extremity tend to grow within a muscular compartment, pushing the femoral vessels or the sciatic nerve aside as they expand. When located in muscle, these tumors frequently extend to the periosteum of the underlying bone. In those instances, removal of the periosteum with the specimen is usually sufficient. The tumors rarely invade bone itself. If they do, then amputation is generally required. In our experience, the addition of irradiation to surgical excision (to be discussed below) has provided sufficient local tumor control so that periosteal involvement has not proved to be a problem.

If the deep femoral venous system is involved, the vein should be included with the resected specimen. It need not be replaced, but every effort should be made in these patients to spare the saphenous vein. It is rare for both of these vessels to be involved. The profunda system is often invaded by tumor, because sarcomas of the thigh derive their blood supply from the profunda femoris artery. If the superficial femoral artery is involved, it should be resected and grafted. If the vascular resection is limited to the thigh, and the distal anastomosis can be placed above the knee, then either a saphenous graft from the opposite leg or a synthetic graft may be interposed. Involvement of the sciatic nerve is best treated by peeling the perineurium off the nerve with the tumor. If deeper nerve involvement exists, then amputation is probably necessary. It is important to preserve those branches of the obturator or femoral nerves that go to the muscles left in place after resection of medial or anterior compartment tumors, respectively, otherwise those muscles will fibrose and fail to function. The randomized trial comparing limb sparing of extremity sarcomas to amputation performed by Rosenberg et al.[2] at the Surgery Branch of the National Cancer Institute (Bethesda, MD) has helped to make the concept of limb sparing more acceptable to surgeons who still believe that amputation is the only safe procedure. The result of this trial indicated no difference in survival between the two patient groups, which were well matched for stage and location of tumor. Proximal thigh tumors were the only ones that had any risk for regional recurrence in that study. Almost all treatment failures were in the form of distant metastases. The use of wide excision as the treatment of choice for lower extremity sarcomas has now been generally accepted by the surgical community, reserving amputation for specific tumors that cannot be encompassed by resection and limb preservation.

Thus, the surgeon must make a choice as to the type of resection, projected borders of excision, and plans for reconstruction, considerations that amputation does not require. This makes pre-operative definition of the anatomical extent of the tumor even more essential. Likewise, careful monitoring of the excision site with physical examination and CT or MR in the post-resection period becomes an important task. If recurrence appears, CT or MR can identify it much earlier than physical examination, especially in irradiated tissues. Early diagnosis of recurrence with re-excision may permit a limb to remain functional. As will be seen from the subsequent presentation of results of treatment, local-regional recurrence is now relatively rare. As combined modality treatment has evolved, local control is the rule. Although most patients with regional recurrence after proper primary treatment will require amputation, occasionally it is possible to successfully resect such recurrences even if they are high-grade sarcomas.

The surgeon has an important responsibility during the conduct of the primary operation to define the extent of the tumor with the pathologist and mark out the areas of greatest risk for recurrence for the radiotherapist. It is our policy to add radiation therapy to all resections for high-grade sarcomas of the lower extremity. Marker clips should be placed to define both the full resection borders and also the area of closest surgical margins. Because the steel clips interfere with the accuracy of subsequent CTs, it is ideal to use titanium clips. These also show up well on plain films but do not produce the "star burst" effect on CTs. Whenever possible, the radiotherapist should be invited to the operating room to see the tumor bed in situ. Decisions for either brachytherapy with catheter placement for afterloading of radioactive implants or intra-operative radiation therapy can be made jointly.

THE ROLES OF RADIOTHERAPY AND CHEMOTHERAPY

Each of these modalities can contribute an additional increment of therapy for the patient with a lower extremity sarcoma. Whereas radiation therapy adds to local-regional control, chemotherapy would presumably increase both local and distant disease-free survival. In each case, there is the opportunity for either pre-operative or postoperative administration, and one or both treatment forms may be used.

The potential advantages of pre-operative irradiation are (1) shrinkage of tumor volume to be resected, (2) reduced seeding of tumor cells from the surface of the sarcoma at the time of resection, particularly in the case of high-grade, more radiosensitive tumor cell populations, (3) the possibility of less extensive resection to accomplish the same result, and (4) reduced vascularity of the tumor. The disadvantages are as follow: (1) irradiated skin flaps must be used for dissection at the time of surgery; (2) if response is not achieved with irradiation, the tumor will be larger at the time of resection; and (3) it is more difficult to effectively treat the initial larger tumor mass, both for dose delivery and for accuracy in localizing therapy. Because limb salvage is the general approach to resection at this time, the surgeon must be concerned about maintenance of function. Treating the most well-defined field and sparing a longitudinal strip of skin will limit edema and fibrosis in the extremity. For this reason, we prefer postoperative irradiation at the Brigham and Women's Hospital and the Dana-Farber Cancer Institute (Boston, MA). However, in all probability, there is little difference in end results with expert radiation therapy given either before or after surgical resection. This is a complex form of radiotherapy to administer, and careful treatment planning with the use of supervoltage equipment, including electron beam, is essential.

Intra-operative irradiation and localized therapy with implants have been mentioned. Each of these approaches attempts to provide a portion of the total therapy with reduced injury to adjacent normal tissues. The implants are particularly valuable for patients who have already had external beam therapy to the tumor area, where the skin cannot tolerate additional radiation. The final verdict on intra-operative irradiation will require experience with more patients and longer follow-up. Because of the high growth fraction of many sarcomas, the use of intra-operative irradiation is appealing, particularly for retroperitoneal tumors. These lesions are much more difficult to resect in their entirety and treat with postoperative radiation therapy. Another innovative concept may be the association of hyperthermia with irradiation. This technique is still a highly experimental one, and is most applicable to recurrent tumors.[10] However, it is conceivable that the combination of local therapy might further increase our ability to spare the limbs when tumors adjacent to the pelvic bone are encountered.

The primary exponents of pre-operative adriamycin chemotherapy for extremity sarcomas have been Eilber and associates at the University of California at Los Angeles[11, 12] and Lehti and colleagues at the University of Oregon.[13] This type of chemotherapy may be combined with irradiation or used alone. The theoretical advantages of such treatment are better local tumor control and a higher resectability rate with more frequent limb salvage. However, the local control rate is extremely high with surgery and irradiation, with or without postoperative chemotherapy.[3–5] In general, this type of pre-operative intra-arterial chemotherapy has not gained general acceptance.[6]

The value and justification of postoperative adjuvant chemotherapy are the subject of extensive debate. In fact, its use is still under investigation at this time. At the National Cancer Institute (NCI), Rosenberg et al.[3] have reported a significant benefit for adjuvant Adriamycin (doxorubicin), Cytoxan, and high-dose methotrexate for extremity sarcomas. Improvement in both overall survival (95% versus 74%) and disease-free survival (92% versus 60%) were obtained. The Dana-Faber Cancer Institute/Massachusetts General Hospital (DFCI/MGH) study showed a benefit from adriamycin alone at a lower dose than did the NCI group, but the differences failed to be significantly different.[4] The local control rate was 100% in each study in the chemotherapy group and 93% in the control arms. In the DFCI/MGH study, the disease-free survival rate was 100% versus 76% (treated versus control), and the overall survival rate was 100% versus 75%.

One of the major concerns with a chemotherapy protocol containing adriamycin is the risk of myocardial toxicity. Careful monitoring by ultrasound ventriculography can identify myocardial functional abnormalities before congestive heart failure is seen. In the NCI series, there was an incidence of 14% of patients showing congestive heart failure, and another 52% had abnormalities determined by noninvasive testing. Adriamycin in this series was given in a cumulative dose of 550 mg/m^2. For the DFCI/MGH series, 10% myocardial toxicity was seen with an Adriamycin cumulative dose of 450 mg/m^2. These are serious complications, particularly because it is not clear that giving chemotherapy prophylactically is any better than using it therapeutically, once recurrence is identified. This is particularly important when one realizes that only one of four patients not receiving adjuvant chemotherapy suffered recurrence in our series. These questions are being refined, and more data should be forthcoming.

INTERACTIONS OF THE SURGEON AND PATHOLOGIST

With the universal adoption of the American Joint Committee on Cancer Staging System for soft-tissue sarcomas,[1, 14] there is an additional burden on the pathologist and surgeon to coordinate their efforts. This holds true for the interpretation of initial biopsies, slides, specimens of primarily resected sarcomas, and the course of the operative procedure itself. Failure to achieve a collaborative relationship with the pathologist will prevent the most appropriate treatment decisions from being made. The pathologist must recognize the need of the surgeon to have the grade and type of sarcoma well defined prior to resection. Slides must frequently be reviewed to define disease stage, and the surgeon must provide adequate tissue at the time of incisional biopsy. The surgeon must insist that the pathologist define the margin status of the resected specimen of primary sarcomas. This is best accomplished by "inking" the surface of the specimen after any biopsies or sections are taken. Metastatic nodules in the lung or liver or recurrent tumor in the local area must also be properly handled to define the margin status. Intra-operative frozen sections may be useful for defining borders of resection and in separating scar tissue from sarcomas in re-operations. This may be difficult on occasion, and careful sampling for biopsy is essential. For surgeons seeing patients in consultation, review of pathology material by their collaborating pathologist should be a requirement.

RESULTS OF THERAPY

Although soft-tissue sarcomas constitute one of the relatively rare tumors in the United States, their management has generated broad interest among oncologists because of the continually improving results of therapy. There are clearly a multitude of factors responsible for this change in outcome. Better staging and pre-operative evaluation define patients who already have metastatic disease, particularly in the form of pulmonary nodules. Recognition of the surgical principles of resection has reduced the incidence of local-regional recurrence. Likewise, modern radiotherapy techniques have lowered the risk for local-regional recurrences, and with them, distant metastases.[15] Chemotherapy has a definite potential to obtain responses for patients with metastatic disease,[16] as does resectional surgery for patients with finite numbers of pulmonary nodules.[17] All of these features serve to lengthen disease-free survival times and lower mortality.

The risk of recurrence and death increases with increasing grade and stage of tumor. For patients with low-grade tumors, adequate local excision with histologically negative markings should achieve virtually 100% freedom from recurrence and mortality.[9] If recurrence has taken place, it is usually at the border of the previous resection and remains low grade. The category of low-grade tumor in this context includes those classified as IA, IB, and IIA. For patients with resectable high-grade tumors (IIB–IVA, inclusive), the risk of local recurrence increases from the least in stage IIB patients to the greatest with stage IVA tumors. There is also a progressive increase in risk for distant metastases with advanced stage. For example, we have seen a greater increase in distant recurrence in stage IIIB and IVA patients than in stage IIB and IIIA patients. Obviously, one must stratify the subsets of high-grade sarcomas in any prospective trial to be certain that they are equally distributed in treatment arms.

THE PATIENT WITH LOCAL RECURRENCE

With adequate primary therapy, there should be a low incidence of local recurrence in patients with extremity sarcomas. This is true whether lesions are high or low grade. The greatest risk for local recurrence in lower extremity sarcomas occurs when the primary tumor is located most proximally. Adequate resection margins are more difficult to achieve when the femoral vessels or the sciatic nerve must be peeled from the tumor surface. Even in those circumstances, local recurrence after the addition of radiation therapy to the initial surgical approach, or when radiotherapy is given prior to resection, should be infrequent. In our experience, the involved margins of low-grade lesions are less likely to be "sterilized" by added radiotherapy.

When local recurrence is expected, usually because of the presence of a new mass or local pain, it is necessary to prove the presence of recurrent sarcoma and restage the patient. Biopsy must be carried out, usually under local anesthesia. Needle biopsy may be useful in this situation, more so than for the primary biopsy in which grade and type of disease are required information. Recurrent tumor nodules may be located in a site difficult to reach by open biopsy; one is particularly reluctant to perform extensive dissection to reach a recurrent nodule if this might interfere with a definite and curative subsequent procedure. On the other hand, scar tissue may be confused with tumor recurrence, hence adequate tissue is needed to differentiate them. Cytological diagnosis with fine-needle aspiration is rarely sufficient. Core-needle biopsy is likely to be successful. If neither of these techniques is positive initially, and one fails to identify recurrent sarcoma when suspected, then open biopsy is necessary. It may be possible to carry out biopsy at the time of definite reresection, with frozen section diagnosis used for confirmation. On occasion, a highly suspicious and enlarging nodule can be presumed to be recurrent tumor and treated as such without histological confirmation pre-operatively. However, under *no* circumstances should amputation be performed without microscopic proof of recurrence.

Restaging should consist of an evaluation of regional and distant metastatic sites. Computed tomography of the area of the extremity, the pelvis, and the chest will be the most important study. The advantage of having an early postoperative CT or MR of the resection area is to use it for comparison should subsequent scans raise the possibility of recurrence. Extension into the true pelvis, through the sciatic, femoral, or obturator canals, completely alters the operative approach for any extremity recurrence. Should pelvic recurrence take place, then abdominal CT is necessary to rule out peri-aortic nodal disease or hepatic metastases. Computed tomography of the chest is the best technique for defining pulmonary metastases. Obviously, a chest CT from the time of initial primary treatment permits more accurate diagnosis of recurrence by comparative evaluation. A bone scan might be considered, because on some occasions soft-tissue sarcomas can spread to the skeleton. Usually, however, there is little added benefit from radionuclide scanning or arteriography. Lymphangiography may help determine whether enlarged lymph nodes contain metastatic disease.

Treatment must be directed at control of the local recurrence as well as of any identified distant disease. If distant lesions are found, and the patient has not received Adriamycin, then it is our policy to start with systemic Adriamycin-based chemotherapy. Tumor response to chemotherapy can then be defined. Chemotherapy by itself can rarely be curative, although on some occasions we have had long-term control of metastases with this regimen: however, resection of recurrent local and distant disease should still be the surgical objective. If no response occurs to measurable disease with two to three courses of chemotherapy, then resection of the local recurrence and the distant metastases should be attempted. If the local recurrence cannot be controlled, then it is inappropriate to attack the distant metastases surgically. These same concepts will be discussed further in the next section.

If there is no distant disease, then the surgeon must plan the attack on the recurrent site. Wide local excision should be attempted, as with the untreated primary tumor. Frozen sections should be used to assist the surgeon in defining resection margins. Biopsy of the tumor bed is essential to this approach. The surgeon must take care not to sample just the necrotic tissue in the search for residual tumor and clear margins. The resection of recurrent disease is far more difficult than the initial operation. Anatomy is distorted, and the cancer does not necessarily follow anatomical planes. Multiple recurrent nodules may be found, making full resection more difficult. If the patient has had no previous radiotherapy, use of this modality can be especially valuable for adding effective control to surgical resection. If previous external beam irradiation has been given, then there is the possibility of using regional brachytherapy. The radiotherapist should be invited to the operating room to evaluate tumor volume, treatment geometry, and catheter placement for afterloading of radiation implants.

If neither external beam radiation therapy nor brachytherapy can be employed, and there is no evidence of distant disease, then amputation may be the only option. This is why full staging is essential prior to operation on recurrent disease. The patient must be made aware of the possibility of amputation whenever recurrent disease is operated on. The site of amputation is obviously dictated by the location of the recurrence. In most patients with lower extremity sarcomas, recurrence will be in the proximal thigh or buttock, hence the operation often required for lower extremity recurrence is hemipelvectomy. Occasionally, disarticulation of the hip is possible. These procedures are described in Chapter 24.

PATIENTS PRESENTING WITH STAGE IVB DISEASE

Stage IVB sarcoma is defined as any primary lesion with M1 (distant metastatic) disease. For lower extremity sarcomas, M1 disease will almost always be pulmonary metastases. Occasionally, intrapelvic and retroperitoneal metastases or liver nodules will be found, but rarely so. Such patients must not be considered untreatable or be denied a chance for long disease-free survival. Whether or not they can be "cured" is uncertain, but that possibility must be kept in mind. Because the lung is a targeted organ, it may be the site of the first and only metastases. Sometimes these are solitary and remain so. When up to four nodules are found, then resection should be considered.[18] Several nodules in both lung fields militate against resection, unless chemotherapy controls all but a few lesions.

The logistics of this approach are by no means standard or simple. It has been my plan to first treat the metastatic disease with systemic chemotherapy containing Adriamycin. This will serve to demonstrate the responsiveness of the tumor to drugs and may also eliminate the most high-grade and aggressive cellular populations. This then can be followed by surgical resection, first of the primary and then of residual metastatic foci. Finally, chemotherapy should be continued postresection for a full course. The key factor is the ability of the surgeon to control the primary tumor, a basic principle of all surgical oncology.

If the primary tumor cannot be removed with an adequate margin, or if surgery and radiotherapy cannot be given, then it is better to consider treating the tumor with aggressive chemotherapy alone. The disability and morbidity associated with an unsuccessful resection in the face of distant metastases is not justified. New and more experimental therapeutic approaches, such as hyperthermia in conjunction with radiation and/or chemotherapy, would be most appropriate for such patients. Likewise, arterial infusion of chemotherapy or new radiotherapy techniques can be considered.

CONCLUSION

This chapter has provided a plan for therapy of lower extremity soft-tissue sarcomas based on accurate diagnosis and staging of the disease, careful treatment planning, and liberal use of a combined modality therapy. These concepts have served to improve greatly the therapeutic outlook and the quality of life for patients with these rare tumors.

REFERENCES

1. Beahrs OH, Hensen DE, Hutter RVP, et al (eds): *Manual for Staging of Cancer*, ch 20, 3rd ed. Philadelphia, J. B. Lippincott, 1988, pp 127–131.
2. Rosenberg SA, Kent H, Costa J, et al: Prospective randomized evaluation of the role of limb-sparing surgery, radiation therapy, and adjuvant chemoimmunotherapy in the treatment of adult soft-tissue sarcomas. *Surgery* 1978; 84:62.
3. Rosenberg SA, Tepper J, Glatstein E, et al: Prospective randomized evaluation of adjuvant chemotherapy in adults with soft tissue sarcomas of the extremities. *Cancer* 1983; 52:424.
4. Antman K, Suit H, Amato D, et al: Preliminary results of a randomized trial of adjuvant doxorubicin for sarcomas: Lack of apparent difference between treatment groups. *J Clin Oncol* 1984; 2:601.
5. Antman K, Amato D, Lerner H, et al: Pooled results of two randomized trials of adjuvant doxorubicin for sarcomas: An Eastern Cooperative Oncology Group and Dana-Farber Cancer Institute/Massachusetts General Hospital study, in Jones SE, Salmon SE (eds): *Adjuvant Therapy of Cancer*, 4th ed. New York, Grune & Stratton, 1984, pp 611–620.
6. Wilson RE, Antman KH, Brodsky G, et al: Tumor cell heterogeneity in soft tissue sarcomas defined by chemo-radiotherapy. *Cancer* 1984; 53:1420.
7. Morton DL, Eilber FT, Townsend CM Jr, et al: Limb salvage from a multidisciplinary treatment approach for skeletal and soft tissue sarcomas of the extremity. *Ann Surg* 1976; 184:268.
8. Eilber FR, Grant TT, Sakai D, et al: Internal hemipelvectomy: Excision of the hemipelvis with limb preservation. *Cancer* 1979; 43:806.
9. Devereux DF, Wilson RE, Corson JM, et al: Surgical treatment of low grade soft tissue sarcomas. *Am J Surg* 1982; 143:490.
10. Gerard H, VanEcho DA, Whitacre M, et al: Doxorubicin, cyclophosphamide, and whole body hyperthermia for treatment of advanced soft tissue sarcoma. *Cancer* 1984; 53:2585.
11. Eilber FR, Mirra JJ, Grant TT, et al: Is amputation necessary for sarcomas? A seven-year experience with limb salvage. *Ann Surg* 1980; 192:431.
12. Eilber FR, Morton DL, Eckardt J: Limb salvage for skeletal and soft tissue sarcomas. Multidisciplinary preoperative therapy. *Cancer* 1984; 53:2579.
13. Lehti PM, Moseley HS, Janoff K, et al: Improved survival for soft tissue sarcoma of the extremities by regional hyperthermic perfusion, local excision and radiation therapy. *Surg Gynecol Obstet* 1986; 162:149–152.
14. Russell WO, Cohen J, Enzinger F, et al: A clinical and pathological staging system for soft tissue sarcomas. *Cancer* 1977; 40:1562.
15. Suit HD, Russell WO, Martin RG: Sarcoma of soft tissue: Clinical and histopathologic parameters and response to treatment. *Cancer* 1975; 35:1478.
16. Blum BH, Corson JM, Wilson RE, et al: Successful treatment of metastatic sarcomas with cyclophosphamide, Adriamycin, and DTIC (CAD). *Cancer* 1980; 46:1722.
17. Ramming KP: Surgery for pulmonary metastases. *Surg Clin N Am* 1980; 60:815.
18. Roth JA, Putnam JB Jr, Wesley MN, et al: Differing determinants of prognosis following resection of pulmonary metastases from osteogenic and soft tissue sarcoma patients. *Cancer* 1985; **55:** 1361–1366.

Chapter 19

Peripheral Nerve Sheath Tumors

Thomas W. Bauer
Melinda L. Estes

The peripheral nervous system consists of nerve fibers, ganglia, and specialized sense organs. Whether myelinated or unmyelinated, every axon is surrounded, throughout most of its length, by a sheath of cytoplasm belonging to Schwann cells. Early neuroanatomists used the term *neurilemma* in reference to the covering of a nerve fiber. It is now recognized that this covering consists of the cytoplasm of Schwann cells (Schwann sheath, or *neurolemma*) with adjacent basement membrane and collagen fibers (often called the *neurilemma*). Small groups of fibers are surrounded by a delicate layer of connective tissue (endoneurium), and these fascicles are contained within perineurium. Larger nerves are surrounded by a somewhat more prominent fibrous sheath, the epineurium.

A wide variety of tumors and tumor-like lesions, many of which are listed in Box 19–1, may arise from peripheral nerves. To a large extent, this spectrum reflects the differentiation potential of Schwann cells. Tumors of the autonomic nervous system (e.g., neuroblastoma) are not discussed in this chapter.

NOMENCLATURE

A major problem in understanding the classification of benign and malignant nerve and nerve sheath tumors has been the evolution of their nomenclature. Most early investigators used the term *neuroma* in reference to all tumors of peripheral nerves. In 1863, Virchow distinguished *true neuromas* (e.g., traumatic neuroma or ganglioneuroma) from *false neuromas* (nerve sheath tumors). Masson[1] was an early proponent of the Schwann cell origin of nerve sheath tumors while other authors, including Mallory,[2] argued that because these tumors contained collagen, they must be derived from perineural fibroblasts. In 1940 Murray and Stout[3] demonstrated the in vitro production of collagen by Schwann cells and, although still controversial, most investigators now agree that nerve sheath tumors derive from Schwann cells.

In 1935, Stout proposed the term *neurilemmoma* for benign tumors of nerve sheath origin.[4] Strictly speaking, this term should refer to a tumor of basement membrane origin, while the

BOX 19–1.
Tumors and Tumor-Like Lesions of Peripheral Nerves

I. Neuroma
  A. Traumatic
  B. Morton's
II. Schwannoma (neurilemmoma, neurolemmoma)
III. Neurofibroma
  A. Solitary
  B. Pacinian
  C. Plexiform
IV. Granular cell tumor (granular cell neurofibroma)
V. Intraneural lipoma
  A. Solitary intraneural lipoma
  B. Lipofibromatous hamartoma
VI. Nerve sheath myxoma
VII. Malignant schwannoma (Neurogenic sarcoma, neurofibrosarcoma)
VIII. Glandular schwannoma
IX. Neuroepithelioma (primitive neuroectodermal tumor)

term *neurolemmoma* more precisely reflects origin from the Schwann cell itself. Nevertheless, *neurilemmoma* remains an acceptable and widely used diagnostic term. Alternatively, the term *schwannoma* is equally appropriate for a benign tumor of nerve sheath origin. The term *neurofibroma* refers to another benign tumor containing Schwann cells, and because of similarities in the histological appearance and origin, some authors have proposed a unified classification system. Hajdu, for example, considers each a subset of *collagenous schwannomas.*[5] Although in occasional tumors the distinction between a schwannoma and neurofibroma may be somewhat arbitrary, the clinical and histological features are sufficiently distinct in most cases to allow their separation (see below).

The terminology of malignant tumors of nerve sheath origin has also been complex. At the present time, the most popular term to describe a sarcoma of nerve sheath origin is *malignant schwannoma.* This may be confusing, however, because benign schwannomas rarely, if ever, give rise to malignant tumors. Sarcomas arise much more commonly in neurofibromas, especially in patients with neurofibromatosis, so some authors prefer the term *neurofibrosarcoma.* Because some of these sarcomas fail to demonstrate definite Schwann cell differentiation, the terms *neurosarcoma, neurogenic sarcoma,* or *malignant tumor of nerve sheath* are also used.

TRAUMATIC NEUROMA

When a peripheral nerve is injured, damage may occur both proximally and distally. Retrograde degeneration often occurs, at least to the margins of the next Schwann cell, and if damage is severe enough the entire cell may die. Simultaneously, the axon distal to the injury disappears and Schwann cells in the immediate region of the injury may also degenerate. Schwann cells distal to the injury, however, often remain intact and, if the damage is not severe, regenerating axon fibers may grow distally and eventually find their way through the residual myelin to re-innervate the original end organ. Many fibers, however, often grow in the wrong direction and, with associated fibrous tissue and proliferating Schwann cells, form a recognizable mass lesion, a neuroma, or traumatic neuroma. Symptomatic neuromas most commonly occur following an amputation, but they can follow other surgical procedures or nonsurgical trauma. Other factors that may influence the development of traumatic neuromas include patient age, type of injury, and distance between severed ends of the nerve. The lesions are usually firm, well-circumscribed but unencapsulated nodules associated with a peripheral nerve, and contain axons, Schwann cells, and fibrous tissue growing in a haphazard fashion. Because traumatic neuromas represent a proliferative response to injury, either accurate reapposition of cut nerve segments or complete closure of the perineurium will tend to prevent their occurrence. Once present, symptomatic neuromas may be excised, often with retraction of the proximal nerve segment away from the previous scar.

MORTON'S NEUROMA

Morton's neuroma[6] is a fusiform enlargement of a plantar digital nerve, usually between the third and fourth toes. It is usually unilateral, occurs most often in women, and is probably the result of repeated compressive injury. Although often considered a variant of a traumatic neuroma[7,8] some authors have emphasized the prominence of degenerative, rather than regenerative, changes in these lesions,[9] including prominent edema and perineural and perivascular fibrosis. Morton's neuromas are usually treated by simple excision.

SCHWANNOMA (NEURILEMMOMA, NEUROLEMMOMA)

The solitary, benign schwannoma is most common in young adults, but can occur in patients of any age and may be slightly more common in women. It occurs most commonly in the head and neck region, and next most commonly in the upper and lower extremities. Tumors frequently involve the auditory nerve (*acoustic neuroma*) and usually present as unilateral tinnitis and hearing loss. Compressive effects in the cerebellopontine angle can be a late complication. Schwannomas involving spinal nerves appear to have a predilection for sensory nerves.[10] Some patients may have multiple schwannomas, and those with bilateral acoustic nerve tumors may have von Recklinghausen's disease (see von Reckinghausen's Neurofibromatosis, below). Schwannomas are also relatively common in the posterior mediastinum and the retroperitoneum. They are usually slow-growing neoplasms; patients most often present with a mass or with symptoms of compression of adjacent structures. Pain is uncommon, but radicular pain or paresthesia distal to the tumor may occur.

Although plexiform schwannomas have been described[11] most schwannomas tend to be lobulated, sharply circumscribed, and encapsulated (Fig. 19–1). They are often pale yellow, and may show areas of cystic degeneration and calcification ("ancient change"). A peripheral nerve may be identified on the surface, but the tumor itself does not contain axons. In large nerves it may be possible to resect the tumor and preserve the nerve trunk.

Histologically, schwannomas may show a range of differentiation, but the characteristic finding is alternating areas of dense cellularity (Antoni A) with loosely cellular and fibrous areas (Antoni B). The Antoni A areas consist of compact bundles of spindle-shaped cells with palisading nuclei and fibrillar, pink cytoplasmic processes. Oval-shaped whorls of nuclei around central bundles of pink cytoplasm are common and are called "Verocay bodies." Mitotic figures are rare. Nuclear palisading is characteristic of Antoni A areas of schwannomas, but is not specific (Fig. 19–2). Other tumors, especially leiomyomas, also may show prominent nuclear palisading. Schwannomas consisting of essentially only Antoni A-type tissue but lacking prominent nuclear palisading have been termed *cellular schwannomas* and may be mistaken for sarcomas.[12]

Antoni B areas consist of more loosely arranged spindled cells without recognizable growth pattern, separated by an intervening myxoid or watery matrix with delicate bundles of collagen. Lymphocytes and macrophages are common; mast cells are also present but in

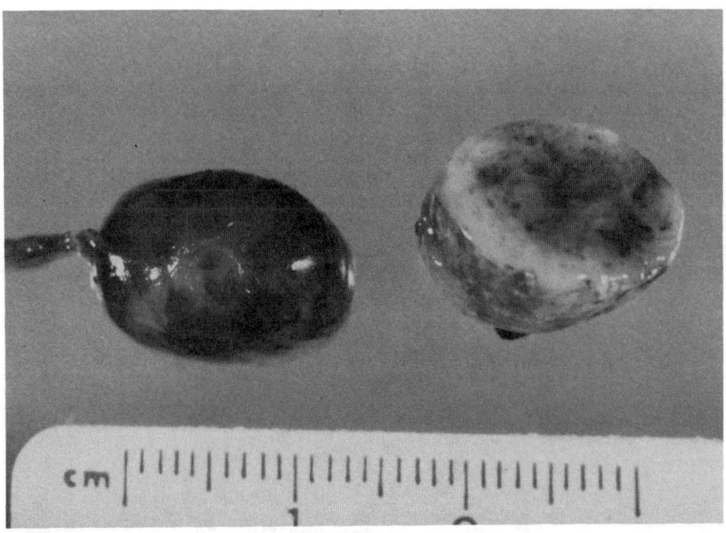

FIG 19–1.
Specimen photograph of a small, benign schwannoma. The lesion appears to be well encapsulated and a peripheral nerve may be identified at one end of the specimen. On cut section, small areas of hemorrhage may be seen.

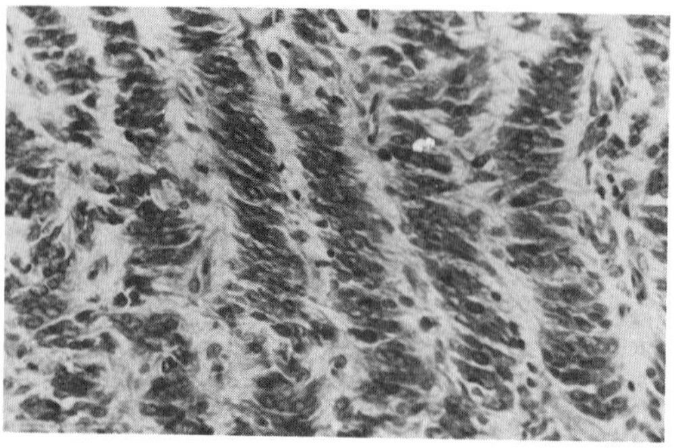

FIG 19–2.
Photomicrograph of schwannoma. The tendency of the nuclei to form long rows separated by pink, fibrillar cytoplasm (nuclear palisading) is a characteristic histological feature, but is not specific. (Hematoxylin-eosin; original magnification, ×128.)

smaller numbers than in neurofibromas. Within Antoni B areas hyalinized blood vessels are characteristic and may be thrombosed (Fig. 19–3). Larger schwannomas may show degenerative changes, including calcification, hemorrhage, hyalinization, and cyst formation. Occasional nuclei in these areas may be large and atypical, and rare mitoses may be identified, but tumors with these areas of ancient change are still benign.[13, 14]

The immunohistochemical localization of S-100 protein, and perhaps other antigens, may be helpful in the diagnosis of tumors of nerve sheath origin. S-100 is an acidic protein that is widely distributed in the central and peripheral nervous system. It can be detected within the Antoni A and Antoni B areas of most schwannomas, and is also present in most neurofibromas, about 50% of malignant schwannomas, and most granular cell tumors.[15] Staining is not limited to nerve sheath tumors, however, so positive staining must be correlated with histological findings.

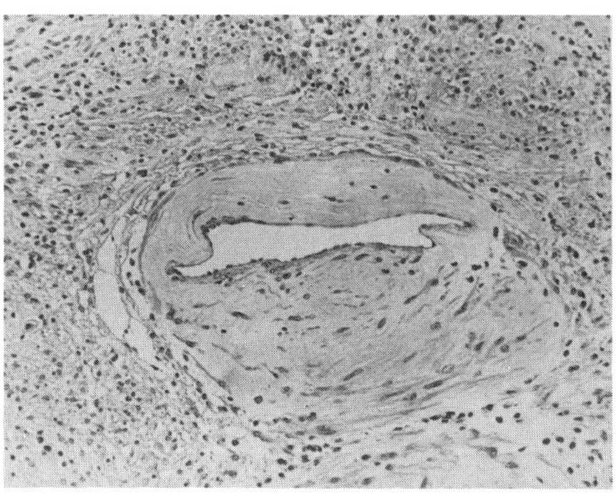

FIG 19–3.
Photomicrograph of schwannoma. Blood vessels with thick, hyalinized walls are another characteristic histological feature of this benign tumor. The irregularly shaped lumen suggests previous thrombosis with organization. (Hematoxylin-eosin; original magnification, ×32).

Schwannomas are benign tumors and complete excision is usually possible, often with preservation of the associated nerve trunk. Retroperitoneal and mediastinal tumors may attain a large size before recognition, but size is not correlated with aggressive behavior in this tumor. Although sarcomas arising in solitary schwannomas have been reported[16] this is a rare event, and difficult to document.

SOLITARY NEUROFIBROMA

Solitary neurofibromas often arise in subcutaneous tissue of young adults. They present as small (1–4 cm), painless masses, are less well circumscribed than schwannomas, and are not encapsulated. Neurofibromas are often white on cross-section and may have a gelatinous or myxoid appearance. Histologically, these tumors consist of a mixture of spindle-shaped cells with wavy or twisted nuclei separated by collagen fibers. All elements of peripheral nerves are present, including Schwann cells, nerve fibers, and fibroblasts. The stroma may be quite myxoid and contain numerous mast cells, as well as lymphocytes and macrophages. Some tumors contain considerable melanin and may be grossly pigmented (Fig. 19–4). Mitoses are rare. Verocay bodies do not occur, and hyalinized vessels are uncommon, but in some lesions the distinction between a neurofibroma and the Antoni B component of a schwannoma may not be possible.

A rare variant of the solitary neurofibroma may contain areas resembling pressure receptors (pacinian corpuscles) and may be termed a *pacinian neurofibroma*.[17] These tumors tend to occur in patients without neurofibromatosis and appear to be benign.

PLEXIFORM NEUROFIBROMA

When involving major nerve trunks, neurofibromas tend to grow along the length of the nerve, creating multinodular, fusiform expan-

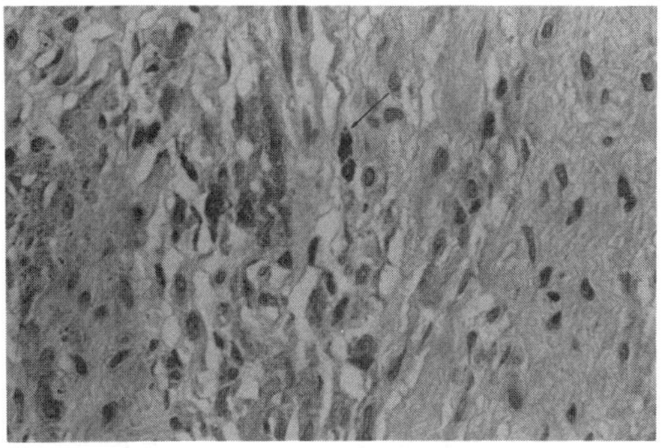

FIG 19–4.
Photomicrograph of a solitary, subcutaneous, pigmented, neurofibroma. In these lesions, melanin can be identified within tumor cells (*arrow*). (Hematoxylin-eosin; original magnification, ×80).

sions. The nerve tends to form a coiled or "wormlike" mass and is designated a *plexiform neurofibroma* (Fig. 19–5). This tumor is often considered to be pathognomonic of von Recklinghausen's neurofibromatosis[18] (see von Recklinghausen's Neurofibromatosis, below). Histologically, plexiform neurofibromas differ from other neurofibromas only in their nodular (plexiform) growth pattern (Fig. 19–6).

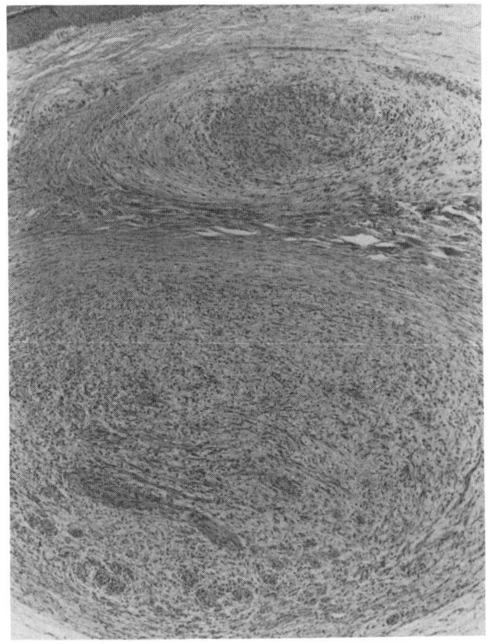

FIG 19–6.
Photomicrograph of a plexiform neurofibroma. The nodular growth pattern associated with a peripheral nerve is a distinctive histological feature. (Hematoxylin-eosin; original magnification, ×32).

GLANDULAR SCHWANNOMA

The glandular schwannoma appears to be a rare tumor, usually found in patients with von Recklinghausen's disease.[5, 19, 20] These lesions consist of cellular neurofibromas with rare nonciliated, mucinous glands. Although fewer than a dozen cases have been reported, it appears that the biological behavior may be estimated by evaluation of the stromal component of the

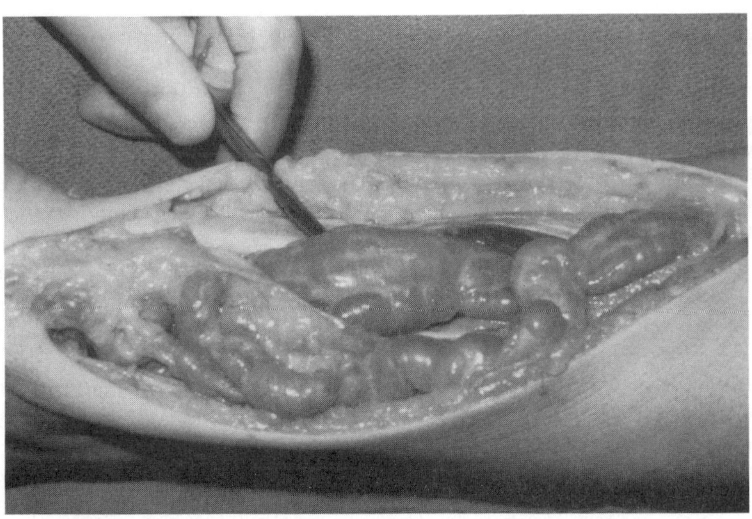

FIG 19–5.
Gross photograph of a plexiform neurofibroma in a patient with von Recklinghausen's neurofibromatosis. The lesions extend along multiple peripheral nerves.

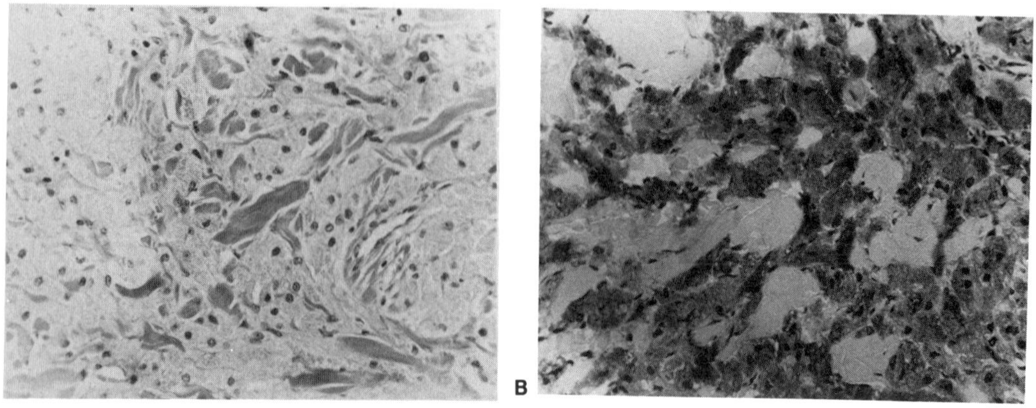

FIG 19–7.
A, photomicrograph of a granular cell tumor obtained from the subcutaneous tissue of the vulva. The lesion consists of large, polygonal cells with central, round nuclei. (Hematoxylin-eosin; original magnification, ×80). **B,** immunohistochemical stains for S-100 protein are strongly positive in tumor cells. (Original magnification, ×80).

tumor using criteria similar to those for malignant schwannomas. Several of these tumors have proved to be malignant,[5] and may be best classified as malignant schwannomas with heterologous elements (see Malignant Schwannomas, below).

GRANULAR CELL TUMOR (GRANULAR CELL NEUROFIBROMA)

Although the granular cell tumor was originally described as originating from muscle (granular cell myoblastoma),[21] it is now well accepted that this common tumor is of Schwann cell origin.[22] Granular cell tumors may present at any age and are slightly more common in females. The tumor is most common in subcutaneous tissue and in the lamina propria or submucosa of the oropharynx or respiratory tract, but may be found in virtually any location. Granular cell tumors are usually less than 2 cm in diameter and tend to be poorly circumscribed. Histologically, the large eosinophilic cells have well-defined borders, small, dark, central nuclei, and tend to grow as cords infiltrating the surrounding fibrous tissue. The pink cytoplasm may show granules that stain positively with periodic acid-Schiff stain (PAS), and the cells are strongly positive for S-100 protein (Fig. 19–7) and myelin basic protein.[23] The epithelium overlying granular cell tumors frequently shows pseudopitheliomatous hyperplasia and must be distinguished from invasive squamous carcinoma.

Some authors use the term *granular cell neurofibroma* in reference to a tumor with the overall growth pattern of a neurofibroma, but in which the cells are similar to a granular cell tumor.[9] Others do not clearly distinguish granular cell neurofibromas from granular cell tumors.[24]

INTRANEURAL LIPOMA AND LIPOFIBROMATOUS HAMARTOMA

Although adipocytes are not a normal constituent of peripheral nerves, benign fatty tumors occasionally occur, most commonly involving the median nerve. Whether these are derived from adipocytes or reflect yet another line of Schwann cell differentiation is unclear. These tumors can usually be classified as either well-defined intraneural lipoma or diffusely infiltrative lipofibromatous hamartoma, often associated with macrodactyly. Well-defined intraneural lipomas are rare, and reported cases involve only the median and sciatic nerves.[25] They tend to occur in adult women and present as a painless mass lesion. Histologically, intraneural lipomas are identical to lipomas elsewhere, consisting of mature adipocytes separated by occasional delicate strands of fibrous tissue.

Lipofibromatous hamartomas of nerve are also rare, and again most commonly involve the median nerve. This diffusely infiltrative lesion is less well encapsulated within the nerve and contains prominent perineural and epineural fibrosis as well as fat.[26] Patients usually present under age 25 and may complain of pain or of symptoms of compression neuropathy. Lesions of this type are more difficult to excise completely, but decompression of the nerve by release of the carpal ligament or other epineural fibrous tissue is usually satisfactory. The significance of macrodactyly in many of these patients is unclear.

VON RECKLINGHAUSEN'S NEUROFIBROMATOSIS

Neurofibromatosis (NF) is a progressive autosomal dominant disorder involving the skin, skeletal system, central and peripheral nervous systems, and occasionally other organs. In 1882 von Recklinghausen recognized the clinicopathological significance of the disorder that now bears his name. Neurofibromatosis may be divided into two major types: classical or peripheral NF, and central NF. In addition, at least two less common forms of NF have been reported: segmental NF, and multiple cutaneous café au lait spots without other manifestations.

Classical or peripheral NF is an autosomal dominant disorder with variable expressivity but virtually complete penetrance. It is a common disorder, occurring in approximately one in 3,000 to 3,200 births,[27] and is worldwide in distribution without sex or ethnic predilection. The disease has a high new mutation rate; over 50% of cases apparently represent spontaneous mutations.[27, 28] Classical NF is defined by three clinical features: (1) café au lait spots, (2) neurofibromas, and (3) Lisch nodules.[29]

Café au lait spots are seen in 99% of patients with NF, and Crowe et al.[27] regard six or more café au lait spots of greater than 1.5 cm in diameter as diagnostic of NF. They usually consist of lightly pigmented cutaneous spots with smooth, delicate margins (Fig. 19–8), are frequently present at birth, and increase in size and number during the first decade. They are widely distributed in all areas of the body with the exception of the face, where only a small number of café au lait spots occur.[29]

The second defining feature of classical NF is the neurofibroma. These tumors occur in the skin, peripheral nerves, and nerve roots and may be discrete, sessile, or pedunculated nodules or appear as diffuse lesions (Fig. 19–9).

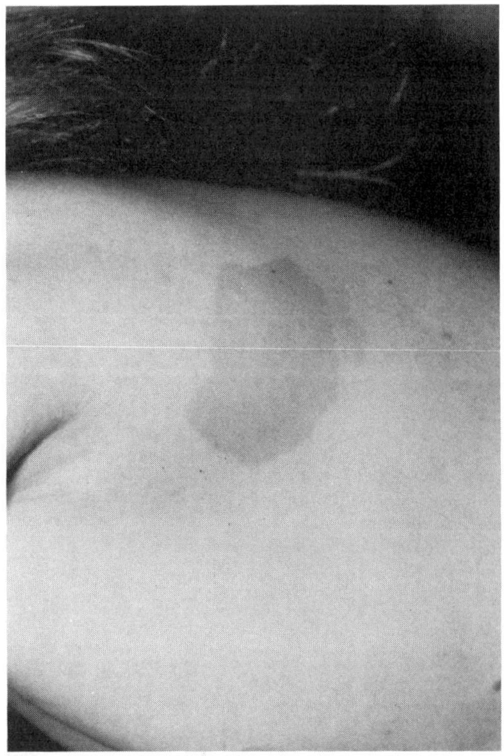

FIG 19–8.
Café au lait spot on a patient with von Recklinghausen's neurofibromatosis.

Neurofibromas most commonly involve the median, radial, orbital, and tibial nerves. The so-called "dumbbell" neurofibroma occurs frequently in the thoracic region of the spinal cord.[30] Schwannomas also occur in classic NF; they arise from spinal and cranial nerve roots and are the most common solitary extramedullary spinal tumor in NF.

The third defining lesions of NF is the Lisch nodule.[31] Ninety-four percent of NF patients over 5 years of age have these pigmented iris hamartomas (Fig. 19–10).[32] The lesions are not seen in central NF.[32]

Central NF is characterized by bilateral acoustic neuromas that produce bilateral hearing loss in up to 50% of patients.[30] Less common symptoms include unilateral hearing loss, tinnitus, balance difficulties, and headache. Sixty-one percent of Eldridge's patients with central NF had mild peripheral manifestations, including café au lait spots and peripheral neurofibromas.[30] Meningiomas also occur in central NF, may be multiple, and arise from the

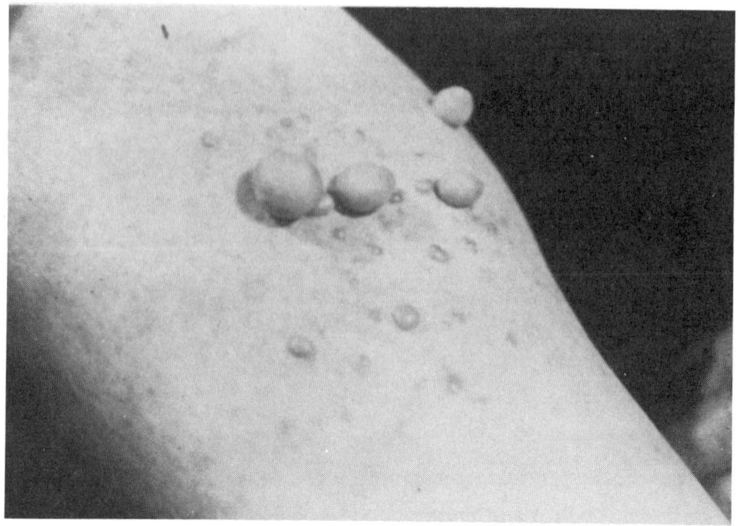

FIG 19–9.
Cutaneous neurofibromas from a patient with neurofibromatosis.

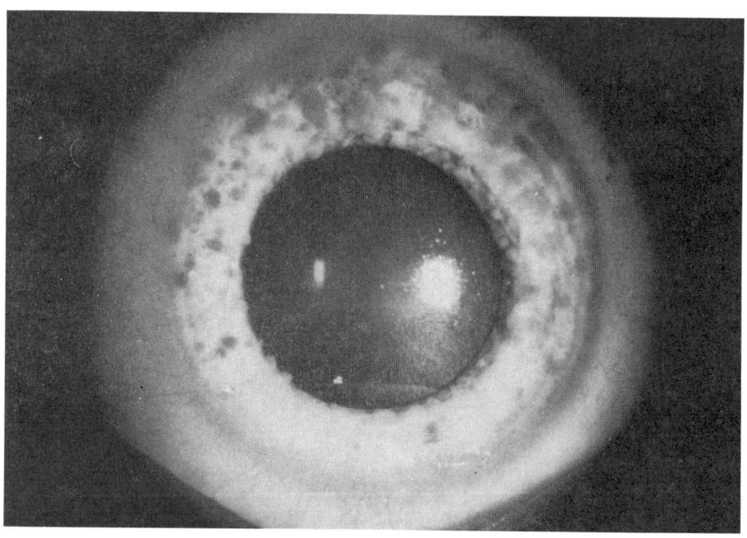

FIG 19–10.
Lisch nodules in a patient with neurofibromatosis. These pigmented hamartomas of the iris are common in patients with peripheral ("classic") neurofibromatosis.

parasagittal region, sphenoid ridge, olfactory groove, and choroid plexus.[29] Gliomas, including astrocytomas and ependymomas, occur in central NF and may be multiple. Optic nerve gliomas occur frequently in NF, and the association of optic nerve glioma with NF is so strong that some investigators have suggested that an optic nerve glioma occurring in the first two decades of life be regarded as a *forme fruste* of NF.[33] Nerve growth factor activity may be useful in distinguishing central NF from classical or peripheral NF. The level of nerve growth factor is markedly increased in central NF and normal in peripheral NF.[34] Multiple other clinical manifestations of NF are common, although not diagnostic, and reflect the combination of neoplasia, dysplasia, and hyperplasia that characterizes NF. These include macrocephaly, central nervous system tumors, segmental hypertrophy, pheochromocytoma, scoliosis, congenital pseudoarthrosis, malignancy, short stature, and intellectual handicaps. A complete list of these clinical manifestations has been detailed by Riccardi.[31]

Benign and malignant tumors of the nervous system are the most readily recognized neoplasms in NF, but other types of tumors also appear to be increased in NF. These include tumors of presumed neural crest origin such as neuroblastoma, pheochromocytoma, medullary carcinoma of the thyroid gland, and melanoma, but patients with NF also appear to have an increased incidence of rhabdomyosarcoma, Wilms' tumor, and leukemia.[35] While patients with NF are clearly at increased risk of malignant tumors, reliable estimates of tumor incidence are unavailable. The authors of a review concerning malignancies in NF concluded that (1) the mean age at diagnosis of a malignant tumor is 38 years for patients with NF compared with 65 in the general population; (2) multiple primary malignancies occur in many patients with NF; and (3) tumor types in patients with NF are atypical, with a high frequency of brain tumors and malignant schwannomas.[35]

The high frequency of neural crest-derived neoplasms has led to the suggestion that NF is principally a disorder related to the maldevelopment of the neural crest and its derivatives (*neurocristopathy*).[36]

MALIGNANT SCHWANNOMA

The reported incidence of malignant schwannoma varies according to the criteria used for its diagnosis. Some authors, applying relatively liberal diagnostic criteria, reported malignant schwannoma to be among the most common types of soft-tissue sarcoma,[37] while others suggested that documentation of origin from a nerve or a neurofibroma is imperative for diagnosis.[38] More recently, most authors have taken an intermediate approach,[9] recognizing that certain histological features allow the recognition of malignant schwannomas that cannot necessarily be proved to arise from a nerve or neurofibroma. In addition, the immunohistochemical identification of certain tumor antigens (e.g., S-100 protein) may also be helpful in obtaining the diagnosis of malignant schwannoma.

Malignant schwannomas may occur in patients with or without von Recklinghausen's NF. The proportion of tumors in each group depends on the criteria used for the diagnosis. Using strict criteria, Stout estimated that about 50% of malignant schwannomas arise in patients with NF.[39] Combining the results of several other large studies,[5, 40–44] 104 of 298 patients (35%) with malignant schwannomas were found to have NF.

Patients with malignant schwannomas may present at any age, but most patients who also have von Recklinghausen's disease present in their late 20's or 30's. Although some authors have noted a later presentation for patients without NF,[45] others have found the mean age at presentation to be similar in both groups.[9] At the Cleveland Clinic Foundation the mean age at presentation for patients with malignant schwannomas and NF is 27.2 years, while the age for those without NF if 46.2 years. There is no definite sex predominance.

Malignant schwannomas tend to arise from large nerve trunks, most commonly the sciatic nerve and the brachial plexus.[9] Origin in the head and neck is fairly uncommon.[42] Most patients present with a painless mass or a recent change in the size of a pre-existing mass, but symptoms of peripheral neuropathy may also be present.

The gross appearance of a malignant schwannoma is similar to that of other malignant soft-tissue tumors (Fig. 19–11). It is usually large, gray or white, and may be partially necrotic. Origin from a nerve is sometimes evident, and if the patient has von Recklinghausen's disease, then an associated plexiform neurofibroma may be recognizable grossly.

Malignant schwannomas vary widely in their histological appearance. In some tumors, the parallel arrangement of tumor cells with associated extracellular collagen closely resembles a fibrosarcoma, in other tumors a storiform growth pattern and marked nuclear pleomorphism are suggestive of malignant fibrous histiocytoma (Fig. 19–12). Hajdu has emphasized more prominent collagen type I fibers in tumors arising in patients with NF than in patients without von Recklinghausen's disease.[5] Additional histological features that may be helpful in diagnosis include extracellular hyalin bands and nuclear palisading.[9] Approximately 50% of malignant schwannomas will stain positively for S-100 protein.[15]

Another interesting histological finding in some malignant schwannomas is the presence of heterologous elements. Rare tumors have been described that contain areas of bone and

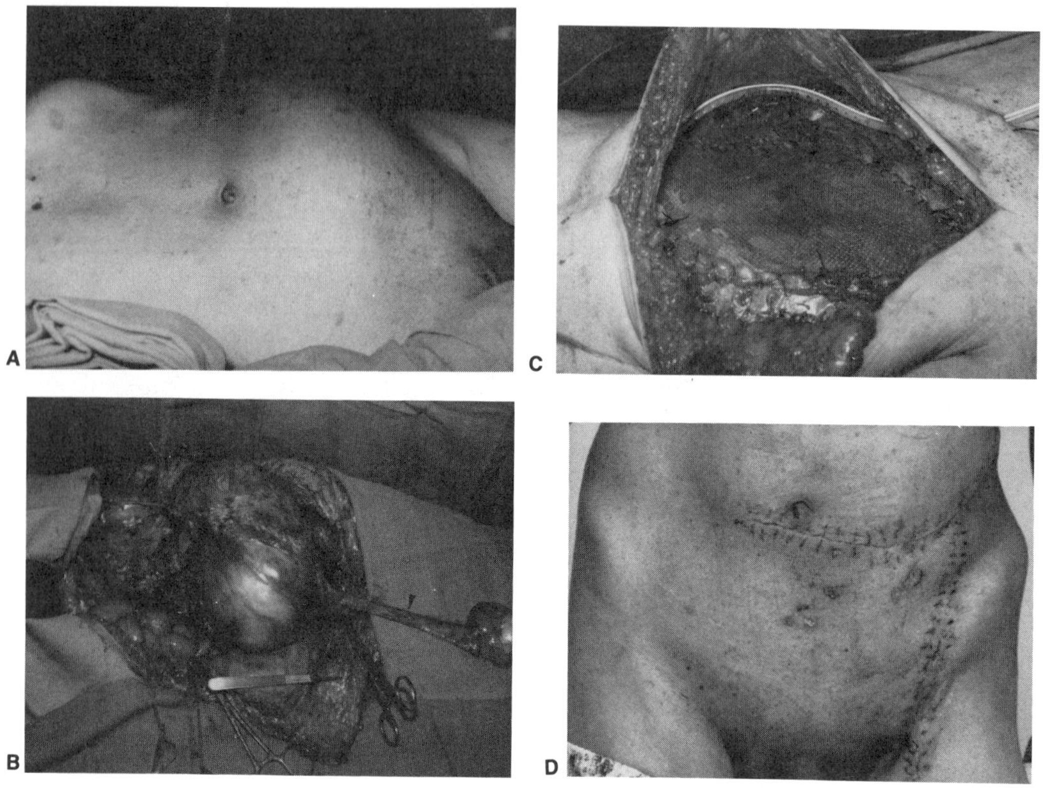

FIG 19–11.
A 30-year-old Spanish American male with classical von Recklinghausen's neurofibromatosis developed a mass in the left lower quadrant of his abdomen. Biopsy showed malignant schwannoma. Following preoperative radiation therapy, the large tumor involving all layers of the abdominal wall and inguinal ligament was resected. **A,** at operation, the patient was placed in a left-side-up lateral position. **B,** all viscera were dissected free of the mass except for the left spermatic cord (*arrowhead*), which was sacrificed. **C,** the abdominal wall was reconstructed using Marlex mesh. **D,** healing and recovery were uncomplicated; the patient received adjuvant chemotherapy.

cartilage formation as well as rhabdomyosarcomatous,[46] glandular,[19, 20] angiomatous,[47] or epithelioid[48] differentiation. Masson and Martin originally used the term *Triton tumor,* postulating that the neural components of this tumor could induce myogenesis, analogous to regenerating limb buds of the Triton salamander.[49] In a study by Woodruff et al.[46] seven of nine patients with malignant Triton tumors died of the disease within 3 to 20 months of diagnosis, suggesting an especially poor prognosis for this variant. A more recent study from the Mayo Clinic,[47] however, found no significant difference in prognosis between malignant schwannomas with heterologous elements, including those with rhabdomyosarcomatous differentiation, and malignant schwannomas without heterologous elements.

Most malignant schwannomas are high-grade neoplasms, have a poor prognosis, and, like other high-grade malignancies, can be shown to contain numerous cells with aneuploid DNA content (Fig. 19–13). Histological criteria often helpful in grading malignant tumors, such as nuclear anaplasia and infiltrative growth pattern, have not been helpful in further defining prognosis for this type of tumor. The number of mitoses[5] and extent of necrosis,[50] however, may be of prognostic significance. Most studies have suggested that the prognosis is worse when the tumor is present in a patient with von Recklinghausen's NF,[9, 41, 42] although one study found no difference in prognosis between these two groups.[40]

The treatment of malignant schwannomas is based on radical excision. Unfortunately, local

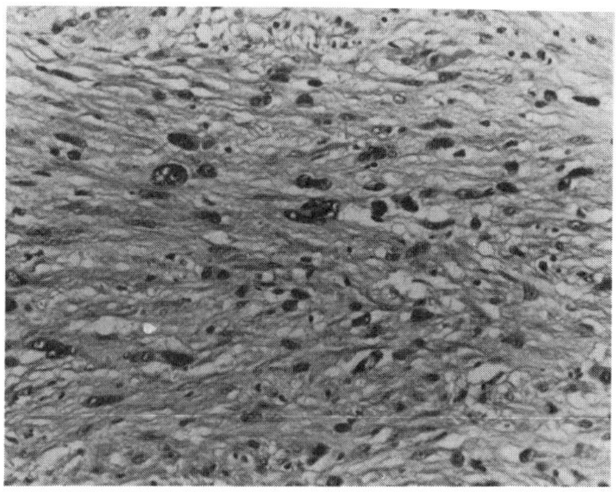

FIG 19–12.
Photomicrograph of a malignant schwannoma, arising in a patient with neurofibromatosis. Histological features include prominent nuclear pleomorphism and high cellularity. These lesions also frequently show numerous mitoses and areas of necrosis (Hematoxylin-eosin; original magnification, ×80.)

recurrence and distant metastases are common. The application of adjuvant radiation and chemotherapy to high-grade sarcomas is discussed elsewhere in this volume and in the literature.[51–53]

PRIMITIVE NEUROECTODERMAL TUMORS (PNET)

Rare tumors of neuroectodermal origin, unrelated to typical nerve sheath tumors, may be seen in either children or adults. These tumors may be divided into two groups: (1) peripheral

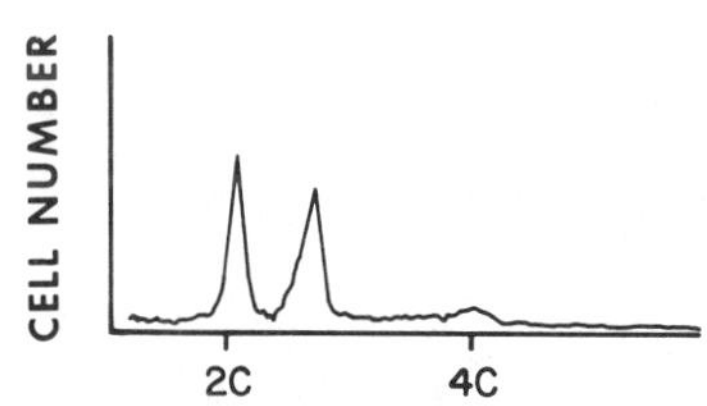

FIG 19–13.
Histogram showing the relative DNA content of cells from a malignant schwannoma. This histogram was obtained by quantitating the intensity of propidium iodide-stained cells by flow cytometry. The 2C peak represents diploid cells and the 4C peak indicates tetraploid cells in mitosis. The intravening peak represents tumor cells with an aneuploid (hyperdiploid) DNA content.

medulloepithelioma and (2) peripheral primitive neuroectodermal tumor. Medulloepitheliomas are extremely rare in the peripheral nervous system; only four cases have been reported.[10] The tumors histologically resemble the medullarly epithelium of the neural tube. This epithelium is capable of differentiating to produce any cell type derived from the neural tube. Central medulloepitheliomas are also rare neoplasms with a malignant course; they occur in children and have no sex predilection.

The peripheral primitive neuroectodermal tumor (neuroepithelioma) is a rare neoplasm arising in association with peripheral nerves.[54, 55] The tumors are densely cellular, composed of small hyperchromatic cells with scant cytoplasm, and may show evidence of neuroblastic differentiation, that is, Homer-Wright rosettes. The tumors are more common in children and are aggressive malignancies.[56–58] The tumors must be differentiated clinically from metastatic neuroblastoma or medulloblastoma.

RERERENCES

1. Masson NP: Experimental and spontaneous schwannomas (peripheral gliomas). *Am J Pathol* 1932; 8:367–416.
2. Mallory FB: *The Principles of Pathologic Histology.* Philadelphia, W. B. Saunders, 1914.
3. Murray M, Stout AP: Schwann cell versus fibroblast in origin of specific nerve sheath tumor; observations upon normal nerve sheath and neurilemmomas *in vitro. Am J Pathol* 1940; 16:41–60.
4. Stout AP: The malignant tumors of the peripheral nerves. *Am J Cancer* 1935; 25:1.
5. Hajdu SI: Tumors of Peripheral Nerves, in *Pathology of Soft Tissue Tumors.* Philadelphia, Lea & Febiger Co., 1979, pp 427–482.
6. Morton TC: A peculiar and painful affection of the fourth metatarsophalangeal articulation. *Am J Med Sci* 1876; 71:37.
7. King LS: Note on the pathology of Morton's metatarsalgia. *Am J Clin Pathol* 1946; 16:124–128.
8. Hauser EDW: Interdigital neuroma of the foot. *Surg Gynecol Obstet* 1971; 133:265–267.
9. Enzinger FM, Weiss SW: *Soft Tissue Tumors.* St. Louis, C. V. Mosby, 1983, pp 580–657.
10. Woodruff JM, Morten BC, Erlandson RA: Pathology of peripheral nerves and para-

gangliomas, in Silverberg SG (ed): *Principles and Practices of Surgical Pathology*, vol. II. New York, John Wiley & Sons, 1983, pp 1503–1520.

11. Woodruff JM, Fundhouser JW, Marshall ML, et al: Plexiform (multinodular) schwannoma. A tumor simulating a plexiform neurofribroma. *Am J Pathol* 1983; 7:691–697.
12. Woodruff JB, Susin M, Godwin TA, et al: Cellular schwannoma. A variety of schwannomas sometimes mistaken for a malignant tumor. *Am J Surg Pathol* 1981; 5:733.
13. Ackerman LV, Taylor FH: Neurogenic tumors within the thorax. A clinicopathologic evaluation of 48 cases. *Cancer* 1951; 4:669–691.
14. Dahl I: Ancient neurilemmoma (schwannoma). *Acta Pathol Microbiol Scand* 1977; 85:812–818.
15. Weiss SW, Langloss JM, Enzinger FM: Value of S-100 protein in the diagnosis of soft tissue tumors with particular reference to benign and malignant Schwann cell tumors. *Lab Invest* 1983; 49:299–308.
16. Yousem SA, Colby TV, Urich H: Malignant epithelioid schwannoma arising in a benign schwannoma. A case report. *Cancer* 1985; 55:2799–2803.
17. Prichard RW, Custer RP: Pacinian neurofibroma. *Cancer* 1952; 5:297.
18. Harkin JC, Reed RJ: Tumors of the peripheral nervous system, in *Atlas of Tumor Pathology*, 2nd series, fasc 2. Washington, D.C., the Armed Forces Institute of Pathology, 1968.
19. Uri AK, Witzleben CL, Raney RB: Electron microscopy of glandular Schwannoma. *Cancer* 1984; 53:493–497.
20. Woodruff JM: Peripheral nerve tumors showing glandular differentiation (glandular schwannomas). *Cancer* 1976; 37:2399–2413.
21. Abrikossoff A: Uber Myome, ausgehend von der quergestreiften willkürlichen Muskulatur. [On myomas originating from transversely striated voluntary musculature.] *Virchow's Arch Pathol Anat* 1926; 260:215.
22. Fisher ER, Wechsler H: Granular cell myoblastoma—a misnomer. *Cancer* 1962; 15:936–954.
23. Penneys NS, Adachi K, Ziegelo-Weissman J, et al: Granular cell tumors of the skin contain myelin basic protein. *Arch Pathol Lab Med* 1983; 107:302–303.
24. Abell MR, Hart WR, Olson JR: Tumors of the peripheral nervous system. *Hum Pathol* 1970; 1:503–551.
25. Chiao HC, Marks KE, Bauer TW, et al: Intraneural lipoma of the sciatic nerve. *Clin Orthop Rel Res* 1987; 221:267–271.
26. Silverman TA, Enzinger FM: Fibrolipomatous hamartoma of nerve. A clinicopathologic analysis of 26 cases. *Am J Surg Pathol* 1985; 9:7–14.
27. Crowe FW, Schull J, Neel AV: *A Clinical, Pathological and Genetic Study of Multiple Neurofibromatosis*. Springfield, Charles C Thomas, 1956.
28. Riccardi VM: Neurofibromatosis: An overview. *Adv Neurol* 1981; 29:1–8.
29. Lott IT, Richardson EP: Neuropathologic findings in the biology of neurofibromatosis. *Adv Neurol* 1981; 29:23–32.
30. Eldridge R: Central neurofibromatosis with bilateral acoustic neuroma. *Adv Neurol* 1981; 29:57–65.
31. Riccardi VM: Von Recklinghausen neurofibromatosis. *New Engl J Med* 1981; 305:1617–1627.
32. Lewis RA, Riccardi VM: Von Recklinghausen's neurofibromatosis: Incidence of iris hamartomata. *Ophthalmology* 1981; 88:348–354.
33. Davis FA: Primary tumors of the optic nerve (a phenomenon of von Recklinghausen's disease). *Arch Opthalmol* 1954; 23:735–821, 957–1022.
34. Rubenstein AE, Mytilineoau C, Yahr MD, et al: Neurological aspects of neurofibromatosis. *Adv Neurol* 1981; 29:11–21.
35. Hope DG, Mulvihill JJ: Malignancy in neurofibromatosis. *Adv Neurol* 1981; 29:33–56.
36. Bolande RP: The neurocristopathies. A unified concept of disease arising in neural crest maldevelopment. *Hum Pathol* 1974; 5:409–429.
37. Geschickter, CF: Tumors of the peripheral nerves. *Am J Cancer* 1935; 25:377.
38. Stout AP: The peripheral manifestations of the specific nerve sheath tumor (neurilemmoma). *Am J Cancer* 1935; 24:751.
39. Stout AP: Tumors of the peripheral nervous system, in *Atlas of Tumor Pathology*, series 1, sect 2, fasc 6. Washington, D.C., Armed Forces Institute of Pathology, 1949.

40. Bojsen-Moller M, Myhre-Jensen O: A consecutive series of 30 malignant schwannomas. *Acta Pathol Microbiol Immunol Scand* 1984; 92A:147–155.
41. Ghosh BC, Ghosh L, Huvos AG, et al: Malignant schwannoma. A clinicopathologic study. *Cancer* 1973; 31:184–190.
42. Nambisan RN, Rao U, Moore R, et al: Malignant soft tissue tumors of nerve sheath origin. *J Surg Oncol* 1984; 25:268–272.
43. Storm FK, Eilber FR, Mirra J, et al: Neurofibrosarcoma. *Cancer* 1980; 45:126–129.
44. Trojanowski JQ, Kleinman GM, Proppe KH: Malignant tumors of nerve sheath origin. *Cancer* 1980; 46:1202–1212.
45. D'Agostino AN, Soule EH, Miller RH: Primary malignant neoplasms of nerves (malignant neurilemmomas) in patients without manifestations of multiple neurofibromatosis (von Recklinghausen's disease). *Cancer* 1963; 16:1003–1014.
46. Woodruff JM, Chernik NL, Smith MC, et al: Peripheral nerve sheath tumors with rhabdomyosarcomatous differentiation (malignant "Triton" tumors). *Cancer* 1973; 32:426–439.
47. Ducatman BD, Scheithauer BW: Malignant peripheral nerve sheath tumors with divergent differentiation. *Cancer* 1984; 54:1049–1057.
48. McCormack LJ, Hazard JB, Dickson JA: Malignant epithelioid neurilemoma (schwannoma). *Cancer* 1954; 7:725–728.
49. Masson P, Martin JF: Rhabdomyomes des nerfs. *Bull Assoc Fr Cancer* 1938; 27:751–767.
50. Costa J, Wesley RA, Glastein E, Rosenberg SA: The grading of soft tissue sarcomas. *Cancer* 1984; 53:530–531.
51. Eilber FR, Eckhardt J, Morton DL: Advances in the treatment of sarcomas of the extremity. Current status of limb salvage. *Cancer* 1984; 54:2695–2701.
52. Rosenberg SA: Prospective randomized trials demonstrating the efficacy of adjuvant chemotherapy in adult patients with soft tissue sarcomas. *Cancer Treat Rep* 1984; 68:1067–1078.
53. Tepper JE, Suit HD: Radiation therapy of soft tissue sarcomas. *Cancer* 1985; 55:2273–2277.
54. Bolen JW, Thorning D: Peripheral neuroepithelioma: A light and electron microscopic study. *Cancer* 1980; 46:2456–2462.
55. Stout AP: A tumor of the ulnar nerve. *Proc NY Pathol Soc* 1918; 18:2–11.
56. Mackay B, Luna MA, Butler JJ: Adult neuroblastoma. Electron microscopic observations in nine cases. *Cancer* 1976; 37:1334–1351.
57. Nesbitt KA, Vidone RA: Primitive neuroectodermal tumor (neuroblastoma) arising in sciatic nerve of a child. *Cancer* 1976; 37:1562–1570.
58. Voss BL, Pysher TJ, Humphrey GB: Peripheral neuroepithelioma in childhood. *Cancer* 1984; 54:3059–3064.

Chapter 20

Extraskeletal Malignant Tumors of Bone

Joseph M. Lane

John H. Healey

Extraosseous osteosarcomas, chondrosarcomas, and Ewing's sarcomas are uncommon soft-tissue malignancies of probable mesenchymal origin.[1] They share histological features with, but are clinically distinct from, the primary bone tumors from which the names are derived. Studies have helped to characterize these clinicopathological entities and to direct therapy. The following discussion will focus on the distinguishing characteristics of these sarcomas and critically review treatment recommendations.

EXTRASKELETAL OSTEOSARCOMA

Extraskeletal osteosarcomas are malignant bone-forming tumors without demonstrable attachments to bone or periosteum. There are three types recognized. The first type resembles classical osteosarcoma. It produces malignant osteoid with variable amounts of chondroid matrix and fibrous stroma. The second type of bone-producing tumor occurs in the viscera. It has been suggested by Fine and Stout[2] that these tumors represent teratomas with proliferation of a single element. In the third type, solid organs, especially breast and testes, may develop secondary osteosarcomas due to radiation. Finally, tumors with multiple malignant mesenchymal lines, such as mesenchymoma, should be excluded despite their ability to produce malignant osteoid.

Epidemiology

Extraosseous osteosarcoma makes up about 1% of all soft-tissue sarcomas. There are approximately 170 cases reported in the literature. The Joint Commission subgroup of soft-tissue sarcoma, in a 13-center study, found six soft-tissue osteosarcomas among 1,215 tumors, an incidence of 0.5%.[3] Allan and Soule reported 26 soft-tissue osteosarcomas among 2,100 soft-tissue sarcomas, an incidence of 1.2%.[4] This constituted 4% of all osteosarcomas seen at their institution. Similarly, Rao et al. reported that 4.6% of osteosarcomas occur in the soft tissues.[5] Slightly lower figures are reported from the Swedish Cancer Registry, where four of 242 osteosarcomas were of the soft-tissue variety.[6] Finally, Sordillo et al. reported 48 cases seen over 33 years at Memorial Sloan-Kettering Cancer Center (New York, NY).[7]

Osteosarcoma of the soft tissue is a disease of middle age. The average age at presentation has been 35 to 59 years in various series.[1, 2, 4–7] Rare cases are reported in children.[8] This age distribution should be contrasted with skeletal osteosarcoma and myositis ossificans, which occur in a younger age group. All investigators have found a slight female predominance.[1]

Clinical Presentation

The presentation differs little from that of other soft-tissue sarcomas. Fifty percent of patients complain of pain. The duration of symptoms is variable, ranging from a few weeks to several months. In the series described by Enzinger and Weiss the mean duration of symptoms was 6.5 months.[1]

The distribution of these tumors is not helpful in distinguishing them from myositis ossificans. They are easily differentiated from skeletal osteosarcoma by their lack of continuity with skeletal bone, The thigh, buttock, and retroperitoneum are the most common sites. Eighty-three percent of the tumors occur in the extremities, particularly in the pelvic and shoulder girdles.[7]

The role of trauma in producing these tumors is contested. Physical injury is occasionally reported to precede development of osteosarcoma. Trauma was implicated as an etiologic factor by Sordillo et al. in six of 48 cases,[7] by Fine and Stout in eight of 26 cases,[2] and by Enzinger and Weiss in zero of 120 cases.[1]

Myositis ossificans may antedate osteosarcoma. Fine and Stout reported two of 12 cases arising in a pre-existant, clinically benign lesion.[2] Cooley reported one case with histological confirmation of myositis ossificans before the development of a soft-tissue osteosarcoma.

The etiology remains obscure in most cases, but specific agents have been well established as causative in some cases. Enzinger and Weiss[1] and Sordillo et al.[7] independently reported that 11% of cases were radiation induced. Hasson has suggested that chemical agents such as Thorotrast (thorium oxide) can produce extraskeletal osteocarsomas. Finally, immunological inocula produced several soft-tissue sarcomas in a therapeutic trial of immunotherapy for skeletal osteosarcoma.[5]

Radiographically, bone involvement is absent. Allan and Soule reported that 16 of 22 cases had soft-tissue masses, and 12 of these 16 masses were calcified.[4] It should be noted that six of 22 cases had no discernable soft-tissue mass and 25% of masses were uncalcified. The absence of a mass or soft-tissue calcification does not exclude the diagnosis of osteosarcoma.

Pathology

Grossly, the tumor is circumscribed but not encapsulated. It occasionally is infiltrative. Vascular invasion was reported to be frequent by Fine and Stout[2] and absent by Rao et al.[5] Histologically it is a malignant spindle cell tumor with a wide variation in pattern. On histological grounds it is indistinguishable from osteogenic sarcoma of bone. Osteoid is always present but is reported to be sparse in at least one half of the cases. The prominent cell type may be chondroblastic, fibroblastic, or osteoblastic. Cellular ultrastructure is reported to be identical to that of the osseous tumors but experience is limited.[1]

Prognosis and Treatment

The prognosis is poor for a patient with extraosseous osteosarcoma (Fig 20–1). The disease reportedly behaves in a virulent fashion, with high rates of local recurrence and metastases. The mortality has been high, particularly in cases treated before chemotherapy was available. Fine and Stout reported that ten of 12 patients died 6 to 22 months after initial treatment.[2] In the series of Allan and Soule, 21 of 26 patients died 1 to 14 years after diagnosis.[4] Of interest was a subset of patients who died after prolonged survival for 7, 9, and 14 years after diagnosis. Sordillo et al. reported that 24 of 35 patients died after a median survival of 31 months. An additional seven patients were alive with metastatic disease at the time of the report.[7] Enzinger and Weiss noted that 76% of 118 patients succumbed to their disease[1] Five-year survival rates have been below 20% in most series.

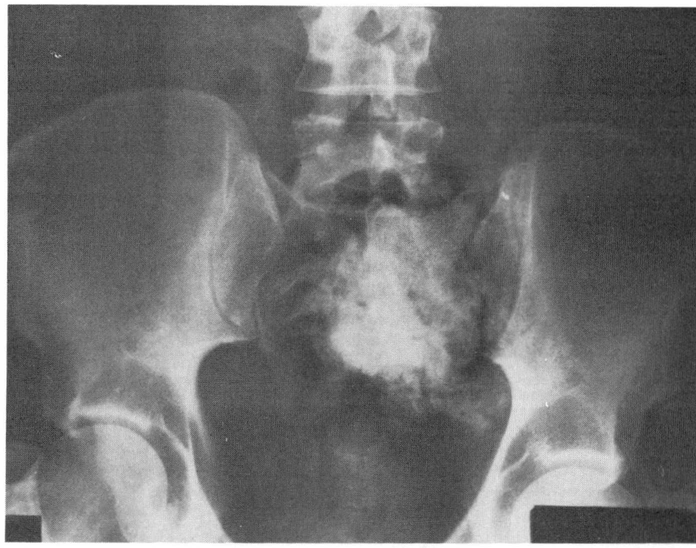

A

B

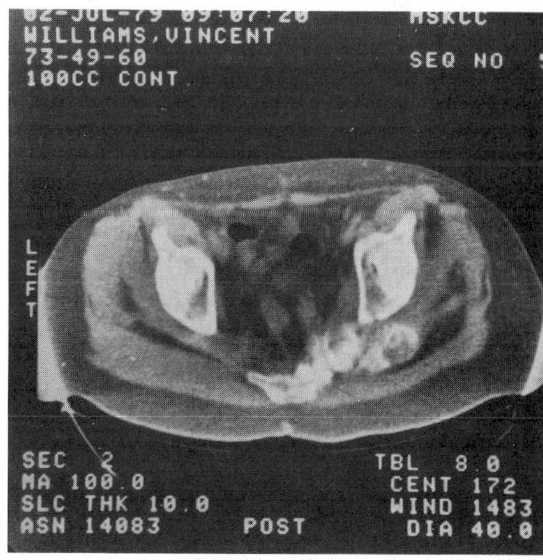

FIG 20–1.
A, a large blastic lesion was seen on the pelvic radiograph of a 41-year-old man with a painful mass in the right buttock. **B,** the soft-tissue location of the tumor was apparent only on CT. Abundant bone formation was present in the soft tissue between the sacrum and ischium. The sacral cortex is irregular and shows reactive bone formation. Despite surgical resection and chemotherapy for this extra-osseous osteosarcoma, the patient died 14 months later.

Extraskeletal osteosarcoma is at least as aggressive as skeletal osteosarcoma and other soft-tissue sarcomas. It is a fully malignant lesion that rapidly metastasizes and recurs locally. Indeed, the poor response to local and systemic treatment was critical in establishing the difference between soft-tissue osteosarcoma and pseudomalignant osseous tumors of soft tissue as discussed by Fine and Stout.[2] Local recurrence has been noted in five of 12 (Fine and Stout[2]), 16 of 21 (Allan and Soule[4]), 31 of 45 (Sordillo et al.[7]), and three of four (Rao et al.[5]) cases after local resection. Amputations have had better success, particularly when performed as a primary surgical procedure. Local recurrence was found in zero of three primary and six of six secondary amputations in one series[4] and in zero of six primary amputations in another series.[7] Rao et al. found that amputation, whether primary or secondary, could effect a cure in their small series.[5] Wide resection could also be successful in preventing local recurrence. Although the number of reported cases was small, recurrent disease was found in zero of four primary[4] and in zero of two secondary[5] cases after wide resection. Other investigators do not distinguish between local and wide excisions, making it impossible to infer the adequacy of surgical margins or to evaluate therapy critically. It may be concluded, however, that wide or radical resection is imperative.

Metastasis usually occurs within the first year after diagnosis and principally involves lung. Secondary metastases have been reported in subcutaneous tissue, liver, bone, and lymph nodes. Resection of pulmonary metastases in combination with systemic chemotherapy has produced an occasional cure.

Nonsurgical methods of treatment are not recommended as primary therapy. Although the treatment specifics were not provided, two patients have been reported who received only radiation therapy. Metastatic disease developed within 6 months and both died after an average of 26 months. One additional patient received radiation therapy without success for an inoperable retroperitoneal tumor.[7]

Adjuvant therapy with a wide variety of agents has been tried, with little standardization of method or objective grading of response. Radiation has provided a temporary, partial response that delays recurrence of disease and prolongs survival, but effects no cures. Immunotherapy has produced no objective benefit; however, soft-tissue osteosarcoma developed in three patients at the site of injection of the irradiated osteosarcoma cells. Adjuvant chemotherapy may be of some benefit. Sordillo et al.[9] reported success in four of five patients who received 9 to 18 months of combination chemotherapy after surgery for recurrent or metastatic disease. A six-drug regimen including doxorubicin, dacarbazine, vincristine, methotrexate, dactinomycin, and Leukeran (chlorambucil) was most effective.[9] Adjuvant chemotherapy may improve the results of the primary surgical therapy, but this has not been investigated. It should be noted that skeletal high-grade osteosarcoma survival improved from 17% to 80+% when treated with adjuvant chemotherapy.

Two acceptable treatment options are apparent from the reports to date. Adequate surgery is fundamental to both approaches. Because most of the tumors are extracompartmental high-grade malignancies (Enneking stage IIB), some investigators claim that radical amputation is necessary, although wide excision alone may be sufficient to obtain adequate resection margins. The option then arises as to whether to use adjuvant chemotherapy immediately or to reserve it for the patients in whom recurrent or metastatic disease develops. Prognosis for patients with extraskeletal osteosarcoma is poor enough to warrant routine use of adjuvant chemotherapy. It has been the practice at Memorial Sloan-Kettering Hospital to use adjuvant chemotherapy and a wide excision or amputation as a minimal surgical procedure. It is unclear whether it is better to use a soft-tissue sarcoma or an osteosarcoma protocol; also unclear is the necessary duration of therapy. Radiation therapy should be limited to cases in which adequate surgery is not possible. These principles of treatment should improve the dismal prognosis in this disease.

EXTRASKELETAL CHONDROSARCOMA

Malignant cartilagenous tumors of soft tissue are of several varieties. Tumors arising in an existing soft-tissue focus of cartilage constitute the first type. Such lesions occur in the respiratory tree [10–12] and in synovial chondromas.[13] The second type include solid-organ chondrosarcomas, which most commonly occur in the bladder and uterus. These lesions most probably develop in teratomas or mixed mesodermal tumors. These categories will not be further considered. The discussion will instead focus on the third variety, primary cartilagenous malignancies of soft tissue. Well-differentiated lesions are rare in soft tissue and should be considered extensions or metastases of bony chondrosarcomas until proved otherwise. Primary soft-tissue chondrosarcomas are poorly differentiated tumors of the cartilage line. The myxoid and mesenchymal varieties will be considered separately. It should be noted, however, that the English literature up to 1970 did not differentiate between these tumors or acknowledge their different clinical behavoir.[11]

Extraskeletal myxoid chondrosarcoma is a neoplasm in the soft tissue of the extremities. It is indistinguishable from the rare myxoid chondrosarcomas of bone, which may morphologically resemble a chordoma. It is a low-grade malignancy capable of recurrence or metastasis and may be cured with adequate surgical resection.

Epidemiology

Extraskeletal chondrosarcoma is a rare tumor. The American Joint Commission Study reported only four extraskeletal chondrosarcomas among 1,215 soft-tissue sarcomas.[3] It was not noted how many were of the myxoid type. Myxoid tumors probably constitute about one third of all soft-tissue chondrosarcomas.

Patients are diagnosed principally in the fifth decade of life, and most are ages 40 to 70 (mean age, 49 years). Rare cases occur in childhood. The youngest reported was a 3-year-old patient with a quadriceps tumor. There is a clear male predominance (65%).[1]

Clinical Presentation

The signs and symptoms are nondiagnostic. A slowly growing mass is the principal complaint. Trauma is reported to be a contributing factor in nearly 25% of cases, but there is no evidence that injury plays a role in the pathogenesis of this lesion.[14, 15] The duration of symptoms varies widely from weeks to years. The lesion usually occurs in the lower extremity (two thirds), and within that limb the thigh and popliteal space (Fig 20–2) are the favored sites.[14] It is usually found in the deep musculature; Enzinger and Shiraki reported only seven of 34 cases to have occurred in the subcutaneous tissue.[14]

Pathology

On gross examination the tumor is lobulated, may be gelatinous or solid, and has a color reflecting the degree of hemorrhage that has occurred. The tumor is well circumscribed and may even have a thick, fibrous pseudocapsule. Microscopically, a nodular pattern is characteristic, with cellular cords in cobweb-like array. Well-differentiated cartilage cells are found in less than half the cases. There is mild hypercellularity. These elongated cells have hyperchromatic nuclei and eosinophilic cytoplasm, and there is a variable intercellular mucinous matrix. Mucin staining of tissue is positive, but of variable intensity. Diastase-sensitive periodic acid-Schiff (PAS) stains demonstrate the glycogen content of the cartilage cells.[1, 14]

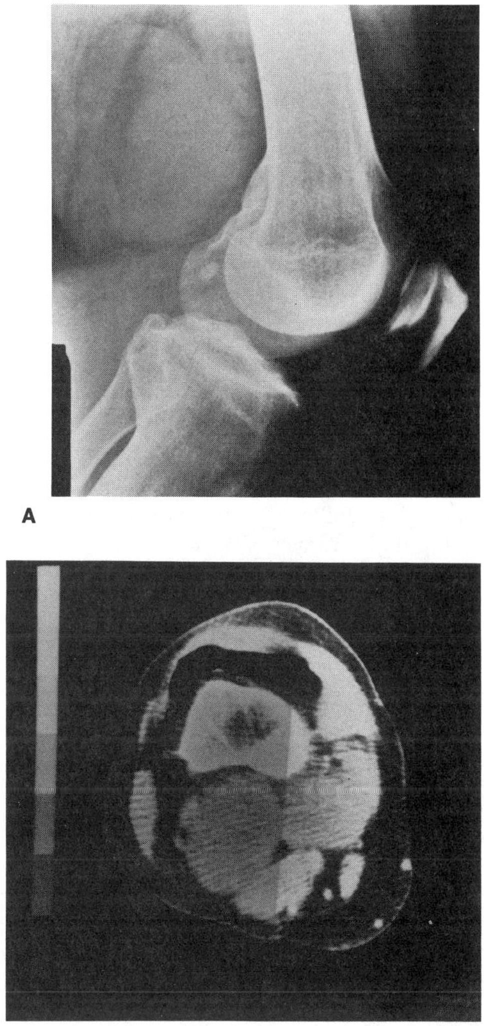

A

B

FIG 20–2.
A, a large, round soft-tissue mass without calcification was present on the lateral radiograph of the knee in a 62-year-old man with poorly differentiated chondrosarcoma of the popliteal space. **B,** computed tomography showed the mass to be close to bone and involving the peroneal nerve and popliteal artery. Six years after an above-knee amputation, the patient is without evident disease and is functioning well.

Differential Diagnosis

Although lesions such as soft-tissue chondroma of the hands[16] and chondromyxoid fibroma may have similar histological appearance, they may be easily excluded from consideration on clinical grounds. Myxoid chondrosarcomas usually have areas of differentiated cartilage with polygonal cells in lacunae, may have multinucleated cells, and lack physaliferous cells.

Myxoid liposarcoma is a major problem in diagnosis, because its clinical behavior is essentially the same as that of myxoid chondrosarcoma. A plexiform vascular pattern and typical lipoblasts at the periphery of the lesion have been reported to be helpful differential points.[1, 14, 17]

Superficial myxoid chondrosarcomas may closely resemble salivary gland tumors. Electron microscopy may be helpful in demonstrating epithelial lines present in mixed tumors. Clinically, the large size and less aggressive behavior characterize myxoid chondrosarcomas.

Prognosis and Treatment

Tumor size correlates poorly with clinical behavior, and the American Joint Commission Staging System does not work well with this lesion. Behavior and prognosis are closely correlated with the cellularity and inversely correlated with the mucin production of these tumors.[1] In a follow-up study of Armed Forces Institute of Pathology (Washington DC) cases after a mean of 3.4 years, 20 of 31 patients were alive, including seven outpatients alive with disease. Seven others had died of unrelated causes. One patient had pulmonary metastases that developed 10 years after tumor resection. Lymph node metastases were more common than in other forms of chondrosarcoma.[1]

Treatment guidelines are difficult to derive from the sparse clinical data presented for cases of myxoid chondrosarcoma. Because most lesions would fit into the Enneking IA or IB stage, wide excision should be definitive. Reports by Wu et al. of two patients free of disease 2 and 11 years after wide resection support this principle.[17] The hypercellular variety of tumor would qualify as stage IIA or IIB and carries a worse prognosis. Adjunctive surgical therapy (radical resection or amputation) and/or adjunctive local radiotherapy or systemic chemotherapy have yet to be shown to be beneficial in preventing local recurrence in distant metastases in these patients.

EXTRASKELETAL MESENCHYMAL CHONDROSARCOMA

Mesenchymal chondrosarcoma in soft tissue is a distinct entity that is fully malignant and routinely metastasizes. The tumor arises from primitive mesenchymal elements. It is most common in the head and neck but it is frequently also seen in the lower extremities. This differs from the distribution of bony mesenchymal chondrosarcoma, which usually occurs in the jaws and ribs.[1, 18, 19]

Epidemiology

Unlike other forms of chondrosarcoma, this tumor usually occurs in late adolescence and early adulthood. It is a rare soft-tissue sarcoma, with an incidence of one third to one sixth that for bone mesenchymal chondrosarcoma and is more common in females.[18, 17]

Clinical Presentation

Tumors arising in the extremity have a nonspecific presentation. They are slowly growing masses of the deep tissues that are occasionally painful. Bone lesions may rarely metastasize to soft tissues and mimic primary soft-tissue tumors. To exclude this possibility, careful evaluation of the skeleton is recommended.[17, 19] Radiographic findings are not specific but consist of focal areas of calcification and/or ossification within a soft-tissue mass.[1, 18]

Pathology

Grossly the tumors are fleshy, lobulated, and circumscribed. They contain less hemorrhage than myxoid chondrosarcoma. Histologically there are two presentations: the small-cell type (one fifth) and the hemangiopericytoma type (four fifths).[18] These cellular elements are mixed with nodules of well-differentiated cartilagenous cells, which may have foci of calcification and ossification. The hemangiopericytoma type has many dilated vascular clefts throughout sheets of poorly differentiated mesenchymal cells.

Differential Diagnosis

The clinical and histological presentation may be the same as for a malignant hemangiopericytoma and synovial sarcoma.

Areas of well-differentiated cartilage, absent intracellular reticulum staining, and cleft-like vascular spaces distinguish mesenchymal chondrosarcoma from hemangiopericytoma. Synovial sarcomas rarely have areas of cartilage formation and usually will have a biphasic pattern demonstrable by reticulum staining.

Prognosis and Treatment

Few reports of treatment appear for this highly malignant tumor. Theoretically, it should be resected with a wide surgical margin, as discussed in Chapter 29 on limb salvage surgery. Adjuvant chemotherapy has not been conclusively shown to be beneficial in soft-tissue chondrosarcoma. Adjuvant radiotherapy may be beneficial, especially when the surgical margin is inadequate, but this has not been established.

EXTRASKELETAL EWING'S SARCOMA

Ewing's sarcoma of soft tissue is an entity distinct from Ewing's sarcoma of bone due to its central axial location and perhaps due to a primitive cellular composition. It has a poor prognosis. Advances in diagnosis have helped to distinguish soft-tissue Ewing's sarcoma from other round cell tumors, and have permitted the use of specific treatment protocols.

Epidemiology

Extraskeletal Ewing's sarcoma is a rare tumor that was not found among the 1,215 soft-tissue sarcomas categorized by the American Joint Commission.[3] Only two substantial series have been reported, and most information is anecdotal. Patients range in ages form 20 months to 63 years, with a mean age at diagnosis of 20 years.[1, 15, 20] As with Ewing's sarcoma of bone, extraskeletal Ewing's sarcoma is more commonly found in men and is not reported in the black population. Ewing's sarcoma of bone almost always has a soft-tissue mass and may resemble primary extraosseous Ewing's sarcoma with bone erosion. The intimate association of the soft-tissue tumor with periosteum, as seen radiographically and pathologically, suggests that some of the soft-tissue tumors are direct extensions of bony tumors. Such an occurrence is strongly contested by several investigators, however.

Neuroblastoma is excluded by the absence of rosette formation in the reticulum staining.[21] In an older age group, possible diagnosis of poorly differentiated bronchogenic carcinoma, reticulum cell sarcoma, or nonhistiocytic lymphomas should be considered. Electron microscopy is helpful in establishing the diagnosis.[21–23]

Clinical Presentation

The distribution of extraskeletal Ewing's sarcoma is different from its osseous counterpart. It occurs principally in paravertebral and intercostal sites (49% as well as in the thigh (Fig 20–3) and pelvic girdle. It presents as a rapidly growing and painful mass, in contrast to the extraosseous bone tumors discussed above. Radiographs confirm the presence of a soft-tissue mass. Bony changes are surprisingly common. Periosteal elevation or cortical thickening was reported in ten of 37 patients and frank erosion of the bone cortex in an additional three of 37 patients.

Pathology

Grossly, the tumor is soft and infiltrative. It is usually attached firmly to the underlying periosteum. Microscopically, immature and monotonous sheets of small cells predominate. The densely packed cells collapse thin-walled vessels. Areas of necrosis and degeneration are common and are associated with thick, dilated vessels. Pseudorosette formation may occur around vascular structures. Histochemical staining is the same as for bone Ewing's sarcoma. Glycogen staining is characteristic, and reticulum staining is absent. The ultrastructure of this soft-tissue lesion closely approximates that of skeletal Ewing's sarcoma. The cell of origin has not been identified for Ewing's sarcoma; however, the ultrastructure appears more suggestive of a mesenchymal than an epithelial origin.

Differential Diagnosis

This tumor closely resembles, and can be difficult to distinguish from, Ewing's sarcoma of bone. Victims of soft-tissue Ewing's sarcoma are slightly older, but this point is of little help in the individual case. The axial location of these tumors can be of diagnostic significance, however.

Areas of well-differentiated cartilage, absent intracellular reticulum staining, and cleftlike vascular spaces distinguish mesenchymal chondrosarcoma from hemangiopericytoma. Synovial sarcomas rarely have areas of cartilage formation and usually will have a biphasic pattern demonstrable by reticulum staining.[18, 19]

Ewing's sarcoma rarely spreads through the lymphatics. Lymph node metastases are suggestive of an alternative diagnosis, such as embryonal rhabdomyosarcoma.[1]

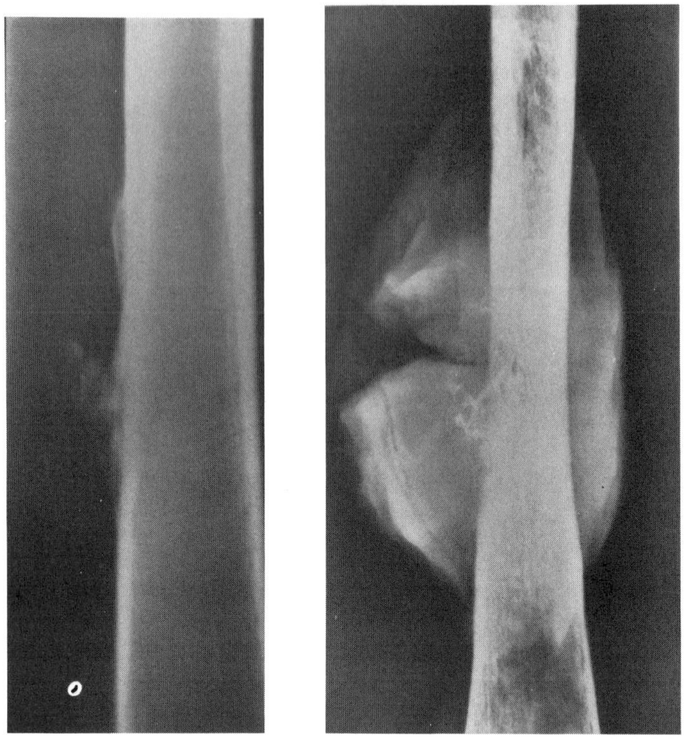

A B

FIG 20–3.
This 22-year-old man had an extra-osseous Ewing's sarcoma of the thigh. **A,** tomograms demonstrated reactive periosteal bone formation and no medullary involvement. Despite hip disarticulation and chemotherapy (bleomycin, Cytoxan [cyclophosphamide], Adriamycin [doxorubicin], and methotrexate), he died 13 months later. **B,** the specimen radiograph demonstrates the large, soft-tissue sarcoma, the reactive bone formation, and the minimal osseous involvement. The actual origin of such tumors remains controversial.

Prognosis and Treatment

The prognosis for this primitive anaplastic tumor is poor. In a review of 37 patients, Angerawall and Enzinger found that 22 had died of the disease 1 month to 14 years after diagnosis. Ten of their patients were alive with no evidence of disease.[20]

A multidisciplinary approach to treatment is recommended. The central location of many of these tumors prevents the surgeon from obtaining a wide resection. Nevertheless, debulking of the tumor may be of benefit. Angerwall and Enzinger found that 33 of their patients were treated surgically, including 25 partial excisions, six wide excisions, and two amputations. Soule et al.[15] reviewed 26 patients with extraskeletal Ewing's sarcoma. All patients received surgery, and in eight there was complete tumor resection with free margins. All patients also received radiation and combination chemotherapy. Twenty of 26 patients had a complete response to therapy; 17 of these patients had no evidence of recurrent disease 10 to 170 weeks after surgery. A complete response occurred in seven of eight patients after complete tumor resection, four of seven patients in whom there was microscopic tumor at the margin of resection, six of eight patients with gross contamination at the resection margin, and zero of three patients who had metastatic disease at the time of presentation.[15] Although the details of treatment were not reported, it may be assumed that the best response would be obtained by using the chemotherapy protocol for Ewing's sarcoma of bone, and high-dose radiation. Gillespie et al.[24] reported successful treatment of three patients who received wide resections, combination chemotherapy, and radiation therapy between 4,000 and 8,400 cGy. However, frequent occurrence of late radiation-induced sarcoma after such high doses of radiation should be noted.

Finally, the central location of these tumors means that there is frequent involvement of the perineural structures and of the spinal cord itself. A combined surgical approach with thoracic, neurosurgical, and orthopedic teams may be best for resecting the tumor and stabilizing the resultant spine defect.

REFERENCES

1. Enzinger FM, Weiss SW: *Soft Tissue Tumors.* St. Louis, C. V. Mosby, 1983, pp 698–744, 801–808.
2. Fine G, Stout AP: Osteogenic sarcoma of the extraskeletal soft tissue. *Cancer* 1956; 9:1027–1043.
3. Russell WO, Cohen J, Enzinger F, et al: A clinical and pathological staging system for soft tissue sarcoma. *Cancer* 1977; 40:1562–1570.
4. Allan CJ, Soule EH: Osteogenic sarcoma of the somatic soft tissues: Clinicopathologic study of 26 cases and review of the literature. *Cancer* 1971; 27:1121–1133.
5. Rao M, Cheng A, Didolker MS: Extraosseous osteosarcoma: Clinicopathologic study of 8 cases and review of the literature. *Cancer* 1978; 41:1488–1496.
6. Lorentzen R, Larsson SE, Boquist L: Extraosseous osteosarcoma: A clinical and histopathological study of 4 cases. *J Bone Joint Surg* 1979; 61B:205–207.
7. Sordillo PP, Hajdu SI, Magill GB, et al: Extraosseous osteogenic sarcoma: A review of 48 patients. *Cancer* 1983; 51:727–734.
8. Kaufman SL, Stout AP: Extraskeletal osteogenic sarcoma and chondrosarcoma in children. *Cancer* 1963; 432–439.
9. Sordillo PP, Magill GB, Shiu MH: Adjuvant chemotherapy of soft part sarcoma with alomad. *J Surg Oncol* 1981; 18:345–353.
10. Morgan HD, Salama FD: Primary chondrosarcoma of the lung. *J Thorac Cardiovasc Surg* 1972; 64:465–468.
11. Stout AP, Verner EW: Chondrosarcoma of the extraskeletal soft tissue. *Cancer* 1953; 6:581–590.
12. Sun CJ, Kroll M, Muller JE: Primary chondrosarcoma of the lung. *Cancer* 1982; 50:1864–1866.
13. Goldman RL, Lichtenstein L: Synovial chondrosarcoma. *Cancer* 1964; 17:1233–1240.
14. Enzinger FM, Shiraki M: Extraskeletal myxoid chondrosarcoma. *Hum Pathol* 1972; 3:42135.
15. Soule EH, Newton W, Moon TE, et al: Extraskeletal Ewing's sarcoma: A preliminary review of 26 cases encountered in the intergroup rhabdomyosarcoma study. *Cancer* 1978; 42:259–264.
16. Chung EB, Enzinger FM: Chondroma of soft parts. *Cancer* 1978; 41:1414–1424.
17. Wu KK, Callon Dg, Guise ER: Extraosseous chondrosarcoma. *J Bone Joint Surg* 1980; 62A:189–194.
18. Huvos AG, Rosen G, Dabski M, et al: Mesenchymal chondrosarcoma: A clinicopathologic analysis of 35 patients. *Cancer* 1983; 51:1230–1237.
19. Salvador AH, Beabout JW, Dahlin DC: Mesenchymal chondrosarcoma: Observations on 30 new cases. *Cancer* 1971; 28:605–615.
20. Angerwall L, Enzinger FM: Extraskeletal neoplasm resembling Ewing's sarcoma. *Cancer* 1975; 36:240–251.
21. Berthold F, Kracht J, Lampert F, et al: The ultrastructural, biomechanical, and cell culture studies of a presumed extraskeletal Ewing's sarcoma with special reference to differential diagnosis from neuroblastoma. *J Can Res Clin Oncol* 1982; 103:293–304.
22. Meister P, Gokel JM: Extraskeletal Ewing's sarcoma. *Virchow's Archiv. A, Pathological Anatomy and Histopathology* (Berlin) 1978; 378:173–179.
23. Wigger HJ, Salazar GH, Blanc WA: Extraskeletal Ewing's sarcoma: An ultrastructural study. *Arch Pathol Lab Med* 1977; 101:446–449.
24. Gillespie JJ, Roth LM, Wells ER, et al: Extraskeletal Ewing's sarcoma. *Am J Surg Pathol* 1979; 3:99–108.

Chapter 21

Soft-Tissue Sarcomas in Children

Susan B. Shurin

Sarcomas in children are far more common than carcinomas, a major difference between cancers in children and adults. The most common sarcomas are rhabdomyosarcoma (embryonal and alveolar), followed by bone sarcomas (Ewing's and osteogenic). Statistically less common, but biologically related and presenting major therapeutic dilemmas, are soft-tissue sarcomas other than rhabdomyosarcoma and extra-osseous Ewing's sarcoma. These are rare diseases that present major management problems for the surgeon, radiation oncologist, and pediatric oncologist. For some of these disorders, surgical cure is feasible. For others, optimal chemotherapeutic and radiation therapeutic management is yet to be defined.

CHEST WALL SARCOMAS (ASKIN TUMOR, EXTRA-OSSEOUS EWING'S SARCOMA)

This group of tumors, which includes malignant small round cell tumor of the thoracopulmonary region of childhood (Askin tumor), extra-osseous Ewing's sarcoma, and primitive neuroectodermal tumors (PNET), originates in the chest wall.[1–4] Local recurrence within the thorax is a major issue for these tumors. Disseminated disease is common in extra-osseous Ewing's sarcoma. Ewing's tumors are so classified largely on the basis of high glycogen content, while Askin tumors are poor in glycogen and have ultrastructural evidence of neuroectodermal differentiation. More recent observations that Ewing's sarcomas primary in bone may have evidence of neuroectodermal differentiation have blurred the distinction between the two pathological entities. Prediction of biological behavior on the basis of pathological classification is fraught with hazard. Long-term survival is uncommon in patients who have not been rendered free of disease surgically, although local control through surgery may be effected following tumor reduction with chemotherapy and radiation therapy.

Patients usually present with either pain or intrathoracic mass causing respiratory symptoms. Extrathoracic masses are uncommon, as is extension through the vertebral foramina. Tumors may originate in the chest wall or in the mediastinum, and may either extend into the lung parenchyma or metastasize to lung. Pathologically, these are malignant small round cell tumors. Special stains including antibodies to desmin, S-100 protein, vimentin, myoglobin, keratin, and periodic acid-Schiff stain for glycogen may assist in classification of these tumors.

When primary tumor excision is possible at the time of diagnosis, it may require partial chest wall excision, and pre-operative chemotherapy and/or radiation therapy may aid in rendering patients resectable with less deforming surgery. Chemotherapy based on that recommended for rhabdomyosarcoma and Ewing's sarcoma has resulted in dramatic tumor shrinkage in patients with measurable disease. Vincristine, adriamycin, cyclophosphamide, and actinomycin D are the bases of most chemotherapy regimens. Current estimates of survival rates for patients presenting without evidence of metastasis for whom local control is feasible with combined therapy is greater than 50%.[4]

FIBROSARCOMA

Primary fibrosarcoma occurs most commonly in young children, and neonatal presentations have been described. Distal extremity primaries are the most usual sites, followed by head and neck, trunk, retroperitoneum, and genitourinary tract.[5] Predisposing disorders that are associated with later onset include previous radiation therapy and von Recklinghausen's neurofibromatosis. In general, children do better than adults with the same histological diagnosis, and younger children do better than adolescents, whose diseases act more like those in adults. The pathological features are those of anaplastic spindle-shaped cells in a herringbone arrangement, prominent mitoses, and high cellularity.

Wide excision is the treatment of choice (Fig 21–1), particularly for younger children.[6] Amputation may be necessary for extremity primaries. Distal metastases are uncommon. Neither radiation therapy nor adjuvant chemotherapy has any clear role in these disorders, and survival after the development of metastatic disease is unusual. Local recurrence, however, may still be followed by long-term survival if repeat resection with an adequate margin is achieved. The course may be quite indolent. Those arising in the retroperitoneal space are frequently unresectable, and are associated with

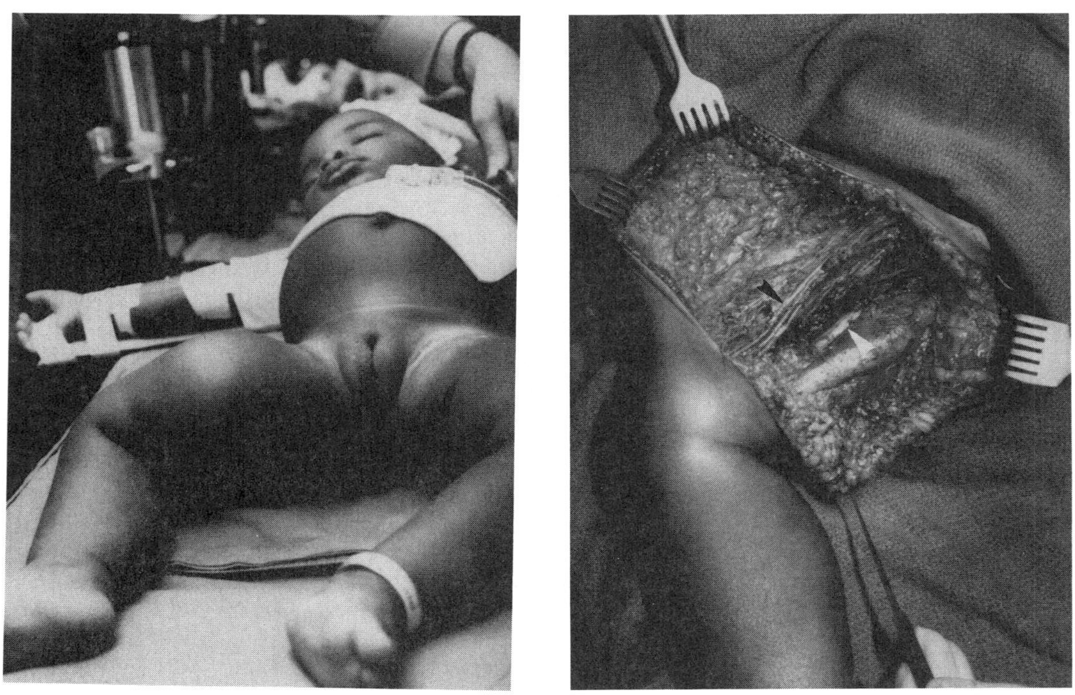

A B

FIG 21–1.
A, pediatric fibrosarcoma in the medial right thigh. **B,** radical resection of the abductor muscles surrounding the tumor has been performed, leaving intact the femoral vessels and nerve (*black arrowhead*) and femur (*white arrowhead*) at the border of the excision.

a particularly poor survival rate due to local invasion.[7]

Variants of fibrosarcoma include neurofibrosarcomas, malignant tumors of neural sheath origin, such as malignant schwannomas (Fig 21–2), and neurolemmomas. These are rarely seen except in patients with von Recklinghausen's disease.[8]

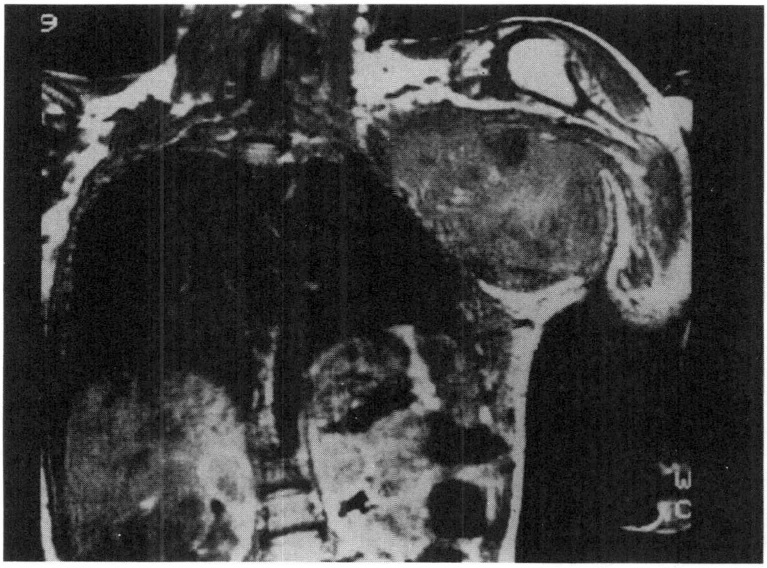

A

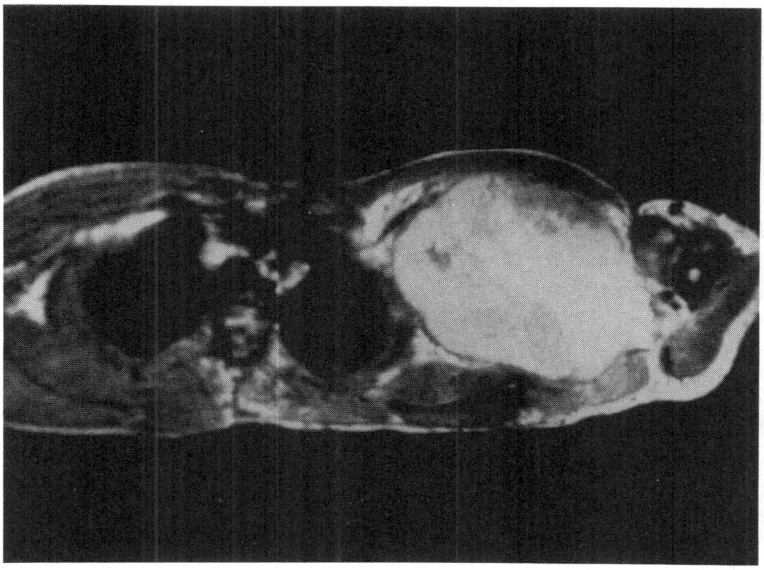

B

FIG 21–2.

A, coronal MRI scan (T_1 weighted) of a malignant schwannoma (neurofibrosarcoma) arising from the brachial plexus of a 19-year-old male with neurofibromatosis. The tumor occupied the axilla and extended into the chest wall and neck; a forequarter amputation was performed. **B,** pre-operative transverse MRI scan (T_2 weighted) of the same patient.

LIPOSARCOMA

Liposarcomas are rare in adults, and vanishingly rare in children. Local control constitutes the major therapeutic challenge. Primary sites in the proximal extremity, particularly the thigh, are most frequent. Other than extremities, primaries in the retroperitoneum, mediastinum and neck have been described. The pathological variants are myxoid, well differentiated, and round cell.[9]

Differentiation from lipoblastomatosis is important; the latter is a biologically benign process that tends to be nodular and circumscribed, rather than tissue invasive, and does not require wide local excision. The only defined role for chemotherapy and/or radiation therapy is in pre-operative shrinkage of the tumor to permit surgical excision in otherwise inoperable tumors.[10]

SYNOVIAL CELL SARCOMA

Synovial cell sarcoma may originate in any joint. Presentation with small primary lesions in the presence of metastatic disease, particularly in the lung, has been described. Lower extremity primaries are the most common, with upper extremity and trunk less frequent. Two pathological patterns, a spindle cell tumor and a pseudo-epithelial tumor, may be found alone or mixed together. The pseudo-epithelial and mixed histologies are thought to predict a better prognosis, as does younger age at presentation.[11]

As with several other rare soft-tissue sarcomas of childhood, the role of adjuvant chemotherapy and/or radiation therapy is not established. The rarity of these tumors, the fact that surgical excision may result in long-term disease-free survival, and the uncommon event of survival in the presence of metastatic disease, even when response to chemotherapy or radiation can be demonstrated, make assessment of such approaches difficult at best. Both late local recurrences and late development of metastatic disease have been described in synovial cell sarcoma, and also complicate assessment of the benefits of therapy.[12]

HEMANGIOPERICYTOMA

Hemangiopericytoma arises in the soft tissues of extremities, head and neck, or retroperitoneum. The cell of origin is the pericyte, which surrounds blood vessels. Infantile or congenital hemangiopericytoma, which is pathologically indistinguishable from that occurring in older children and adults, behaves entirely differently, and surgical excision is usually the definitive treatment.[13] In older children, the behavior is more akin to that in adults, with pulmonary and bony metastases common. Wide local excision usually followed by irradiation if amputation has not been performed, is the first treatment of choice. Metastatic, locally recurrent, and unresectable lesions have responded to a variety of chemotherapeutic agents, including vincristine, cyclophosphamide, adriamycin, and actinomycin. Again, the paucity of extensive experience with children with this disease limits the evaluability of therapy other than addressed at local control.[14]

REFERENCES

1. Askin FB, Rosai J, Sibley RK, et al: Malignant small cell tumor of the thoracopulmonary region in childhood: A distinctive clinicopathologic entity of uncertain histogenesis. *Cancer* 1979; 43:2438–2451.
2. Kumar APM, Green A, Smioth JW, et al: Combined therapy for malignant tumors of the chest wall in children. *J Pediatr Surg* 1977; 12:991–999.
3. Cavazzana AO, Miser JS, Jefferson J, et al: Experimental evidence for a neural origin of Ewing's sarcoma of bone. *Am J Pathol* 1987; 127:507–518.
4. Shamberger RC, Grier HC, Weinsten HJ, et al: Chest wall tumors in infancy and childhood. *Cancer* 1989; 63:774–785.
5. Neifeld JP, Godwin D, Berg JW, et al: Prognostic features of pediatric soft-tissue sarcomas. *Surgery* 1985; 98:93–97.
6. Exelby PR: Surgery of soft tissue sarcomas in children. *Natl Cancer Inst Monogr* 1979; 56:153–157.
7. Crist WM, Raney RB, Tefft M, et al: Soft tissue sarcomas arising in the retroperitoneal space in children. A report from the Intergroup Rhabdomyosarcoma Study (IRS) Committee. *Cancer* 1985; 56:2125–2132.
8. Raney RB, Littmann P, Jarrett P: Results of multimodal therapy for children with neurogenic sarcoma. *Med Pediatr Oncol* 1979; 7:229–236.
9. Enzinger FM, Winslow DJ: Liposarcoma: Study of 103 cases. *Virchow's Arch Pathol Anat* 1962; 335:367–388.

10. Castleberry RP, Kelly DR, Wilson ER, et al: Childhood liposarcoma. Report of a case and review of the literature. *Cancer* 1984; 54:579–584.
11. Raney RB: Synovial sarcoma. *Med Pediatr Oncol* 1981; 9:41–45.
12. Cameron HU, Kostyuik JP: A long term follow up of synovial sarcoma. *J Bone Joint Surg* 1974; 563:613–617.
13. Enzinger FM, Smith BH: Hemangiopericytoma. An analysis of 106 cases. *Hum Pathol* 1976; 7:61–82.
14. Wong PP, Yagoma A: Chemotherapy of malignant hemangiopericytoma. *Cancer* 1978; 41:1256–1260.

Chapter 22

Classic, African, and Acquired Immunodeficiency Syndrome-Associated Kaposi's Sarcoma

Patricia L. Myskowski

Bijan Safai

Kaposi's sarcoma (KS), a rare multifocal neoplasm, was first described by Moritz Kaposi in 1872.[1] In the original description of "idiopathic multiple hemorrhagic sarcoma," Kaposi described the occurrence of violaceous nodules on the skin of the lower legs of three eldery men. In these original three cases, Kaposi noted the progressive and eventually fatal nature of the illness, as all of the patients died within 3 years of diagnosis.[2]

VARIANTS OF KAPOSI'S SARCOMA

Classic Kaposi's Sarcoma—Before 1981, KS had been categorized into three different clinical variants.[3] Classic KS was seen primarily in North America and Eastern Europe as an indolent neoplasm of elderly men. Classic KS is a rare neoplasm with an estimated annual incidence in the United States of 0.021 to 0.061 per 100,000.[4–6] A marked male predominance has also been noted, with the disease being three[7] to ten[8] times more common in men than in women. The disease remains an illness of older individuals with a mean age of 63 years (range 23–90 years in one series).[9] In the United States, a mean survival of 8 to 13 years has been reported, with patients often dying from second malignancies or unrelated causes.[2] An ethnic predominance has been noted in the classic form: Many of the patients were Italians or of Eastern European background, that is, Polish, Hungarian, Russian, and especially Ashkenazic Jewish ancestry.[2–10] A genetic association in HLA gene patterns has also been seen in classic KS, with a significant increase in the incidence of HLA-DR5.[10, 11] HLA-DR5 is also more frequent in Eastern European populations, but its increased incidence in classic KS patients suggests a subgroup of individuals with an increased genetic susceptibility to the disease.[10, 11]

The skin lesion of classic KS usually begins on the lower extremities as a purple patch.[2] The

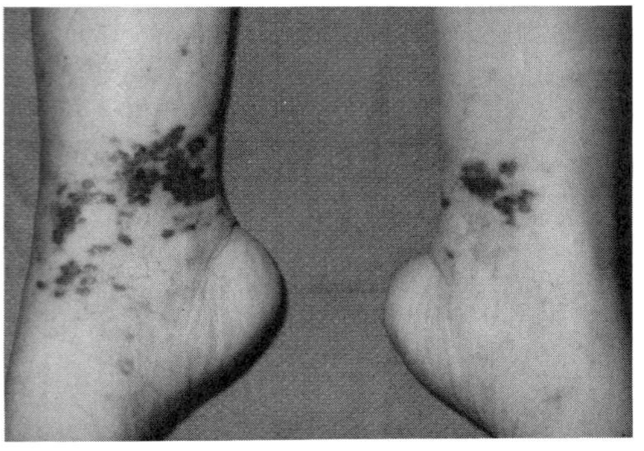

FIG 22–1.
Bilateral initial lesions of classic KS on the ankles.

initial lesions may be unilateral or bilateral (Fig. 22–1), but eventually progress to to more infiltrative and nodular forms. The feet are often initially affected (Fig. 22–2). Reddish-purple patches and plaques may then appear on the legs, then on the hands and arms (Fig. 22–3). Lymphedema of the extremities often appears as a late sign. Violaceous lesions may also be found on the mucous membranes. Lymph node and visceral involvement may occur late in the disease, although this is much less common. When visceral involvement is found, the gastrointestinal tract is the most frequent site, but other organ systems, including the respiratory tract, may be involved by the disease.[11] A striking association in classic KS patients is the development of a second malignancy in up to 37% of patients.[7] These secondary neoplasms are generally of the lymphoproliferative type, and their occurrence may support the relationship between classic KS and immunological alterations.[7]

African Kaposi's Sarcoma.—Another form of Kaposi's sarcoma has been recognized in Africa for many years.[4, 12] In contrast to the rarity of KS in North American populations, this is a relatively common tumor in Central Africa. The geographic distribution of African KS is similar to that of Burkitt's lymphoma. In Uganda in 1962, African KS constituted 9% of all the malignancies diagnosed in that country,[4] and it has continued to be a common neoplasm.[13, 14] African KS is found in four different clinical types,

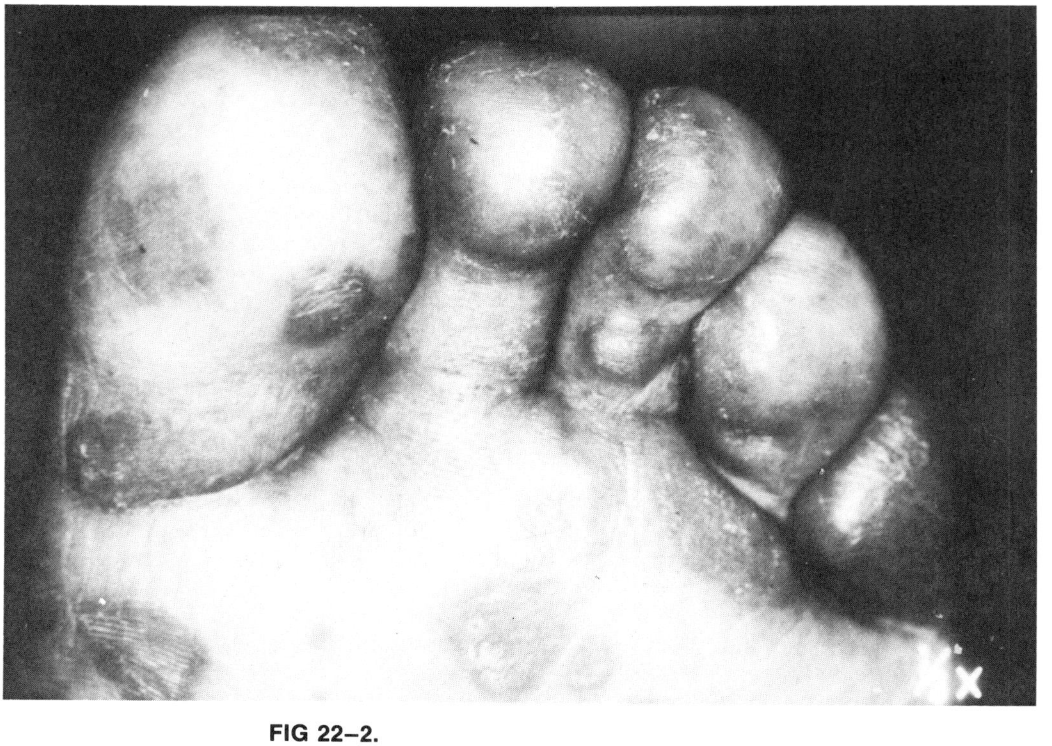

FIG 22–2.
Violaceous skin lesions of classic KS on the feet.

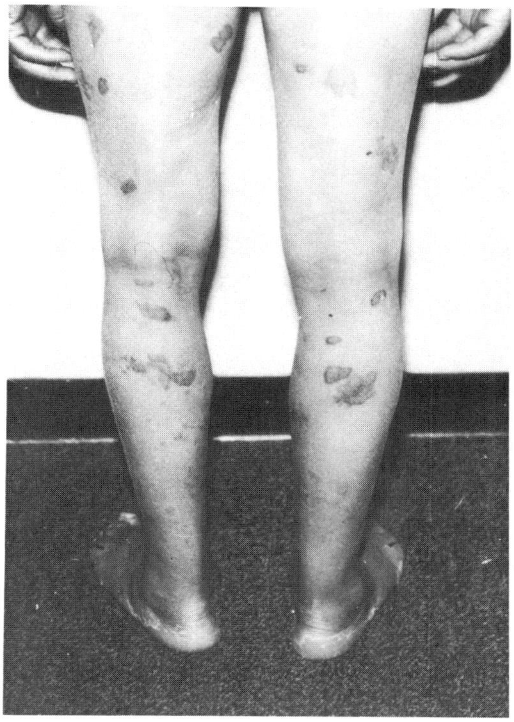

FIG 22–3.
More advanced skin involvement by classic KS.

which have been well described by Taylor et al.[12] The *nodular* type is a relatively indolent variant that occurs in adults and presents in a manner similar to that of classical KS. In the nodular form of African KS, involvement of bone or lymph node is a rare finding. In the *florid* form, locally aggressive tumors are the rule, and may enlarge to form fungating and exophytic masses on the lower extremities. The florid form of African KS also affects adults, and while lymph node involvement is rare, bony involvement is quite common. In the *infiltrative* form of African KS, aggressive infiltrating tumors may rapidly involve the entire feet or hands. Bony involvement invariably accompanies this type, which also affects adults. Finally, there is the *lymphadenopathic* form of African KS, occurring in children and young adults under the age of 25 years. This is an aggressive and widely disseminated form of the disease in which skin lesions are relatively infrequent, but lymph node and visceral involvement is constant. Although the three adult forms of African KS may have a prolonged course, the lymphadenopathic variant in children is usually fatal within a short time.[12]

Kaposi's Sarcoma in Immunosuppressed Patients.—A third form of KS has also been recognized in patients who are immunosuppressed by various medications.[15, 16] This variant has been seen predominantly in renal transplant recipients, and also in patients with collagen vascular diseases such as systemic lupus erythematosus and dermatomyositis.[17] These patients typically give a history of immunosuppressive drug therapy, for example, use of prednisone, azathioprine, and cyclophosphamide. Visceral lesions in these patients may often pursue a more aggressive course than in classic KS patients.[15–17]

Kaposi's Sarcoma Associated with Acquired Immunodeficiency Syndrome.—In 1981, a new group of patients with Kaposi's sarcoma was described in New York City and San Francisco, which marked the beginning of the KS epidemic in acquired immune deficiency syndrome (AIDS).[18] As is now well known, these patients differed from the three previously described groups of KS patients in several important respects.[3, 18, 19] Epidemiological differences were evident in the cluster distribution of these new cases, and by the identification of certain risk groups.[18] While the initial patients were almost exclusively homosexual and bisexual men, other risk groups such as intraveneous drug users, hemophiliacs, Haitians, and blood transfusion recipients soon appeared. AIDS-associated KS is a disease of younger individuals, with a median age of 39 years being seen in at least one series.[19] The clinical presentations are quite varied and differ substantially from those of the classical form of the disease.[3] Reddish-purple, often oval-shaped macules and papules may begin on any part of the body. In particular, the upper part of the body is often initially involved (Fig. 22–4), especially the trunk and arms. Of note is the tendency for these skin lesions to follow the skin lines, similar to the distribution of pityriasis rosea (Fig. 22–5). Mucous membrane, lymph node, and gastrointestinal lesions may also be evident as the early, or even initial, manifestation of the disease. Skin lesions tend to appear rapidly, often over a few weeks or months, in contrast to the slower development of classic KS lesions. The hallmark of KS in AIDS is profound immunosuppression, which is felt to be the direct result of infection by the AIDS-associated retrovirus, HIV-1 (HTLV-III).[20] This immunosuppression is manifested clinically by the frequent, often fatal, develop-

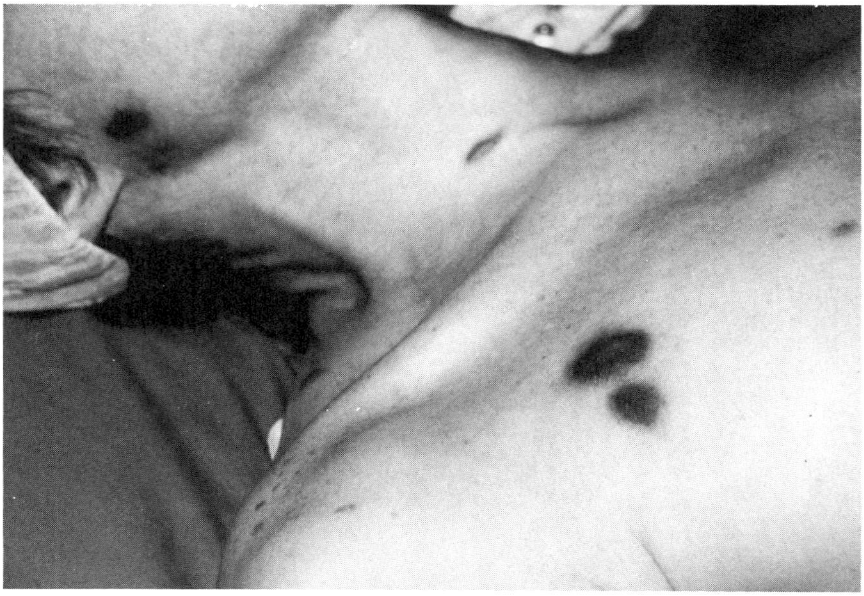

FIG 22–4.
Early skin lesions of AIDS-associated KS in a 39-year-old male.

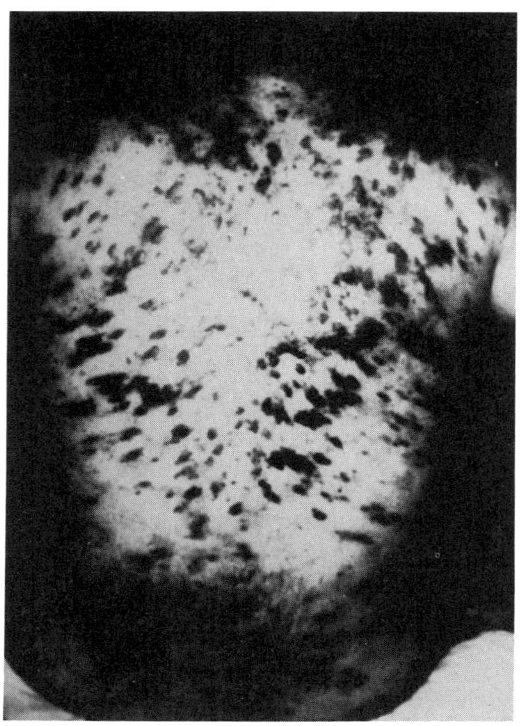

FIG 22–5.
Skin lesions in AIDS-associated KS, following the skin lines.

ment of opportunistic infections, such as *Pneumocystis carinii* pneumonia, atypical mycobacterial infections, aggressive herpes simplex infections, central nervous systems toxoplasmosis, and fungal infections.[18] Profound disturbances in immune factors are also seen, with leukopenia and a marked decrease in helper T lymphocytes being extremely common. Abnormalities in many different immunological functions have been recorded, and may point to the key role of virally induced immunosuppression in AIDS-associated KS.

HISTOPATHOLOGY

The skin lesions of KS begin in the upper dermis.[2, 21] Histopathological findings characteristically include the appearance of interweaving areas of spindle-shaped cells and vascular-appearing structures embedded in a reticular collagen fiber network (Fig. 22–6). The vascular-appearing structures are slitlike clefts that appear between bundles of spindle cells. Extravasated red blood cells are found within the clefts, and hemosiderin-laden macrophages are also commonly seen. Nuclear pleomorphism is another frequent finding within these skin lesions.[13] The histopathological findings of KS in

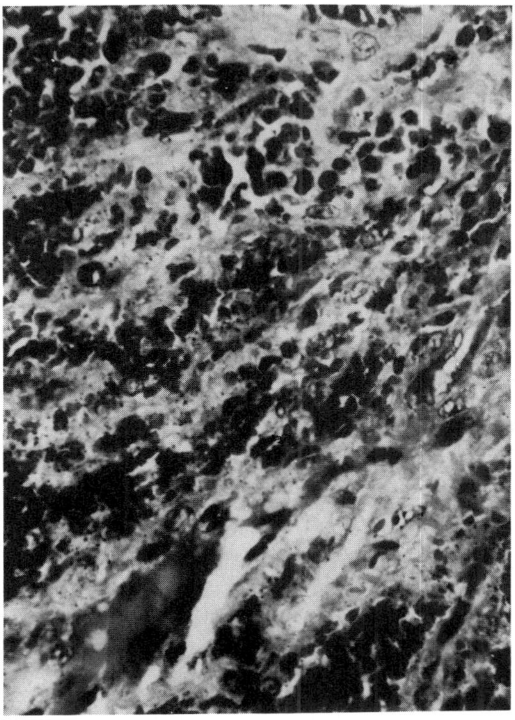

FIG 22–6.
Histopathology of KS. Spindle-shaped cells in dermis with extravasated erythrocytes.

lymph nodes and the gastrointestinal tract are quite similar to those in the skin, with spindle cells, extravasated red blood cells, and clefts all being prominent. Although the different clinical forms of Kaposi's sarcoma may differ substantially, there appears to be no difference between the histological features of classic KS and AIDS-associated KS.[21]

ETIOLOGY

The cell origin in KS is not known. Indeed, it is debated whether KS represents a true malignancy or an abnormal proliferation of endothelial cells in response to certain infectious or antigenic stimuli.[13] Different authors have suggested several various cell types as the origin of the neoplastic cell in KS.[22, 23] A reticuloendothelial origin has been suggested because of the increased association of lymphoreticular malignancies in classic KS.[7] Alternatively, an endothelial origin for KS has gained favor with the demonstration that KS cells appear to stain with anti-factor VIII antibodies.[24, 25] However, the results of all these studies remain tentative.

The role of viruses in the etiology of KS is another area of controversy. Cytomegalovirus (CMV) has been suggested as the agent by several authors. First, Giraldo et al.[26] demonstrated herpes-type viral particles in tissue culture cell lines from African KS patients.[26] There is also a known serological association between CMV infection and both classic[27, 28] and African[29] KS cases. Retroviruses may provide the immunosuppression necessary for the development of KS in AIDS, and may therefore promote the aggressive nature of the illness in this population.[20]

THERAPEUTIC APPROACHES

Therapeutic goals in the various forms of KS may be quite different.[30] In classic KS, treatment is primarily aimed at local control, and aggressive systemic therapy may not be warranted. In the more virulent African forms of the disease, an aggressive systemic approach may be more appropriate because of rapidly progressive skin and bone lesions, and the presence of visceral involvement.[31] In KS associated with renal transplant recipients, removal of the immunosuppressive agents alone may result in the spontaneous regression of the KS lesions.[15, 16] Finally, in AIDS-associated KS, the disseminated nature of the neoplasm warrants a systemic approach, but therapy is complicated by the profound immunosuppression of the disease itself.[30]

Classic Kaposi's Sarcoma

The initial treatment of classic KS is aimed at the management of skin disease. Although surgical removal may be practical when there are only a few isolated lesions, the multifocal nature of the disease limits this modality.[31] Cryosurgery with liquid nitrogen has proved effective for the destruction of tumors, and laser therapy has also been used with some success.[30]

Irradiation is an effective therapeutic modality and, indeed, it may be the primary form of therapy in classic KS.[32] Kaposi's sarcoma is an extremely radiosensitive tumor, and many radiotherapy regimens have proved effective. Individual spot therapy, limited and extended field radiation therapy, and total skin electron beam therapy have all been successful in treating skin disease.[32-36] Borok et al.[33] employed whole-leg radiation therapy for mild to moderate disease, using megavoltage therapy with a total skin dose of 3,000 rads, which was given in 20 fractions during a 4-week period. Lo et al.[34] treated 60 classical Kaposi's sarcoma patients via three different radiotherapy regimens with good results. Twenty patients received megavoltage photons, and 27 patients received a combination of both electrons and photons. These authors reported a response rate of 93% overall, following a single fractioned course of radiotherapy. They noted that a single dose of radiation therapy, of 800–1,200 rads, was necessary for effective treatment of localized skin lesions.[34] Harwood[35] treated 38 classic KS patients with extended field radiotherapy by irradiating at least half of the affected extremity with cobalt 60 radiation. This regimen was also found to be effective. Perhaps the most successful use of localized radiation therapy was reported by Nisce et al.[36] in their use of total skin electron beam therapy. They found a 100% overall treatment response rate in 20 classic Kaposi's sarcoma patients. These patients received 400 rads weekly to the entire skin surface for 6 to 8 weeks with use of a 3.5-MeV electron beam apparatus. In this group, 17 (85%) patients experienced complete remission of skin lesions, with the remainder having a partial response. Median duration of response was 48 months (range 10 to 92 months).[36] Thus, radiation therapy is an effective means of controlling local disease for prolonged periods of time in classic KS.

Chemotherapy has also been effective in classic KS. Although large trials with combination chemotherapy have primarily been conducted in African KS patients,[31] there is a significant amount of experience with single chemotherapeutic drugs in classical KS.[37-42] *Vinca* alkaloids are the most commonly administered chemotherapeutic agents for classical KS.[31, 39] Scott and Voight[37] were the first to use vincaleukoblastine in three American men with KS of the lower extremities with good results. Goldman et al.[38] reported prolonged remissions using systematic vinblastine therapy in five similar patients. Tucker and Winkelman[39] reviewed their own and 18 other cases in the literature of classic KS that had been treated with vinblastine. They concluded that significant tumor regression could be achieved in most patients, and that vinblastine was a relatively nonmyelosuppressive and nontoxic agent when given in a standard intravenous dose of 0.1 mg/kg/week.[39] Klein and co-workers[40] treated 14 classic KS patients with vinblastine, using a number of different routes of administration including intraarterial, intralesional, and systemic (intravenous). Following initial tumor regression, the patients were maintained on a low-dose maintenance regimen; the longer duration of treatment was in a patient who received 900 mg of vinblastine systemically over an 8-year period. Transient leukopenia was the primary side effect of therapy, but was mild in most cases. These authors reported good to excellent results in most patients.[40] Solan et al.[41] also treated four patients with classic KS with long-term intravenous vinblastine, with remissions of 2 to 7 years being achieved. They also felt that this was a nontoxic and relatively safe drug. Vincristine is another *Vinca* alkaloid that has been used (although less extensively) with some beneficial effect in classical KS. Odom and Goette[42] successfully treated KS lesions in a 68-year-old patient with intralesional vincristine sulfate, using injections of 0.4–0.5 mg/lesion. Single-agent chemotherapy, then, appears to be a safe and effective method for the management of skin tumors in classic KS.

Acquired Immunodeficiency Syndrome-Associated Kaposi's Syndrome

The treatment of KS in AIDS has been limited by the profound coincident immunosuppression and the high incidence of opportunistic infections. Whereas all of the treatment modalities effective in classic KS remain effective in AIDS-related KS, the aggressive and disseminated nature of epidemic KS often results in short-lived remissions. In addition, further immunosuppression by chemotherapeutic agents may add to the possibility of severe and potentially fatal opportunistic infections. Therefore, in addition to more traditional antineoplastic regimens, therapeutic approaches in AIDS-associated KS have included the use of biological response modifiers and anti-retroviral agents.[30]

The first immune modulator to be used with some effect in AIDS-related KS was interferon. This agent proved attractive because of its antiviral, antiproliferative, and immune-regulatory actions. Krown et al.[43] were the first to report its efficacy in AIDS-related KS. They treated 13 patients with high-dose recombinant leukocyte A interferon, at a dosage of 36×10^6 units to

54×10^6 units intramuscularly daily, for 28 days. Patients with evidence of tumor regression or stable disease by the end of the first 28 days of therapy were continued on three-times-a-week maintenance at the same dose. Of 12 evaluable patients, five exhibited major objective responses, with three of 12 patients achieving complete remission of KS tumors. Side effects consisted primarily of a flulike syndrome and mild myelosuppression. Opportunistic infections appeared to be infrequent in this initial group of patients.[43] Groopman and colleagues[44] reported the results of a randomized trial of high- versus low-dose recombinant interferon α_2. Twenty patients with AIDS-related KS were randomized and received either low-dose (1×10^6 units/m^2) or high-dose (50×10^6 units/m^2) recombinant interferon α. Treatment was given consecutively for 5 days, on alternate weeks, for three or four treatment cycles. Patients who exhibited some response were then continued on maintenance therapy at the same dose, with interferon being given on five consecutive days, once every 3 to 4 weeks. Patients who did not respond to the low-dose arm of the study were then allowed to cross over and receive high-dose interferon therapy. The higher dose of interferon appeared more efficacious, because an objective response was found in nine of 16 patients treated in this manner, compared with four of ten patients with an objective response in the low-dose arm. Survival and duration of response were beyond 11 months.[44] Opportunistic infections were infrequent, but did develop in four patients who failed interferon therapy.[44] Volberding et al.[45] have observed similar encouraging results with high-dose intravenous recombinant interferon α_2, and noted that opportunistic infections developed in only two of the 20 patients treated.[45, 46] Thus, interferon appears to be a promising agent for some patients with AIDS-related KS and is associated with a relatively low incidence of side effects and opportunistic infection.[46]

Another approach involves the combined use of interferon-alfa and anti-retroviral agents in HIV-associated KS. In a study of interferon-alfa and zidovudine, Krown et al. found tumor response rates exceeding 40%, especially in patients with higher CD4 counts (greater than 200/μl).[46] With this combination, tumor responses were seen at interferon-alfa doses far below those effective in single-agent therapy. Other anti-retroviral drugs, such as dideoxyinosine, are also entering similar trials. Further work is necessary with these and other agents to define their roles in this disease.[46]

Chemotherapy is also useful in the management of AIDS-related KS. As with classical forms of the disease, vinblastine has been the most effective single agent employed.[47] Volberding and co-workers[47] treated 20 patients with weekly intravenous vinblastine and noted an objective response rate of 37%. Opportunistic infections associated with this therapy presented a significant problem, however, with 25% of patients developing this complication.[47] Etoposide, or VP-16, is an investigational podophyllotoxin that has been used extensively by Laubenstein,[48] who reported a 79% response rate in 32 patients with AIDS-related KS who were treated with the drug; nearly half of these patients achieved complete remissions. However, these patients generally had less advanced disease, because individuals were excluded from the study if they had fever, weight loss, night sweats, or visceral involvement. Adverse reactions consisted primarily of mild alopecia and myelosuppression. The median survival and response rate appeared to be at least 10 months in this group.[48]

Combination chemotherapy has also been used in patients with more disseminated forms of AIDS-related KS.[49] Laubenstein et al.[50] treated patients with more advanced KS with Adriamycin (doxorubicin), bleomycin, and vinblastine sulfate (ABV). They observed an 80% response rate in these patients, but unfortunately 75% were partial rather then complete remission. There was, however, an extremely high rate of occurrence of opportunistic infections (50%) in these patients. Volberding[46] reported similar experiences with seven AIDS-associated KS patients, and noted that 6 patients had some objective responses, but four developed concurrent opportunistic infections. Volberding suggested that further trials of combination chemotherapy be postponed, pending the results of single-agent therapy.

Radiation therapy is another palliative measure for AIDS-related KS. Cooper and colleagues[32] have found that AIDS-related KS is extremely radiosensitive, in a manner similar to classic KS lesions. They treated 15 patients with megavoltage, kilovoltage, or a combination of both types of radiation. Doses ranged from 1,800 to 3,000 rads. All patients noted symptomatic improvement and shrinkage of the lesions, which flatten, and a significant decrease in discomfort. No complications were observed from radiotherapy.[32] Although this approach cannot address the multifocal nature of disease, it is a valuable method for palliation and cosmetic improvement.

SUMMARY

Kaposi's sarcoma, in its different clinical variants, represents a spectrum of neoplastic disease.[51, 52] In its most indolent form, classic KS remains primarily a cutaneous disorder. The therapy of classic KS is aimed at local control primarily through radiation therapy, but also through chemotherapeutic agents. At the other end of the spectrum is AIDS-associated KS, for which staging criteria have been proposed.[53] In this aggressive form of KS, effective tumor control is important because of the dissemination of disease. However, antineoplastic therapy may be complicated by severe accompanying immunosuppression. Immune restoration, through the use of biological response modifiers, has been helpful in achieving remissions in some patients. Single-agent and combination chemotherapy has also been used successfully in tumor management. In addition, irradiation is also effective in the treatment of cutaneous disease. Antiviral therapy against retroviruses may hold some promise for future approaches to KS in AIDS.

Many crucial questions remain unanswered. First, there is the elusive nature of the cell of origin in KS. Next, environmental factors, such as other viruses, may play a role in the pathogenesis of the disease. Genetic susceptibility may be an important contributory factor. Finally, there is the critical relationship between KS and the immune system. Further investigation is needed to understand this complex and intriguing neoplasm.

REFERENCES

1. Kaposi M: Indiopathisches multiples Pigmensarkom der Haut. *Arch Derm Syph* 1872; 4:265–273.
2. Safai B, Good RA: Kaposi's sarcoma: A review and recent developments. *Clin Bull* 1980; 10:62.
3. Myskowski PL, Romano JF, Safai B: Kaposi's sarcoma in young homosexual men. *Cutis* 1982; 29:31.
4. Oettle AG: Geographical and racial differences in the frequency of KS as evidence of environmental or genetic causes. *Acta-Unis Internationalis Contra Cancrum* 1962; 18:330.
5. Reynolds WA, Winkelmann RK, Soule EH: Kaposi's sarcoma. *Medicine* 1965; 44:419.
6. Dorn HF, Cutler SJ: Morbidity from cancer in the United States. Part I. Variation in incidence by age, sex, martial status and geographic region. *Public Health Monogr Wash DC* 1955; 29:121.
7. Safai B, Mike V, Giraldo G, et al: Association of Kaposi's sarcoma with second primary malignancies. *Cancer* 1980; 4:1472–1479.
8. Rothman S: Remarks on sex, age and racial distribution of Kaposi's sarcoma and on possible pathogenetic factors. *Acta Un Int Cancer* 1962; 18:322.
9. DiGiovanna JJ, Safai B: Kaposi's sarcoma: Review of ninety cases with particular emphasis on the familial occurrence, ethnic background, and prevalence of other disease. *Am J Med* 1981; 71:779–783.
10. Pollack MS, Safai B, Dupont B: HLA-DR5 and DR2 are susceptibility factors for acquired immunodeficiency syndrome with Kaposi's sarcoma in different ethnic subpopulations. *Dis Markers* 1983; 135–139.
11. Pollack MS, Safai B, Myskowski PL, et al: Frequency of HLA and Gm immunogenetic markers in Kaposi's sarcoma. *Tissue Antigens* 1983; 21:1–8.
12. Taylor JF, Templeton AC, Vogel CL, et al: Kaposi's sarcoma in Uganda: A clinicopathological study. *Int J Cancer* 1971; 8:122.
13. Safai B, Anhalt T: Kaposi's sarcoma. *Semin Dermatol* 1984; 3:69–71.
14. Templeton A, Hutt M: Distribution of tumors in Uganda. *Recent Results Cancer Res* 1973; 41:1–22.
15. Harwood AR, Osoba D, Hofstader SL, et al: Kaposi's sarcoma in recipients of renal transplants. *Am J Med* 1979; 67:759–765.
16. Stribling J, Weitzner S, Smith GV: Kaposi's sarcoma in renal allograft recipients. *Cancer* 1978; 42:442–446.
17. Klein M, Pereira F, Kantor I: Kaposi's sarcoma complicating systemic lupus erythematosus treated with immunosuppression. *Arch Dermatol* 1974; 110:602–605.
18. Centers for Disease Control: Epidemiologic aspects of the current outbreak of Kaposi's sarcoma and opportunistic infections. *N Engl J Med* 1982; 306:248–252.

19. Urmacher C, Myskowski P, Ochoa M, et al: Outbreak of Kaposi's sarcoma in young homosexual men. *Am J Med* 1982; 72:569–575.
20. Gallo RC, Salahuddin SZ, Popovic M, et al: Frequent detection and isolation of cytopathic retroviruses (HTLV-III) from patients with AIDS and at risk for AIDS. *Science* 1984; 224:500–503.
21. Gottlieb GJ, Ackerman AB: Kaposi's sarcoma: An extensively disseminated form in young homosexual men. *Hum Pathol* 1982; 13:882.
22. Hashimoto K, Lever WF: Kaposi's sarcoma: Histochemical and electron microscope studies. *J Invest Dermatol* 1964; 43:549.
23. Becker BJP: The histogenesis of Kaposi's sarcoma. *Acta Un Int Cancer* 1962; 18:477–485.
24. Guarda LG, Silva EG, Ordonex NGF, et al: Factor VIII in Kaposi's sarcoma. *Brief Sci Rep* 1981; 76:197–200.
25. Friedman-Kien AE: Disseminated Kaposi's sarcoma in young homosexual men. *J Am Acad Dermatol* 1981; 5:468–471.
26. Giraldo G, Beth E, Haguenau F: Herpes-type virus particles in tissue culture of Kaposi's sarcoma from different geographic regions. *J Natl Cancer Inst* 1972; 49:1509–1526.
27. Giraldo G, Beth E, Kaurilsky F, et al: Antibody patterns to herpes virus in Kaposi's sarcoma: Serological association of European Kaposi's sarcoma with cytomegalovirus. *Int J Cancer* 1975; 15:839–848.
28. Giraldo G, Beth E, Henle W, et al: Antibody patterns to herpes virus in Kaposi's sarcoma. II. Serological associations of American Kaposi's sarcoma with cytomegalovirus. *Int J Cancer* 1978; 22:126–131.
29. Giraldo G, Beth E, Huang E: Kaposi's sarcoma and its relationship to cytomegalovirus. III. CMV, DNA, and CMV early antigens in Kaposi's sarcoma. *Int J Cancer* 1980; 26:23–29.
30. Krown SE, Myskowski PL, Paredes J: Kaposi's sarcoma medical management of AIDS patients. *Med Clin N Amer* 1992; 76:235–252.
31. Olweny CLM, Toya T, Katongole-Mbiddle E, et al: Treatment of Kaposi's sarcoma by combination of actinomycin-D, vincristine and imidazole carboxamide (NSC-45388): Results of a randomized clinical trial. *Int J Cancer* 1974; 14:649–665.
32. Cooper JS, Fried PR, Laubenstein J: Initial observations on the effect of radiotherapy on epidemic Kaposi's sarcoma. *JAMA* 1984; 252:934–935.
33. Borok T, Farina AT, Leider MA: Radiotherapy for Kaposi's sarcoma. *J Dermatol Surg Oncol* 1979; 5:39–42.
34. Lo TCM, Salzman FA, Smedal M, et al: Radiotherapy for Kaposi's sarcoma. *Cancer* 1980; 45:684–687.
35. Harwood AR: Kaposi's sarcoma: An update on the results of extended field radiotherapy. *Arch Dermatol* 1981; 117:778.
36. Nisce LZ, Safai B, Poussin-Rosillo H: Once weekly total and subtotal skin electron beam therapy for Kaposi's sarcoma. *Cancer* 1981; 47:640–644.
37. Scott WP, Voight JA: Kaposi's sarcoma: Management with vincaleucoblastine. *Cancer* 1966; 19:557–564.
38. Goldman J, Greenwald ES, Schulman PL: Vinblastine therapy of Kaposi's sarcoma. *NY State J Med* 1974; 74:1828–1831.
39. Tucker SB, Winkelmann RK: Treatment of Kaposi's sarcoma with vinblastine. *Arch Dermatol* 1976; 74:958–961.
40. Klein E, Schwartz RA, Laor Y, et al: Treatment of Kaposi's sarcoma with vinblastine. *Cancer* 1980; 45:427–431.
41. Solan AJ, Greenwald ES, Silvay O: Long-term complete remissions of Kaposi's sarcoma with vinblastine therapy. *Cancer* 1981; 47:637–639.
42. Odom RB, Geotte DK. Treatment of cutaneous Kaposi's sarcoma with intralesional vincristine. *Arch Dermatol* 1978; 114:1693–1694.
43. Krown SE, Real FX, Cunningham-Rundles S, et al: Preliminary observations of the effect of recombinant leukocyte A interferon in homosexual men with Kaposi's syndrome. *N Engl J Med* 1983; 308:1071–1076.
44. Groopman JE, Gottlieb MS, Goodman J, et al: Recombinant alpha-2 interferon therapy for Kaposi's sarcoma associated with the acquired immunodeficiency syndrome. *Ann Intern Med* 1984; 100:671–675.
45. Volberding P, Moran T, Abrams D, et al: Recombinant alpha interferon therapy of Kaposi's sarcoma in the acquired immunodeficiency syndrome (abstract). *Blood* 1983; 62(suppl 1):118a.
46. Krown SE, Gold JWM, Niedzwiecki D, et al: Interferon-α with zidovudine: safety tolerance and clinical and virologic effects in patient's with Kaposi's Sarcoma associated with the acquired immunodeficiency syndrome (AIDS). *Ann Intern Med* 1990; 112:812–821.
47. Volberding P, Conant MA, Strickler RB, et al: Chemotherapy in advanced Kaposi's sarcoma. *Am J Med* 1983; 74:652–656.

48. Friedman-Kien AE, Laubenstein LJ, (eds): *AIDS: The Epidemic of Kaposi's Sarcoma and Opportunistic Infections.* (Papers based on an international symposium held at New York University Medical Center in 1983.) New York, Masson Publishing, 1984.

49. Gill PS, Rarick MU, Espina B, et al: Advanced acquired immunodeficiency syndrome-related Kaposi's sarcoma. Results of pilot studies using combination chemotherapy. *Cancer* 1990; 65:1074–1078.

50. Laubenstein LJ, Krigel RL, Odajnyk CM, et al: Treatment of epidemic Kaposi's sarcoma with etoposide or a combination of doxorubicin, bleomycin, and vinblastine. *J Clin Oncol* 1984; 2:1115–1120.

51. Bergfeld WF, Zemtsov A, Lang RS: Differentiation between AIDS-related and non-AIDS-related Kaposi's sarcoma. *Cleve Clin J Med* 1987; 54:315–319.

52. Odajnyk C, Muggia FM: Treatment of Kaposi's sarcoma: Overview and analysis by clinical setting. *J Clin Oncol* 1985; 3:1277–1285.

53. Krown SE, Metroka C, Wernz JC: Kaposi's sarcoma in the acquired immune deficiency syndrome: A proposal for uniform evaluation, response, and staging criteria. *J Clin Oncol* 1989; 7:1201–1207.

PART 3

Treatment: Surgical Techniques

Chapter 23

Methods of Biopsy

James P. Neifeld

Walter Lawrence, Jr.

Biopsy of a soft-tissue mass is done to determine whether it is a neoplasm or not and, if a neoplasm, whether it is benign or malignant. The subsequent definitive resection of the neoplasm would be considerably different for a large benign neurofibroma or intramuscular lipoma than for a fibrosarcoma, although the clinical findings prior to biopsy may be similar. The benign tumor would be properly "enucleated" with preservation of adjacent soft tissues, whereas the definitive procedure for the sarcoma would be radical soft-tissue resection with a truly adequate margin of normal tissue to achieve local control.

The specific type of neoplasm, if malignant, may influence the choice of primary treatment as well. For example, an extranodal lymphoma arising within the soft tissues would be better treated by irradiation than by a major, extensive soft-tissue resection or amputation. It is clear that treatment planning for the proper management of a soft-tissue mass requires a specific histological diagnosis, which must be obtained by some form of biopsy. If a soft-tissue sarcoma is identified by such a biopsy, the histology must also be examined from the standpoint of "grade," because this affects both proper staging and the treatment plan.

Sarcomas have been described in virtually all anatomical locations although, in adults, there is a preponderance of lesions in areas with bulky mesodermal tissue (e.g., the extremities, particularly the thigh). Also, variations in location seem to occur with differing histological classifications. Less often, the clinical presentation may be a dermal nodule (dermatofibrosarcoma protuberans), or a mass arising within a major body cavity (such as sarcomas arising from the mesoderm of the gastrointestinal tract or the retroperitoneum). However, the usual presentation is that of a nonspecific solid mass in the subcutaneous or deeper tissues brought to attention by its physical size and presence, discomfort, or more often by a recent change in size noted by the otherwise asymptomatic patient. The specific technique of biopsy chosen is affected by the anatomical location, but in general one should remember that the undiagnosed mass might be a sarcoma. The approach to biopsy should be planned by the surgeon so that any subsequent therapeutic operation will not be compromised. Except for those unusual lesions arising within the body cavities, this can be accomplished by following the simple principles to be described.

The temptation to enucleate an undiagnosed soft-tissue mass should be studiously avoided because this will often compromise the subsequent definitive resection of the sarcoma once the diagnosis is established. This is true for all sites, and sarcomas on the extremities that are potentially suitable for limb-preserving definitive resections are a patricular case in point. An overly aggressive, inadequate resection performed for biopsy purposes will often seriously jeopardize the subsequent procedure that is intended to retain limb function while achieving inadequate tissue margins around the sarcoma.

Four types of biopsy procedures can be employed to establish the diagnosis of soft-tissue sarcomas: fine-needle aspiration, core-needle biopsy, excisional biopsy, and incisional biopsy. Each of these will be discussed from the standpoint of their suitability and disadvantages under varying clinical circumstances.

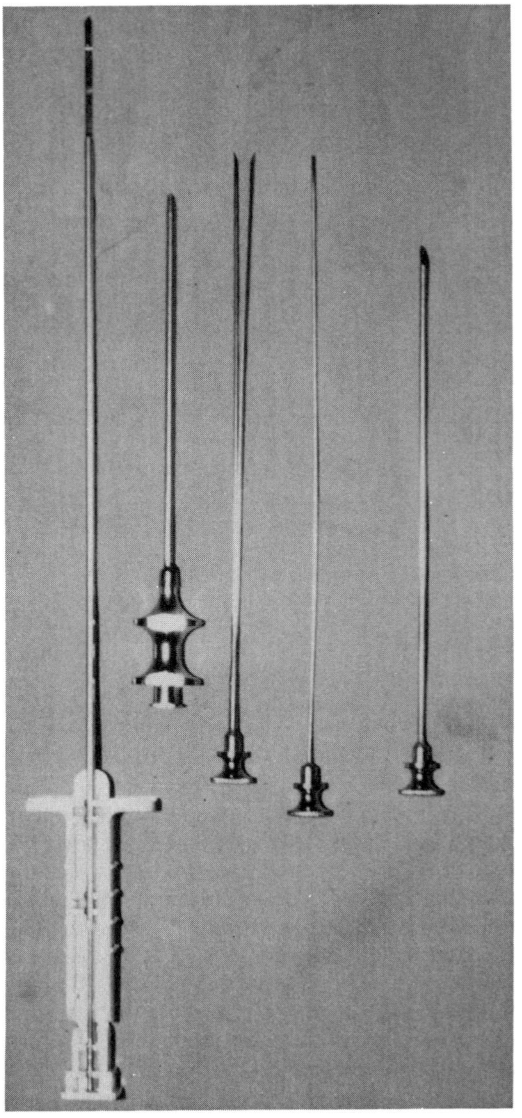

FIG 23–1.
Tru-Cut® (left) and Vim-Silverman (right) needles. These needles are useful in obtaining tissue cores for histological examination.

FINE-NEEDLE ASPIRATION

Fine-needle aspirations have been shown to be useful in the diagnosis of many carcinomas, but they should not be used for the initial definitive diagnosis of soft-tissue tumors. Although an aspiration biopsy of this type may demonstrate certain cytological characteristics consistent with a sarcoma, exact histological classification is difficult, and determining the degree of differentiation (or grade) is essentially impossible. For well-differentiated soft-tissue sarcomas, it may not be possible to differentiate a benign tumor from a malignant sarcoma with confidence. In addition, we have seen benign inflammatory lesions, such as thrombosed varices (which presented as groin masses), misdiagnosed as malignant fibrous histiocytomas by fine-needle aspiration, but incisional biopsy demonstrated the true nature of the mass. Fine-needle biopsy may, however, be useful in documenting locally recurrent or metastatic sarcoma (such as an enlarging pulmonary nodule) after prior treatment, when histological classification of the primary tumor has already been achieved. It should be stressed, then, that *initial* treatment for primary soft-tissue sarcomas should *not* be based on fine-needle aspiration biopsy.

CORE-NEEDLE BIOPSY

A core of tissue may be obtained by a core-needle biopsy obtained with various types of needles designed for this purpose, including the Vim-Silverman and Tru-Cut® needles (Fig 23–1). These special needles have the advantage of providing a true tissue diagnosis, rather than a cytological diagnosis. By obtaining several cores of tissue, one can employ a variety of diagnostic stains that may be helpful in histological characterization of the tumor, and a fragment can be processed for electron microscopic examination as well. The problem with this approach is the inadequacy of the histological material that is sometimes obtained, as well as the usual uncertainty of obtaining a sample at the viable outer edge of the tumor. Because specific histological classification and grading by this biopsy approach tends to be somewhat compromised, we do not consider this the procedure of choice for the biopsy of most sarcomas. Nevertheless, there are instances when this approach is chosen, such as in a child with prostatic rhabdomyosarcoma who will subsequently be treated by a chemotherapeutic program as the initial course of therapy. If operation is to be the initial treatment plan for a suspected extremity or trunk sarcoma, we prefer either incisional or excisional biopsy to this core-needle approach. The core-needle biopsy may be useful in diagnosing deep-seated masses, such as pelvic or retroperitoneal sarcomas, where open biopsy would require a major operation.

OPEN INCISIONAL OR EXCISIONAL BIOPSY

Either incisional or excisional biopsy of most soft-tissue masses is, in our view, the optimal approach to the diagnosis of suspected soft-tissue sarcomas. Many surgeons employ excisional biopsy quite freely, but we believe excision should be rarely performed when a soft-tissue tumor is suspected of being malignant. Except for small soft-tissue lesions, excisional biopsy will usually compromise the adjacent tissue planes for a subsequent adequate soft-part resection. The apparent "capsule" surrounding such a tumor, one that is tempting to use as a plan of excision for the biopsy, is actually a pseudocapsule composed of compressed fibrous tissue containing tumor cells. Merely enucleating such a mass will leave some tumor cells behind in the margin of the wound. This may make it extremely difficult to estimate the full extent of residual tumor at the time of the subsequent definitive operation. Only small tumors can be excised for biopsy without altering the surrounding tissue planes and compromising the subsequent operation. Another disadvantage of enucleation is that the removal of all palpable tumor may cause the patient to think that the tumor has been adequately treated and, therefore, refuse definitive therapy (Fig 23–2). Local recurrence rates following limited local excision approach 90%.

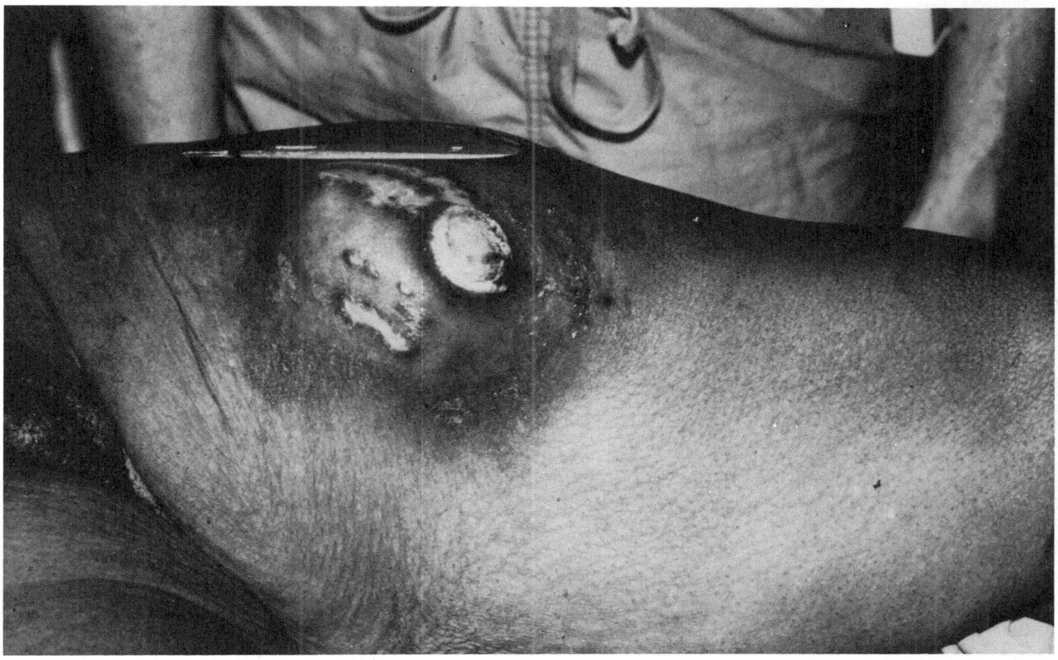

FIG 23–2.
Patient who underwent excisional biopsy of a 2-cm liposarcoma, but refused further surgery or radiation therapy because she thought the tumor had been removed. A recurrent mass became evident 5 months later, and she presented to the hospital 3 months afterward with an 18-cm tumor.

Figure 23–3 demonstrates an inappropriate transverse incision on an extremity to excise a small soft-tissue sarcoma in the biceps area of the arm. When a small soft-tissue tumor in an extremity is suitable for excision for biopsy purposes, the direction of the incision should be longitudinal and in the axis of the involved or underlying muscles. The incision should be short enough so that an appropriate ellipse of skin and underlying tissue can be included with the biopsy wound at the time of the subsequent wider, definitive soft-tissue resection.

Incisional biopsy of a soft-tissue mass is usually the procedure of choice for obtaining a diagnosis because most soft-tissue sarcomas have reached a significant size before they are brought to the attention of a physician. The incision should be carefully placed over the midportion of the tumor and aligned in such a way that the subsequent resection can easily encompass the biopsy wound itself with wide margins. On the extremity, this should be longitudinal in line with the extremity, as described above, for excisional biopsy. It should be placed in a location that will not compromise the subsequent curative procedure by either soft-tissue resection or amputation (if this should be necessary). Occasionally, in a patient with a deep-seated tumor, the midpoint of the mass may be difficult to ascertain by palpation; in this case, computed tomography is useful in delineating the extent of the tumor and aiding in placement of the biopsy incision. Figure 23–4 demonstrates a properly placed incision over a large mass in the medial aspect of the proximal thigh. For other anatomical locations, the placement of the biopsy incision should also be planned with subsequent resection in mind (Fig 23–5).

When incisional biopsy is performed, the incision should be carried directly through the overlying tissues down to the neoplasm and an elliptical portion of the tumor tissue excised by sharp dissection. A large enough specimen of

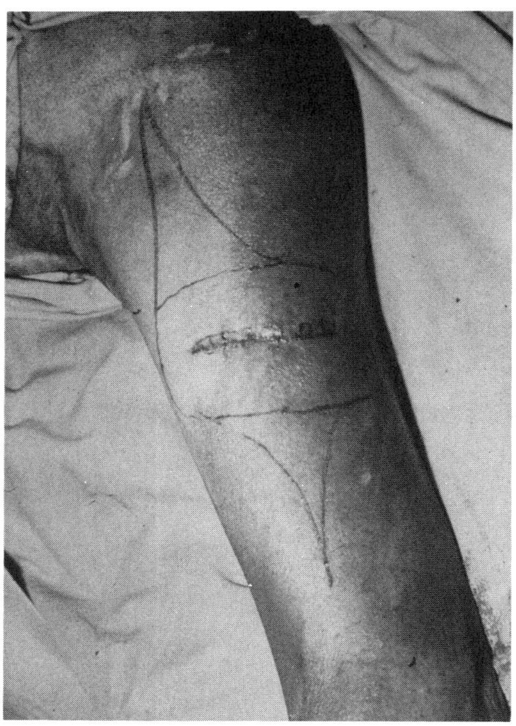

FIG 23–3.
Transverse incision over a sarcoma of the upper arm. This incision was inappropriate, and the definitive resection (outlined) could not be closed primarily due to the location of the biopsy incision.

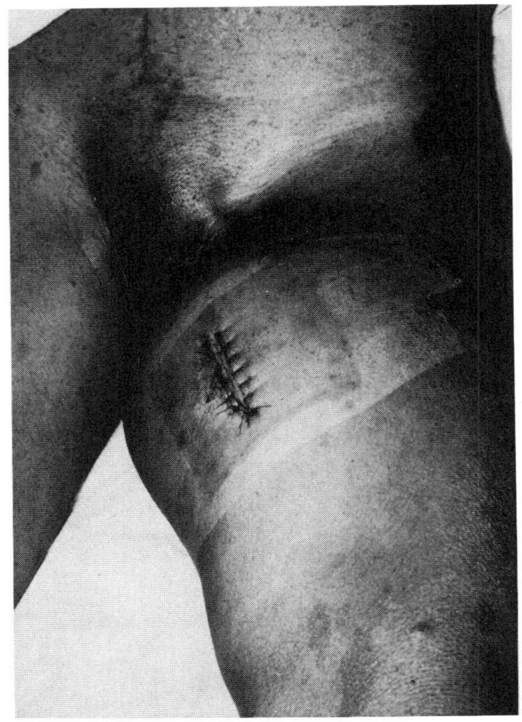

FIG 23–4.
Appropriate direction of biopsy incision over an upper thigh mass. The incision is placed so as not to preclude a definitive soft-tissue resection; the incision is also placed so that if amputation (hemipelvectomy) is required, the skin incisions will be distant from the biopsy incision.

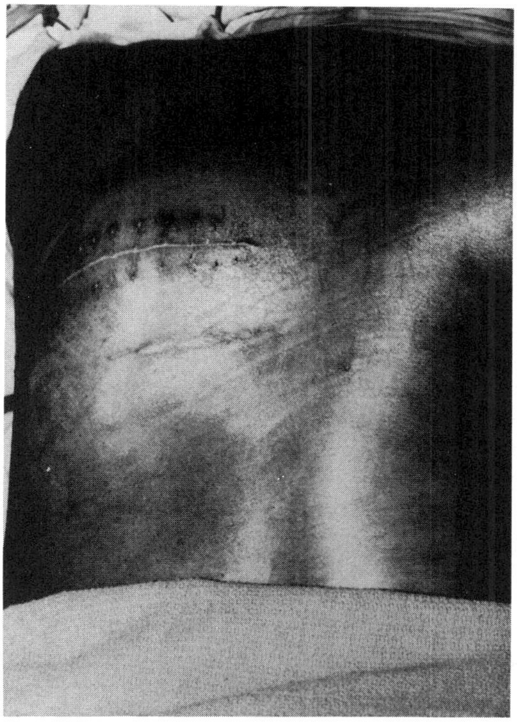

FIG 23–5.
Transverse incision over a liposarcoma overlying the left scapula (patient is lying supine). Although the incision is longer than usually required, its direction is appropriate for subsequent scapulectomy.

tumor tissue should be obtained to provide for appropriate light and electron microscopic studies, and hemostasis can be obtained by approximating sutures through the margins of the tumor tissue itself. We feel it is important to await permanent histological sections and, if necessary, the results of electron microscopy rather than basing treatment on a frozen section of the biopsy tissue. The frozen section diagnosis may be misleading and is certainly less precise than that provided by a more thorough study of the histological findings. Both histological diagnosis and degree of differentiation can be discussed in detail with the pathologist when this course is followed. Appropriate staging and optimal treatment planning are thereby accomplished.

SUMMARY

In summary, optimal treatment planning for soft-tissue masses suspected of being sarcomas requires attention to detail in the initial stage, particularly in performing the biopsy. Adequate tissue for precise diagnosis and staging is mandatory, and the biopsy technique should avoid any compromise of the adequacy of the subsequent operative procedure. If feasible, biopsy should be performed by the surgeon who will subsequently manage the patient by definitive operation.

SUGGESTED READINGS

Barth RJ, Jr, Merino MJ, Solomon D, et al. A prospective study of the value of core needle biopsy and fine needle aspiration in the diagnosis of soft tissue masses. *Surgery* 1992; 112:536–543.

Lawrence W Jr, Neifield JP, Terz JJ: *Manual of Soft-Tissue Tumor Surgery*. New York, Springer-Verlag, 1983.

Mankin HJ, Lange TA, Spanier SS: The hazards of biopsy in patients with malignant primary bone and soft-tissue tumors. *J Bone Joint Surg* 1982; 64-A: 1121–1127.

Sugarbaker PH, Nicholson TH: *Atlas of Extremity Sarcoma Surgery*. Philadelphia, J. B. Lippincott, 1984.

Chapter 24

Surgical Techniques for Extremity Soft-Tissue Sarcomas

Paul H. Sugarbaker

The major determinants for the surgical treatment of a soft-tissue sarcoma are the anatomical location of the primary tumor and its histological grade. The anatomical location of the tumor is found through laboratory and radiological tests that may indicate the presence of systemic metastases; also a careful physical examination, plus radiological and nuclear medicine studies, allow the physician to estimate the anatomical position of the tumor and its relationship to other, normal anatomical structures. Staging of the sarcoma is important because the requirements for a wide or narrow margin are determined by the histological grade of the malignancy. A complete discussion of the surgical considerations included in the assessment of the anatomical location and the histological grade is presented in Chapters 4 and 5. The goal of this chapter is to describe the surgical procedures that are available for removal of primary soft-tissue sarcoma of an extremity.

Wide local excision will be discussed first. This is a definitive treatment for low-grade tumors; however, radiation therapy and/or chemotherapy must be used in addition to surgery in patients with high-grade soft-tissue sarcomas. Next, the muscle group excisions that can be performed in both the upper and lower extremity will be discussed. Muscle group excisions (also commonly referred to as compartmental excisions) are used as the definitive treatment for selected sarcomas located favorably within muscle tissue so that a wide margin of excision is present at all points surrounding the tumor mass. If a satisfactory wide local excision is performed, radiation therapy and chemotherapy need not be added to the local treatment. However, chemotherapy for the adjuvant treatment of systemic disease may be indicated. The third group of procedures to be discussed are the amputations.

Figure 24–1 diagrams the treatment alternatives for extremity soft-tissue sarcoma. Amputation is considered when the other surgical treatments are not appropriate. Amputation should be performed in those patients in whom no

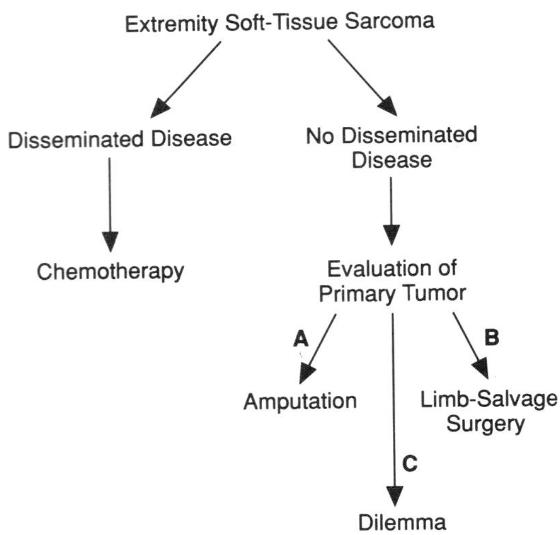

FIG 24–1.
Treatment alternatives for extremity soft-tissue sarcoma. **A,** Amputation indicated if evaluation of primary tumor shows (1) proximal margin of resection positive with limb salvage, (2) major vessel or nerve involved by primary tumor, or (3) major bone involved. **B,** Limb salvage indicated if evaluation of primary tumor shows local treatment failure unlikely. **C,** Problem group of patients exists in whom examinations of primary tumor do not give sufficient precise information. Evaluation suggests that limb-salvage surgery may not give optimal survival in this group.

other treatment alternative seems completely satisfactory. Quality of life data supplied by Sugarbaker and Barofsky[1] definitively showed that patients with major amputations for sarcoma had a good quality of life that was sometimes better than that following limb salvage treatment.

In this study, patients with large tumors of the upper thigh that required extensive surgery and an unusually wide field of irradiation were more satisfactorily treated by hemipelvectomy than by a limb salvage protocol. Wound-healing problems related to the radiation therapy, loss of sexual functioning, loss of reproductive capacity, and pain from radiation neuritis were found with the multimodality treatment (surgery, radiation therapy, and chemotherapy). These long-term problems were not present in the patients undergoing hemipelvectomy. In the era in which we live, with extensive use of the automobile and modern physical therapy methods, the mobility of these patients was equally as good as, often better than, patients receiving the limb-sparing treatment option. A single bothersome long-term feature of hemipelvectomy was phantom limb pain. Research in the treatment of pain needs to be focused on this clinical problem.

Our results with quality-of-life studies led us to suggest the following treatment plan. When managing patients in whom a surgical dilemma occurs, where evaluation of the primary tumor by physical examination and radiological tests does not give the clinician a clear signal as to whether amputation or limb salvage surgery should be selected, amputation should be selected as the treatment of choice. If the surgeon errs on the side of performing too many amputations, there will be no quality-of-life compromise; neither will there be suboptimal surgical results as evidenced by locally recurrent disease. However, if a surgeon performs a wide local excision that results in a local recurrence, the patient's chance for long-term survival has been severely compromised but quality of life has not improved. As diagnostic procedures to evaluate the primary sarcoma become more sophisticated, presumably fewer patients will fall into the dilemma group (Fig 24–1) in which a precise selection of treatment alternatives is impossible. This philosophy reflects the conviction that the overriding consideration is one of survival, and that if one is in doubt the survival consideration should dominate.

REMOVAL OF SOFT-TISSUE SARCOMA BY WIDE LOCAL EXCISION

Approximately 80% of extremity soft-tissue sarcomas can be treated by wide local excision plus wide-field, high-dose irradiation. This should be considered the standard treatment for sarcoma in an extremity.[2] Nearly all soft-tissue sarcomas of the head, neck, and trunk, and also retroperitoneal tumors, are treated by wide local excision. We cannot, of course, discuss anatomical structures that are encountered with tumors in all of these locations. Rather, the principles by which a soft-tissue sarcoma should be removed by wide local excision will be presented.

The overriding surgical principle for all wide local excisions of sarcoma is to *operate only within normal tissues*. To do this, previous biopsy sites and areas that may have been contaminated by hematoma as a result of the biopsy must be excised along with the local tumor. This surgical principle demands that the sarcoma should be removed without visualizing the tumor during the surgical excision. If tumor can be seen at the time of surgical excision, this will greatly increase the possible amount of tumor spillage and result in a greater incidence of local recurrence.

Resection of draining lymph nodes is not necessary to fulfill the surgical principles demanded by wide local excision. For soft-tissue sarcomas, lymph nodes, unless clinically suspected to contain tumor, need not be included within the specimen.[3]

Before operating using a wide local excision, consideration must be given to postoperative radiation therapy. The radiation therapist must be consulted prior to surgery. The structures to be preserved, especially lymphatics and veins, should be discussed so that a swollen and painful extremity will not result from the combined therapy. Also, during the surgery the surgeon must mark the extent of the dissection with metal clips. These metal clips allow the radiation therapist to ensure that all tissues potentially contaminated by tumor that were open at the time of tumor resection are included within the radiation field.

The surgery and subsequent radiation therapy should be planned so as not to jeopardize a subsequent amputation, should that be indicated. Radiation therapy should not heavily treat buttock skin in treating upper thigh sarcomas, because this would make hemipelvectomy for local recurrence difficult or impossible. Also, physical therapy and psychological counseling may be required as a part of this multimodality treatment. Especially if radiation therapy is given across a joint, physical therapy will be mandatory if optimal function is to be achieved.

As an example of a wide local excision, the removal of a liposarcoma located in the anterior thigh between quadriceps and adductor muscle groups is shown (Fig 24–2,A). Planning the excision is of utmost importance. Much thought should go into the resection prior to making a skin incision. First, the anticipated skin incision should be marked out, widely excising the previous biopsy site. Then, the limits of the skin flaps should be marked out on the skin surface. After making the skin incision and dissecting back the skin flaps, the surgeon can better palpate the extent of the tumor mass. At this point, vital structures in the anatomical area are identified and their relationship to the tumor mass determined (Fig 24–2,B). In the medial aspect of the thigh, these include the superficial femoral artery and vein. The extent of these vessels above and below the tumor is located, and then one proceeds to dissect these structures away from the specimen. An attempt to keep 2 cm of normal muscle tissue on the tumor specimen should be made to assure an adequate margin of excision. If this is done, daughter tumor nodules will be kept in the specimen. If an excision is done through the tumor pseudocapsule, there will be tumor seeding of the incision. Also, entering tumor vasculature within the pseudocapsule may result in extensive blood loss. The dissection continues, guided by the extent of the tumor mass but always proceeding from within normal tissue. Repeated palpation of the tumor mass through normal tissues during the dissection is required to keep from entering the tumor mass. After removal, the specimen is sent to the pathologist immediately so that the margins of excision can be assessed. Frequently, questionable margins indicated by the surgeon will be subjected to frozen-section examination. Prior to skin closure, the extent of the soft-tissue dissection is marked with metal clips to help the radiation therapist in treatment planning. Closure of the wide local excision is uncomplicated. The subcutaneous tissue is closed with absorbable suture and the skin is closed using plastic surgical technique. The tissue spaces are eliminated using suction drains.

The surgical principles for excision of a sarcoma on the head, neck, or trunk or in the retroperitoneum are essentially the same as for an extremity. The overriding principle involved in tumor excision is that all dissection is done from within normal tissues. If the dissection strays into the tumor capsule, tumor cells are spilled, and blood loss may become uncontrolled. For head, neck, and trunk sarcomas, the margins of excision are often not favorable. Vital structures such as the vertebral column may be left as a positive margin. These should be carefully marked with metal clips so that high-dose boost radiation fields can be applied. Treatment of these tumors by radiation alone can usually be equated with no treatment at all. For best results a vigorous attempt at a complete surgical excision should be made, positive margins noted, and then radiation therapy used as an adjunct. Intra-operative radiation therapy is currently being explored as an adjunct in patients with positive surgical margins.

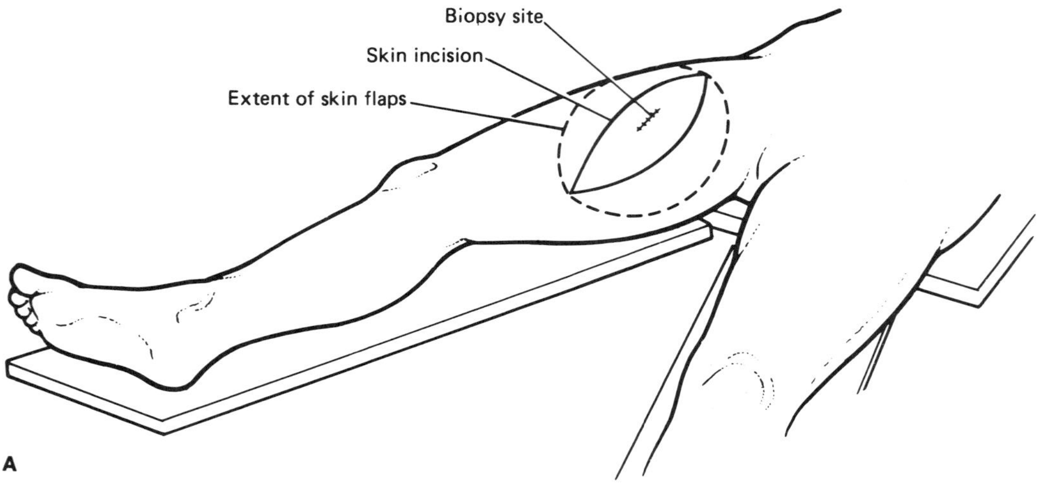

A

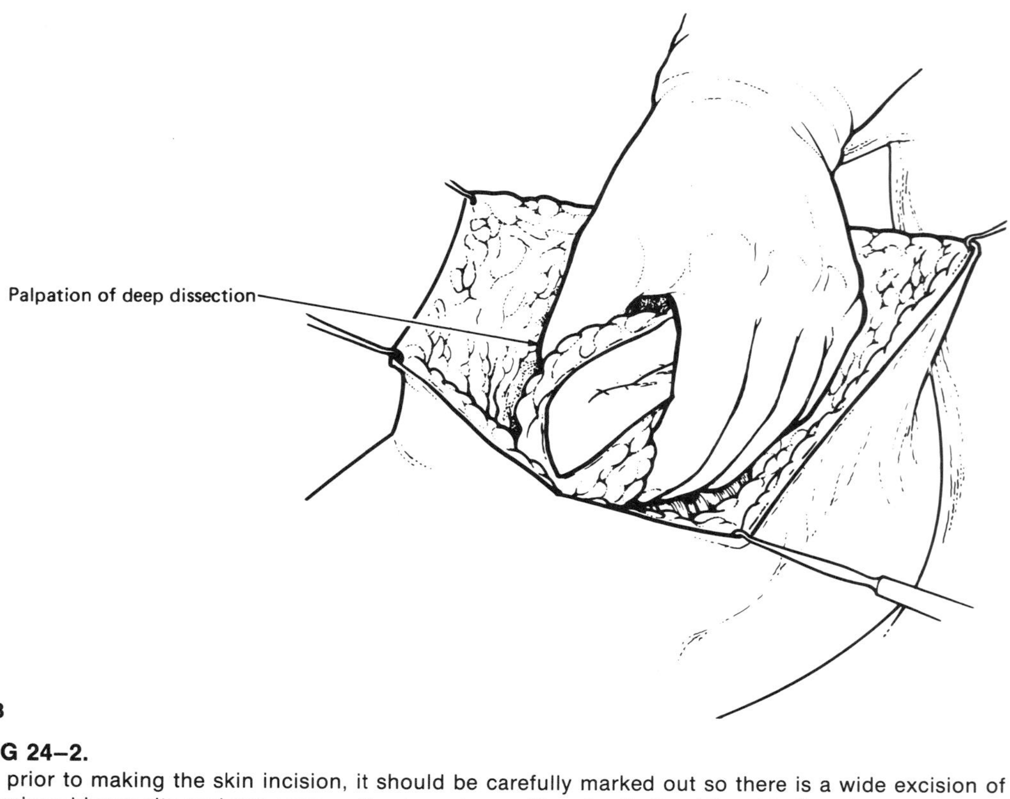

B

FIG 24–2.
A, prior to making the skin incision, it should be carefully marked out so there is a wide excision of the previous biopsy site and any surrounding hematoma. Also, the limits of the skin flap should be indicated. **B,** after making the skin incision and dissecting back the skin flaps, the surgeon can better palpate the extent of the tumor mass. Repeated examination of the tumor mass by palpation through normal tissues during the dissection is required to keep from tearing into the tumor mass and spilling tumor cells.

MUSCLE GROUP EXCISION FOR THE TREATMENT OF EXTREMITY SARCOMA

Several muscle group excisions can be performed for the complete treatment of extremity sarcomas anatomically favorably located. The procedure most frequently performed is the adductor muscle group excision. Quadriceps muscle group excisions are also frequently required. The buttockectomy procedure for sarcomas superficial to or within the gluteus maximus muscle is possible. Also, a muscle group excision of the posterior thigh, anterior compartment of the leg or posterior compartment of the leg is possible.

Adductor Muscle Group Excision.—Successful adductor muscle group excision is accomplished when a tumor of the medial thigh is excised with a wide margin of normal tissue but venous, arterial, and lymphatic supply to the leg is preserved.[4] The structures contained within this compartmental excision are shown diagrammatically in Figure 24–3,A. The patient is placed on an exenteration table, and a long incision from pubic tubercle to medial epicondyle of the tibia is made. Skin flaps are raised medially to the flexor muscles and laterally to the sartorius muscle. The femoral triangle is dissected to visualize the superficial femoral artery and vein but to avoid damage to the superficial inguinal lymphatics and saphenous vein. Also, some loose areolar tissue and lymphatic channels on the superficial femoral artery and vein should be preserved, if possible, to spare some lymphatic channels along these major vessels.

The dissection proceeds from lateral to medial; starting with the pectineus, all the adductor muscles are released from their origins on the superior and inferior pubic rami. Care is taken to preserve the obturator externus muscle. The pelvic bones form the proximal limits of the dissection. The origins of the flexor muscles and the quadratus femoris muscle are left intact as they arise from the ischial tuberosity. The adductor muscles are then released from the shaft of the femur. The superficial femoral artery and vein are traced from proximal to distal and the branches into the adductor muscle group ligated. This includes the profunda femoris vessels (Fig 24–3,B). Distally, the insertions of the muscle are divided at the medial epicondyle of the knee. This releases the specimen, which is carefully oriented for the pathologist. The extent of the dissection is marked with metal clips in case the margins of excision are positive and postoperative irradiation therapy is thought to be required.

Quadriceps Muscle Group Excision.—A quadriceps muscle group excision is appropriate for the definitive treatment of soft-tissue tumors confined within the quadriceps muscle group.[5] It may be the treatment of choice even for low-grade tumors, located distally in the muscle group, that require excision of the patella or patellar tendon. Retaining the quadriceps muscle mass is pointless if muscle function is lost because of patellar tendon removal. The tissue removed in the quadriceps muscle group excision is shown in Figure 24–4,A.

The incision extends longitudinally from the anterior inferior iliac spine to the patella. If the patella is to be removed, the incision should extend down to the anterior tibial tubercle. The incision should be elliptical to encompass the biopsy site widely. Skin flaps are made superficial to the fascia lata; they extend to the adductor group medially and to the greater trochanter and flexor muscles laterally. The dissection begins proximally with exposure of the common femoral artery and vein. The saphenous vein is divided as it enters the fossa ovalis. The inguinal ligament and femoral triangle are unroofed, exposing the common femoral artery and vein and the femoral nerve. Lateral traction is placed on the quadriceps muscle group so that muscular branches of the superficial femoral artery and vein into the quadriceps muscles are placed on traction. These vessels are ligated and divided. Care should be taken in the distal portion of the dissection not to damage the superficial femoral artery as it passes through the adductor canal beneath the sartorius muscle.

Starting proximally, the origins of the quadriceps muscles are released. Electrocautery is used to release the tensor fasciae latae muscle from its origins on the wing of the ilium. The sartorius muscle is released from the anterior superior iliac spine, and the rectus femoris muscle is released from the anterior inferior iliac spine. Transections of these muscles are through their tendinous portions to keep blood loss at a minimum (Fig 24–4,B). The origins of the vastus lateralis, vastus intermedius, and vastus medialis on the femur are transected from the bone using electrocautery. Strong upward traction on the muscle group facilitates this dissection. Moving from proximal to distal

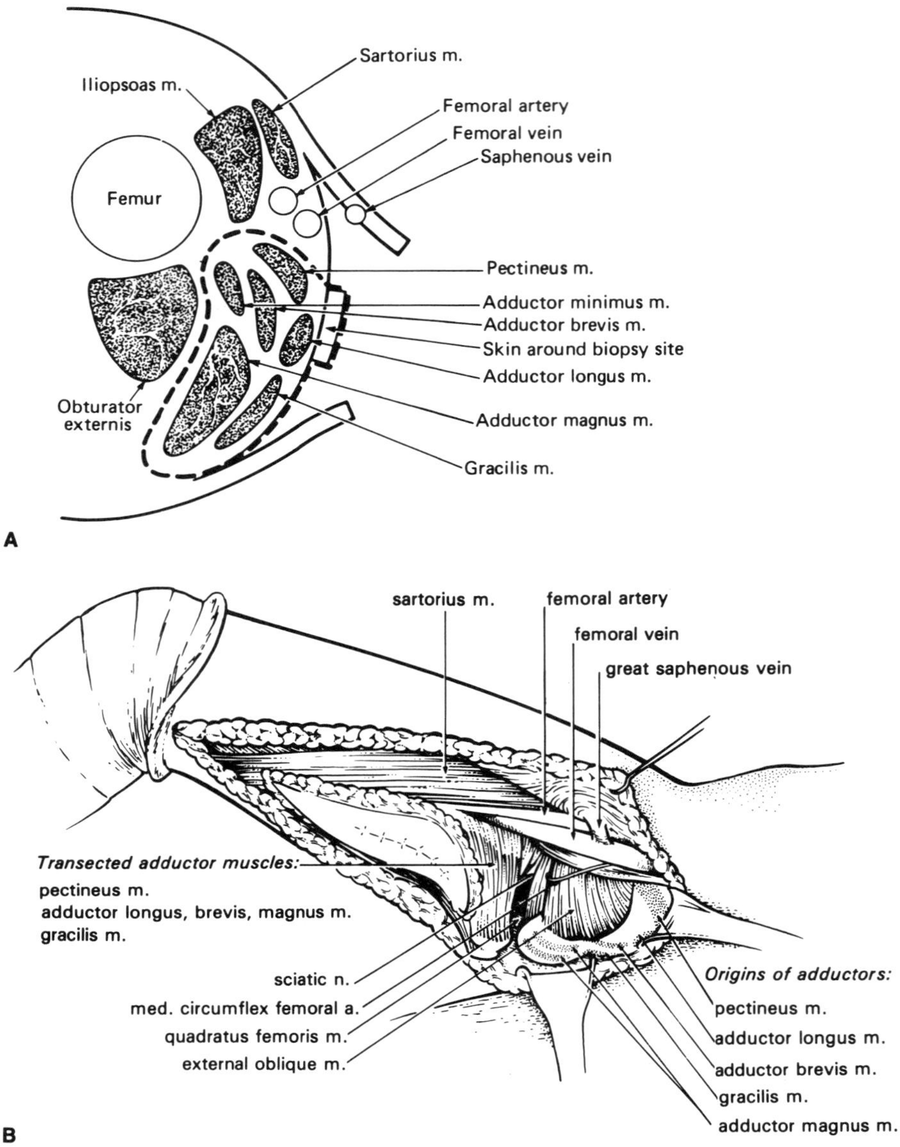

FIG 24–3.
A, structures of the medial thigh excised in performing an adductor muscle group excision. **B,** dissection of the superficial femoral artery and vein after release of the adductor muscles from the pubic rami; branches of the femoral artery to the adductor muscle are isolated, ligated, and divided. This includes the profunda femoris artery. The superficial femoral artery and vein are dissected free of the specimen down to the area of the adductor canal.

FIG 24–4.
A, tissue to be excised in a quadriceps muscle group excision. **B,** transection of quadriceps muscle insertions from the pelvis. After visualization of the superficial femoral artery and vein, multiple branches from these vessels to the quadriceps muscles are isolated, ligated, and divided. The femoral nerve is ligated and divided. This allows division of the sartorius muscle from the anterior superior iliac spine, the tensor fasciae latae muscle from its tendinous origin, and the rectus femoris muscle from the anterior inferior iliac spine. The origins of the other quadriceps muscles are on the femur itself. **C,** comparison of the extent of muscle excision in a wide local excision (dotted line of excision) versus a quadriceps muscle group excision (dashed line of excision). **D,** cross-section comparing the extent of muscle excision in a wide local excision and in a quadriceps muscle group excision.

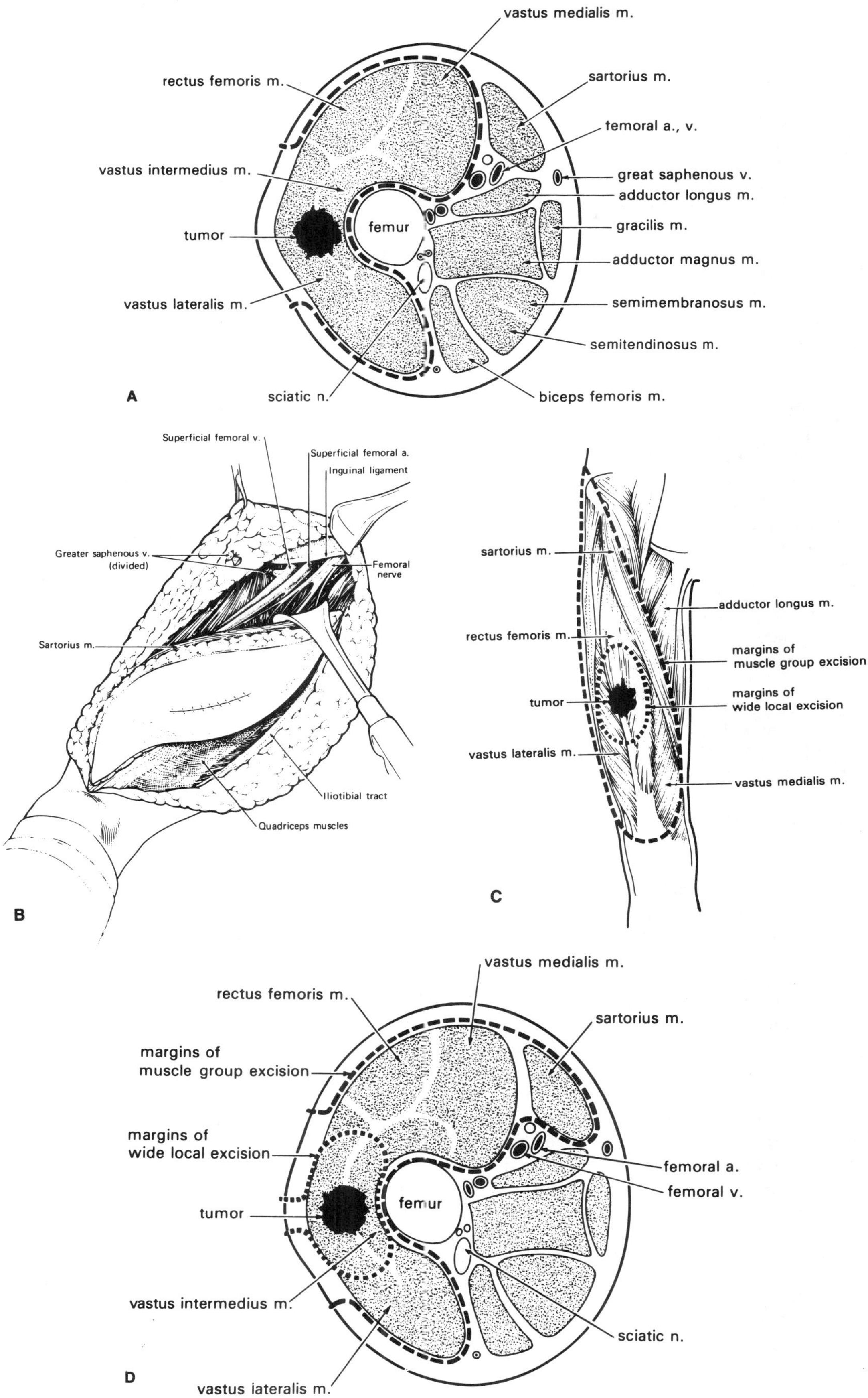

vastus medialis m.
rectus femoris m.
sartorius m.
femoral a., v.
vastus intermedius m.
great saphenous v.
adductor longus m.
femur
tumor
gracilis m.
adductor magnus m.
vastus lateralis m.
semimembranosus m.
semitendinosus m.
A
sciatic n.
biceps femoris m.
Superficial femoral v.
Superficial femoral a.
Inguinal ligament
Greater saphenous v.
(divided)
Femoral
nerve
Sartorius m.
Iliotibial tract
Quadriceps muscles
B
sartorius m.
adductor longus m.
rectus femoris m.
margins of
muscle group excision
tumor
margins of
wide local excision
vastus lateralis m.
vastus medialis m.
C
vastus medialis m.
rectus femoris m.
sartorius m.
margins of
muscle group excision
margins of
wide local excision
femoral a.
femoral v.
femur
tumor
vastus intermedius m.
sciatic n.
D
vastus lateralis m.

the entire quadriceps muscle mass is dissected free; transection of tissues through the prepatellar and postpatellar bursae allows elevation of the specimen. The patella should be left behind if possible. To do so, the specimen is delivered by incising through the patellar tendon in its tendinous portion.

To facilitate rehabilitation and help provide stability to the knee, the gracilis muscle medially and the short head of the biceps muscle laterally are used in reconstruction. These muscles are divided through their tendinous insertions on the medial and lateral collateral ligaments and transplanted to the patellar tendon. If the patella is excised, this muscle reconstruction is not possible. Suction drainage is achieved with catheters beneath the skin flaps. The subcutaneous tissue is closed with absorbable sutures and the skin is closed using a plastic surgery skin closure technique. An ankle-foot orthosis is provided in the postoperative period. This blocks dorsiflexion of the ankle and maintains five or more degrees of plantar flexion, and prevents flexion of the knee on contact with the floor.[6] Patients should continue to use a cane in their contralateral hand.

Figures 24–4,C and 24–4,D illustrate the differences in wide local excision and muscle group excision. For a tumor in the midportion of the anterior thigh, a wide local excision would remove the tumor and 2 to 3 cm of normal muscle tissue on either side of the malignancy. Following this, the entire quadriceps muscle group would be treated with radiation therapy. For a muscle group excision, the entire quadriceps mechanism is removed from origin to insertion. No postoperative radiation therapy is required.

Buttockectomy.—The buttockectomy is an en bloc resection of the gluteus maximus muscle and is usually performed for low-grade tumors in this anatomical site.[7, 8] The patient is placed in the supine position on an exenteration table with the legs slightly separated. A generous incision encompassing the biopsy site and tumor is outlined. Six to 8 cm of skin can be sacrificed and yet close the skin, primarily because of the excess skin provided by the gluteal fold. The skin flaps are dissected superiorly to the crest of the ilium, medially to the midline, inferiorly to the gluteal fold, and laterally to the greater trochanter. The skin flaps are tapered so they become progressively thicker toward their base (Fig 24–5,A). The gluteal fascia should be left on the specimen. After dissecting the superior and inferior skin flaps, the lower rolled edge of the gluteus maximus muscle is located. The insertion of this muscle is released from the iliotibial tract and greater trochanter. This dissection begins exposure of the deep margin of the muscle. Continuing in a clockwise direction, for a left buttock tumor, the origins of the gluteus maximus muscle on the crest of the ileum are divided from lateral to medial. This allows elevation of the muscle from the sciatic nerve and allows visualization of the superior and inferior gluteal vessels that are present above and below the piriformis muscle (Fig 24–5,B). To complete the removal of the specimen, the origins of the gluteus maximus muscle on the sacrum, iliotibial tract, and coccyx are divided. The excision site is copiously irrigated and any further bleeding points secured. Suction drainage is secured beneath the skin flaps. The subcutaneous tissue is closed with absorbable sutures, and the skin is closed using a plastic surgical technique.

Muscle Group Excision of the Posterior Thigh.—Occasionally, a tumor located within the hamstring muscles can be curatively removed with a muscle group excision of the posterior thigh. However, usually high-grade tumors in this region are intimately associated with the sciatic nerve. When this occurs, a wide local excision with stripping of the tumor from the sciatic nerve is required for removal of the sarcoma. For large tumors, a hemipelvectomy may be required. Alternatively, high-dose radiation therapy to the excision site, covering the positive margin on the sciatic nerve, has resulted in good rates of local control. An exception to this is sarcomas of neural origin arising in the posterior thigh. These tumors intimately involve the sciatic nerve and require excision of this nerve if the extremity is to be spared (Fig 24–6). Surprisingly, a flexor muscle group excision that includes the sciatic nerve gives rather good function results.

Excision of the Anterior Compartment of the Leg.—The muscle and soft tissue to be removed are shown in Figure 24–7. A longitudinal incision is made from the head of the fibula down to the level of the malleoli. Skin flaps are dissected back to the tibia medially and to the fibula laterally. Working from medial to lateral, the anterior tibial artery is isolated, ligated, and divided. Superficial and deep branches of the peroneal nerve also must be divided. As the muscle is removed from proximal to distal (Fig

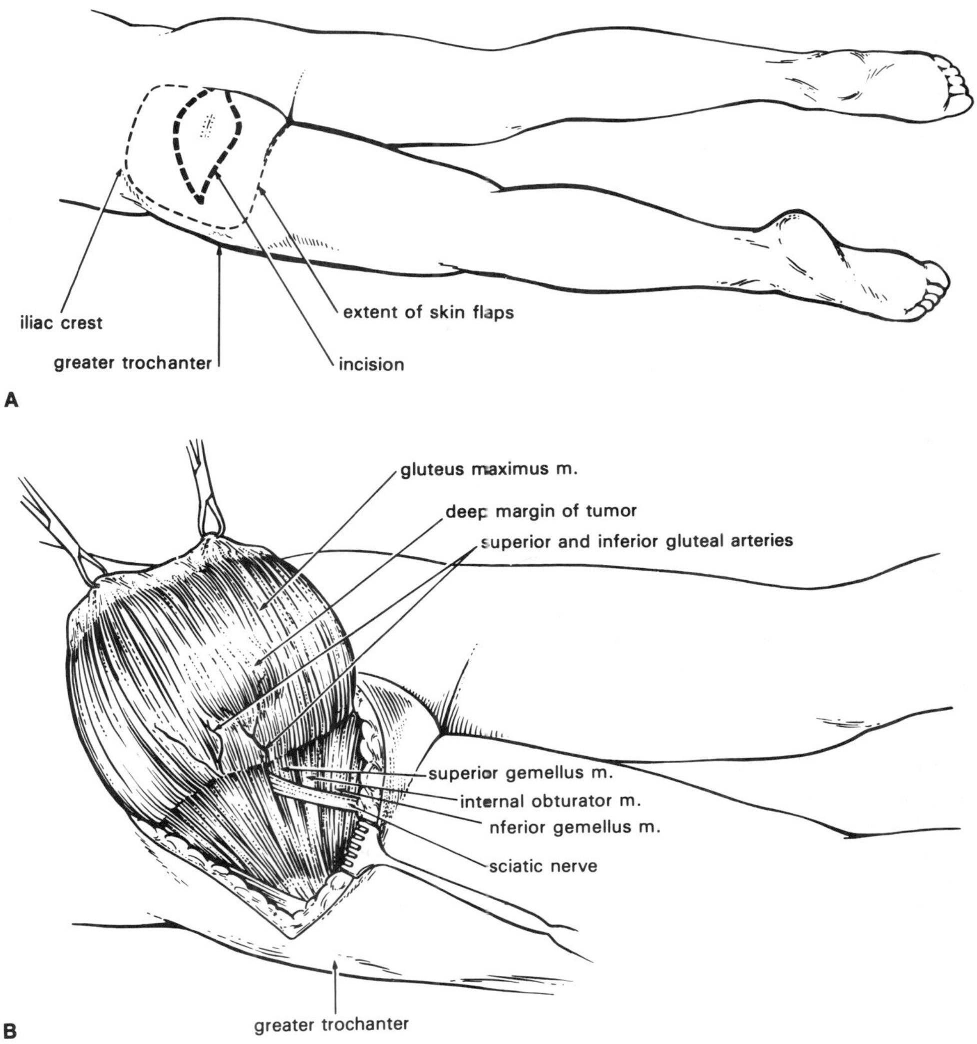

FIG 24–5.
A, line of incision and extent of the skin flaps for the buttockectomy procedure. **B,** elevation of the specimen from lateral to medial allows visualization of the sciatic nerve, superior gluteal vessels, and inferior gluteal vessels. These large vessels are present above and below the piriformis muscle.

24–7), the tendons that must be divided are identified; these are sutured to the fascial edge so they do not retract down into the foot. The extent of the dissection is marked with metal clips, the subcutaneous tissue is closed with absorbable sutures, and the skin is closed using a plastic surgical technique. Suction drainage is achieved with catheters brought out through stab incisions at the most proximal portion of the dissection.

An excision of the proximal portion of the fibula is often an appropriate procedure for osteosarcoma of the proximal fibula; this procedure is rarely, if ever, indicated for a soft-tissue sarcoma.

Muscle Group Excision of the Posterior Leg.—For tumors within the calf, a muscle group excision of the entire posterior compartment may be adequate. The medial and lateral gastrocnemius muscles, the soleus muscle, posterior tibial, and popliteal muscles can be removed from origin to insertion (Fig 24–8). The peroneal artery and vein and the tibial nerve

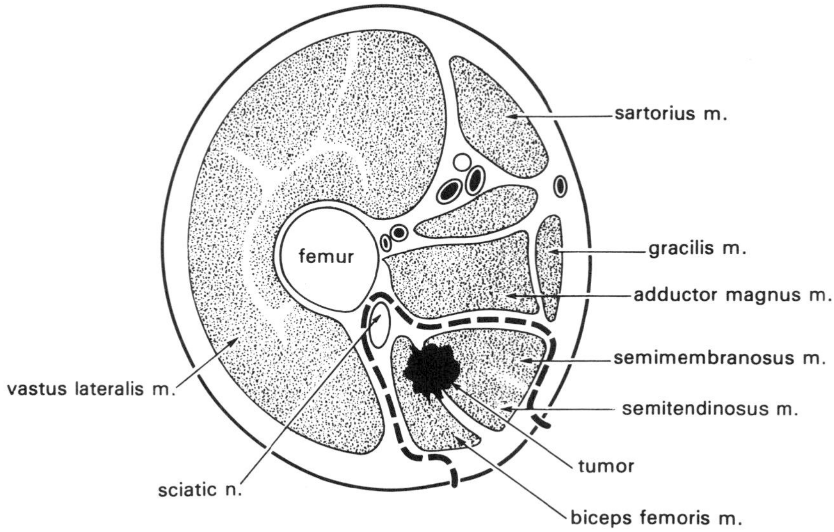

FIG 24–6.
The resection of a soft-tissue sarcoma of the posterior thigh involves excision of the biceps femoris, semitendinosus, and semimembranosus muscles. If the tumor is intimately involved with the sciatic nerve or arises from it, the nerve must be sacrificed with the specimen. In some situations, a positive tumor margin on the sciatic nerve may be treated with postoperative radiation therapy.

must be sacrificed. The anterior tibial artery and vein and the common peroneal nerve in the anterior compartment are left to supply the remaining leg and foot. An orthotic device is required postoperatively, but the mobility required for walking is usually preserved.

Several other muscle group excisions for extremity soft-tissue sarcoma are occasionally possible. Excisions of the biceps or triceps muscles have been performed. Usually when tumors occur in these areas, a wide local excision supplemented by wide-field, high-dose radiation

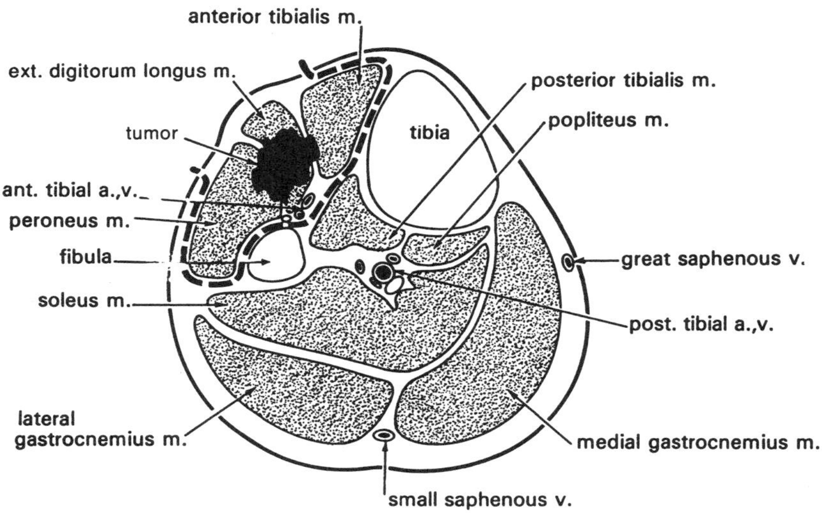

FIG 24–7.
Excision of the anterior compartment of the leg.

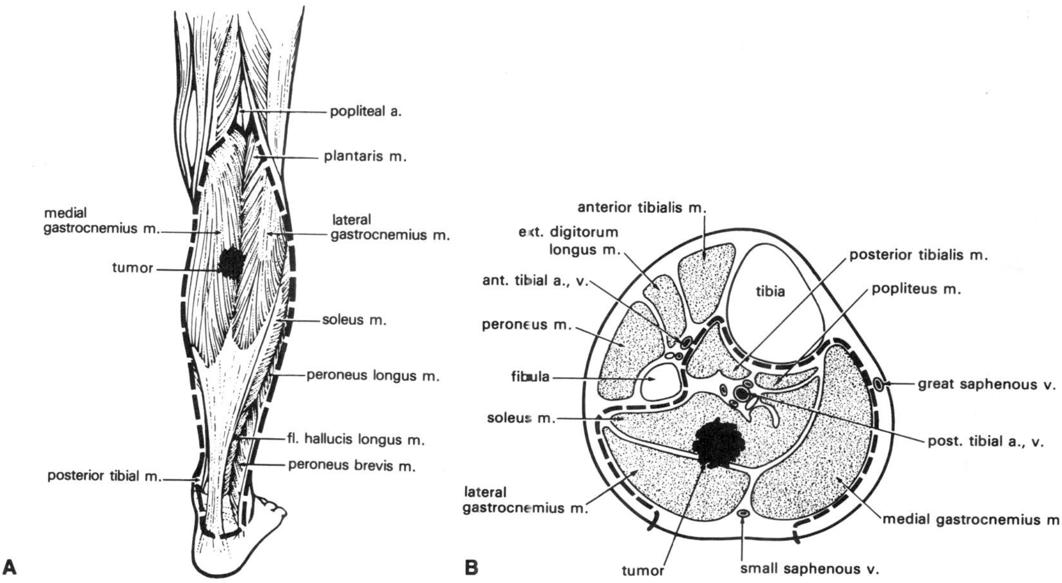

FIG 24–8.
A, posterior leg illustrating the extent of a muscle group excision of the calf muscles. **B,** transverse section through the leg illustrating the radical resection of gastrocnemius, soleus, popliteus, and posterior tibial muscle.

therapy gives a better functional result without compromising the local control of tumor. Also, small tumors in the flexor or extensor muscle groups of the forearm are best treated by wide local excision plus postoperative radiation therapy. In the upper extremity, where radiation therapy to high doses is well tolerated, wide local excision is usually a superior treatment to muscle group excision.

Scapulectomy.—Scapulectomy is indicated for soft-tissue tumors located superficial to the scapula and for primary malignant tumors of this bone.[9] The patient is placed in the prone position with the arm resting in 90° abduction on an arm board. The arm should be draped free so that an assistant can move the arm as required during the operation. A skin incision is made encompassing the tumor and previous biopsy site. It extends from the tip of the acromion obliquely to below the tip of the scapula. Skin flaps are constructed so that the medial and lateral borders of the scapula can be easily palpated (Fig 24–9,A). The attachments of the neck and back muscles to the posterior and superior portion of the scapula are divided. Superiorly, the attachment of the deltoid muscle to the lateral tip of the scapular spine is similarly divided. Muscles divided include the rhomboids, latissimus dorsi, trapezius, and levator scapulae muscles. The proximal portion of the trapezius and levator scapulae muscles should be tagged with a suture so they are easily located for use in reconstruction. If the tip of the scapula is retracted downward, the back muscles to be transected are stretched and can then be divided bloodlessly using electrocautery. A straight towel clip through the tip of the scapula is helpful to complete this maneuver. If the inferior tip of the scapula is elevated, the contents of the axilla can be identified. The neurovascular bundle is dissected off the specimen anteriorly and protected. The lateral muscles attached to the scapula include the teres major, teres minor, and the long head of the triceps. These are transected through their tendinous portions near the scapula. Next, supraspinatus and infraspinatus tendons and attachments of the serratus anterior muscles are released from the scapula. The shoulder joint is exposed from beneath the skin flap. The scapular spine is divided near the acromion by using an osteotome. The only muscle remaining attached to the scapula is the subscapularis. This is transected from the chest wall, leaving the major portion of the muscle on the specimen (Fig 24–9,B).

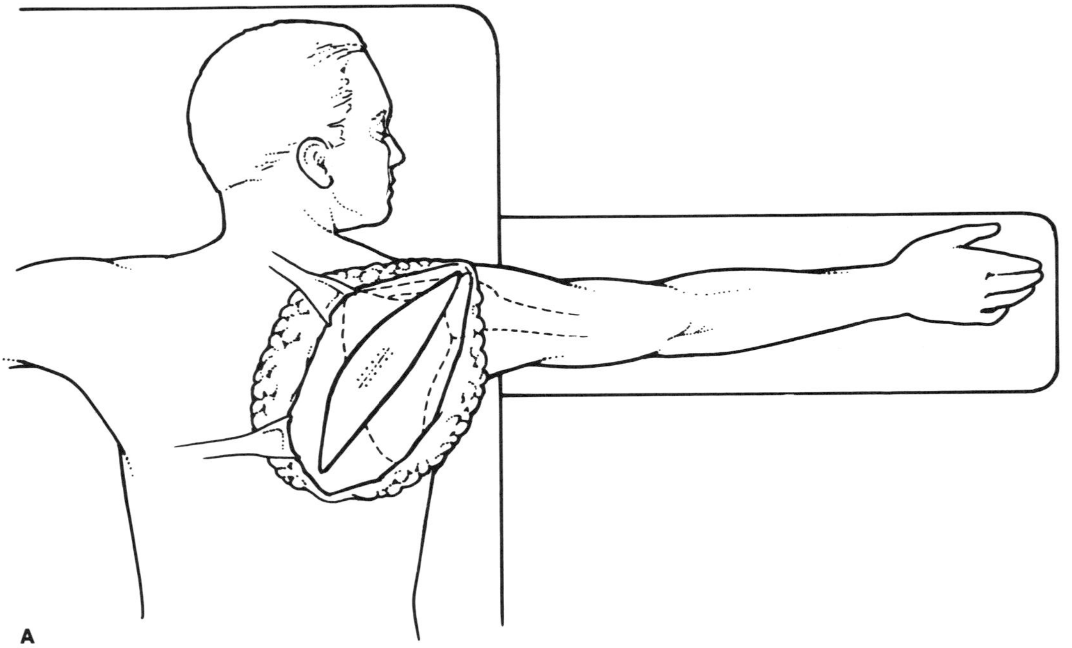

A

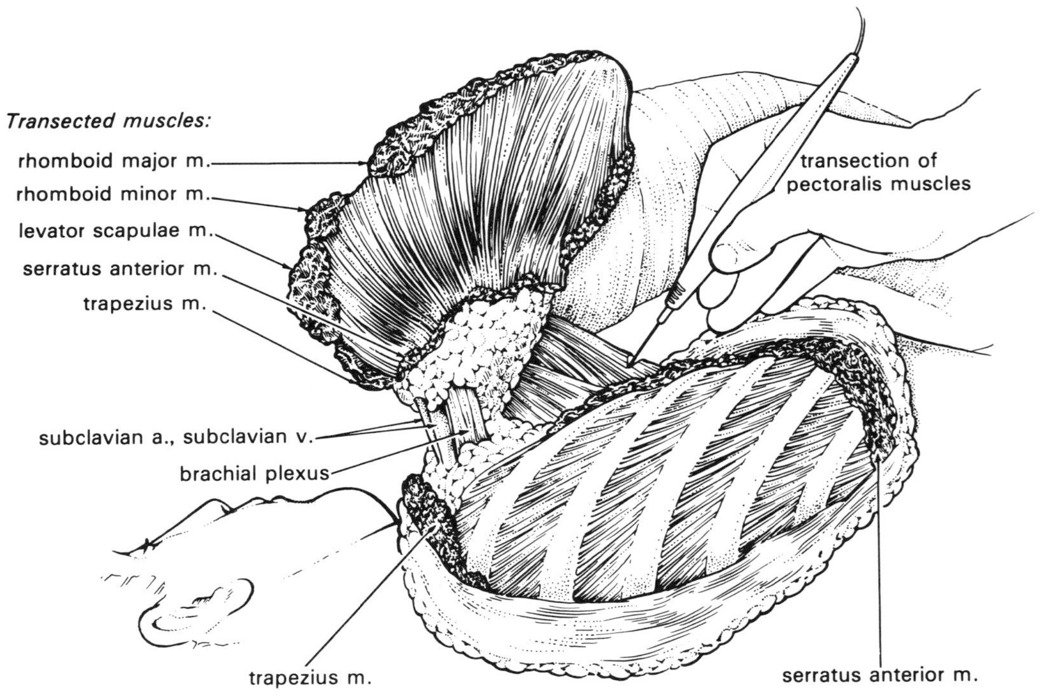

B

FIG 24–9.
A, incision and extent of skin flaps for a scapulectomy. **B,** release of muscular attachments of the scapula in a scapulectomy. The medial attachments of the scapula are first divided, then the lateral muscles are transected. Finally, the glenohumeral joint is transected. To prevent traction on neurovascular structures postoperatively, the trapezius muscle should be secured to the tendinous portion of the rotator cuff that has been preserved on the humerus.

An osteotomy through the neck of the scapula may be used to release the specimen, or the glenohumeral joint can be transected. The position for this incision is determined by the anatomical location of the tumor. If the osteotomy is through the neck of the scapula, a Gigli saw is passed around the scapula and used to divide the bone through its neck.

Reconstruction through muscle transplants greatly improves the functional result of this procedure. The tendinous portions of the trapezius and levator scapulae muscles should be secured to the glenohumeral joint capsule to suspend the arm. If this can be done, an orthosis need not be used postoperatively to support the extremity. Also, remnants of the deltoid muscle may be sutured to the residual scapula or glenohumeral joint to help support the upper extremity postoperatively. Remnants of back muscles, including the rhomboids, latissimus dorsi, teres major, and teres minor muscles, are sutured to the chest wall. Suction catheters are brought out through stab incisions at the most proximal or distal portions of the skin incision. The subcutaneous tissue is closed with absorbable sutures and the skin closed using plastic surgical technique.

AMPUTATIONS FOR EXTREMITY SOFT-TISSUE SARCOMA

Because soft-tissue sarcomas tend to spread along fascial planes and between muscle bundles, the complete muscle group involved by tumor should be removed with the amputation. When an amputation is required, it should be performed above the joint proximal to the tumor mass. Therefore, for tumors in the forearm, a transarm amputation above the elbow is recommended. For tumors of the upper arm, a forequarter amputation is generally recommended. A shoulder disarticulation can be performed, but is of no functional or cosmetic advantage compared to the forequarter amputation. High-grade tumors at the shoulder girdle are usually treated by forequarter amputation. However, a Tikhoff-Linberg procedure should be considered. Also, tumors overlying the scapula may be treated by scapulectomy in selected patients.

Tumors below the ankle are treated by below-knee amputation. Tumors of the leg are treated by above-knee amputation. Tumors of the adductor muscle group that cannot be removed by the adductor muscle group excision or wide local excision are treated using a modified hemipelvectomy. All other large tumors of the proximal thigh requiring amputation are treated by the standard posterior flap hemipelvectomy. The hip disarticulation procedure is rarely if ever performed for a patient with soft-tissue sarcoma of the lower extremity. Tumors of the buttock that penetrate down to the sciatic nerve or pelvic bones should be treated by anterior flap hemipelvectomy.

Forequarter Amputation.—Forequarter amputation is performed for aggressive tumors of or surrounding the shoulder girdle and tumors of the proximal portion of the upper arm. Unless the patient has a disfiguring tumor mass, a mold of the involved shoulder is made preoperatively. This simplifies construction of a suitable shoulder prosthesis postoperatively. The forequarter amputation as described by Littlewood[10] is performed for nearly all tumors in this area. An exception is a large tumor overlying the scapula; tumors located posteriorly are better approached from the anterior rather than the posterior aspect of the patient. The patient should be placed in a full lateral position. A racket-shaped incision is started over the midportion of the clavicle. It is continued anteriorly and posteriorly around the arm to meet below the axilla. All the axillary hair should be shaved (Fig 24–10,A). The incision can be varied to create either a long anterior or long posterior flap if this helps in the complete removal of the primary tumor and biopsy site. Posteriorly, skin flaps are constructed back to the posterior border of the scapula. The anterior skin flap is elevated back to the anterior axillary line. The posterior muscular attachments of the scapula are divided, including the rhomboids, trapezius, and levator scapulae. In the superior portion of the incision, the structures of the supraclavicular triangle are divided between hemostats. In this tissue are found the transverse cervical and transverse scapular arteries, many lymphatic channels, and the omohyoid muscle. Anterior traction is exerted on the scapula, which is moved anteriorly to stretch the serratus anterior muscle; this muscle is divided at its origin on the chest wall, clearly exposing the neurovascular bundle (Fig 24–10,B).

Anteriorly, the pectoralis major and pectoralis minor muscles are divided at a convenient site. Elevation of the inferior angle of the scapula allows these muscles to be divided under tension using electrocautery for minimal blood loss.

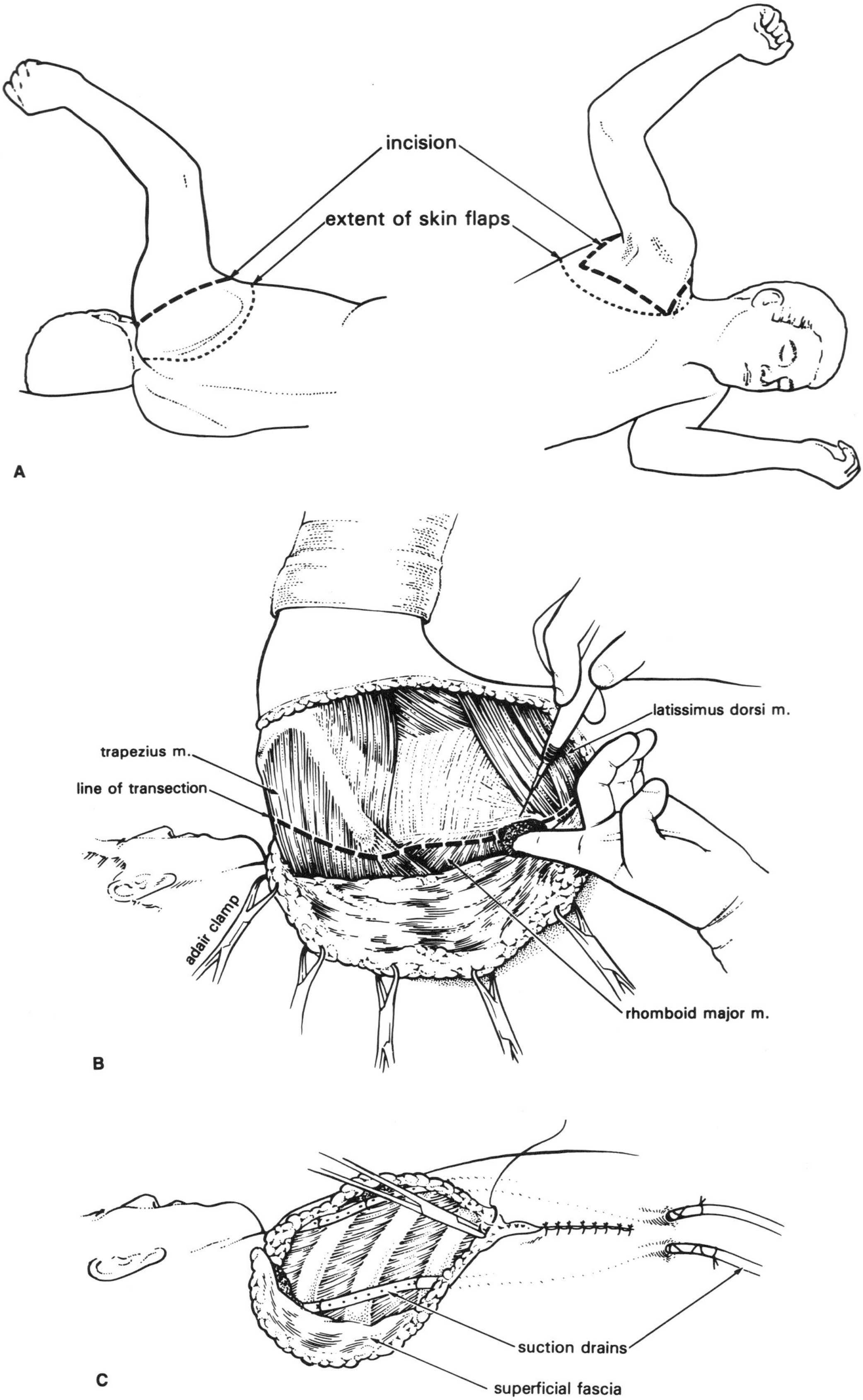
incision
extent of skin flaps
A
latissimus dorsi m.
trapezius m.
line of transection
adair clamp
rhomboid major m.
B
suction drains
superficial fascia
C

The clavicular head of the sternocleidomastoid muscle is severed from the clavicle. Then the clavicle can be disarticulated from its sternoclavicular joint. Now the specimen is attached only by the neurovascular bundle. The subclavian artery, subclavian vein, and nerves of the brachial plexus are ligated and divided under direct vision.

A careful closure is required to obtain a satisfactory cosmetic result. The posterior skin flap will be nearly twice the length of the anterior skin flap. Marked redundancy of the skin may present an unacceptable cosmetic appearance unless careful approximation of the skin flaps occurs. The midportion of the long posterior flap is closed to the midportion of the anterior flap. Halving the closure in this way pleats the posterior flap and prevents unsightly folds of skin (Fig 24–10,C). A two-layered closure of superficial fascia and then skin is used. Suction drainage should be secured.

Radical Forequarter Amputation With Chest Wall Resection.—If the tumor is adherent to the chest wall, a resection is still possible in selected patients. A potentially curative procedure involves removal of a portion of the chest wall. Before starting the chest wall resection, a thoracotomy is performed through a convenient interspace so one can palpate the extent of tumor within the chest and at the thoracic outlet. If a curative resection is possible, the scapular attachments of the back muscles are divided as in a forequarter amputation. The intercostal neurovascular bundles are secured posteriorly and the ribs divided. Anteriorly, the bone incision can be made through the costal cartilages or through the sternum (Fig 24–11). The strap muscles and sternocleidomastoid muscles must be released from the clavicle and first rib. The innominate vein, subclavian artery, and brachial plexus are dissected free and divided from within the chest. Division of the anterior, medial, and posterior scalene muscles allows removal of the specimen. Reconstruction of the chest wall may be with prosthetic mesh or by simple closure with the skin flaps. Suction drainage through a chest tube is secured.

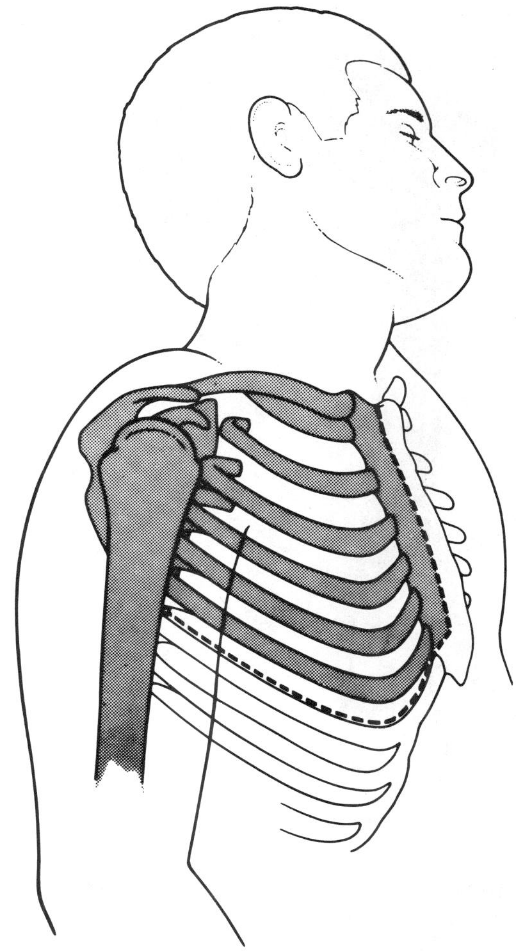

FIG 24–11.
Diagram of the skeleton, indicating the extent of a resection in a forequarter amputation with chest wall resection.

Tikhoff-Linberg Procedure.—The Tikhoff-Linberg procedure is rarely used for sarcomas of the shoulder girdle. The resection, if it is performed, involves removal of the bony structures indicated in Figure 24–12. The procedure is most commonly used for resection of osteosarcoma of the proximal humerus.[11]

FIG 24–10.
A, skin incision and extent of skin flaps in a forequarter amputation. **B,** posterior (Littlewood) approach to forequarter amputation. By releasing the posterior attachments of the scapula, the specimen is rolled anteriorly. This allows clear visualization of the major vessels and nerves so that blood loss during their transection is prevented. **C,** closure of a forequarter amputation. Notice that the posterior skin flap is pleated so that cosmetically unacceptable folds of skin do not occur.

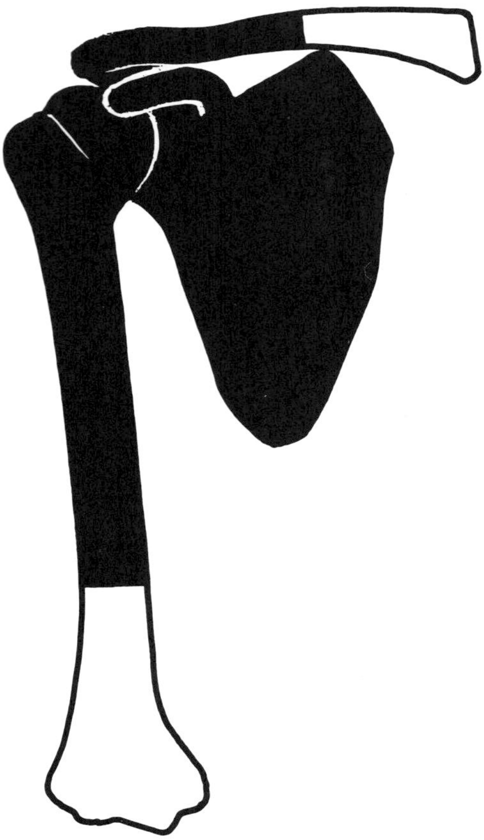

FIG 24–12.
Bone resected in a Tikhoff-Lindberg procedure performed for soft-tissue sarcoma.

Hemipelvectomy.—Hemipelvectomy using a standard posterior subcutaneous skin flap is indicated for large tumors of the upper anterior thigh.[12, 13] The patient is placed in a lateral position on the operating table, with iliac crest over the point of flexion of the operating room table. The opposite extremity is wrapped with an elastic bandage to prevent venous pooling. The extremity to be removed is draped free so that during the procedure it can be manipulated to facilitate muscle transections. The incision should be drawn out carefully so that an adequate posterior flap is created. Anteriorly, the incision extends from 2 in. (5 cm) above the anterior superior iliac spine in a curvilinear fashion to the pubic tubercle. Laterally, the incision courses over the greater trochanter and then parallel to the gluteal crease around the inner thigh to the pubic tubercle (Fig 24–13,A). In a large patient with an extensive anterior-posterior dimension of the pelvis, the skin incision may need to be below the gluteal crease. The previous biopsy site must be widely excised and included in the operative specimen.

The incision is first developed anteriorly. The common iliac artery and vein are ligated just below the aortic bifurcation. Next, the branches of the internal iliac vessels that lie over the sacral nerves in the pelvis must be divided. This allows bloodless transection of the sacral nerve roots (Fig. 24–13,B).

At this point, the posterior skin incision is made and the skin flap constructed back to a line connecting the posterior superior and posterior inferior iliac spine. Care must be taken not to thin out the skin flap posteriorly. The flap is gradually thickened and dissection continued into the posterior portion of the gluteus maximus muscle so that the blood supply to the skin flap from the most proximal portion of this muscle is preserved. Back and abdominal musculature must be released from the wing of the ileum (Fig 24–13,C).

The psoas muscle is transected in the depths of the incision. Also, the genital femoral nerve, which lies superficial to the psoas muscle, and the obturator and femoral nerves, which lie deep to it, are transected. The two lumbosacral nerve trunks just lateral to the L5 vertebral body should also be transected.

FIG 24–13.
A, incisions used in a standard posterior flap hemipelvectomy. **B,** vessels secured anteriorly in a hemipelvectomy. The common iliac artery and vein are secured just below the aorta. The multiple visceral branches of the internal iliac artery that overlie the sacral nerve roots are ligated and divided. **C,** posterior skin flap in a hemipelvectomy. The posterior skin flap is dissected until a line is seen between the posterior superior and posterior inferior iliac spine. If one goes beyond this point the blood supply to the long posterior flap is severely jeopardized. **D,** transection of the sacral nerve roots. With release of the pubic symphysis and the sacro-iliac joint, the pelvis can be widely opened. The sacral nerve roots are divided, and the pelvic diaphragm is clearly visualized. **E,** skin closure of a posterior flap hemipelvectomy. Because the posterior skin flap is longer than the anterior portion of the incision, the skin stitches gather the skin of the posterior flap to avoid cosmetically unacceptable skin folds.

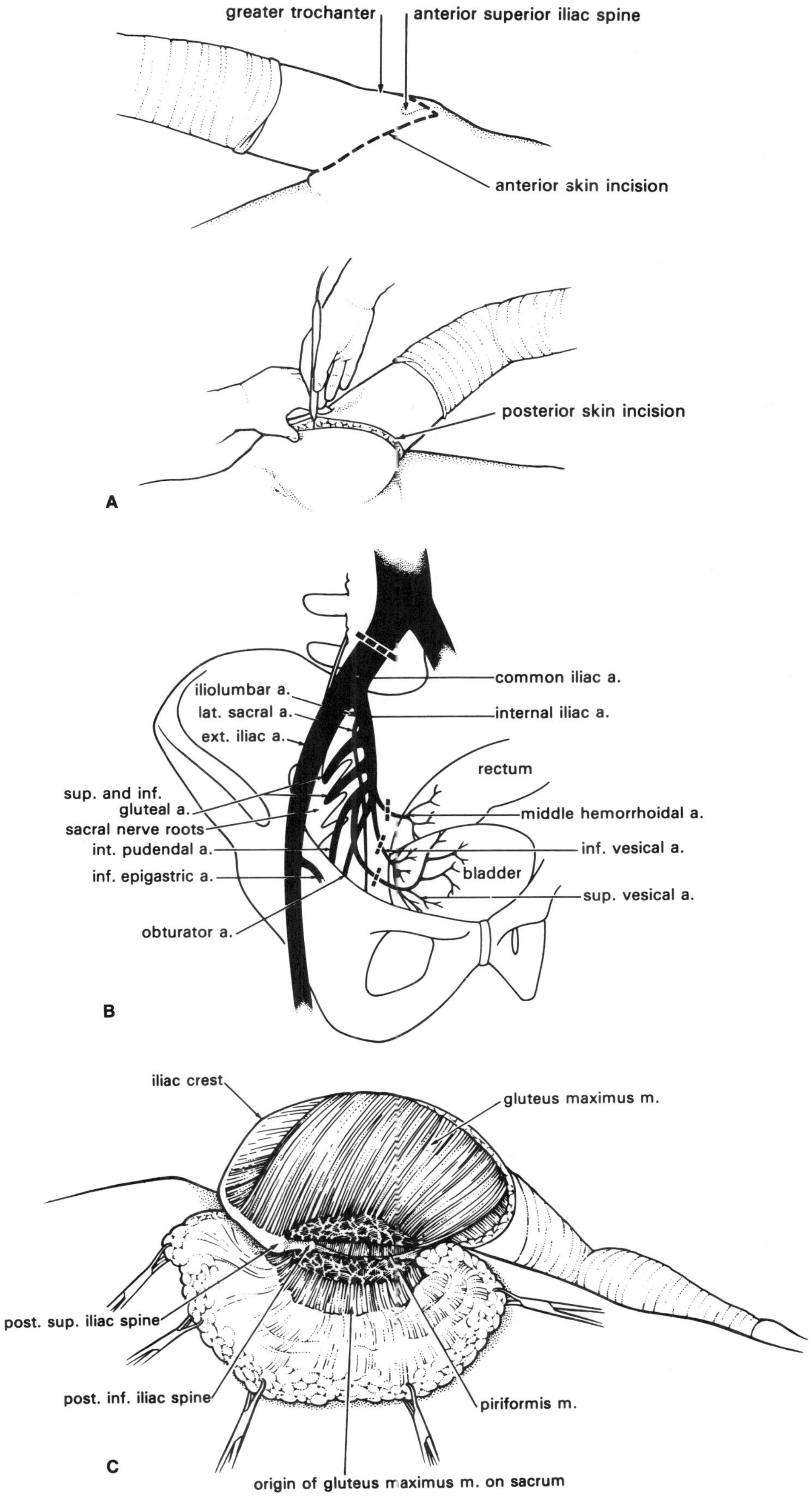
greater trochanter
anterior superior iliac spine
anterior skin incision
posterior skin incision
A
common iliac a.
iliolumbar a.
lat. sacral a.
internal iliac a.
ext. iliac a.
rectum
sup. and inf.
gluteal a.
sacral nerve roots
middle hemorrhoidal a.
int. pudendal a.
inf. vesical a.
bladder
inf. epigastric a.
sup. vesical a.
obturator a.
B
iliac crest
gluteus maximus m.
post. sup. iliac spine
post. inf. iliac spine
piriformis m.
C
origin of gluteus maximus m. on sacrum

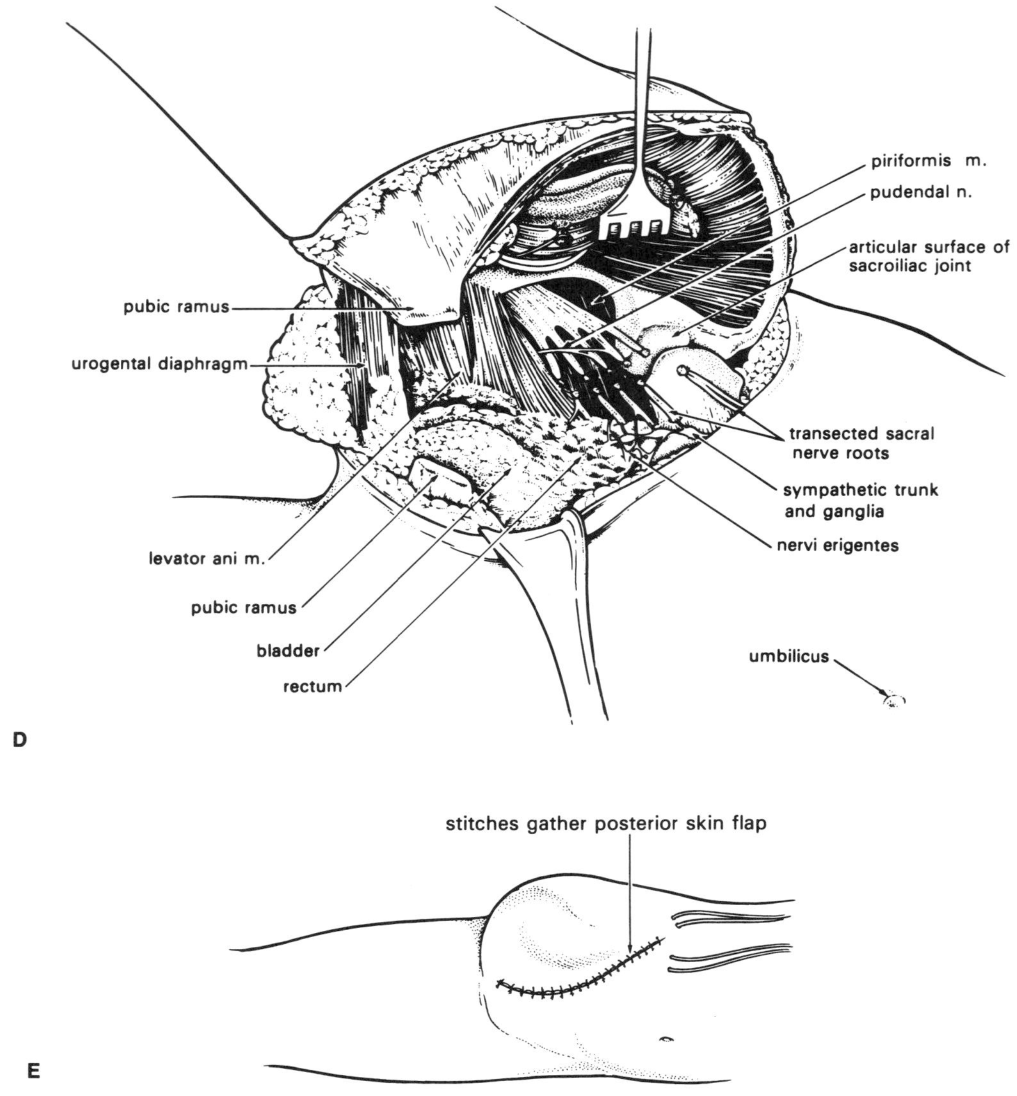

FIG 24–13.—*Continued*

The pubic symphysis is divided, and this allows the hemipelvis to open approximately 1 in. (2.5 cm). This improved exposure allows the sacral nerve roots to be ligated and then transected approximately 2 cm from the ventral foramina. If possible, the nervi erigentes that course from the sacral nerve roots to the pelvic plexus should be identified and preserved. This ensures minimal sexual and bladder dysfunction postoperatively. The iliolumbar ligament between the transverse process of the fifth lumbar vertebra and the sacrum is divided. The anterior capsule of the sacroiliac joint is divided with a scalpel. This allows the hemipelvis to open wide (Fig 24–13,D).

Strong upward traction is placed on the extremity that is to be removed. This lifts the specimen away from bladder and rectum. The urogenital diaphragm, piriform muscle, and levator ani muscles are stretched and divided bloodlessly using electrocautery. A few slips of the sacro-iliac joint capsule posteriorly are divided to deliver the specimen.

The area is then copiously irrigated and hemostasis achieved. Suction drainage is secured. The subcutaneous tissue is closed to the anterior abdominal wall with absorbable suture, and the skin is closed using a plastic surgical technique (Fig 24–13,E). Postoperatively, pressure is kept off the sacral region. A trapeze over the patient's bed is often useful. The Foley catheter should remain in place until the patient is ambulatory. Because much bone marrow is lost in the specimen, blood transfusion in the postoperative period may be required.

Anterior Flap Hemipelvectomy.—In an anterior flap hemipelvectomy, the tumor is generally located in the buttock or high in the posterior thigh.[14] In this procedure, extensive buttock skin is replaced by a myocutaneous flap constructed from the quadriceps femoris muscle and overlying skin and subcutaneous tissue. The superficial femoral artery is preserved to sustain the myocutaneous flap. The incision should be mapped out carefully to assure that there is adequate coverage of the large posterior defect (Fig 24–14,A).

The incision should be begun posteriorly. Usually with buttock tumors, the medial margin of the tumor is the closest one to the line of excision. If there is any doubt as to the adequacy of the margin, tissue specimens for cryostat sectioning should be requested. The posterior incision is continued down to the midsacral spine and the gluteus maximus and erector spinal muscles are divided from their origins on the sacrum. The incision is extended anteriorly so that the back muscles can be released from the iliac crest (Fig 24–14,B). With the extremity flexed at the hip the tissue overlying the ischiorectal space is stretched. After extending the incision up to the pubic tubercle the ischiorectal fossa is opened so the pelvis can be entered posteriorly.

Next, the anterior incisions along the medial and lateral aspect of the thigh are made. The quadriceps muscle is divided down to bone and the superficial femoral artery ligated and divided at Hunter's canal. The entire quadriceps muscle is elevated from the femur. The superficial femoral artery forms the most dependent portion of the myocutaneous flap. Multiple small branches of the superficial femoral vessels into adductor muscles are carefully clamped, divided, and ligated. As the myocutaneous flap is elevated at the level of the inguinal canal, the rectus femoris muscle must be released from the anterior inferior iliac spine and the sartorius muscle from the anterior superior iliac spine. The femoral sheath overlying the hip joint is divided, and the left rectus abdominis muscle is released from the pubic bone. At this point, firm traction medially on the myocutaneous flap allows full access to the pelvis. Some abdominal muscle insertions into the wing of the ilium laterally must be cut in order to divide the attachments completely between the patient and the hemipelvis (Fig 24–14,C).

The pubic symphysis should be divided, taking care to protect bladder and urethra. The internal iliac artery and vein are divided at their point of origin from the common iliac vessels. Multiple visceral branches of the internal iliac vessels that cross the sacral nerve routes are divided. Strong medial traction on the viscera will help expose these vessels. The psoas muscle is divided near its junction with the iliacus muscle; the obturator and genital femoral nerves are also divided. Care is taken to preserve the femoral nerve, which supplies the myocutaneous flap. The lumbosacral and sacral nerve routes are ligated and divided close to their ventral sacral foramina (Fig 24–14,C).

The extremity to be removed is placed under strong upward traction so that the pelvic diaphragm is stretched. The urogenital diaphragm, levator ani, and piriform muscles are divided near their pelvic attachments.

The sacrum is divided through the neural foramina to free the specimen. The surgeon posterior to the patient locates the neural foramina from within the sacrum. The osteotome is then directed toward this structure using the opposite hand. The assistant drives the osteotome through the bone with mallet. In this manner, a clean and accurate osteotomy is performed (Fig 24–14,D).

The operative site is copiously irrigated and hemostasis achieved. The fascia of the quadriceps femoris muscle is sutured to the muscles of the anterior abdominal wall, to the back muscles, to the sacrum, and pelvic diaphragm. The skin is closed with interrupted sutures. Suction drainage is achieved (Fig 24–14,E).

Alternative Approaches to Hemipelvectomy.—If a patient has a large tumor high in the adductor muscle group, a modified hemipelvectomy is indicated. In this procedure the pelvis is transected through the symphysis pubis and sciatic notch. This leaves the iliac crest in place. The posterior skin flap is constructed until an imaginary line coursing between the anterior superior iliac spine and the tip of the coccyx is reached. The dissection within the pelvis is similar except that branches of the internal iliac artery are divided just proximal to the sciatic notch. A Gigli's wire saw is used to transect the

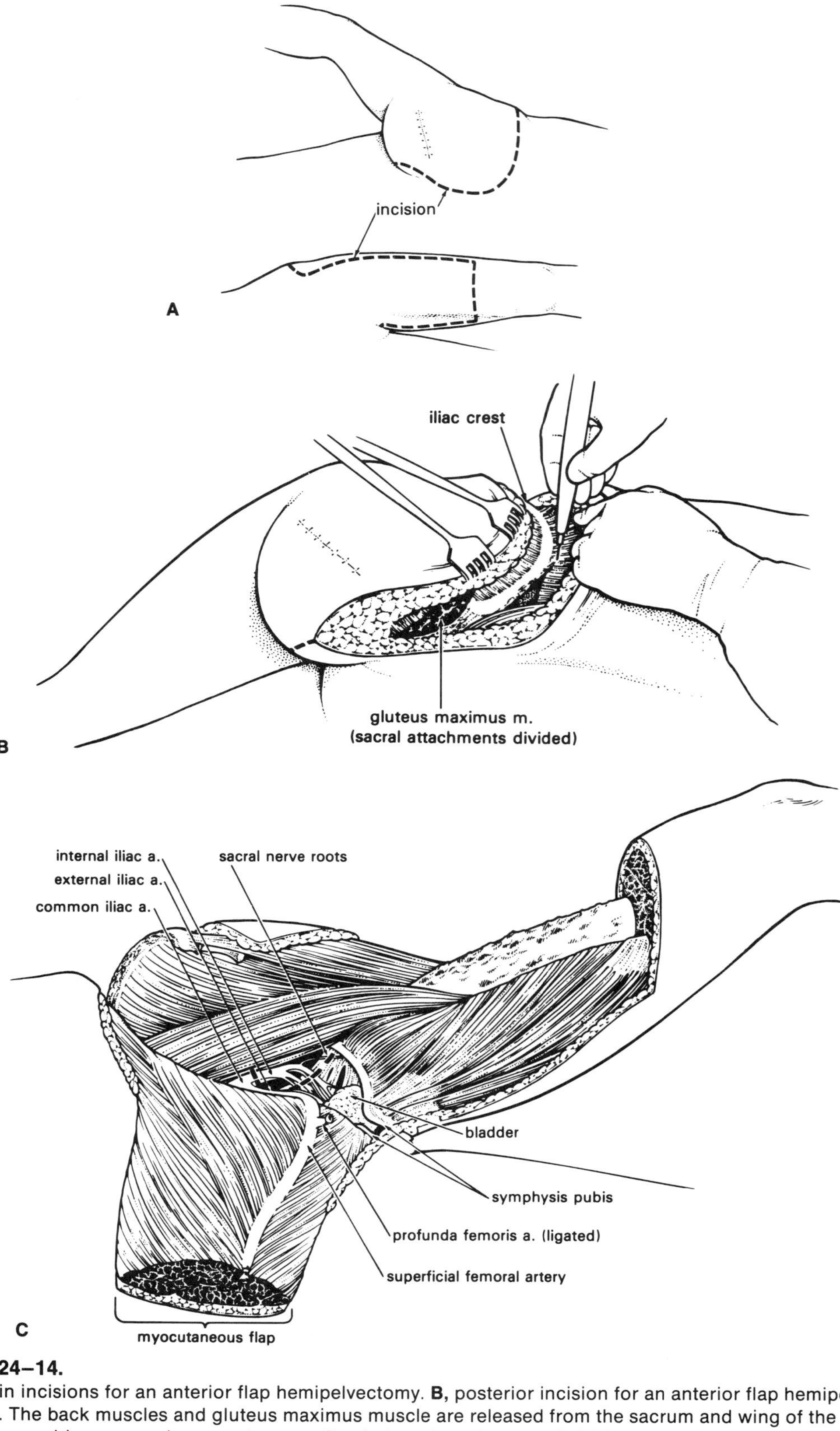

FIG 24–14.
A, skin incisions for an anterior flap hemipelvectomy. **B,** posterior incision for an anterior flap hemipelvectomy. The back muscles and gluteus maximus muscle are released from the sacrum and wing of the ilium. **C,** the quadriceps muscle myocutaneous flap is based on the superficial femoral artery. It is dissected up off the femur and allows access to the pelvis. The internal iliac artery is divided at its origin from the common iliac artery. Its visceral branches are divided as they pass over the sacral nerve roots. **D,** an osteotome is used to divide the sacrum between the posterior sacral foramina. **E,** skin closure following an anterior flap hemipelvectomy.

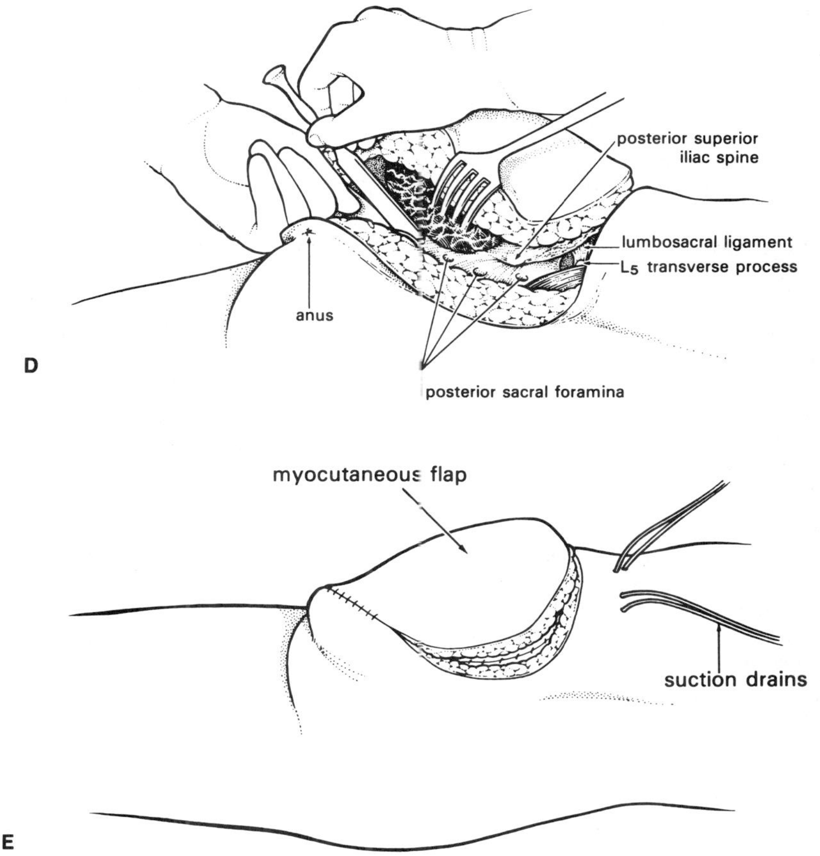

FIG 24–14.—*Continued*

pelvis. Blood supply to the posterior skin flap is generous, and ischemia of this flap does not occur.

In extended hemipelvectomy, the osteotomy is through the sacral neural foramina rather than the sacro-iliac joint. This procedure is indicated for tumors involving the bony pelvis. These tumors rarely extend through the sacro-iliac joint and, therefore, a clean margin of resection can be achieved if the osteotomy is above this joint.

Occasionally, an intraperitoneal approach to hemipelvectomy is indicated. This is usually used for large tumors that extend into the pelvis and may be of questionable resectability. It may be easier to secure the iliac vessels over such a large tumor if one is working from within the peritoneal cavity.

A compound hemipelvectomy involves excision of bladder, rectum, and female internal genitalia or other viscera along with the hemipelvis and lower extremity.

An internal hemipelvectomy can sometimes be performed without sacrifice of the entire extremity. Enneking, [15] Eilber et al.,[16] and Karakousis[17] have described several variations of the internal hemipelvectomy.

Hip Disarticulation.—Hip disarticulation[18, 19] is rarely performed for a soft-tissue sarcoma. Its usual indication is a large osteosarcoma of the distal or middle femur.

REFERENCES

1. Sugarbaker PH, Barofsky I, Rosenberg SA, et al: Quality of life assessment of patients in extremity sarcoma clinical trials. *Surgery* 1982; 91:17–23.
2. Lawrence W Jr, Baker LH, Balch CM, et al: Consensus conference: Limb-sparing treatment of adult soft-tissue sarcomas and osteosarcomas. *JAMA* 1985; 254:1791–1794.

3. Weingrad DN, Rosenberg SA: Early lymphatic spread of osteogenic and soft-tissue sarcomas. *Surgery* 1978; 84:231–240.
4. Mentzer SJ, Sugarbaker PH: Adductor muscle group excision. *Surgery* 1982; 91:662–668.
5. Sugarbaker PH, Lampert MH: Excision of quadriceps muscle group. *Surgery* 1983; 93:462–466.
6. Lehmann JF: Biomechanics of ankle-foot orthoses: Prescription and design. *Arch Phys Med Rehab* 1979; 60:200–207.
7. Bowden L, Booher RJ: Sarcoma of the buttock, in Pack GT, Ariel IM (eds): *Tumors of the Soft Somatic Tissues, a Clinical Treatise,* ch 29. New York, Hoeber-Harper, 1958.
8. Sugarbaker PH, Chretien PA: A surgical technique for buttockectomy. *Surgery* 1982; 91:104–107.
9. Das Gupta TK: Scapulectomy, in Sugarbaker PH, Nicholson TH (eds): *Atlas of Extremity Sarcoma Surgery,* ch 13. Philadelphia, J. B. Lippincott, 1984.
10. Littlewood H: Amputation at the shoulder and at the hip. *Br Med J* 1922; 1:381–383.
11. Malawer MM, Sugarbaker PH, Lampert M, et al: The Tikhoff-Linberg procedure: Report of ten patients and presentation of a modified technique for tumors of the proximal humerus. *Surgery* 1985; 97:518–528.
12. Pack GT, Ehrlich HE: Exarticulation of the lower extremities for malignant tumors: Sacro-iliac disarticulation (hemipelvectomy). *Ann Surg* 1946; 124:1–27.
13. Chretien PA, Sugarbaker PH: Surgical technique of hemipelvectomy in the lateral position. *Surgery* 1981; 90:900–909.
14. Sugarbaker PH, Chretien PA: Hemipelvectomy for buttock tumors utilizing an anterior myocutaneous flap of quadriceps muscle. *Ann Surg* 1983; 197:106–115.
15. Enneking WF: Local resection of malignant lesions of the hip and pelvis. *J Bone Joint Surg* 1966; 48-A:991–1007.
16. Eilber FR, Grant TT, Sakai D, et al: Internal hemipelvectomy—excision of the hemipelvis with limb preservation. *Cancer* 1979; 43:806–809.
17. Karakousis CP: Internal hemipelvectomy. *Surg Gynecol Obstet* 1984; 158:279–282.
18. Pack GT, Ehrlich HE: Exarticulation of the lower extremities for malignant tumors: Hip joint disarticulation (with and without deep iliac dissection). *Ann Surg* 1946; 123:965–984.
19. Sugarbaker PH, Chretien PB: A surgical technique for hip disarticulation. *Surgery* 1982; 90:546–553.

Chapter 25

Hemicorporectomy for Advanced Pelvic Cancer

Theodore R. Miller

EDITORIAL COMMENT

Dr. Theodore R. Miller, for many years Chief of the Bone Service at Memorial Sloan-Kettering, New York, provides a provocative account of a now almost extinct surgical procedure, hemicorporectomy. His own experience, perhaps the largest in the world, involved 11 patients operated on between 1964 and 1981. Most physicians today will differ with his view that such aggressive surgery should be in the armament of all oncological surgeons, or that extirpation of the breast, ovaries, prostate, and uterus should be widely used for cancer prevention. Nonetheless, Dr. Miller provides a strong argument that hemicorporectomy may represent a chance for cure in the rare patient with unresectable low-grade cancer of the pelvis (perhaps a sarcoma), and this operation can improve the quality of life in the setting of paraplegia and pelvic osteomyelitis.

John H. Raaf, M.D.

INTRODUCTION

With the increased ability to diagnose cancer earlier and to treat it with chemotherapy, the need for radical surgery has generally been thought to have diminished. However, adequate surgical procedures are still necessary to cure some types of cancer. The tendency to use modifications of the operations that have been designed and developed to cure cancer and the resultant increase in recurrent disease have led to renewed salvage efforts for treatment failures. The local excision of soft-part sarcomas and bone tumors too often is followed by recurrence. It is still possible to cure advanced cancer with radical surgery after failure of multiple inadequate operations, vigorous chemotherapy, and radiation therapy. Unfortunately, the chance of cure diminishes with each unsuccessful attempt at eradication. Most soft-part sarcomas and other tumors show an increase in malignancy with each recurrence, making salvage less likely. Procedures such as pelvic exenteration, interscapulothoracic amputation, hemipelvectomy, and hemicorporectomy can extend useful life and even offer a chance of cure to patients with advanced or recurrent cancer.

The operation called hemicorporectomy or translumbar amputation is often considered salvage surgery, although there are some tumors so located that they can be treated for cure only by this extensive procedure, such as sacral chordoma, tumors involving the midline of the bony pelvis or the sacrum, and soft-part sarcomas involving the pelvic structures. In these cases, the operation must be considered therapeutic.

Major surgery should be considered for all patients who have recurrent cancer if there is a reasonable chance of cure or palliation. Recurrent cancer often follows limited surgery for a small tumor (the present tendency in surgical circles), which is often performed even though the chance of cure by further surgery is greatly diminished. Fungation, intractable pain, persistent hemorrhage, and ulceration are all problems in the management of recurrent tumors. If the recurrent disease is limited to an extremity, major amputation can even cure. If the tumor involves a pelvic organ and is fixed or invades the pelvic wall on one side, hemipelvectomy with pelvic exenteration can provide salvage. Other salvage operations include pelvic exenteration, total cystectomy and node dissection, the so-called "Andy Grump" operation for head and neck cancer, extended total gastrectomy, extended pancreatectomy, extended radical mastectomy, right or left hepatectomy for solitary hepatic metastasis, and hemicorporectomy. All of these operations can relieve pain, permit a reasonable degree of rehabilitation, and extend a useful and comfortable life.

Intractable pain, necessitating frequent and large doses of narcotics, can be controlled by salvage surgery. Most of the cases of hemicorporectomy reported here involved severe dependence on analgesics for pain. When the pain was relieved, the need for drugs was eliminated, and the drug dependence was easily controlled. This, in itself, added to the quality of life.

The ideal approach to the management of cancer is, of course, prevention, both epidemiologically and surgically. According to data from the American Cancer Society,[1] about 1,040,000 new cases of cancer are estimated to occur annually in the United States. Of these cases, approximately 50% are expected to survive 5 years. Of the cured cases, 65% will be cured by surgery alone. Surgery can also be preventive, in that a premalignant lesion can be excised. This also implies that organs susceptible to cancerous change, such as the breasts, ovaries, prostate, and uterus, should be removed once their function has been served. If both breasts were removed in all women over 40, 93% of breast cancer could be prevented.[2] The same is true of ovarian, uterine, cervical, and prostatic cancer. The best example of preventive surgery is circumcision, which appears to prevent cancer of the penis. Pack[3] and others have suggested that women who have had unilateral radical mastectomy for cancer should have the other breast removed by simple mastectomy, because cancer will develop in the remaining breast in 9% to 21% of these cases. The removal of normal organs would certainly be prophylactic, but considering the approach to the smoking problem by the public and the government, it is unlikely that people would accept this form of prevention. Kennedy[4] advocated vaginal hysterectomy and removal of both ovaries in all women past child-bearing age. Certainly, the surgeon who knowingly removes a malignant tumor of one ovary and conserves the remaining ovary is vulnerable to criticism. Because of the frequency of second colonic cancers, Lillehei and Wangensteen[5] have advocated subtotal colectomy for patients who have had two or more polyps or a carcinoma of the colon. However, less than 10% of such patients have a second tumor.

Fortunately, bilateral cancer of paired organs, one of which is essential for life (such as kidney or lung), is rare. Bilateral cancer in paired endocrine organs that have important functions (such as adrenals and testes) is also infrequent.

INDICATIONS

The prime indication of translumbar amputation is advanced, recurrent cancer of the pelvic organs, still limited to the pelvis and without distant metastases. The tumor should be low-grade, as indicated by its slow evolution.[6]

Cancer of the cervix, recurrent after pelvic exenteration or exenteration and hemipelvectomy, might be cured by translumbar amputation because in 35% of all patients dying of cervical cancer, the disease is still limited to the pelvis. Patients with recurrent vaginal, penile, bladder, prostatic, and colonic cancer after abdominoperineal resection are all candidates. Sacral chordoma is usually a slow-growing tumor and can rarely be eradicated by anything short of translumbar amputation. Patients with chondrosarcoma of the perineum are prime candidates. The carcinoma occurring in decubitus ulcers in the paraplegic also lends itself well to this operation.[7] A much more common indication for the operation is paraplegia due to trauma or meningomyelocele with advanced osteomyelitis of the pelvis.[6]

Of the 11 cases reported here (Figs. 25–1 to 25–5), two hemicorporectomy procedures were done for benign conditions in paraplegics and nine for advanced cancer. Of these nine, three were rendered free of cancer, and one is alive 15 years later and supporting himself in his own electronics firm. Two of the cancer patients died of postoperative complications: one of renal failure due to advanced amyloidosis, the other due to internal hydrocephalus. These two were free of cancer at postmortem examination. The remaining six patients, who had advanced cancer, died of metastatic disease in the liver and lungs. Only one of the six had locally recurrent disease. These six cancer patients lived from 3 to 24 months, in various stages of rehabilitation, and were able to care for themselves and were free of pain. The last patient was a 44-year-old male who had a far-advanced chrondrosarcoma and was completely bedridden and dependent on analgesic drugs. He returned to his work with computers, free of pain, but died of pulmonary metastases 24 months after amputation.

Five of the 11 patients were paraplegics; six were still able to move their legs but were unable to walk because of pain. The presence of paraplegia makes the operation more acceptable. All the cancer patients described in Tables 25–1 and 25–2 were in an advanced state, had undergone surgery, and were given all the radiation and chemotherapy that was possible.

My experience with the 11 patients indicates that translumbar amputation is safe and can yield good palliation and a reasonable chance of cure.

TECHNIQUE

Hemicorporectomy can be done in one or two stages. It is probably best initially to do exploratory surgery to determine the extent of the disease and to do the fecal and urinary diversions. Then, any problems involved can be presented to the patient and family. Five of the 11 cases were done in one stage and six in two stages. An advantage of the two-stage procedure is that it allows the patient to recover from the fecal and urinary diversions before amputation, and reduces the operative time of the second stage.[6]

After studies and exploration have established that there are not distant metastases, and the diversions have been constructed, the operation begins with the patient in the supine position. After adequate anesthesia is attained, a central venous catheter and other monitoring devices are placed. A Czerny-type incision is used, reflecting the anterior abdominal wall in full thickness upward (Fig. 25–6). All previous operative scars should be excised, where possible. The lymphoid and fatty tissue is then dissected from the duodenum downward. The common iliac arteries are doubly ligated, and the vena cava is similarly cleared and a ligature placed (Fig. 25–7). The patient is then put in the Trendelenburg position and the central venous pressure monitored until it rises to 13 cm H_20 or is stable for 3 minutes. The vena cava is ligated and all three vessels divided. The posterior or lateral flaps are developed and the musculature cleared from the crest of the ileum. The spine is then divided through the appropriate lumbar interspace, and after the pedicles are fractured with an osteotome the dura and cauda equina are divided. The lower half of the body is then removed, and the spinal canal plugged with a piece of muscle taken from the abdominal wall or psoas, to avoid spinal fluid leak (Fig. 25–8). The flaps are then brought together, anchoring the posterior one to the vertebral stump to prevent herniation of the viscera between the flaps and the vertebra. The wound is approximated with through-and-through sutures of heavy silk, with a sump drain in place. Little blood replacement is needed because of the reduction in blood volume. In fact, care should be exercised to prevent overloading the circulation.[6]

Two amputations were performed through the L3–4 interspace, five through the L4–5 interspace, and four through the L5–S1 interspace.

COMPLICATIONS

Wound problems were encountered because most of these patients had longstanding severe infection and massive ulceration in the portion of the body to be amputated. With the use of pre- and postoperative antibiotics, this complication was easily managed.[6]

Phantom pain was not a problem. In fact, many of these patients who had been dependent on opiates because of pain found that withdrawal was not a problem.

Fluid balance should be carefully monitored, because the blood volume is reduced about 50%. Meningitis was not a problem, in spite of the fact that the dural canal was opened in a contaminated field. Plugging the canal with muscle avoids spinal fluid leak, and pre- and postoperative antibiotic therapy protected the

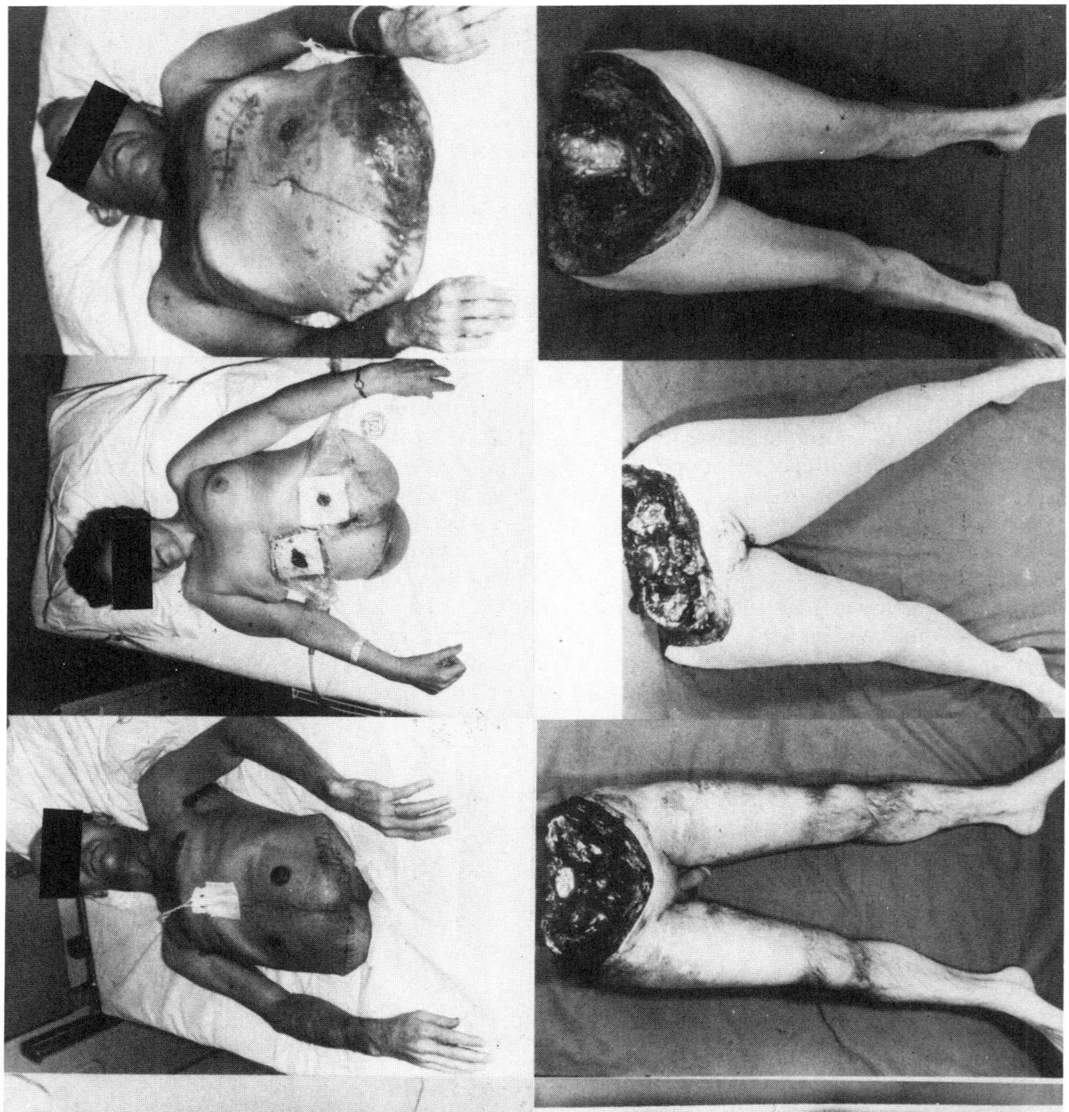

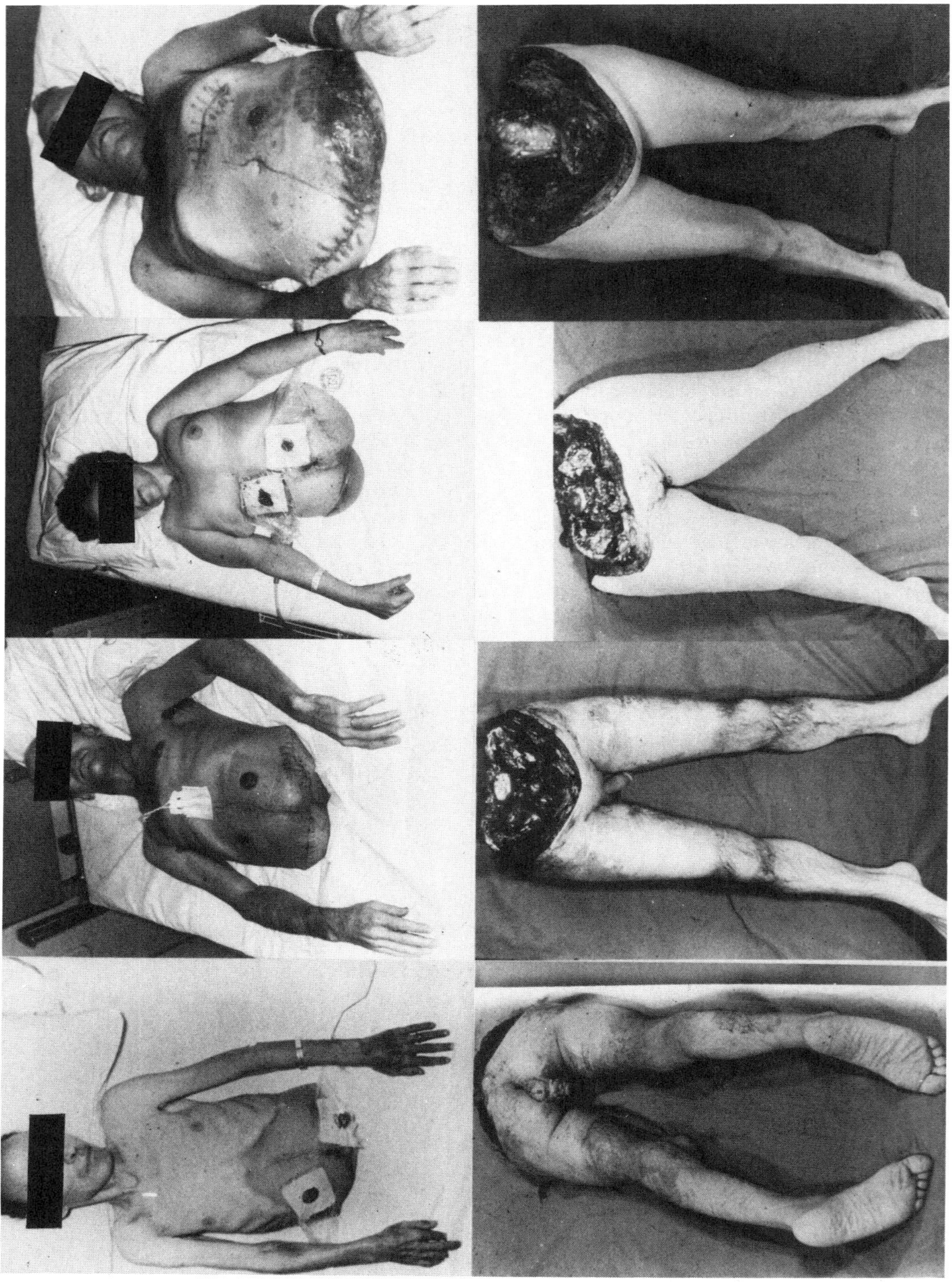

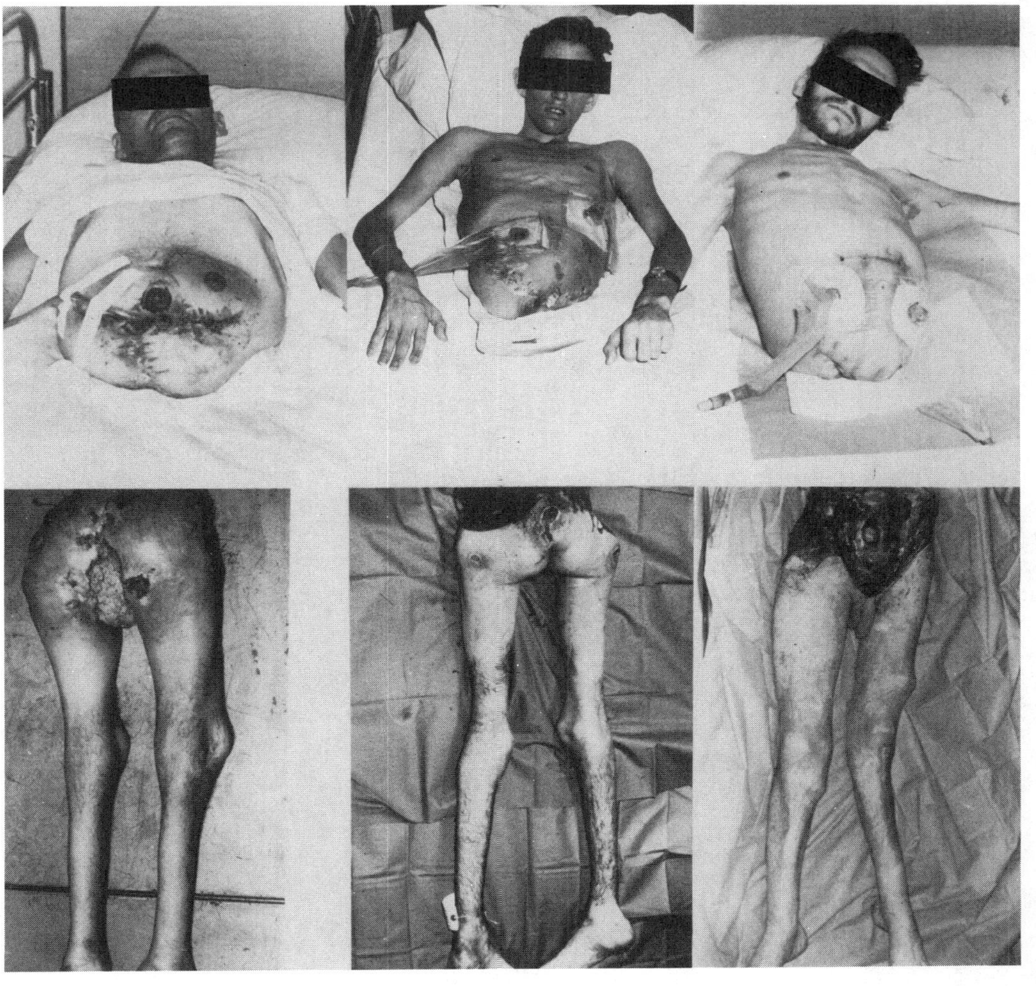

FIG 25–2.
Patients 5–7 (see Tables 25–1 and 25–2). (From Miller TR: *Prog Clin Cancer* 1982; 8:227–236. Used by permission.)

patient. One of our patients (No. 5), a paraplegic due to meningomyelocele, died free of his squamous cell carcinoma of the anus 3 months after the operation, due to an internal hydrocephalus. Patients with such a problem should be carefully examined by a neurologist, and shunting should be performed before the amputation is attempted.

PHYSIOLOGICAL ALTERATIONS

About 45% of the body weight is removed by the operation, reducing the blood volume sharply. Oxygen consumption is reduced by only about 10 to 11%, because the liver and brain remain intact.[8]

Although "team therapy" has been highly

FIG 25–1.
Patients 1–4 (see Tables 25–1 and 25–2). (From Miller TR: *Prog Clin Cancer* 1982; 8:227–236. Used by permission.)

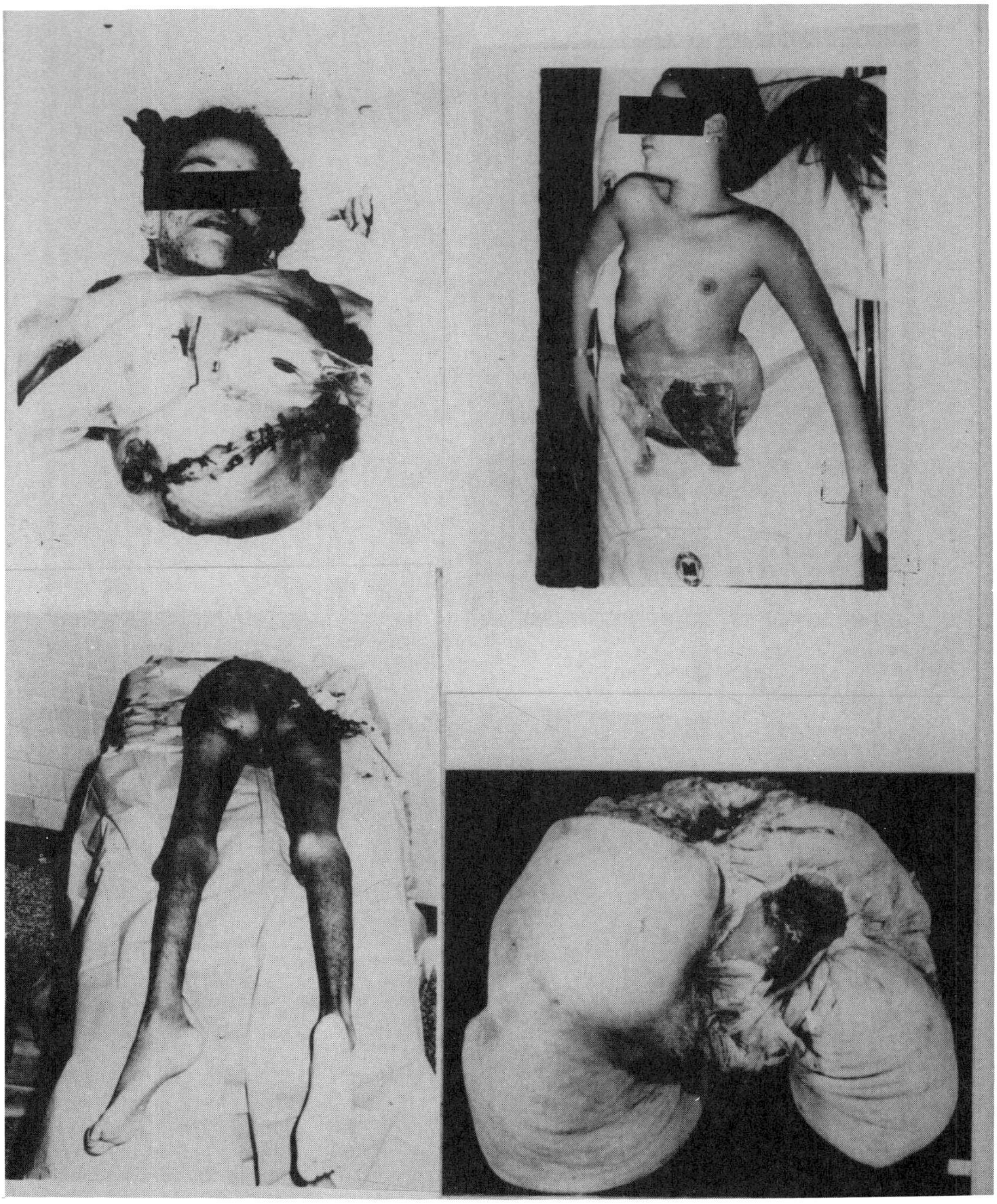

FIG 25–3.
Patients 8 and 9 (see Tables 25–1 and 25–2). (From Miller TR: *Prog Clin Cancer* 1982; 8:227–236. Used by permission.)

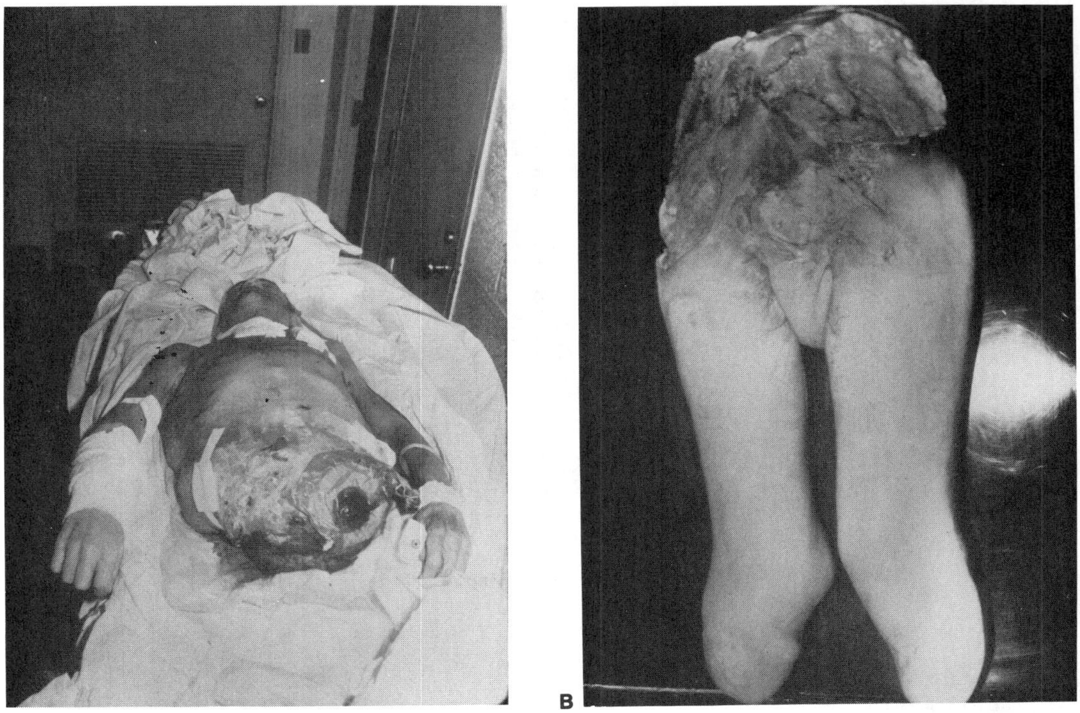

FIG 25–4.
Patient 10 (see Tables 25–1 and 25–2).

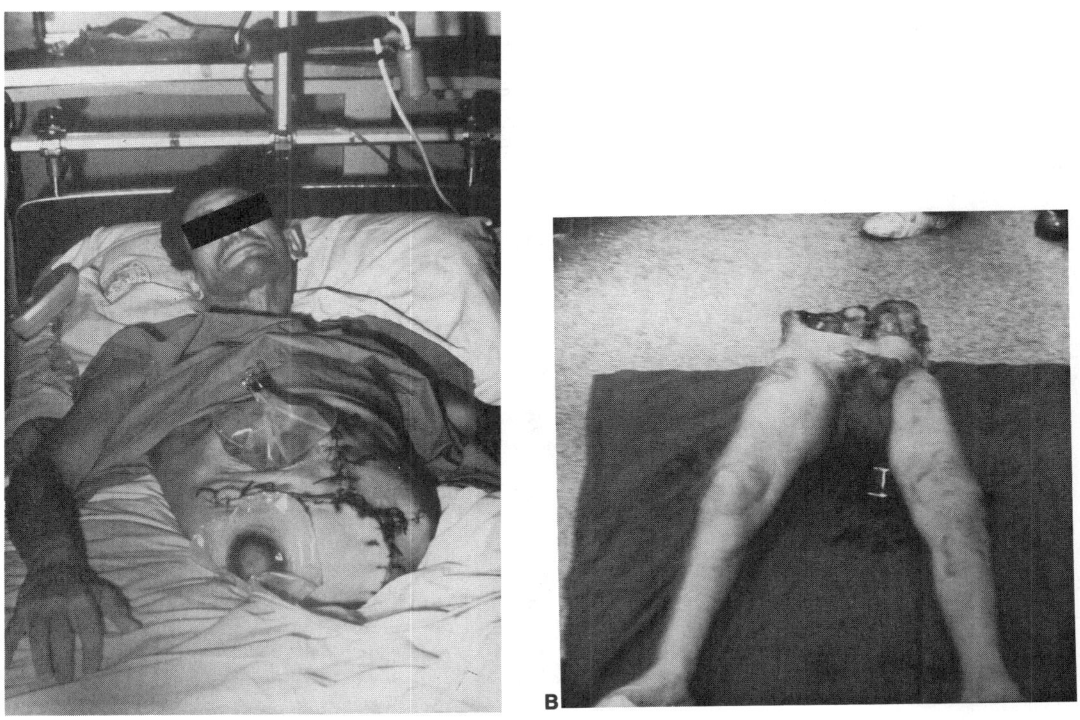

FIG 25–5.
Patient 11 (see Tables 25–1 and 25–2).

TABLE 25–1.
Patients

Patient Number	Age (yr)	Sex	Paraplegic	Diagnosis	Date of Operation	Length of Life After Operation	Date of Death	Cause of Death
1	48	M	No	Carcinoma of bladder	9/23/64	19 yr	—	Living and well, NED*
2	39	M	No	Carcinoma of bladder	1/6/65	1 yr	1/13/66	Local recurrence, liver metastases
3	46	F	No	Carcinoma of vagina	7/21/65	9 mo	4/4/66	Liver metastases
4	41	M	No	Sarcoma of prostate	8/4/65	7 mo	3/20/66	Pulmonary metastases
5	43	M	Yes	Squamous carcinoma of anus	6/5/65	2 mo	8/10/65	Internal hydrocephalus (NED at postmortem)
6	19	M	Yes	Osteomyelitis	6/26/68	15 yr	—	Living and well, NED
7	26	M	Yes	Chondrosarcoma	2/12/69	3 mo	5/12/69	Pulmonary metastases
8	22	F	No	Osteogenic sarcoma	4/9/73	19 mo	11/24/74	Pulmonary metastases
9	20	F	Yes	Osteomyelitis	10/8/74	68 mo	4/26/80	Cardiac arrest
10	51	M	Yes	Squamous carcinoma in decubitus	4/12/77	7 days	4/19/77	Renal failure, amyloidosis (NED at postmortem)
11	44	M	No	Chondrosarcoma	8/18/81	2 yr	8/6/83	Pulmonary metastases

** NED = no evidence of disease.*

TABLE 25–2.
Procedures

Patient Number	Operative Stages	Fecal Diversion	Urinary Diversion	Level of Amputation	Operative Time (hr)	Blood Loss (cc)	Complications	Hospital Days After Amputation
1	2	Terminal colostomy	Ileal bladder	L4 and L5	3	500	Wound healing	78
2	2	Terminal colostomy	Sigmoid conduit	L5 and S1	$2\frac{1}{2}$	1,950	Stress ulcer	28
3	1	Terminal colostomy	Sigmoid conduit	L5 and S1	$3\frac{1}{2}$	1,400	None	33
4	1	Terminal colostomy	Wet colostomy	L4 and L5	$2\frac{1}{2}$	1,000	Ruptured spleen	98
5	1	Terminal colostomy	Sigmoid conduit	L3 and L4	$4\frac{1}{2}$	2,500	Hydrocephalus	71
6	2	Terminal colostomy	Ileal bladder	L4 and L5	$2\frac{1}{4}$	1,500	None	21
7	2	Colostomy	Ileal bladder	L5 and S1	4	1,500	Ollier's disease	59
8	1	Terminal colostomy	Ileal bladder	L5 and S1	5	1,500	Pulmonary resection for metastases	21
9	2	Terminal colostomy	Ileal bladder	L4 and L5	$3\frac{1}{4}$	4,000	Wound healing	38
10	1	Terminal colostomy	Skin ureterostomies	L3 and L4	3	4,500	Amyloid disease, renal failure	7
11	1	Colostomy	Sigmoid conduit	L4 and L5	4	1,200	None	44

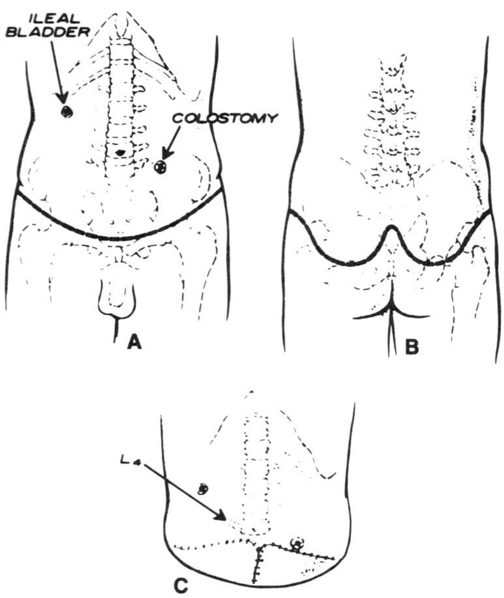

FIG 25–6.
Outline of incisions, (**A** and **B**, and closure, **C**. (From Miller TR: *Prog Clin Cancer* 1982; 8:227–236. Used by permission.)

touted, it cannot replace the support of the individual physician. If ever the surgeon needs to resume the role of "family doctor" or to continue to work with the family doctor, it is in the lifetime management of these patients. I have cared for all of these patients personally, from start to finish.

SUMMARY

Despite the simplicity of this operation, its magnitude[9] precludes its use as a palliative procedure. Evidence that there are no metastases or extension beyond the tissue to be excised should be determined before surgery is undertaken. The patient and family should be fully apprised of the consequences of this operation, and the patient's general physical condition and mental attitude should be well enough to tolerate the intensive rehabilitation and training that must follow. It is perhaps unwise to attempt this procedure unless adequate rehabilitation therapy is available.

Of 33 patients I found suitable for this procedure, only the 11 reported here accepted the operation. I have been able to locate only 14 other reported hemicorporectomies, done by 12 different surgeons. The 11 in this series brings the total number of reported cases to 25.

Hemicorporectomy has been done largely as a salvage procedure, in desperate cases. It should be in the armament of any oncologic surgeon in this day of inadequate and compromise surgery. The quality of life after hemicorporectomy is compatible with comfortable existence and even self-support; two of my patients drove automobiles (even in New York City), and three returned to productive work (Figs. 25–9 and 25–10). Because the operation is safe and the indications are clear, it is my view that this major amputation should be done earlier and more frequently than has been done in the past.

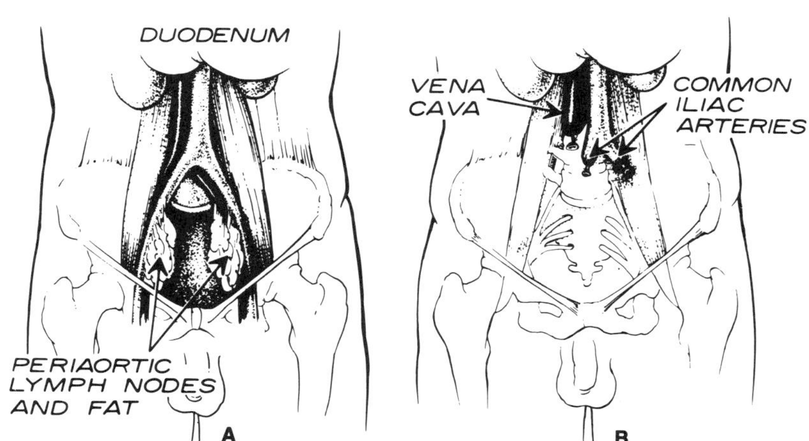

FIG 25–7.
(**A** and **B**), dissection prior to amputation. (From Miller TR: *Prog Clin Cancer* 1982; 8:227–236. Used by permission.)

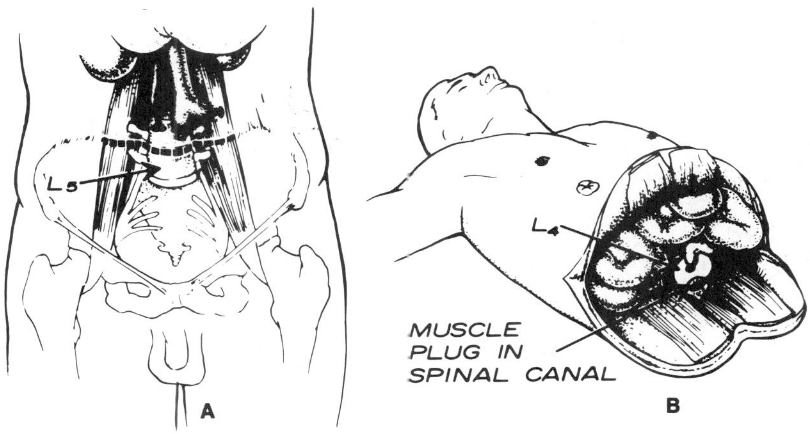

FIG 25–8.
A, level of amputation. **B,** patient prior to closure. (From Miller TR: *Prog Clin Cancer* 1982; 8:227–236. Used by permission.)

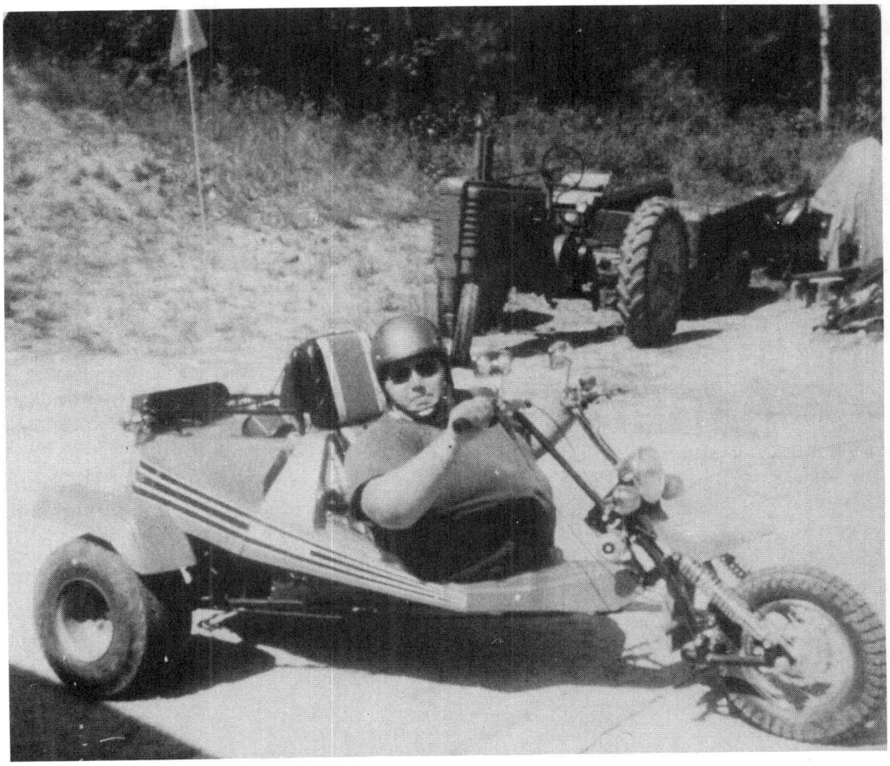

FIG 25–9.
Patient 6 on motor tricycle, designed and built by himself. (From Miller TR: *Prog Clin Cancer* 1982; 8:227–236. Used by permission.)

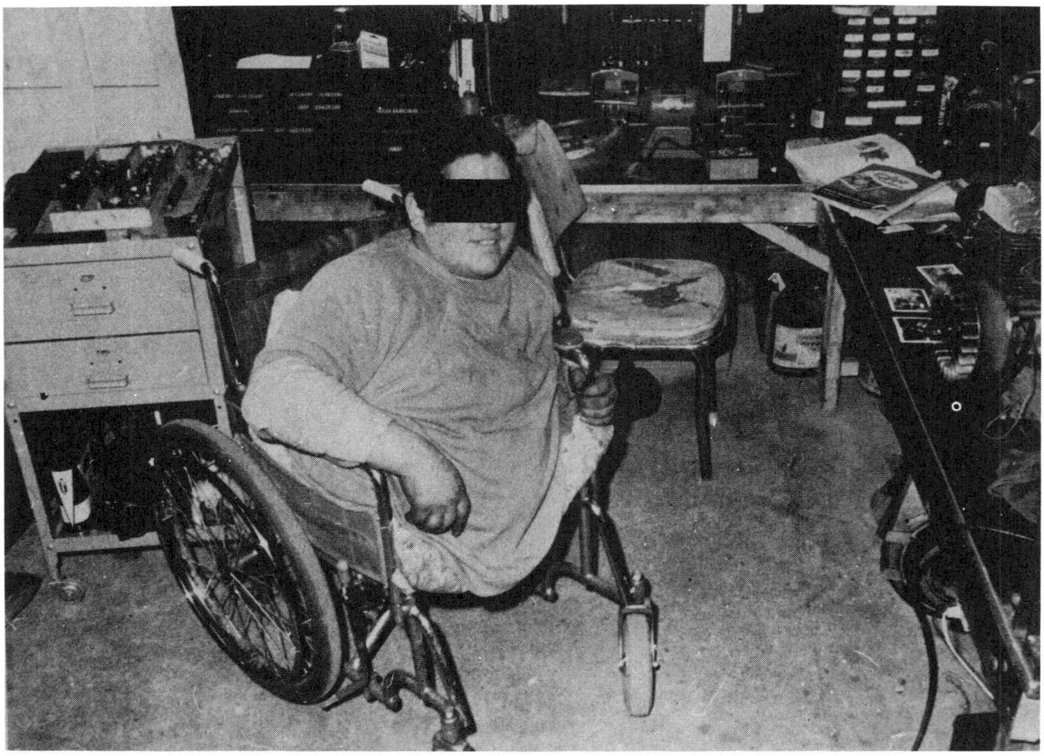

FIG 25–10.
Patient 6 at work in the laboratory of his electronics business.

REFERENCES

1. American Cancer Society: *Cancer Facts & Figures—1990.* Atlanta, GA, American Cancer Society, Inc.
2. Allen JG: *Surgery: Principles and Practice.* Philadelphia, J. B. Lippincott, 1957.
3. Pack GT: Argument for bilateral mastectomy (editorial). J Surg 1951; 29:929.
4. Kennedy J: Personal communication with author at Joseph Price Hospital, Philadelphia, 1931.
5. Lillehei RC, Wangensteen OH: Bowel function after colectomy for cancer, polyps and diverticulitis. *JAMA* 1955; 159:163–170.
6. Miller TR: Translumbar amputation. *Prog Clin Cancer* 1982; 8:227–236.
7. Pearlman NW, McShane RH, Jochimson PR, et al: Hemicorporectomy for intractable decubitus ulcers. *Arch Surg* 1976; 111:1139–1143.
8. Miller TR, Mackenzie AR, Randall HT. Translumbar amputation for advanced cancer: Indications and physiologic alterations in four cases. *Ann Surg* 1966; 164:514–519.
9. Shafir M, Abel M, Tausk H, et al: Hemicorporectomy—Perioperative management: A case presentation and review of literature. *J Surg Oncol* 1984; 26:79–82.

Chapter 26

The Abdomino-inguinal Incision in the Management of Pelvic Sarcomas

Constantine P. Karakousis

Tumors located in the midline of the pelvis without lateral fixation usually do not present difficulties in resection. Tumors located in or extending to the wall of the pelvis with apparent fixation are usually called unresectable or are treated with hemipelvectomy. The reason for the alleged unresectability of these tumors, or the necessity to resort to hemipelvectomy, is inadequacy of exposure of the pelvis by conventional abdominal incisions.

The pelvis may be subdivided into the lesser pelvis below the pelvic brim and the greater pelvis above the pelvic brim. At exploration, the pelvic brim is not directly visible, but its approximate location is indicated by the medial margin of the psoas muscle, and the iliac vessels coursing on this muscle.

A tumor located in the area of the distal portion of iliopsoas cannot be removed through a midline, paramedian, or low oblique incision above the inguinal ligament because there is not sufficient distal exposure to permit a safe and deliberate resection. The iliopsoas muscle extends into the upper thigh and inserts into the lesser trochanter. The femoral nerve proximally lies deep within the muscle fibers of psoas muscle and cannot be easily identified. The common iliac vessels can be dissected proximally through an abdominal incision, but the exposure over the distal portion of external iliac vessels is inadequate and does not easily permit distal vascular control. In the past, tumors in this area have been managed with hemipelvectomy.

In the case of a tumor with fixation to the wall of the lesser pelvis, similar problems arise. Proximal vessel control is easily accomplished through abdominal incisions, but vascular control is lacking. Adequate exposure is crucial in this area. Most tumors in this region are abandoned as unresectable due to the high risk of exsanguinating bleeding from large veins in the wall of the pelvis. Because it is usually not possible to obtain a wide margin medically due to the proximity of ureter, bladder, and rectosigmoid, hemipelvectomy has not been commonly employed for these tumors. To further compound the problems, some tumors extend anteriorly to involve the anterior abdominal wall.

From the foregoing discussion, it is apparent that an abdominal incision that provides simultaneous exposure of the abdomen, the pelvic wall structures, and the groin in one continuous field (the abdomino-inguinal incision), is needed for these tumors. Given the requirement for exposure and versatility and desirability of leaving the peritoneum on the surface of the tumor to be resected, it follows that the abdominal portion of the incision should be a transperitoneal approach. Because midline incisions provide great versatility and exposure, and considering the anatomical area that we are interested in, the abdominal portion of the incision should be a lower midline incision from just above the umbilicus to the pubic symphysis. Because the groin and femoral vessels on the involved side are to be exposed in continuity with the iliac vessels, the lower end of the midline incision should be extended laterally to the approximate level of the femoral vessels and then inferiorly for about 5 cm. The ipsilateral rectus muscle should be divided close to the pubic crest and the inguinal ligament near the pubic tubercle. The inferior epigastric vessels originate from the terminal portion of the external iliac vessels just above the inguinal ligament and travel to the posterior surface of the rectus abdominis muscle. These vessels, therefore, should be ligated and divided near their origin from the external iliac vessels to allow mobilization of the inferior abdominal wall, which may be facilitated further by dissecting the lateral third of the inguinal ligament off the iliac fascia.

With the preceding discussion, we were able to deduce a method for allowing adequate exposure, to permit safe dissection and removal of pelvic tumors with lateral fixation. This technique was developed in practice due to the necessity for exposure of low pelvic tumors, but was aided by the background knowledge of our technique of radical groin dissection, which also involves division of the inguinal ligament (lateral to the femoral artery) and of the inferior epigastric vessels.[1]

TECHNIQUE

With the patient supine on the operating table a lower midline incision from just above the umbilicus to the pubic symphysis is performed. The linea alba is incised and the peritoneum opened (Fig. 26–1). The transperitoneal approach provides better exposure, versatility, the chance to explore the rest of the abdominal cavity to rule out metastatic disease, and the opportunity to leave the posterior parietal peritoneum on the surface of the pelvic tumor for greater margin. A low oblique incision on the side of involvement, even if made to extend into the groin and to transect the inguinal ligament to provide complete exposure of the vessels, cannot provide adequate exposure for dealing with the ureter, bladder, and rectosigmoid.

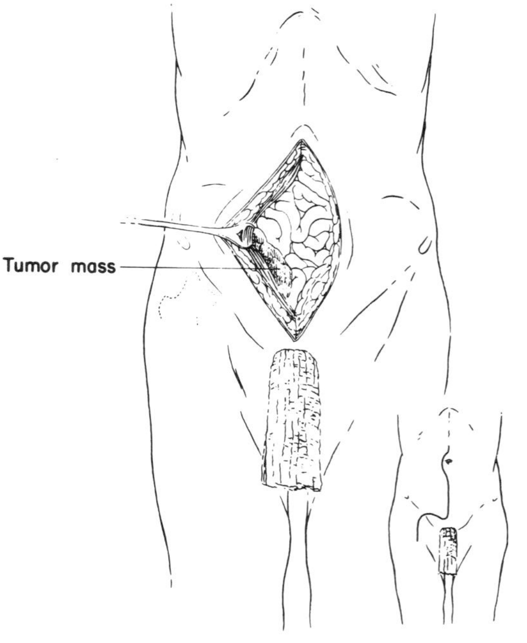

FIG 26–1.
A lower midline incision is first performed to assess the extent of the tumor and its relation to the midline structures. The complete incision is shown in the inset. (From Karakousis CP: *Cancer* 1984; 54:2543–2548. Used by permission.)

The area of tumor is then approached, and dissection may be performed to separate the ureter, rectosigmoid, and bladder from the tumor. This is done provided the dissection is easy and these structures are not involved by tumor. If they are involved, the nature of the tumor to be resected (i.e., whether primary or metastatic and according to its histology) should determine whether removal of structures such as the ureter, rectosigmoid, and bladder, to be followed by the appropriate reconstruction, would be warranted.

Fixation of the tumor does not imply unresectability; the psoas muscle itself is not movable on palpation, yet it is resectable. If the iliac or ischiac portions of the innominate bone are not involved on the basis of a prior pelvic X-ray and bone scan, one should be able to proceed with the resection. The pubic bone, if involved, is removed easily with the abdomino-inguinal incision.

After the decision to proceed with the resection has been made, the lower end of the abdominal incision is continued transversely to the same groin as the side of pelvic fixation of the tumor. At the point of pulsation of the femoral artery, or roughly the middle of the inguinal ligament, the incision is carried inferiorly for about 6 cm. Through this vertical portion of the incision, the common femoral vessels are exposed, and vessel loops are passed around them (Fig. 26–2). If large lymph nodes are present in the obturator area, the vertical portion of the incision may be continued caudally to almost the apex of the femoral triangle. Skin flaps are raised, and dissection of the inguinal nodes, as in superficial groin dissection, is accomplished. The femoral canal nodes should be removed in continuity with the deep iliac nodes, which is the way the procedure was originally described, that is, as a combination with groin dissection.[2] However, inguinal node dissection is not necessary for most pelvic tumors (particularly sarcomas), and only the exposure of the femoral vessels is necessary.

The anterior rectus sheath is then divided within a few millimeters from the pubic crest, leaving only enough on the crest to permit the placement of sutures and reconstruction of this sheath at the end of the operation. The rectus muscle is also divided near the crest. The inguinal ligament is then divided near the pubic tubercle. It seems best to divide the ligament at this point because it is then mobilized completely with the rest of the lower abdominal wall. If the inguinal ligament were to be divided more laterally, for example, near its middle, exposure over the femoral canal area or for removal of the pubic bone would be inadequate, and the plane of dissection would certainly not be anatomical.

After the inguinal ligament has been divided at the pubic tubercle, dissection continues cautiously on its undersurface until the inferior epigastric vein and artery are exposed, ligated, and divided (Fig. 26–3). The lateral third of the inguinal ligament is then sharply dissected off the iliac fascia to which it is normally fused. This allows complete mobilization of the lower abdominal wall, with the rectus muscle now retracted above the level of anterior superior iliac spine (Fig. 26–4).

In the male patient, the spermatic cord encountered at the level of the external inguinal ring is encircled with umbilical tape, the external oblique aponeurosis is opened in the direction of its fibers to the level of the internal inguinal ring, and the posterior inguinal wall is opened

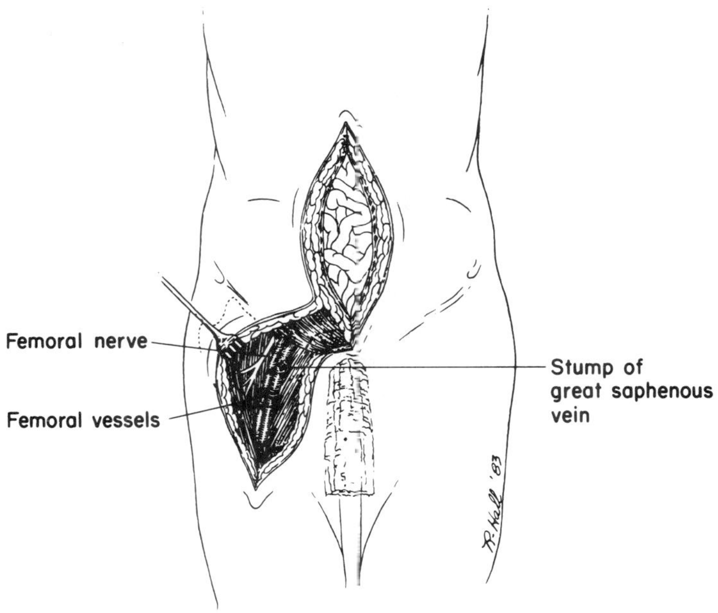

FIG 26–2.
The femoral vessels are exposed and, if necessary for a laterally located tumor, the femoral nerve. (From Karakousis CP: *Cancer* 1984; 54:2543–2548. Used by permission.)

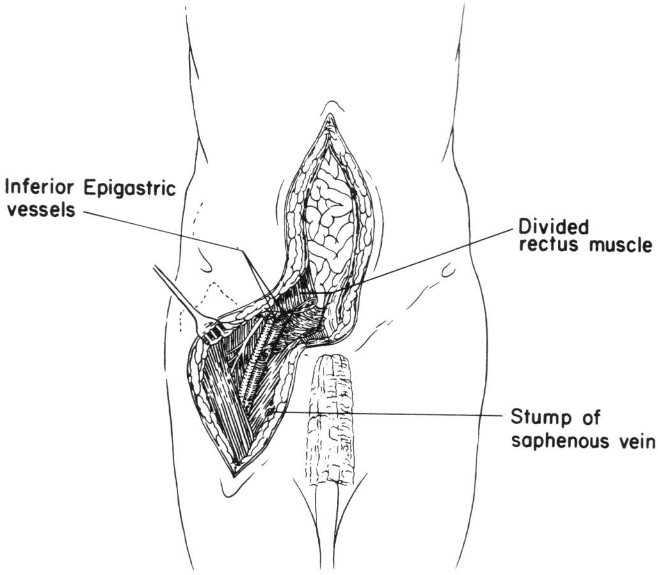

FIG 26–3.
The ipsilateral rectus sheath and muscle have been divided as well as the inguinal ligament near its attachment to the pubic tubercle. The inferior epigastric vessels are dissected so they can be ligated and divided. (From Karakousis CP: *Cancer* 1984; 54:2543–2548. Used by permission.)

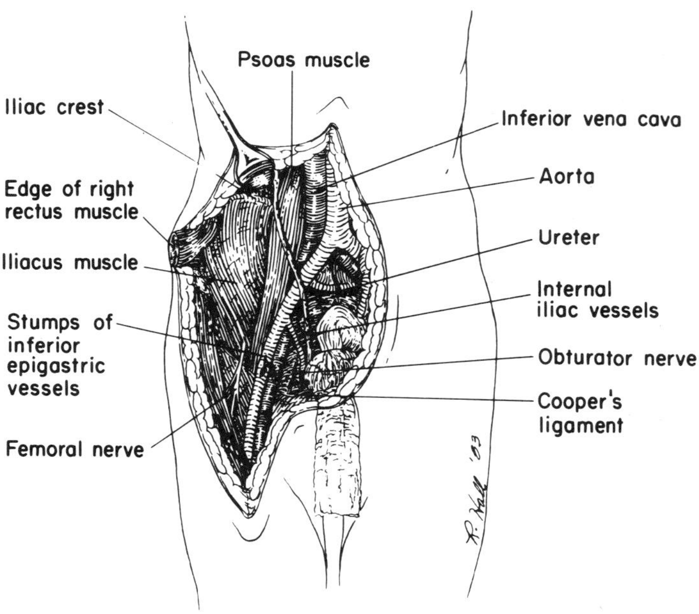

FIG 26–4.
The inferior epigastric vessels have been divided and the lateral third of the inguinal ligament detached off the iliac fascia. There is now full exposure of the pelvis on the side of the abdomino-inguinal incision. (From Karakousis CP: *Cancer* 1984; 54:2543–2548. Used by permission.)

in the same direction. At this point, the internal spermatic vessels may be divided deep to the level of the internal inguinal ring and the vas deferens displaced more medially and out of harm's way; the other alternative is simply to ligate and divide the spermatic cord at the level of the internal ring. Either procedure permits preservation of the viability of the ipsilateral testis as long as the latter has not been mobilized out of its scrotal bed. The inguinal ligament is then divided at the pubic tubercle, and the dissection is continued as previously described.

More recently, we have used a third method for extricating the spermatic cord from the inguinal canal. As the rectus muscle and sheath are divided off the pubic crest and the spermatic cord is approached, visualization of the internal ring from within the peritoneal cavity is easy. An incision then on the inner side of the abdominal wall, from the level corresponding to the external ring to the internal ring, divides the floor of the inguinal canal and permits medial retraction of the vas deferens and the spermatic vessels when the latter are not involved proximally. This maneuver leaves the external oblique aponeurosis undisturbed.

After the lower abdominal wall and inguinal ligament have been mobilized laterally, the lower abdomen and the groin on the side of involvement are exposed in one field. Vessel loops may be passed around the common iliac vessels proximally and, if not obstructed by the tumor, around the internal iliac vessels.

The dissection then proceeds according to the location of the tumor. For a tumor located in the greater pelvis, the femoral nerve should be identified. It is found most easily lateral to the femoral artery, one plane behind the level of the artery, at the point where it starts dividing into branches. It is then traced proximally behind the iliac fascia, between the psoas and iliacus muscles, to the origin at the lumbar spine. Near its origin, the femoral nerve splays out to the lumbar roots (L2–L4), which contribute to its formation. If during dissection of the femoral nerve it is found to be involved by tumor, it may be sacrificed. The resulting deficit in extension of the knee is something the patient can learn to cope with and overcome by physical therapy, so that walking with the use of a cane may be expected. The iliopsoas muscle may be removed completely from origin to insertion through this approach, a procedure that does not result in any apparent deficit in ordinary activity (Fig. 26–5).

Dissection of the iliac vessels, or occasionally even removal of a tumor-involved iliac vessel and replacement with a graft, can be accomplished. For complete removal of a tumor located in the lesser pelvis, the external iliac vein, obturator nodes, distal portion of the ureter, a portion of the wall of the bladder, the rectosigmoid and the uterus and ipsilateral ovary and Fallopian tube may have to be resected (Figs. 26–6 and 26–7). The obturator nerve may be removed if involved (Fig. 26–8). Observations of patients with resection of the entire adductor group of muscles, or deliberate sacrifice of the obturator nerve above the obturator foramen, suggest there is no appreciable deficit in ordinary walking; no crutch or cane support is needed. However, when lying supine with the thigh abducted, the patient may have to sit and use hands to adduct the leg.

The closure of this incision is accomplished by approximating the inguinal ligament to the iliac fascia lateral to the vessels and to Cooper's ligament medial to the vessels, using nonabsorbable interrupted sutures. The rectus sheath and muscle are approximated to the pubic crest (Fig. 26–9).

A suction drain may be placed in the inguinal area, the subcutaneous fat is approximated with interrupted chromic catgut sutures, and the skin is approximated with interrupted monofilament sutures. If the inguinal nodes have been removed in continuity with large deep nodes, and the inguinal flaps were thin, the femoral vessels should be covered with the sartorius muscle as in a groin dissection.[1] The abdominal portion of the incision is a routine fashion.

If the tumor extends anteriorly to involve the deep layers of the anterior wall, several choices are available. If the tumor is attached to the transverse abdominis muscle, a plane may be developed between the internal oblique and external oblique muscles and the two deep muscles attached to (in order to be removed with) the tumor can be left, while the external oblique aponeurosis and inguinal ligament are mobilized as explained before.

If the tumor invades more extensively anteriorly, a plane may be developed between the subcutaneous fat and the external oblique aponeurosis, resecting the appropriate portion of the anterolateral abdominal wall muscles with the tumor; this implies removal of the inguinal ligament, and the resulting defect may be repaired later with polypropylene (Marlex) mesh.

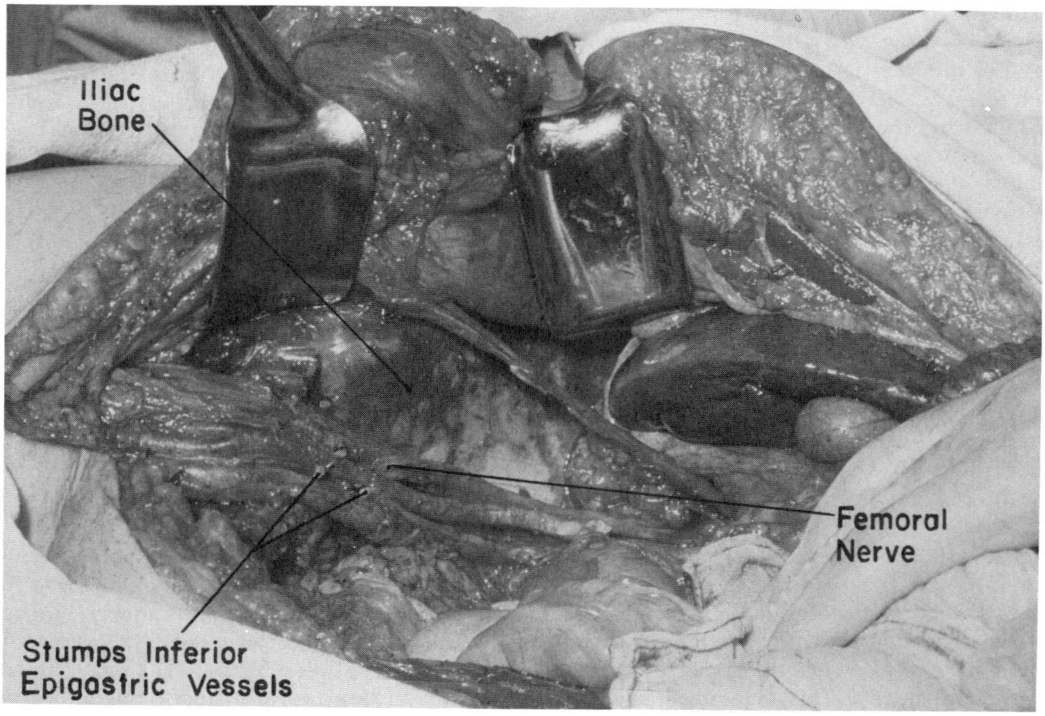

FIG 26–5.
The iliopsoas muscle has been removed. The femoral nerve and iliofemoral vessels are visible. (From Karakousis CP: *Cancer* 1984; 54:2543–2548. Used by permission.)

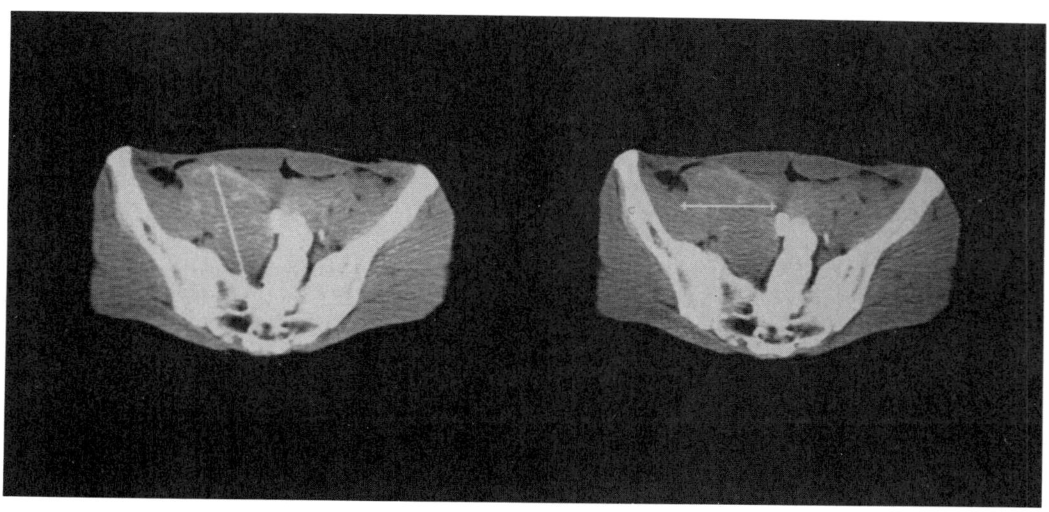

FIG 26–6.
Computed tomography showing desmoid tumor in the area of the lesser pelvis.

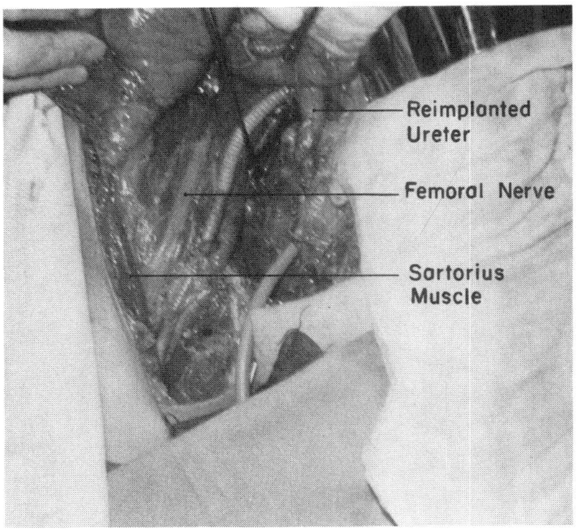

FIG 26–7.
View of the pelvis following resection of tumor together with right salpingo-ophorectomy, hysterectomy, resection of involved portion of distal ureter and proximal re-implantation in the bladder, and Dacron graft replacement of right iliac artery.

This is sutured superiorly to the edge of the available fascia and inferiorly to the iliac fascia lateral to the femoral vessels or to Cooper's ligament medial to the femoral vessels. If the pubic bone is to be resected along with a soft-tissue mass, the pubic symphysis is divided with a Gigli saw and the adductor muscles divided near their origin from the pubic bone. The superior and inferior pubic rami are also divided with a Gigli saw, and the medial portion of the pubic bone is removed (Fig. 26–10). Finally, if a full thickness of the lower abdominal wall including the skin needs to be removed, the resulting defect in this area may be covered with a myocutaneous tensor fasciae latae flap.[3–5]

DISCUSSION

In the period 1979 to 1983, the abdomino-inguinal incision has been used in 24 patients to expose various tumors situated in the pelvis that had lateral fixation, precluding safe dissection and removal through an abdominal incision.[6, 7]

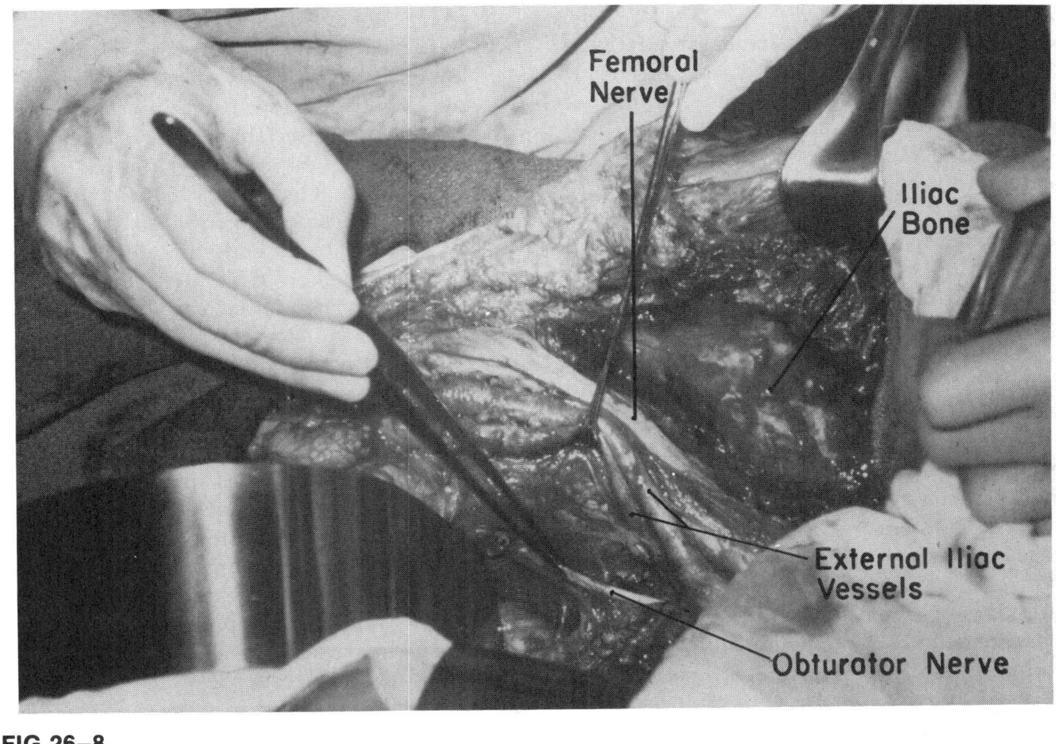

FIG 26–8.
A recurrent liposarcoma in the right iliac fossa has been removed. The femoral nerve and vessels are exposed. The obturator nerve was preserved because it was not involved with tumor.

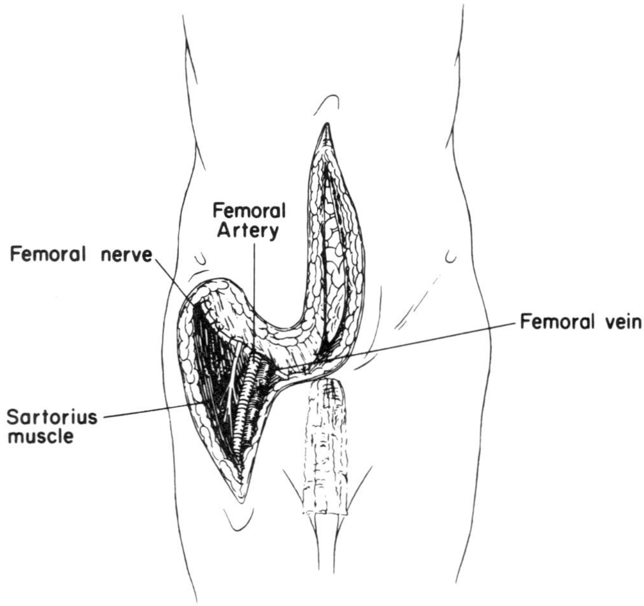

FIG 26–9.
At closure, the inguinal ligament is approximated to the iliac fascia and Cooper's ligament, leaving sufficient space in between for the passage of the femoral vessels and femoral nerve. (From Karakousis CP: *Cancer* 1984; 54:2543–2548. Used by permission.)

In nine of 16 patients with sarcomas of soft tissue or osseous origin, the tumor was locally recurrent and considered unresectable on one of more explorations at another institution. There has been one local reccurence in a patient with malignant fibrohistiocytoma. At the writing of this report, 11 of the 16 patients remained well, with a mean follow-up of 23 months (range, 3 to 56 months).

There was a clearcut local recurrence in only one patient, whereas two patients developed intraperitoneal tumor in the upper abdomen without definite evidence of recurrence in the iliac fossa. Two patients with chondrosarcomas in the lesser pelvis had the tumor resected through the abdomino-inguinal incision, four other patients had metastatic tumor in iliac lymph nodes removed through this incision. These patients usually present with further metastases later; therefore, resection of these large metastatic nodes may have only palliative value. In two patients with radiation necrosis of the inguinal area, the abdomino-inguinal incision was used to resect the radiation-induced ulcer and adjacent tissues. In these patients, the external iliac artery was first exposed and controlled in the retroperitoneum. Finally, this incision was used successfully in removing an unclassified tumor in the left groin and a sigmoid adenocarcinoma with fixation to the iliac fascia previously called unresectable.

In patients with tumors situated in the lesser pelvis with lateral fixation, there are additional benefits besides improved exposure that may be provided by the abdomino-inguinal incision. Bilateral ligation of the internal iliac arteries can be performed to decrease bleeding during the dissection. Also, the plane of dissection can be kept away from the tumor and may include, for example, an adjacent portion of rectosigmoid. A better margin is thus obtained, and there is less bleeding. In the plane between the tumor and adjacent tissues, there are usually numerous blood vessels precluding a clean, accurate dissection. Adjacent organs to be removed depend on the judgment of the surgeon as to the necessity for a greater margin and the functional sequelae to the patient following the removal of the particular organ. Finally, most of the deep pelvic dissection can be carried out under direct vision. With large tumors situated in the lesser pelvis, there comes a point where sharp dissection posteriorly must be accomplished with palpatory guidance only.

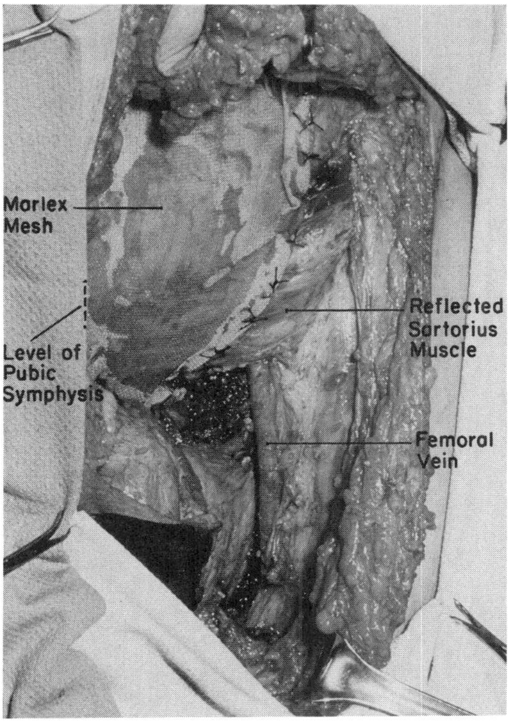

FIG 26–10.
Marlex mesh is replacing the removed portion of the lower abdominal muscles and the left inguinal ligament. In this patient, the medial portion of the left pubic bone has been removed and the defect covered with the Marlex mesh, which is sutured inferiorly to the perineal fascia.

If the internal iliac arteries are bilaterally ligated, there should not be brisk arterial bleeding, but exsanguinating venous bleeding may still occur from the pelvic wall. In most cases, it should be possible to control the bleeders with suture ligatures. If the venous bleeding exceeds the capacity of the suctioning apparatus to keep the field dry for suture ligation, the alternative is to pack the lesser pelvis tightly with large vaginal packs. The packs are removed in 48 hours and if there is still some oozing, this can be controlled with gel-foam packing or other hemostatic material. This procedure has been used successfully in two instances.

The abdomino-inguinal incision takes $1\frac{1}{2}$ hours for opening and closure and is accomplished with minimal blood loss. There have been no wound infections or incisional hernias. In one patient whose tumor had been approached previously through a transverse abdominal incision, a small area of skin-edge necrosis developed in the corner of the skin near the pubic symphysis. This area was debrided and a skin graft applied. This occurrence is easily explained because the upper transverse incision had interrupted the superior epigastric vessels and possibly lumbar branches, whereas the abdomino-inguinal incision routinely interrupts the inferior epigastric vessels. In a patient who has had a previous lower oblique incision, skin flap ischemia may be avoided by making the transverse portion of the abdomino-inguinal incision within the lower oblique incision scar. A narrow piece of skin between two parallel incision is thus avoided. Following resection of the lower abdominal muscles and inguinal ligament, due to involvement by the tumor, a mesh may be used for reconstruction, but care should be taken that direct contact between the mesh and the femoral vessels is avoided by interposing the mobilized sartorius or rectus femoris muscle. One of our patients, with previous radiation elsewhere, presented with bleeding 2 weeks postoperatively from the distal external iliac artery, which at re-exploration appeared to be due to erosion of the artery by the mesh. In situations involving resection of the lower abdominal wall, we have used for coverage (more recently) the contralateral rectus abdominis muscle based on the inferior epigastric vessels, which appears to be the method of choice.

There is little question that the abdomino-inguinal incision provides greater opportunities than abdominal incisions for the removal of pelvic tumors with lateral fixation. It should be used for smaller tumors if a more adequate margin is needed, or for larger tumors in combination with adjuvant irradiation to control microscopic residual disease.

For lateral pelvic tumors with involvement of the iliac bone, the procedure of internal hemipelvectomy with limb preservation may be used,[8] and for large tumors involving the iliac bone in addition to the iliofemoral nerve, the usual posterior flap hemipelvectomy may be used.[9]

SUMMARY

The abdomino-inguinal incision, a method for exposure and resection of pelvic tumors with lateral fixation, has been used in 24 patients with a variety of tumors, including 14 patients with soft-tissue sarcomas. These tumors, previously considered unresectable, were removed through this incision, which should increase the rate of resectability of tumors in this area and decrease the need for hemipelvectomy.

REFERENCES

1. Karakousis CP: Ilioinguinal lymph node dissection. *Am J Surg* 1981; 141:299–303.
2. Karakousis CP: Exposure and reconstruction in the lower portions of the retroperitoneum abdominal wall. *Arch Surg* 1982; 117:840–844.
3. Nahai F, Hill HL, Hester TR: Experiences with the tensor fascia lata flap. *Plast Reconstr Surg* 1979; 63:788–799.
4. Hill HL, Hester R, Nahai F: Covering large groin defects with the tensor fascia lata musculocutaneous flap. *Br J Plast Surg* 1979; 32:12–14.
5. Airhart RA, deKernion JB, Guillermo EO: Tensor fascia lata myocutaneous flap for coverage of skin defect after radical groin dissection for metastatic penile carcinoma. *J Urol* 1982; 128:599–601.
6. Karakousis CP: Utility of the abdominoinguinal incision in the resection of abdominal tumors. *J Surg Oncol* 1984; 26:176–182.
7. Karakousis CP: The abdominoinguinal incision in limb salvage and resection of pelvic tumors. *Cancer* 1984; 54:2543–2548.
8. Karakousis CP: Internal hemipelvectomy. *Surg Gynecol Obstet* 1984; 158:279–282.
9. Karakousis CP: The technique of major amputations for malignant tumors. *J Surg Oncol* 1983; 23:43–55.

Chapter 27

Surgical Treatment of Soft-Tissue Sarcoma Pulmonary Metastasis

Clifton F. Mountain

Pulmonary metastasis from primary sarcomas of the soft tissues is a common event, often occurring within a year or two of the primary treatment. In fact, during the initial period of their natural history, soft-tissue sarcomas metastasize virtually exclusively to the lungs.[1] The prevalence of blood-borne metastasis from these tumors is related to the intimate association of the sarcomas to their vascular channels, with large and small vessel invasion being frequently described in the more rapidly growing tumor types.[2] The potential for success of a surgical approach is based on the premise that for a time, that cannot be precisely quantitated, the metastatic disease apparently is confined to the lungs and is amenable to complete resection. This is confirmed by reports in the literature of (1) autopsy series in which the lungs are the only site of metastasis, (2) studies of patterns of metastatic spread,[3–5] and (3) the many references giving 5-year survival rates from the date of pulmonary surgery of 20% to 50% for patients with specific tumor types.[6–10]

The scientific rationale for the resection of pulmonary metastatic disease is supported by the work of Weiss et al.[11, 12] in experimental animal tumor systems. This work proposes that metastasis of metastases is a key feature of the natural history of cancer in humans, and that many tumors first metastasize to "generalizing" sites from which further metastases arise. Although target organ preference does not always relate to anatomical considerations, the most frequent organ location of distant metastasis in many types of cancer appears to be the first capillary bed encountered by the circulating cells, for example, sarcomas metastasizing to lungs, lung cancer metastasizing to brain, and colorectal tumor disseminating to liver.[13] Skipper[14] has recently reviewed earlier work on tumor cell kinetics which indicated that the reduction of total body burden of tumor may provide an enhanced setting for the use of adjuvant treatment to control micrometastasis.

CRITERIA FOR SELECTION OF PATIENTS

The objective of resection as primary modality treatment for pulmonary metastatic disease is to eradicate all tumor and render the patient disease free. The extent to which this may be successfully accomplished depends on adherence to simple, but strict, selection criteria that are generally agreed on by the thoracic surgical community: first, the primary cancer must be fully controlled with no recurrent or metastatic disease, other than the lung metastasis; second, a reasonable potential exists for complete resection of all known tumor by the planned surgical procedure(s); and third, the patient must be physiologically able to tolerate the planned surgery and loss of pulmonary tissue. If these basic criteria apply, lesions appearing sequentially and bilateral disease may be successfully treated.

With the advent of more effective chemotherapy for soft-tissue sarcoma,[15] selected patients may undergo operation for pulmonary metastasis as adjuvant therapy in a multimodal schema aimed at achieving complete remission status.[16]

Several investigators have examined the prognostic significance of a number of tumor and host characteristics. Tumor doubling time, disease-free interval from primary treatment to detection of pulmonary metastasis, number and size of pulmonary tumors, site of the primary lesion, and histology are reported to have a significant impact on survival.[17–21] Not all authors agree that all factors are significant. Casson et al.[19] reported that a multivariate analysis of tumor doubling time, number of nodules on preoperative computed tomography, number of nodules resected, extent of resection, histology, laterality, and disease-free interval showed the most significant prognostic indicator to be four or more nodules on computed tomography (CT) scan. All other factors became nonsignificant, indicating an interdependence with four or more nodules on CT scan. The data of most authors consistently confirm a significant survival advantage for complete removal of all pulmonary disease. Investigators from various areas with differing referral patterns report similar survival rates, using the basic selection criteria, whether or not additional factors are a part of the selection process. Reported differences in prognostic elements may relate to the types of cases included in a particular series and the numbers of patients in specific subsets. The results that are achieved reflect the impact and limitations of surgery, or surgery plus adjuvant therapy on the process of disease progression in specific situations.

DIAGNOSIS AND EVALUATION

In our practice, careful screening for clinical or biochemical signs of disseminated disease or diffuse seeding in the lungs is the first stage of the selection process. Studies of diagnostic imaging in metastatic lung disease prove that CT is the most sensitive screening method for detecting pulmonary metastases.[21, 22] Although specificity is diminished because the technique does not reveal nodules smaller than 2 to 3 mm in diameter, this factor is related to clinical circumstances and a high specificity can be anticipated for tumors with a high propensity for metastasizing to the lungs. Pass et al.[23] reported that 95% of CT-depicted nodules in selected osteogenic and soft-tissue sarcoma patients represented metastasis. During the time frame of the series of patients reported in this chapter, few patients underwent computed tomography; however, in today's practice we consider CT to be imperative in the work-up of all patients who are candidates for surgical treatment of pulmonary metastasis. When CT is not available or feasible, full-chest linear tomography is obtained. Liver and brain scans are performed only if abnormalities in the biochemical profile or bone scans are found. If both diagnosis and treatment are to be accomplished at thoracotomy, needle biopsy is seldom performed. Mediastinoscopy usually is not indicated in patients with pulmonary metastasis from primary sarcomas. Spirometry, arterial blood gas analysis, and xenon 133 regional function studies are obtained to evaluate predicted postoperative lung function.

CONTRIBUTION OF SURGICAL TREATMENT

To evaluate precisely the contribution of surgical treatment or of surgical treatment plus planned adjuvant therapy to the control of pulmonary metastasis, we reviewed our own experience from 1947 through 1980 at the M. D. Anderson Cancer Center (Houston, Texas).[24] Seven hundred and seventy-two resections were performed on 556 patients with a surgical mortality rate of 1.5%. A selection of 443 patients was made that excluded patients that died within 30 days of the operation, that did not meet the selection criteria, and whose first pulmonary metastasis was treated definitively by other modalities. The overall cumulative 5-year survival rate from the date of the first pulmonary resection was 35%. Survival calculations were made according to the method of Gehan.[25] Included in this set of data were 49 patients with sarcoma originating in the soft tissues, 76 patients with primary skeletal tumors, and 17 patients with sarcoma in miscellaneous other sites, such as skin, peritoneum, and male and female genital tract. The survival rate for the soft-tissue sarcoma group was not significantly different from that for patients with primary skeletal tumors, although the rate was lower. Patients with miscellaneous other primary sarcomas had a significantly poorer prognosis than was observed for those with soft-tissue or skeletal sarcoma (Fig. 27–1).

Twelve histological entities were treated (Table 27–1). Pulmonary metastasis was controlled by surgery, with and without adjuvant therapy in 41% (20/49) of the patients; however, further distant metastatic disease was documented in three patients, 15% (3/20) of the group that had full control of all lung disease. In the 29 patients whose pulmonary disease was not controlled, 16 patients, 55% (16/29), had further distant metastasis or relapse of the primary. Although the numbers of patients are too small for valid assessment of the influence of histological type on the outcome, synovial sarcoma and rhabdomyosarcoma were the least favorable tumor types. In all other categories with more than one patient, 40% or more had all lung disease controlled by the surgical approach. Malignant fibrous histiocytoma has become the most commonly diagnosed soft-tissue sarcoma in most cancer centers[6]; however, because of the biological behavior of this tumor, few patients with tumors of this cell type are included in this report.

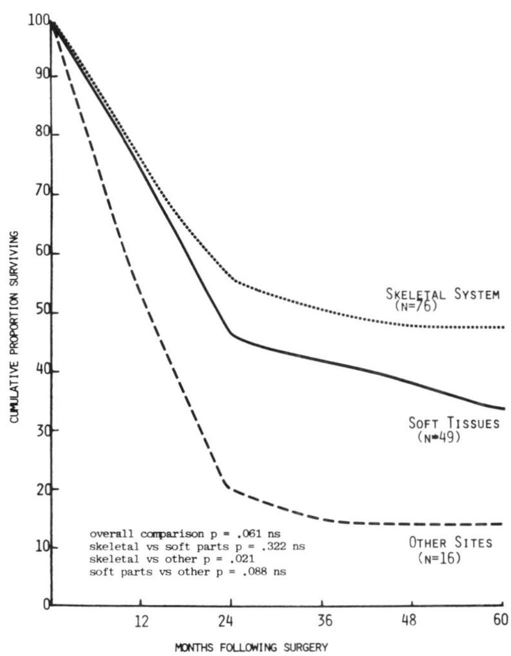

FIG 27–1.
Cumulative proportion of patients surviving after apparent complete resection of pulmonary metastasis from primary soft-tissue sarcoma according to anatomical site (M. D. Anderson Cancer Center, 1955 to 1980).

SURGICAL PROCEDURE

The majority of patients referred for surgical treatment have peripheral solitary lesions as the first manifestation of disease; therefore, conservative surgery is a feasible approach. Wedge or segmental resection is the procedure of choice, if all known disease can be encompassed by these operations. Conservation of lung tissue is important to permit bilateral thoracotomy or to allow for resection of subsequent metastatic nodules, should they appear.

Multiple and bilateral lesions at first presentation were more common in the sarcoma patients than in those with carcinoma. Thirty-three percent (16/49) of the soft-tissue sarcoma patients had multiple lesions, most of them involving more than one lobe, and six presented with bilateral disease (Table 27–2). One third of the group underwent lobectomy as the first operation, another third had multiple wedge excisions, and one-fourth had single wedge or segmental resections. Five patients had planned bilateral thoracotomy and two patients underwent pneumonectomy. Planned pneumonectomy is not indicated, however, in view of the biological behavior of the disease and the evidence for preserving lung function to allow subsequent resection if it is required. Median sternotomy has been advocated as the most suitable approach for resection of pulmonary metastasis because bilateral disease not shown pre-operatively may be identified and its use eliminates a second surgical procedure.[26, 27] In our practice median sternotomy is used selec-

TABLE 27–1.
Control* of Pulmonary Metastasis According to Histological Type†

Histological Type	*N*	Pulmonary Metastasis: Controlled	Pulmonary Metastasis: Not Controlled
Fibrosarcoma	12	5	7
Neurofibrosarcoma	4	3	1
Sarcoma NOS‡	6	3	3
Liposarcoma	6	3	3
Synovial sarcoma	5	1	4
Fibrohistiocytoma	5	2	3
Rhabdomyosarcoma	4	1	3
Chondrosarcoma	2	1	1
Leiomyosarcoma	2	1	1
Hemangiosarcoma	1	0	1
Mixed mesodermal sarcoma	1	0	1
Angiosarcoma	1	0	1
Total	49	20 (40.8%)	29 (59.2%)

* *Full control of all disease in the lungs.*
† *M. D. Anderson Cancer Center, 1955 to 1980.*
‡ *NOS = not otherwise specified.*

tively, depending on the location of the lesions, for example, those in the right lung and left upper lobe.

The first observed pulmonary metastasis was a solitary nodule in 55% (27/49) of the patients with primary soft-tissue sarcomas. Thirty-three percent (16/49) had ipsilateral multiple lesions, involving more than one lobe in all but one patient, and 12% (6/49) had bilateral tumors. A markedly poorer survival rate was observed for the ipsilateral–multiple-lesion group than for patients with solitary tumors or bilateral disease. The difference was statistically significant between the patients with ipsilateral multiple lesions and the small number with bilateral disease (Fig. 27–2). Local failure was a major problem in the 16 patients treated initially for ipsilateral multiple tumors; in 80% of these patients full control of the lung disease was not achieved. Included in this group were five patients with unfavorable histological findings (Table 27–1) and the two patients who required pneumonectomy.

Figure 27–3 illustrates the survival pattern according to the number of thoracotomies performed. These data support the principle that if all known malignant disease can be removed, resection is a valid option in patients with tumors appearing sequentially, as well as for those with bilateral disease. Sixteen patients had more than one thoracotomy (ten patients, two thoracotomies; four patients, three thoracotomies; two patients, four thoracotomies). The survival rate for these patients was slightly higher than for patients with one operation, but the difference was not significant. This does not imply that bilateral tumors and local recurrence are a good thing, but that in selected patients these

TABLE 27–2.
Appearance of First Observed Pulmonary Metastasis*

First Observed Pulmonary Metastasis	Number	Percentage
Solitary lesion, < 3 cm	12	24.5
Solitary lesion, > 3 cm	15	30.6
Multiple lesions, one lobe	1	2.1
Multiple lesions, more than one lobe (one hemithorax)	15	30.6
Bilateral	6	12.2
Total	49	100.0

* *M. D. Anderson Cancer Center, 1955 to 1980.*

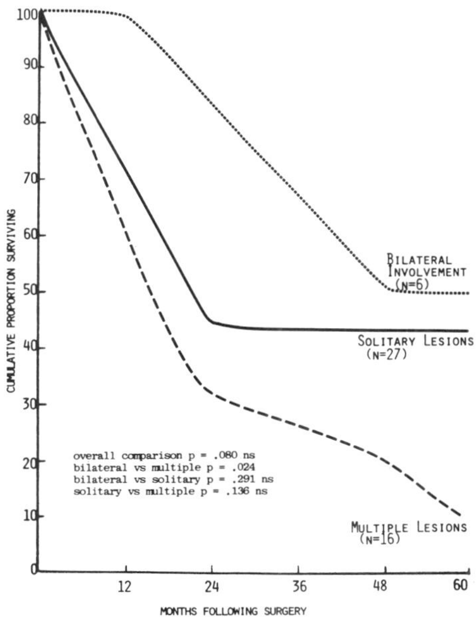

FIG 27–2.
Cumulative proportion of patients surviving after apparent complete resection of pulmonary metastasis from primary soft-tissue sarcoma, according to appearance of first observed pulmonary metastasis (M. D. Anderson Cancer Center, 1955 to 1980).

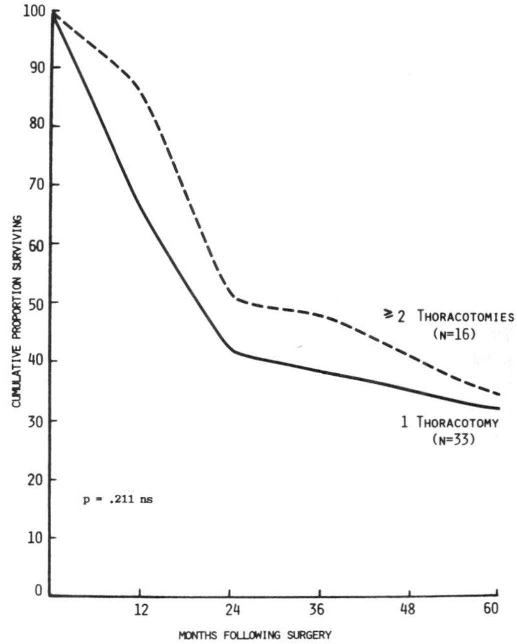

FIG 27–3.
Cumulative proportion of patients surviving after apparent complete resection of pulmonary metastasis from primary soft-tissue sarcoma, according to number of thoracotomies performed (M. D. Anderson Cancer Center, 1955 to 1980).

situations can be successfully managed, as long as the initial selection criteria are applied.

DURATION FROM PRIMARY TREATMENT TO FIRST OBSERVED PULMONARY METASTASIS

Pulmonary metastasis was detected in 39% (19/49) of patients within the first year following primary treatment (Table 27–3). Metastases were observed in another 31% (15/49) in the second and third years and in 31% (15/49) after 3 years. Figure 4 shows that there was no significant difference in the outcome according to this disease-free interval. The 5-year cumulative survival rate ranged from 28% for patients with pulmonary metastasis detected within the first year of primary treatment to 37% for those patients with disease detected after 3 years. Included in the less-than-1-year group are three patients whose pulmonary metastasis was present at the time of the primary treatment or discovered before the primary was treated. One patient with fibrous histiocytoma, who had bilateral disease at first presentation, remained tumor free 3½ years after the second thoracotomy; a second patient had no evidence of disease 6 years after pulmonary resection with en bloc removal of involved diaphragm. This patient had a fibrosarcoma of the shoulder that was treated pre-operatively with chemotherapy with no response. In a third patient with unclas-

TABLE 27–3.
Duration From Primary Treatment to First Observed Pulmonary Metastasis*

Duration (mo)	Number	Percentage
0	3	6.1
1–12	16	32.7
13–24	6	12.2
25–36	9	18.4
37–48	8	16.3
49–60	2	4.1
>60	5	10.2
Total	49	100.0

* *M. D. Anderson Cancer Center, 1955 to 1980.*

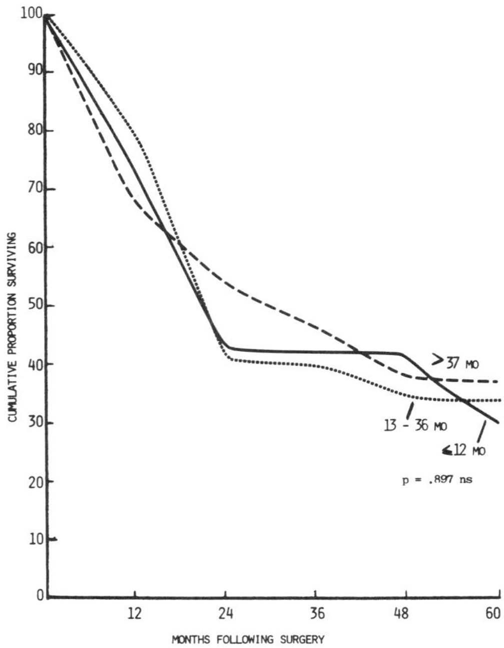

FIG 27–4.
Cumulative proportion of patients surviving after apparent complete resection for pulmonary metastasis from primary soft-tissue sarcoma, according to disease-free interval from primary treatment to first observed pulmonary metastasis (M. D. Anderson Cancer Center, 1955 to 1980).

sified sarcoma and a pulmonary lesion present at the time of primary treatment, the lung disease was not controlled. Although the findings in these three patients are anecdotal, based on our whole experience we consider the disease-free interval as a variable element related to the biology of the particular tumor and, probably, growth-modulating factors in the host. Patients having pulmonary metastasis detected within the first year of primary treatment are not excluded from surgical consideration on this basis alone, if the other selection criteria are met.

ROLE OF ADJUVANT THERAPY

In the present series of patients used to illustrate the applications of surgery for pulmonary metastasis from primary soft-tissue tumors, all known disease in the lungs was completely resected at each operation; however, about 60% (29/49) of these patients ultimately succumbed to the disseminated and uncontrolled growth of tumor cells. Thirty-one patients were treated with planned surgical adjuvant therapy; 19 underwent chemotherapy, eight chemoradiation and three chemoimmunotherapy, and one patient underwent planned chemoimmunoradiation. The outcome was superior for the patients treated with planned adjuvant treatment; 36% were expected to survive 5 years compared with 28% for the group of 18 patients undergoing surgery alone or surgery plus other unplanned treatment (Fig. 27–5). The difference is not significant. These results contrast with results for a total group of sarcoma patients ($N = 141$) undergoing resection for pulmonary metastasis. Statistically significant improvement was shown in this set of data for patients who received adjuvant therapy.[24] At present, trials are underway to evaluate the role of combination chemotherapy as initial treatment followed by surgery for patients with pulmonary metastatic disease. The same principles used for treatment of primary soft-tissue sarcoma are now applied to patients with metastatic disease.[16] The use of chemotherapy preoperatively has the obvious advantage of

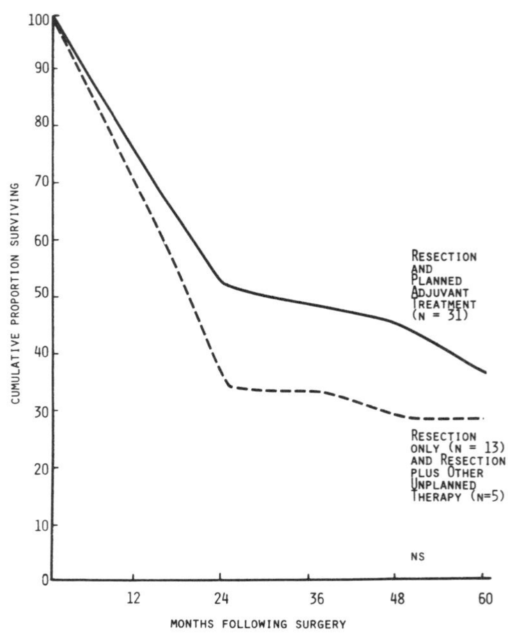

FIG 27–5.
Cumulative proportion of patients surviving after apparent complete resection for pulmonary metastasis from primary soft-tissue sarcoma, according to treatment regimen (M. D. Anderson Cancer Center, 1955 to 1980).

assessing the sensitivity of the tumor (in vivo) to specific drug regimens. In the present series, ten patients (20%, 10/49) had a partial response to pre-operative chemotherapy and were referred for resection of residual pulmonary disease. In current practice a larger proportion of patients now fall in this category. We are evaluating a protocol using a trial of two courses of pre-operative chemotherapy followed by resection and postoperative chemotherapy in those responding to the drugs.

ACKNOWLEDGMENTS

This project was supported by the Herman Neel Hipp Fund for Research in Thoracic Surgery and the Clifton F. Mountain Fund. The author acknowledges the contribution of K. E. Hermes to the research and writing of this chapter.

REFERENCES

1. Rosenberg SA: Adjuvant chemotherapy of adult soft tissue sarcomas, in Baker LH (ed): *Soft Tissue Sarcomas.* Boston, Martinus-Nijhoff Publishers NE Kluwer Academic, The Hague, Dordrecht, Lancaster, 1983, pp 85–99.
2. Willis RA: *The Spread of Tumors in the Human Body,* 3rd ed. London, Butterworths, 1973, p 12.
3. Farrell JT: Pulmonary metastasis; A pathological, clinical, roentgenologic study based on 78 cases at necropsy. *Radiology* 1935; 24:444–451.
4. Huth JF, Eilber FR: Patterns of metastatic spread following resection of extremity soft tissue sarcomas and strategies for treatment. *Semin Surg Oncol* 1988; 4:20–26.
5. Potter DA, Glenn J, Kinsella T, et al: Patterns of recurrence in patients with high grade soft-tissue sarcomas. *J Clin Oncol* 1985; 3:353–366.
6. Pezzi CM, Rawlings MS, Esgro JJ, et al: Prognostic factors in 227 patients with malignant fibrous histiocytoma. *Cancer* 1992; 69:2098–2103.
7. Steward J, Carey JA, Merrill WH, et al: Twenty year's experience with pulmonary metastasectomy. *Am Surg* 1992; 58:100–103.
8. Vogt-Moykopf I, Meyer G, Merkle NM, et al: Late results of surgical treatment of pulmonary metastasis. *Thorac Cardiovasc Surg* 1986; 34:143–148.
9. McCormack P: Surgical resection of pulmonary metastasis. *Semin Surg Oncol* 1990; 6:297–302.
10. van Dongen JA, Hart AM, Jonk A, et al: Resection of pulmonary metastasis. *Thorac Cardiovasc Surg* 1986; 34:140–142.
11. Weiss L, Ward PM, Holmes JC: Liver to lung traffic of cancer cells. *Int J Cancer* 1983; 32:79–83.
12. Weiss L, Ward PM: Effects of metastatic cascades on metastatic patterns: Studies on colon-26 carcinomas in mice. *Int J Cancer* 1988; 41:450–455.
13. Liotta LA, Stetler-Stevenson WG: Principles of molecular cell biology of cancer metastasis, in Devita VT, Hellman S, Rosenberg SA (eds): *Cancer, Principles and Practice of Oncology.* Philadelphia, J. B. Lippincott, 1989, pp 98–115.
14. Skipper HE: Tumor differences, drug differences, treatment design difference, and effects on therapeutic outcome (degree and duration of therapeutic response), in *Effects of Therapy and Kinetics of the Residual Tumor, Part A: Pre-Clinical Aspects.* New York, Wiley-Liss, 1990, pp 81–98.
15. Eilber FR, Huth JF, Mirra J, et al: Progress in the recognition and treatment of soft tissue sarcomas. *Cancer* 1990; 65:660–666.
16. Antman KH, Eilber FR, Shiu MH: Soft tissue sarcomas: Current trends in diagnosis and management. *Curr Prob Cancer* 1989; 13:337–367.
17. Jablons D, Steinberg SM, Roth J, et al: Metastasectomy for soft tissue sarcoma. *J Thorac Cardiovasc Surg* 1989; 97:695–705.
18. Pastorino U, Valente M, Gasparini M, et al: Lung resection for metastatic sarcomas: Total survival from primary treatment. *J Surg Oncol* 1989; 40:275–280.
19. Casson A, Putnam JB, Natarajan G, et al: Five-year survival after pulmonary metastasectomy for adult soft tissue sarcoma. *Cancer* 1992; 69:662–668.
20. Morton DL, Joseph WL, Ketcham AS, et al: Surgical resection and adjunctive immunotherapy for selected patients with multiple pulmonary metastases. *Ann Surg*1973; 178:360–366.
21. Dinkel E, Mundinger A, Schopp D, et al: Diagnostic imaging in metastatic lung disease. *Lung* 1990; 168(Suppl):1129–1136.
22. Davis SR: CT evaluation for pulmonary me-

tastases in patients with extrathoracic malignancy. *Radiology* 1991; 180:1–12.

23. Pass HI, Dwyer A, Makuch R, et al: Detection of pulmonary metastasis in patients with osteogenic and soft-tissue sarcomas: The superiority of CT scans compared with conventional linear tomograms using dynamic analysis. *J Clin Oncol* 1985; 3:1261–1265.
24. Mountain CF, McMurtrey MJ, Hermes KE: Surgery for pulmonary metastasis: A 20-year experience. *Ann Thorac Surg* 1984; 38:323–330.
25. Gehan EA: Estimating survival functions from life table. *J Chron Dis* 1969; 21:629.
26. Pogrebniak HW, Roth JA, Steinberg SM, et al: Reoperative pulmonary resection in patients with metastatic soft tissue sarcoma. *Ann Thorac Surg* 1991; 52:197–203.
27. Rizzoni WE, Pass HI, Wesley MN, et al: Resection of recurrent pulmonary metastases in patients with soft-tissue sarcomas. *Arch Surg* 1986; 121:1248–1252.

Chapter 28

Primary Soft-Tissue Sarcomas of the Chest Wall

Clifton F. Mountain

The object of surgical treatment for primary chest wall sarcoma is to provide full control of local disease. This is accomplished through treatment planning that incorporates understanding first of anatomical and histological variables that have prognostic implications and, second, the therapeutic contribution of radiotherapy and chemotherapy in specific clinical situations.

The opportunity for cure of this disease depends on the completeness of the initial resection. For this reason wide or radical excision is advocated. In those patients with bony invasion, adjacent uninvolved ribs, sternum, portions of vertebral bodies, and organs that may be adherent to the tumor must be included in the chest wall resection to ensure that no microscopic disease is left behind. Intra-operative microscopic assessment of adequate excision is essential for ensuring an optimal resection.

Depending on the size and anatomical location of the tumor, pre-operative irradiation may be used for converting an initially inoperable tumor to resectable status. Primarily resected tumors with microscopic residual disease may be effectively treated by postoperative irradiation. Selected sarcomas have been shown in national clinical trials[1] and other studies[2] to be chemosensitive. In such instances pre- and postoperative adjuvant chemotherapy and possible cytoreductive operation may have a role in the management of chest wall tumors.

DIAGNOSIS AND EVALUATION

Although the majority of patients initially seeking treatment for an enlarging soft-tissue mass are asymptomatic, patients with primary chest wall tumors often have chest pain as a presenting symptom if underlying structures such as intercostal nerves or periosteum are involved. It is possible for chest wall tumors to attain considerable size before significant discomfort prompts a patient to seek medical attention.

If history, physical findings, and clinical judgment cannot rule out the question of malignancy, a complete work-up and histological diagnosis should be obtained for a patient presenting with a persistent soft-tissue mass overlying the thoracic cage. The location, size, shape, consistency, mobility, tenderness, and warmth of the tumor are all important physical findings; however, they may be unreliable for predicting malignancy.

Biopsy of a questionably malignant soft-tissue tumor of the chest wall should be planned by the surgeon who is prepared to execute the definitive surgery. A biopsy should be treated as an integral part of the definitive operative procedure.[3] If incisional biopsy is to be performed, placement of the incision is critical and must be done so that the incision will be amenable to en bloc resection by any subsequent surgical procedure. Although primary soft-tissue sarcoma of the chest wall is infrequent, and seldom encountered in general medical practice, it should be remembered that excisional biopsy or an inadequate local excision may well compromise a patient's chance for cure. Not only are such approaches to initial management extremely ill advised, but they also unnecessarily complicate definitive surgical resection. The use of true-cut (trephine) needle biopsy, when it is applicable, is preferred by many oncological surgeons. Such biopsy should be performed at or near the time of definitive resection. In the majority of tumors true-cut biopsies will at the least provide the surgeon with essential minimal information: "Is the lesion malignant or benign and, if malignant, is lymphoma ruled out"? If imaging guidance is necessary, the surgeon should work closely with the consulting radiologist.

Careful evaluation to determine the clinical extent of disease should be completed before biopsy is performed, including thorough imaging to delineate the relation of the tumor to the underlying soft tissue, muscle, and bones of the thorax, scapula, and spine. The most valuable examination for this purpose is computed tomography (CT). Magnetic resonance imaging (MRI) is useful for evaluating tumors adjacent to vertebral bodies to rule out extension to the spinal cord. Reports[4, 5] demonstrate the utility of MRI for defining the extent of soft-tissue sarcoma and the advantage of multiplane imaging. In addition to anteroposterior and lateral radiographs, skeletal survey and bone scans may be appropriate, depending on the clinical picture. Wide excision or full-thickness chest wall resection may present particular problems related to planning reconstruction or skin coverage. It is essential that these needs be determined preoperatively.

SURGICAL TREATMENT OF ANTERIOR AND POSTERIOR CHEST WALL SOFT-TISSUE SARCOMA: THE M. D. ANDERSON CANCER CENTER (1958–1982)

From 1958 through 1982, 180 patients with primary soft-tissue sarcoma of the chest wall were treated at the M. D. Anderson Cancer Center (MDACC), Houston, TX. Sixty-nine patients, 38% (69/180), underwent surgical treatment. Thirty-nine patients, 56.5% (39/69), had tumors of the anterior chest wall, and 30 tumors, 43.5% (30/69), were posterior.

The clinical status of these patients on admission is shown in Table 28–1, which reflects the nature of referrals to a categorical institution. One-fourth (18/69) of the patients had gross disease, not previously treated and no biopsy performed. The remainder had undergone biopsy, incomplete local excision, or had recurrent disease following prior surgical treatment. In some patients, such as those with grade I fibrosarcoma of the desmoid type, as many as four recurrences had been treated prior to their referral. Accordingly, in my personal experience during the time frame of this study, relatively

TABLE 28–1.
Primary Soft-Tissue Sarcoma of the Chest Wall*

Clinical Status on Admission		Number	Percentage
Gross untreated disease		18	26.1
Biopsy only		14	20.3
Residual disease after incomplete excision		15	21.7
Recurrent disease		22	31.9
	Total	69	100.0

* *M. D. Anderson Cancer Center, University of Texas, 1958–1982.*

few patients were suitable for an integrated plan of total management from the outset.

Nature of the Operation and End Results

In 45 patients the initial surgical procedure at MDACC was a wide excision. In an additional 24 patients a full-thickness chest wall resection, including involved or adjacent structures such as portions of the sternum, clavicles, ribs, or vertebral bodies, was performed. Table 28–2 shows the final outcome according to disease status following the operation. An apparent complete resection was accomplished in 51 patients, 73.9% (51/69). In eight patients, 15.7% (8/51), the disease ultimately was incurable, and in 43 patients, 84.3% (43/51), the disease was completely controlled. Residual disease remained following the operation in 18 patients, 26.1% (18/69); however, it is important to note that in three of these patients complete control of all disease was achieved through subsequent further operation and adjuvant radiation in one patient, and adjuvant radiation and chemotherapy in another. Of the remaining 15 patients undergoing incomplete resection, five had pulmonary metastasis present at the time of MDACC operation and surgical control was attempted in four. One patient, who initially responded to chemotherapy, had surgery performed after the failure of the chemotherapy to control persistent disease. In all but two patients, multimodality attempts to control the disease were made. These treatments provided survival from 13 months to 3½ years for six patients. Five patients who had residual tumor and who subsequently died of their disease underwent complete resection and multimodality treatment with survival of 16 months to 6 years.

Histological Type, Grade, and Disease Control

Twelve histological entities were treated and are documented in Table 28–3 according to the final disease status (minimum follow-up, 2 years). In forty-six patients, 66.7% (46/69), all disease was ultimately controlled. The median survival time of this group was 90 months. Sixty-three percent survived longer than 5 years. Because of the time frame of the series and the proportion with primary tumors removed prior to admission, definitive assessment of elements related to tumor grade is precluded; however, if this information was available, it is indicated (Table 28–3). The largest groups treated were patients with fibrosarcoma and unclassified sarcoma. The best outcome was achieved for patients with fibrosarcoma, which would be expected given that over three fourths of the group were classified as having grade I or desmoid-type tumors. In all of the other histological subsets containing two or more patients, at least 50% had all of the disease controlled, except for two patients with rhabdomyosarcoma, who died of the disease.

Tumor grade is accepted as the dominant prognostic variable for soft-tissue sarcoma.[6] Gordon et al.[7] and van Haelst-Pisani et al.[8] studied the experience of surgery for soft-tissue sarcoma at Memorial Sloan-Kettering Cancer Center (New York, NY) from 1948 to 1988 and reported a significant difference in survival based on tumor grade; patients with low-grade

TABLE 28–2.
Primary Soft-Tissue Sarcomas of the Chest Wall*: Disease Control by Operation Status and Procedure

Operation Status		Chest Wall Resection	Wide Excision	Total
Complete resection†				
Disease controlled		11	32	43
Not controlled		1	7	8
	Total	12	39	51
Incomplete resection				
Disease controlled		3	0	3
Not controlled		9	6	15
	Total	12	6	18

** M. D. Anderson Cancer Center, University of Texas, 1958–1982.*
† Apparent complete resection: margins negative, no other residual or known metastatic disease.

TABLE 28–3.
Disease Control by Histological Type*

Histological Type	Disease Controlled (*N* = 46)	Percentage of Total	Disease Not Controlled (*N* = 23)
Fibrosarcoma	17	85.0	3
Grade I desmoid	(8)		(1)
Other			
Grade I	(5)		
Grade II	(2)		(1)
Grade III			(1)
No grade	(2)		
Unclassified sarcoma	10	55.6	8
Grade I	(1)		
Grade II	(2)		
Grade III			(2)
No grade	(7)		(6)
Malignant fibrous histiocytoma	8	61.5	5
Grade I	(2)		
Grade II	(2)		
No grade	(4)		(5)
Neurofibrosarcoma	3	100.0	—
Grade I	(1)		
Grade II	(1)		
No grade	(1)		
Liposarcoma	2	50.0	2
Grade I	(2)		
Grade II			(1)
Grade III			(1)
Neurogenic sarcoma	2	100.0	—
Grade I	(1)		
No grade	(1)		
Malignant schwannoma	—	—	1
No grade			(1)
Alveolar soft-part sarcoma	1	100.0	—
No grade	(1)		
Angiosarcoma	1	100.0	—
Rhabdomyosarcoma	—	—	2
Grade II			(1)
No grade			(1)
Embryonal Rhabdomyosarcoma	1	50.0	1
No grade	(1)		(1)
Leiomyosarcoma	1	50.0	1
No grade	(1)		(1)

* *M. D. Anderson Cancer Center, University of Texas, 1958–1982.*

sarcomas had a higher survival, 90% and 82% at 5 and 10 years, respectively, than was observed for high-grade tumors, 49% and 39% surviving 5 and 10 years, respectively.

SURGICAL TREATMENT PLAN

Specific and individualized planning of the surgical procedure from the biopsy stage through reconstruction is required due to the variety of tumor types and particular problems associated with different location sites. It cannot be overemphasized that initial extensive resection that includes 5 cm of normal tissue beyond palpable tumor margins, if this is anatomically feasible, is the most important single factor in effecting control of the primary tumor. Perry et al.,[9] reporting the outcome of 28 patients undergoing resection for high-grade sarcoma at the Surgery Branch of the National Cancer Institute (Bethesda, MD) from April 1977 through January 1988, showed that patients with positive margins had a mean survival of 6 months and those with negative margins had a 67% survival at 5 years. Suit, reporting on patterns of failure following surgery for soft-tissue sarcoma in all sites, showed that the local failure rate following adequate radical excision is only 5%.[10] With the newer methods of repair and reconstruction, including the use of myocutaneous flaps, virtually any size chest wall defect can be satisfactorily repaired.

Primary Surgery

Primary tumors of the chest wall are no exception to the growth pattern of soft-tissue sarcomas in other sites. The tumor cells grow and extend along muscle bundles, fascial planes, and nerve sheaths beyond the palpable tumor mass.[11] Thus even apparently small tumors of low histological grade and anticipated nonaggressive behavior may require wide excision. Soft-tissue sarcomas of the chest wall may invade the underlying thoracic cage or may arise in the intercostal structures. In such patients radical en bloc resection of the chest wall should be performed. The essence of chest wall resection is to ensure tissue margins that are microscopically free of tumor. Ribs and associated intercostal tissue, sternum, and portions of vertebral bodies may require en bloc resection to effect this complete tumor removal. Such extensive surgery, along with required reconstruction of the chest wall, is well within the capabilities of modern thoracic surgical techniques. Further, such surgery, although it appears radical, is physiologically well tolerated and is cosmetically acceptable.

The surgical approach is defined by the size and location of the primary tumor. At MDACC, the approach is through a lateral thoracotomy incision distal to the tumor site. This permits the best assessment of gross tumor extent both intrapleurally and with respect to overlying soft tissues. The pleural space is entered superiorly and inferiorly through the periosteal bed of the second rib distal to the palpable tumor. The anterior-posterior limits of resection are then defined by 5 cm of grossly normal rib and intercostal muscle. Accordingly, the tumor and appropriate surrounding normal tissues are removed en bloc.

Reconstruction of the Chest Wall

Methods for restoration of the bony chest wall, if that is needed, are many and varied, and their efficacy is the subject of some debate. The objectives of chest wall reconstruction are to effect normal ventilatory mechanics, create stability of the chest wall, and to effect a satisfactory cosmetic appearance. The size of the defect that will have to be created in patients who may have had prior radiation therapy is not always obvious pre-operatively and includes both the surface area and the depth of the chest wall. Wide excision will be necessary to achieve sound healing in these patients.

For many years surgeons at MDACC have favored and used Marlex® (Bard, Inc., Billerica, MA), plastic mesh to effect chest wall stability with excellent anatomical and physiological results. Advantages of this material, in addition to its ready availability, are its incorporation by dense fibrous tissue and minimal foreign body reaction. As noted by Goffney and Morton,[12] Marlex fulfills virtually all of the requirements for a prosthetic for chest wall resection. When Marlex mesh is used, the mesh must be "drumhead" tight when the chest wall closure is completed.[13] The prosthesis is secured to the bony structures and muscles surrounding the defect. The edges of the Marlex sheet are turned over to give an approximately 0.5-in. (1.3 cm) margin of double thickness around the entire periphery of the prosthesis. This folded cut edge is placed external to the thoracic cavity. The high tensile strength of the material allows it to be stretched across the surgical defect, thus ensuring a stable thoracic repair. In most instances these tumors do not extensively invade the skin and subcutaneous structures. Accordingly, primary closure of the skin is generally possible. It is of interest that this prosthetic procedure is entirely suitable in pediatric patients because the remaining thoracic structures permit adjustment to growth without significant deformity. Other synthetic material, such as Gore-Tex® (W. L. Gore, Inc., Flagstaff, AZ), are also in use.

The following case illustrates several points regarding complete resection and the use of Marlex mesh for repair of chest wall defects. A 16-year old girl was referred for treatment of recurrent fibrosarcoma, grade I desmoid type. The first resection was done 9 years previously and was followed by three recurrences and subsequent resections. All of these procedures were performed prior to her admission to MDACC. Three years after the last resection she presented with massive tumor involvement of the anterior chest wall. The consensus was that complete resection would represent the best, if not the only, course of action to control this disease. At exploration the tumor was 15 × 15 × 15 cm and involved the sternum, the pericardium, and medial superior aspect of the diaphragm. Resection of the left anterior chest wall mass with removal of anterior ribs 3–10 and part of the sternum, part of the diaphragm, and part of the pericardium was accomplished with replacement of diaphragm and anterior chest wall with Marlex mesh (Figs 28–1 and 28–2). No significant postoperative complications occurred. She had no further recurrence and subsequently continued to lead a normal life with no evidence of recurrence—she married and has had two children.

If adequate resection requires sacrifice of major areas of skin, subcutaneous tissues, and muscles, or if the tumor has ulcerated and become infected, alternate techniques of closure are required. The development of myocutaneous flaps affords an excellent solution in these patients. The flaps may be developed from the several muscles of the chest wall that have broad bases and that have a reliable vascular supply.[14] The technique permits immediate closure of thoracic wall defects. The creation of these flaps has been described by Larson et al.,[15] McKenna et al.,[16] and others.[17–19] The latissimus dorsi, shown in Figure 28–3, is the most commonly used. The muscle has a long pedicle, which affords it a wide arc of rotation that effectively allows the tissue to reach almost any part of the anterior aspect of the hemithorax. The pectoralis major flap is shown in Figure 28–4. Its main advantage is closure of anterior chest wall defects, including the sternum. The rectus abdominus flap is illustrated in Figure 28–5. This muscle provides a bulky flap, when based on the superior epigastric artery, and can reach most of the anterior chest wall. Such flaps are dependent, however, on a patent internal mammary artery.[20] When this type of resection and reconstruction is contemplated, coordinated pre-operative planning between the thoracic surgeon and plastic surgeon is required.

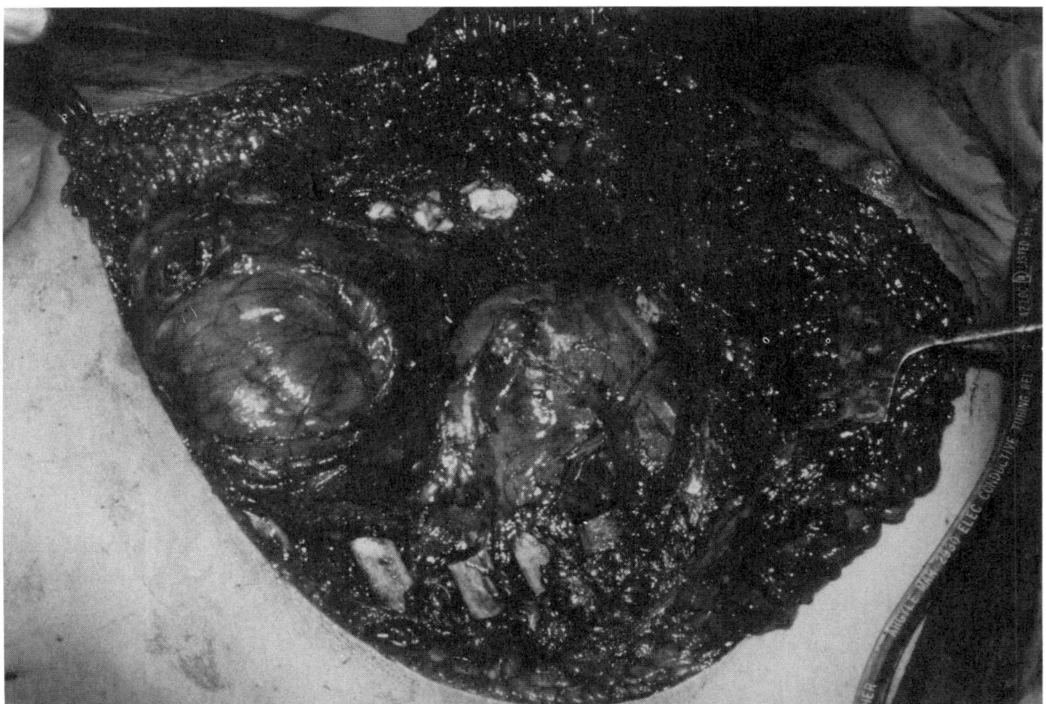

FIG 28–1.
Operative defect following en bloc chest wall resection of fibrosarcoma involving anterior chest wall, diaphragm, and pericardium.

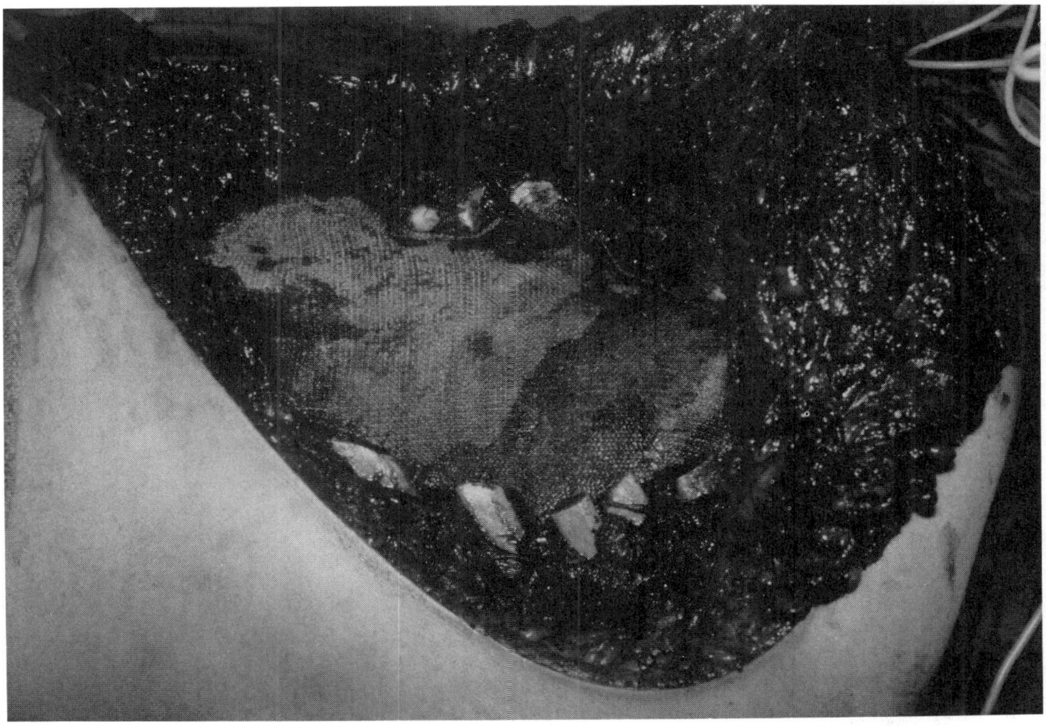

FIG 28–2.
Marlex mesh prostheses in place for repair of chest wall defect.

DISCUSSION

Primary soft-tissue sarcoma of the chest wall is a rare malignancy. A variety of treatment plans were used in the present series of patients; therefore, only small numbers of patients had similar disease and treatment characteristics. Based on this experience, highly specific recommendations for care cannot be made. Nevertheless, the data clearly illustrate that surgical resection with adequate margins provides a significant opportunity for cure. The disease was completely controlled in approximately 85% of the patients who underwent an apparent complete resection.

To place the role of adjuvant modalities in perspective with respect to soft-tissue sarcoma of the chest wall, the experience developed from soft-tissue sarcomas and their response to radiation and chemotherapy may be relevant. Lindberg et al.[21] reported the effectiveness of postoperative irradiation and conservative operation to control these tumors. The absolute 5-year survival rate for all patients (168 eligible patients treated from 1963 to 1974) was 61.3%. In 1971 a clinical study of the benefit of pre-operative irradiation in patients with massive soft-tissue sarcomas was initiated by this group. Due to the size and location of the tumor these patients were not candidates for conservative surgery and thus received pre-operative radiation treatment followed 4 to 6 weeks later by conservative excision. Nineteen patients (of 50) had a minimum of 5 years of follow-up in 1976 and 73.7% of them were reported alive and disease free.[22] In general, the present approach at MDACC for the treatment of extremity lesions is as follows: in high-grade, large tumors, pre-operative chemotherapy, with or without radiation therapy, is given. This treatment is followed by wide excision. In similar patients who have undergone resection prior to their admission to MDACC, postoperative chemotherapy and radiation therapy are given.

In patients with primary soft-tissue sarcoma of the chest wall, the location of the majority of tumors would preclude pre-operative irradiation in the dose range used for the treatment

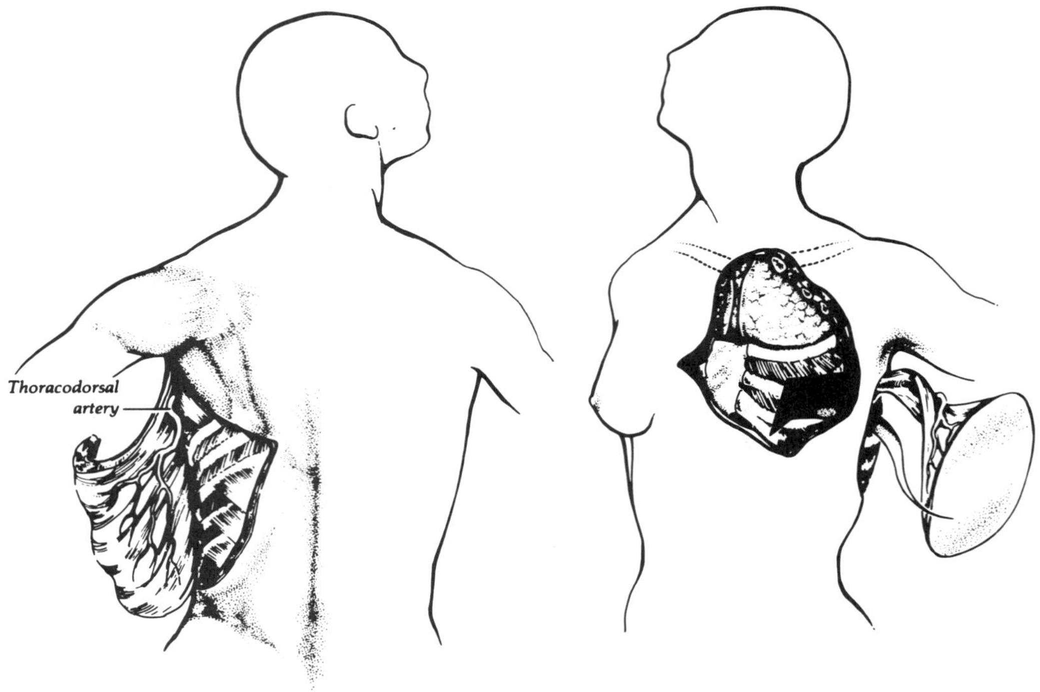

FIG 28–3.
Latissimus dorsi musculocutaneous flap; schematic drawing shows path of flap rotation and identifies blood supply. (From Larson D, McMurtrey M, Howe J, et al: *Cancer* 1982; 49:1286–1293. Reprinted by permission.)

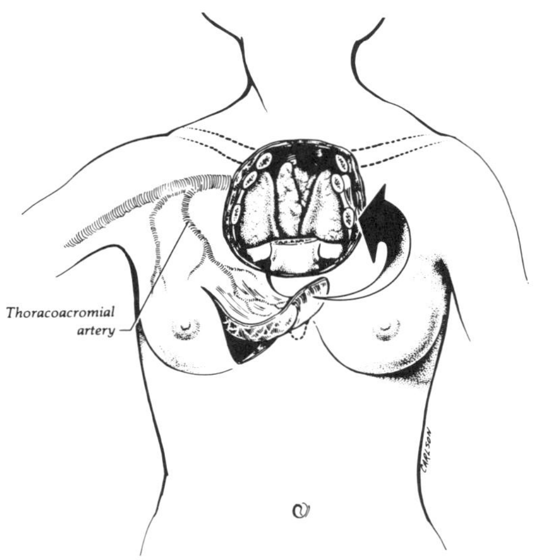

FIG 28–4.
Pectoralis major musculocutaneous flap; diagram shows flap and its accompanying blood supply. (From Larson D, McMurtrey M, Howe J, et al: *Cancer* 1982; 49:1286–1293. Reprinted by permission.)

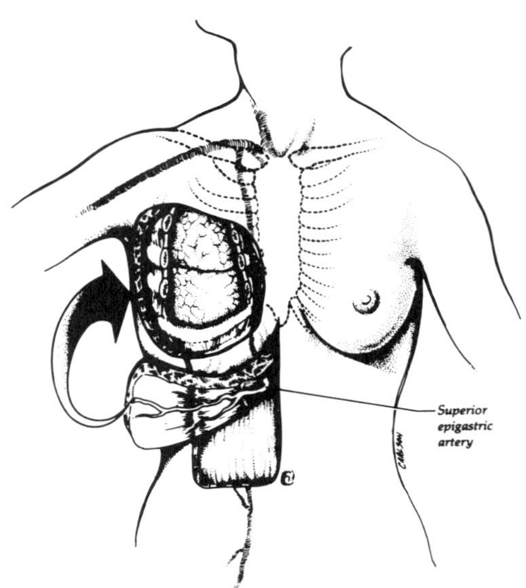

FIG 28–5.
Rectus abdominus musculocutaneous flap; diagram illustrates blood supply and arc of rotation of flap. (From Larson D, McMurtrey M, Howe J, et al: *Cancer* 1982; 49:1286–1293. Reprinted by permission.)

of extremity lesions (5,000 to 6,000 cGy) because of potential damage to the lungs. We have successfully induced and maintained pneumothorax during the course of pre-operative irradiation to exclude the lung from the field of therapy. This technique might be extended to a greater range of applications, thus permitting full-dose irradiation with preservation of ventilatory function.

Our present recommendation for the surgical treatment of primary sarcoma of the chest wall is based on the philosophy that the initial resection should encompass all known disease. Adjuvant therapies are selected and planned for those patients for whom such treatment may be appropriate and where reasonable expectations of benefit can be determined, for example, in the following situations: (1) pre-operative irradiation should be considered when the size and location of the tumor places the probability of complete resection in doubt, or in those instances where shrinkage of the tumor might permit a less radical resection, (2) postoperative irradiation should receive primary consideration if surgical margins are either tumor positive or doubtful due to their proximity to the tumor, (3) in those instances where the morphology of the tumor is known to be highly responsive to chemotherapy, it would seem rational to include such therapy in the multimodal plan.[2, 8, 23]

ACKNOWLEDGMENTS

This project was supported by the Herman Neel Hipp Fund for Research in Thoracic Surgery and the Clifton F. Mountain Fund. The author acknowledges the contributions of K. E. Hermes to the research and writing of this chapter.

REFERENCES

1. Mertens WC, Branwell VHC: Adjuvant chemotherapy for soft tissue sarcomas, in Pinedo HM, Verweij J, Suit HD (eds): *Soft Tissue Sarcomas: New Developments in the Multidisciplinary Approach to Treatment.* Boston, Kluwer Academic Publishers, 1991, pp 93–103.
2. Pezzi CM, Pollock RE, Evans HL, et al: Preoperative chemotherapy for soft tissue sarcomas of the extremities. *Ann Surg* 1990; 213:187–188.
3. Bains MS, Pomerantz A, McCormack PM, et al: Soft tissue sarcomas of the chest wall, in Shiu MH, Brennan MF (eds): *Surgical Management of Soft Tissue Sarcoma.* Philadelphia, Lea & Febiger, 1989, pp 137–146.
4. Pettersson H, Herrlin K: Diagnostic imaging, in Pinedo HM, Verweij J, Suit HD (eds): *Soft Tissue Sarcomas: New Developments in the Multidisciplinary Approach to Treatment,* Boston, Kluwer Academic Publishers, 1991, pp 11–35.
5. Collins JD, Shaver M, Batra P, et al: Magnetic resonance imaging of chest wall lesions. *J Natl Med Assoc* 1991; 83:352–360.
6. Antman K, Eilber FR, Shiu MH: Soft tissue sarcomas. Current trends in diagnosis and management. *Curr Prob Cancer* 1989; 13:340–367.
7. Gordon MS, Hajdu SI, Bains MS, et al: Soft tissue sarcoma of the chest wall. Results of surgical resection. *J Thorac Cardiovac Surg* 1991; 101:843–854.
8. van Haelst-Pisani CM, Buckner JC, Reiman HM, et al: Does histologic grade in soft tissue sarcoma influence response rate to systemic chemotherapy? *Cancer* 1991; 68:2345–2358.
9. Perry RR, Venzon D, Roth JA, et al: Survival after surgical resection for high grade chest wall sarcomas. *Ann Thorac Surg* 1990; 49:363–369.
10. Suit HD: Patterns of failure after treatment of sarcoma of soft tissue by radical surgery or by conservative surgery and radiation. *Cancer Treat Symp* 1983; 2:241–246.
11. Chang AE, Rosenberg SA, Glatstein EJ, et al: Sarcomas of soft tissues, in Devita VT Jr, Hellman S, Rosenberg SA (eds): *Cancer, Principles and Practice of Oncology.* Philadelphia, J. B. Lippincott, 1989, p 1361.
12. Goffney WH, Morton DL: Sarcomas of the chest wall and trunk, in Eilber FR, Morton DL, Sondak VK, et al (eds): *The Soft Tissue Sarcomas.* New York, Grune & Stratton, 1987, pp 159–168.
13. Humphrey EW: *Manual of Pulmonary Surgery.* New York and Heidelberg, Springer-Verlag, 1982, pp 158–163.
14. le Roux BT, Shama DM: Resection of tumors of the chest wall. *Curr Prob Surg* 1983; 20:349–386.
15. Larson D, McMurtrey M, Howe J, et al: Major chest wall reconstruction after chest wall irradiation. *Cancer* 1982; 49:1286–1293.
16. McKenna RJ, McMurtrey MJ, Larson DL, et al: A perspective on chest wall resection in

breast cancer patients. *Ann Thorac Surg* 1984; 38:482–487.

17. Arnold PG, Pairolero PC: Use of pectoralis major muscle flap to repair defects of anterior chest wall. *Plast Reconstr Surg* 1979; 205:63.

18. Boyd AP, Shaw WW, McCarthy JG, et al: Immediate reconstruction of full-thickness chest wall defects. *Ann Thorac Surg* 1981; 337:32.

19. Mathes GJ, Bostwick J: Rectus abdominus myocutaneous flaps to reconstruct abdominal wall defects. *Br J Plast Surg* 1977; 282:30.

20. Robbins TW: Rectus abdominus myocutaneous flap for breast reconstruction. *Aust NZ J Surg* 1979; 527:49.

21. Lindberg RD, Martin RG, Romsdahl MM, et al: Conservative surgery and postoperative radiotherapy in 300 adults with soft tissue sarcomas. *Cancer* 1981; 47:2391–2397.

22. Martin RG, Lindberg RD, Russell WO: Preoperative radiation therapy for sarcoma of soft tissue, in *Management of Primary Bone and Soft Tissue Tumors*. Chicago, Year Book Medical Publishers, 1977, pp 299–307.

23. Young MM, Kinsella TJ, Miser JS, et al: Treatment of sarcomas of the chest wall using intensive combined modality therapy. *Int J Radiat Oncol Biol Phys* 1989; 16:49–57.

Chapter 29

Orthopedic Considerations in Limb-Sparing Surgery

Joseph M. Lane

John H. Healey

Limb preservation has always been the preferred goal in the treatment of extremity sarcomas. In the past, it has been unsuccessful in cases of high-grade malignancy because of an unacceptable local recurrence rate. Advances in the utilization of adjuvant radiotherapy and chemotherapy not only have significantly increased survival rates for extremity sarcomas but also have enabled use of closer surgical margins.[1–13] Significant diagnostic advances in definition of tumor boundaries and pre-operative staging have permitted more exact surgical planning. This process has enabled the surgeon to anticipate more clearly the extent of the surgical resection as well as to use specific adjuvant tools to "sterilize" the potentially contaminated margins. This chapter will discuss surgical staging techniques, other concepts of limb preservation, and various techniques of reconstruction when osseous structures are within the tumor field. Specific anatomical sites will also be discussed.

STAGING

Staging systems and methods of defining surgical margins are required to make reasonable comparisons of treatment modalities. A number of these systems exist. The method advocated by Enneking et al.[14] appears to be especially suitable for tumors that involve osseous structures. The technique involves histological characterization of the tumor as high grade or low grade, the definition of whether the tumor is within a given anatomical compartment or has invaded more than one, and last, the presence of regional and/or distant metastases. Tumors that have a low mitotic rate and a low propensity for distant metastasis are classified as low grade. Conversely, lesions that have a high mitotic rate, marked atypia of the cells, and a great propensity for distant metastasis would be defined as high grade. Desmoplastic fibromas would be classified as low-grade lesions, whereas biphasic synovial sarcomas would be high grade.

Anatomical compartments usually are circumscribed areas with clear fibrous or osseous boundaries. The quadriceps, gastrocnemius, and medullary areas of the femur are all compartments. Lesions that are completely within such a compartment would be classified as intracompartmental. Lesions that have broken through the osseous cortex or have extended through the fascia and compartment boundary would be extracompartmental. An example would be a quadriceps lesion extending through the iliotibial tract and the lateral fascia into the posterior compartment of the thigh. Similarly, lesions located in poorly defined anatomical areas such as the popliteal space or Hunter's canal would be extracompartmental.

Utilizing these three general criteria, Enneking et al.[14] have established the following staging system (Table 29–1). Stage IA lesions are low-grade tumors histologically and are located within a definable anatomical compartment, without evidence of regional or distant metastases. Stage IB lesions are low-grade tumors histologically and have extended out of a single anatomical compartment, but do not have regional or distant metastases. Stage IIA lesions have high-grade histological characterizations, are located within a definable anatomical compartment, and do not have regional or distant metastases. Stage IIB lesions are high grade histologically, are not located within a definable anatomical compartment, but do not have regional or distant metastases. Stage III lesions are either low grade or high grade histologically, either within or without a definable anatomical compartment, and do have regional and/or distant metastases.

SURGICAL EXCISION

When considering limb preservation, definition of the surgical margins is important[14] (Table 29–2). Four methods of surgical excision are possible. Intralesional procedures involve surgery entering the tumor, purposely or incidentally. Examples would include curettage of a giant cell tumor or a debulking procedure. A marginal procedure is one in which one surface of the tumor is dissected at its pseudocapsule, such as a "shell-out" of a lipoma. Our studies have indicated that 98% of the patients with malignant sarcoma so treated surgically without adjuvant therapy will have local recurrence. A wide excision refers to a procedure in which all margins of the tumor are completely resected with a cuff of normal tissue interposed on all boundaries. Wide excisions can be performed within the anatomical compartment or across all the anatomical compartments involved by the tumor. However, at least one of the anatomical compartments containing the tumor is entered. The extent of wide excision may not be critical and whether a 1-or 3-cm margin is used does not seem to affect prognosis. Last, a radical resection involves excision of the tumor outside all anatomical compartments containing the tumor; an example would be a complete resection of the quadriceps mechanisms for a lesion lying within the vastus lateralis.

Amputations, per se, are not necessarily wider than resections in terms of surgical margins. An amputation through the tumor is an incisional intralesional amputation. An amputation adjacent to a pseudocapsule is a marginal amputation. An amputation through the compartment with normal tissues separating the tumor from the amputation line would be a wide amputation. Last, an amputation that removes all tumor-containing compartments in their entirety would be a radical amputation.

A 3-cm lesion within the vastus lateralis, treated with either a debulking procedure or an amputation through the lesion, would involve an intralesional procedure. If the resection or amputation was located at the border of the pseudocapsule, it would be a marginal procedure. If the resection or transfemoral amputation had several centimeters of normal muscle around the tumor in all directions, it would be a wide procedure. Last, a complete resection of the quadriceps mechanism or a disarticulation of the hip would be a radical procedure.

Using this technique Enneking et al.[14] reported a 70% cure rate and less than 10% local recurrence rate for high-grade lesions treated by

TABLE 29–1.
Surgical Stages of Musculoskeletal Sarcoma*

Stage	Histological Grade	Anatomical Extent	Metastases
IA	Low	Intracompartmental	None
IB	Low	Extracompartmental	None
IIA	High	Intracompartmental	None
IIB	High	Extracompartmental	None
III	High or low	Intra- or extracompartmental	Distant or regional

* *From Enneking WF, Spanier SS, Goodman MA: Clin Orthop Rel Res* 1980; 153:106–120.

TABLE 29–2.
Surgical Margins*

Excision	Margin	Potential Local Residual Tumor
Intralesional	Intralesional	Macroscopic
Marginal	Pseudocapsule	Microscopic
Wide	Normal cuff tissue; within compartment	Skip
Radical	Extracompartmental	None

* *From Enneking WF, Spanier SS, Goodman MA: Clin Orthop Rel Res* 1980; 153:106–120.

a radical resection or amputation but no adjuvant chemotherapy or radiotherapy. More limited procedures, such as wide excisions or wide amputations for high-grade tumors, require additional treatment modalities to provide comparable survival. Use of adjuvant radiotherapy together with wide excision can achieve cure rates without local recurrence that are equal, if not superior, to radical surgery alone.

Careful pre-operative evaluations are critical. Arteriography, computed tomography (CT), magnetic resonance (MR), radionuclide studies (using gallium or technetium), selective lymphangiography, plain tomography, and systemic evaluation are important in aiding the surgeon to develop a treatment plan.

LIMB PRESERVATION PROCEDURES

The key element in limb preservation procedures is complete resection of the tumor and then reconstruction of the skeletal structures, using the above principles.[2–5, 12] The tumor must be removed by at least a wide excision. There is a high chance of local recurrence unless additional therapy is used. Radiotherapy is particularly useful for local ablation of the tumor. This treatment, however, will significantly impair osteosynthesis, which may be required for limb reconstruction, and will significantly damage the adjacent muscles. Inadequate surgery will lead to local recurrence.

Limb preservation requires both maintenance of skeletal continuity following the removal of the tumor and functional reconstruction of the muscular elements. Soft-tissue lesions that are resected without destroying the skeletal continuity are obviously amenable to limb preservation. Specifically, muscle transfer (based on principles derived from poliomyelitis experience), bracing, and appropriate physical therapy often will compensate for such lesions. This chapter, however, will discuss those lesions that are amenable to limb preservation but that may involve discontinuity of the skeletal framework. The continuity can be maintained despite skeletal resection in some circumstances. A curettage or partial resection of a hemicondyle or the removal of single bone in a double-boned limb (Fig. 29–1) will allow skeletal continuity. When only part of a hemicortical longitudinal segment of the bone is resected (Fig. 29–2) the bone is significantly weakened and must be protected with bracing until the anatomical continuity has been re-established. Bone grafting, particularly with cancellous bone, is most advantageous. Supplemental internal fixation with a plate or intramedullary rod may be necessary.

Most resections that involve the skeleton, however, lead to a discontinuity of the limb.[2–5] These resections have been divided into intercalary and osteochondral resections. An intercalary resection usually involves removing a part of the diaphysis of the bone without disruption of the adjacent joints. Osteochondral resection involves the distal or proximal end of the bone, including part of the joint.

There are multiple options for skeletal reconstruction after limb preservation tumor resections.[4, 5] One choice is no reconstruction but allowing a small discontinuity to be protected with bracing or external supports. An example would be a girdle stone resection about the hip in which, after femoral head and neck resection, the intratrochanteric area of the proximal femur will articulate with the acetabulum and the outer wall of the iliac wing (Fig. 29–3). Arthrodesis offers another choice, in which osteosynthesis is achieved between the proximal and distal ends of the resection.[15] Shortening of the limb is often necessary to bridge the defect, and if a joint has been removed, the motion will be sacrificed for stability. Following resection

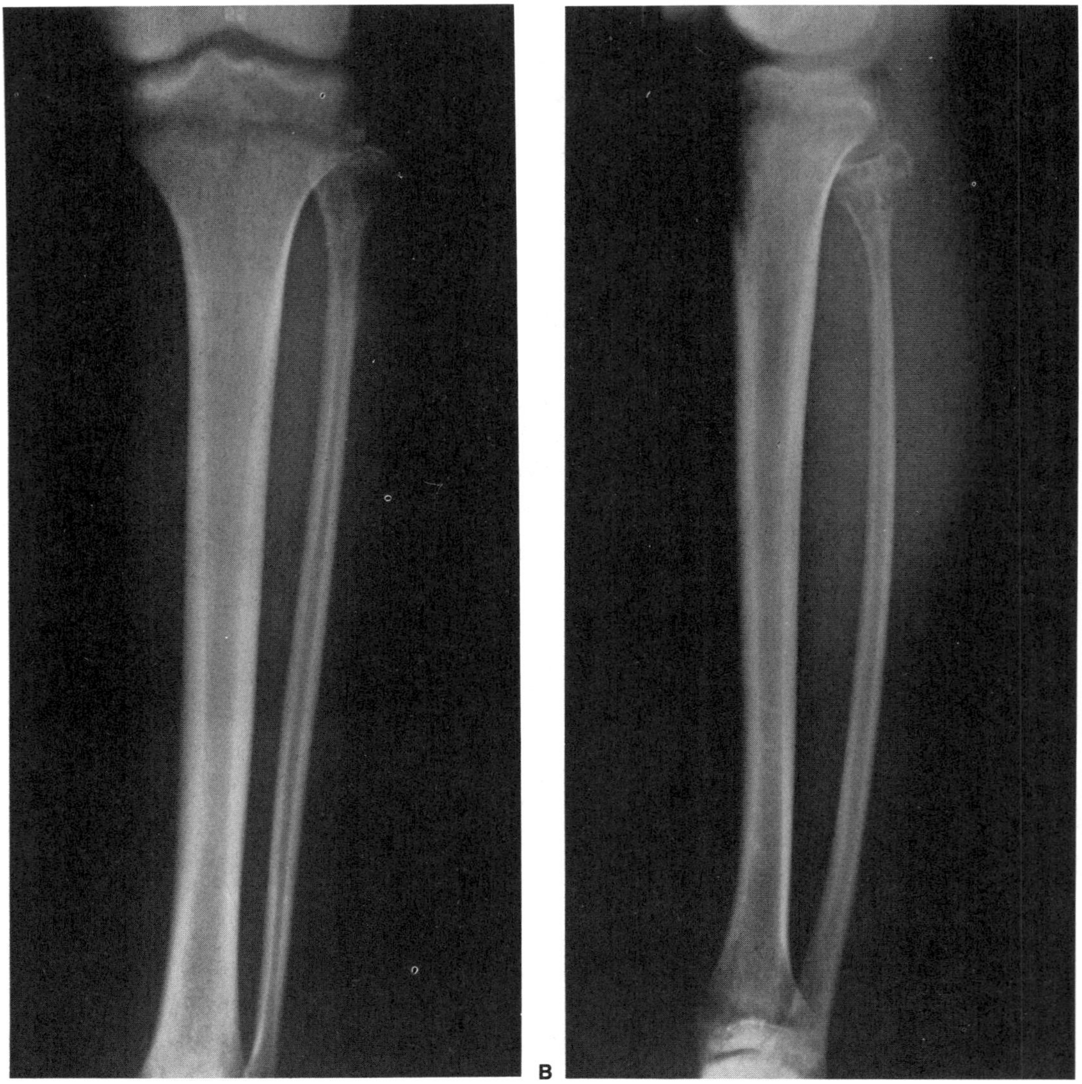

A B

FIG 29–1.
A, Anteroposterior and **B,** lateral views of an embryonal rhabdomyosarcoma of the proximal fibula. The patient underwent an en bloc resection of the proximal 80% of the fibula (**C,** anteroposterior and **D,** lateral views). The patient was tumor-free 1 year following combined resection, radiotherapy, and chemotherapy.

about the hip, direct arthrodesis to the ischial tuberosity with no significant shortening may be possible (Fig. 29–4). The gap can be closed with various forms of grafts, as discussed below.

Most bone defects can be filled with an autograft.[16, 17] This involves the transplantation of cancellous, cortical, or combined cancellous/cortical bone. These grafts are basically nonviable, and only small segments of the marrow cells may be revascularized in sufficient time to maintain their viability. Most recently, free vascularized grafts have been used, in which the blood supply to the bone is maintained and can also include overlying muscles, subcutaneous tissue, and skin. Typical examples of the vascularized autograft include the vascularized fibula using the peroneal artery (Fig. 29–5), the anterior iliac crest using the superficial and deep circumflex iliac artery, and the rib graft using the intercostal artery. Nonosseous vascularized

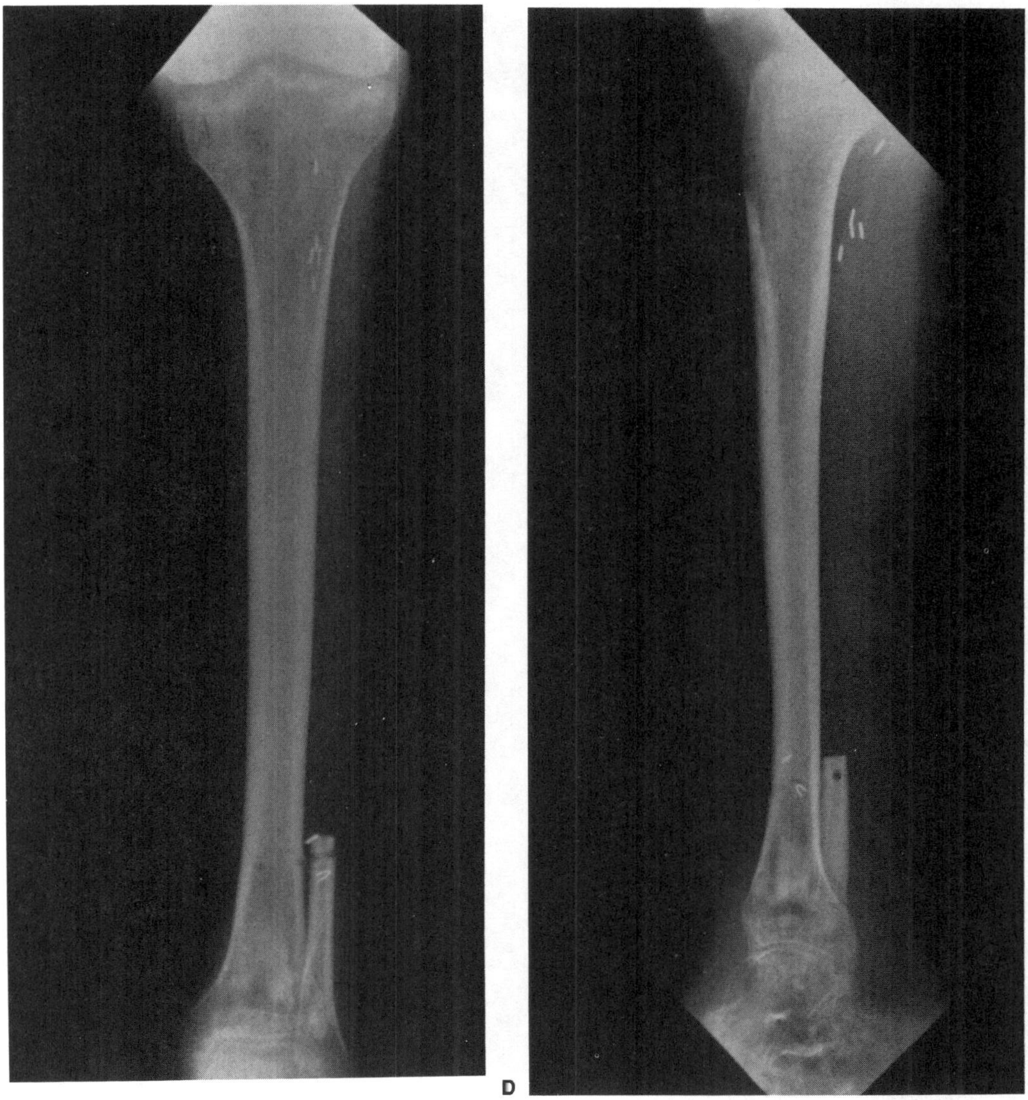

FIG 29–1.—*Continued*

grafts most commonly include the latissimus dorsi and the gracilis. In these grafts, approximately 80% to 90% of the bone remains viable and osseous union and remodeling are achieved more quickly. In special locations, pedicle grafts such as gracilis, latissimus dorsi, and quadratus femoris (the latter with bone segment) are suitable.

The autograft has many advantages.[4, 5, 17] Remodeling will result in an osseous structure closely resembling the preresection state of that bone. Autografts contain osteoinductive substances that induce the reparative process and have osteoconductive properties that provide an environment suitable to bone formation. Cancellous bone is most efficacious but lacks structural strength. Cortical bone provides structural advantages at the expense of decreased osteoinductive properties. Nonviable autografts are excellent for defects of less than

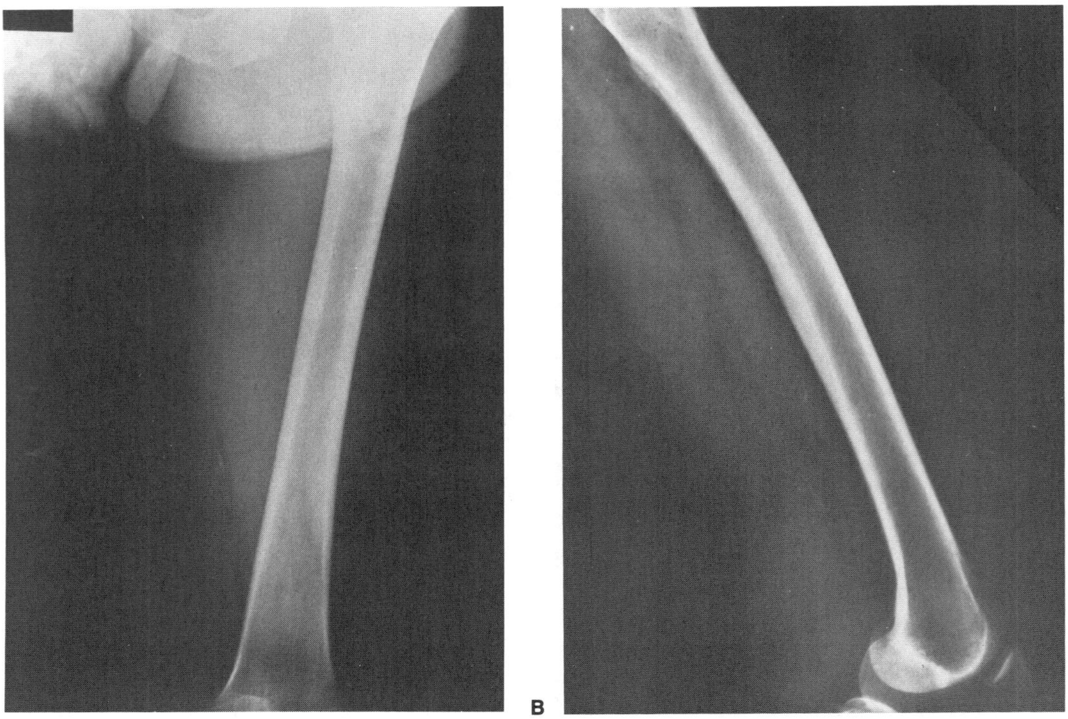

A B

FIG 29–2.
Quadriceps malignant fibrohistiocytoma. The **A,** anteroposterior and **B,** lateral radiographs do not clearly show the tumor, but the **C,** CT demonstrates it. Due to the placement adjacent to the anterior femur, a cortical segment was removed at the time of en bloc resection, **D**. The cortical defect was stabilized with a plate and screws.

12 cm.[16] However, in defects of greater length, 58% of patients have nonunion or delayed stress fractures. Also, if these autografts are not stressed they have a tendency to atrophy with time. Autografts provide excellent transplants for intercalary defects but do not tolerate chemotherapy and radiotherapy well, nor are they ideal for osteochondral defects. However, the proximal head of the fibula has been used to replace the distal radius.

The vascularized graft provides a viable osseous matrix that can bridge large gaps relatively easily.[17] It has a high osteosynthesis rate and has all the advantages of the autograft plus increased incorporation and remodeling rates. It hypertrophies with time in response to load. Stress fractures and nonunion are significantly less frequent than in nonvascularized grafts. It can be used along with chemotherapy and radiotherapy, and can survive despite infection or inadequate skin coverage. Fixation, however, can be difficult, particularly near the end of a joint. External fixators have been used quite successfully in that circumstance until union of the graft and host bone occurred.

Allografts have only recently become successful, although the first ones were performed in 1905 by Lexer in Russia.[18] These allografts consist of either osseous diaphyseal segments (Fig. 29–6) or composite osteochondral segments (Fig. 29–7). Although the bone is dead and maintained in a deep-frozen state to decrease antigenicity, 10% to 70% of cartilage viability can be maintained by cryopreservatives, most notably 10% glycerol or dimethyl sulfoxide (DMSO).

Allografts have the advantage of providing exact replicas of the resected material. They achieve good osteosynthesis and will be slowly replaced. Antigenic sensitization to grafted tissue continues throughout life. Replacement is never completely accomplished. Difficulties include a 13% infection rate, an ~7% fracture rate, and nonunion. Relative contraindications to us-

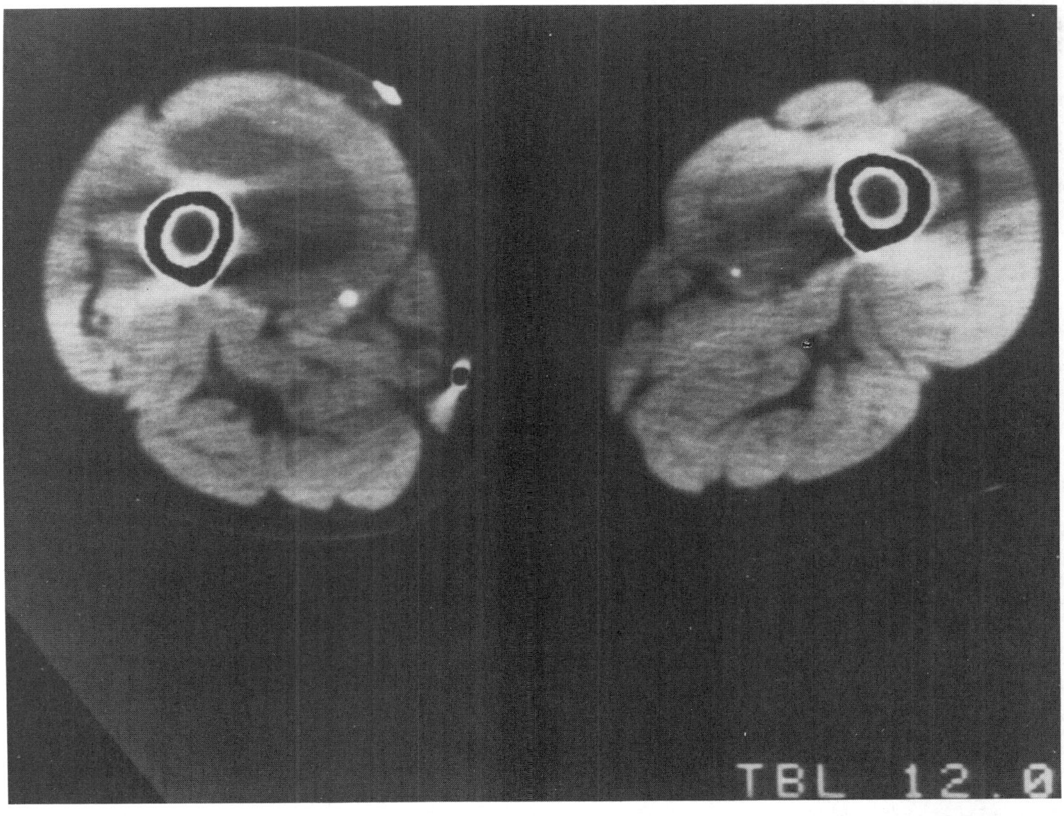

C

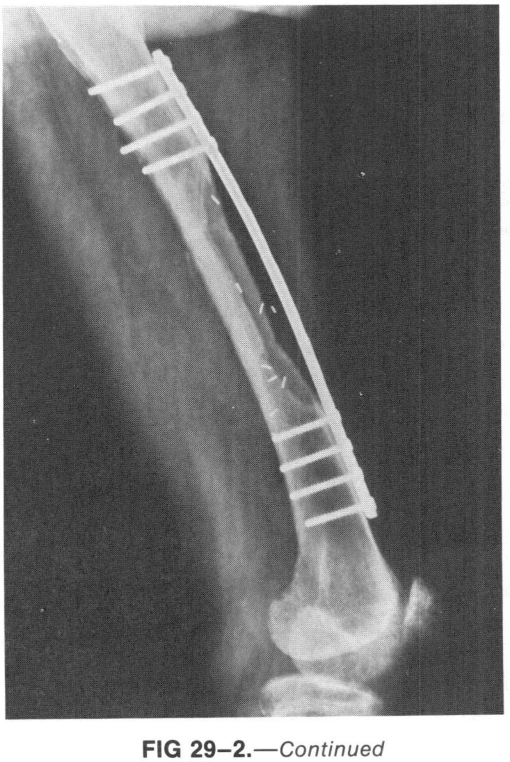

D

FIG 29–2.—*Continued*

ing the allograft include prior infection, radiation, and postoperative adjuvant chemotherapy. Ideal conditions for allografts are after resection of aggressive, benign tumors and low-grade malignant tumors when adjuvant modes of therapy are not being used. Allografts cannot, however, be used on both sides of a weight-bearing joint and are most successful as hemicondyles (Fig. 29–7) and proximal humerus. When used for the distal femur, there is a significant degree of instability, which can be partially protected with muscle strengthening and braces.

Most recently, artificial implants of ceramic or metals have been used.[2–5, 12] These implants can be joined directly to bone with polymethylmethacrylate, and more recently by biological means, using porous ingrowth by host bone cells (Fig. 29–8). The implants provide joints and have largely been developed based on experience with prosthetics using implants for reconstruction following degenerative arthritis of the hip and the knee. Cement provides immediate implant fixation while porous ingrowth promises durable, biological prosthetic fixation. At

A

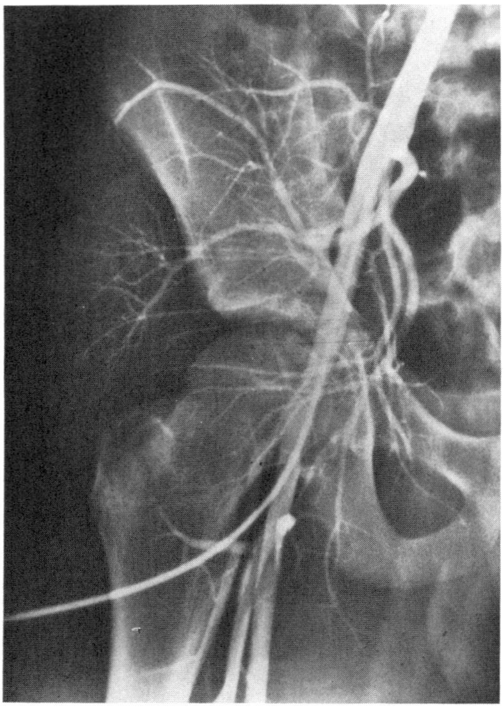

FIG 29–3.
Osteogenic sarcoma of the medial aspect of the acetabulum and proximal ischium, **A**. The patient was successfully treated with chemotherapy and internal hemipelvectomy, **B**. The pubic ramus, acetabulum, and femoral head were removed en bloc. The patient was tumor free after 50 months and was able to ambulate with a single cane and a 2 in. (5-cm) lift.

B

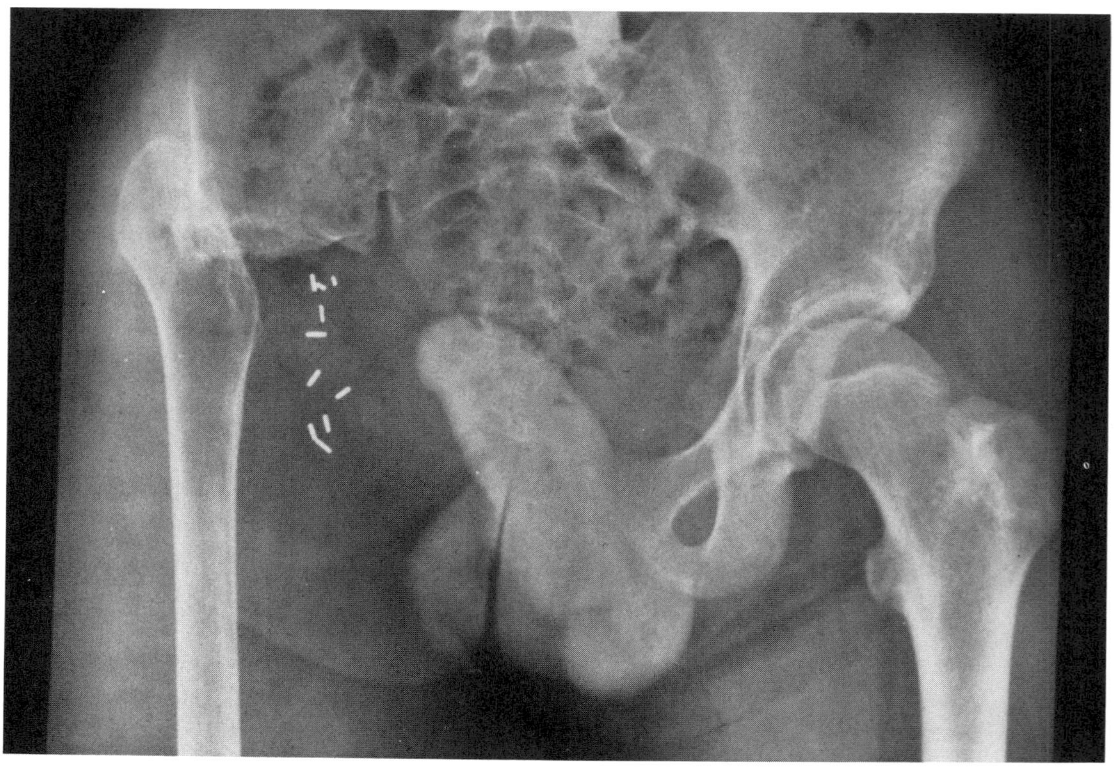

this time, implants spanning two joints for distances well over 40 cm have been constructed and have been quite successful. Critical elements in making the choice are the anatomical site, the span of skeletal resection to be bridged, the age of the patient, health of the surrounding normal tissues, and whether or not the patient has received or will receive localized radiation and/or adjuvant chemotherapy.

Artificial implants are ideal for replacing large segments and providing instantaneous fixation. They can compensate for any muscle resection. The current metals used are a cobalt-chromium alloy (Vitallium) and titanium (Fig. 29–8); the latter is becoming more popular because of better biocompatibility and increased durability. Originally, a high rate of breakage and loosening presented significant problems. With better alloys the breakage rate has significantly decreased, although there has been difficulty with late loosening of the devices. Unlike allografts and autografts, the device has continued to fail with time rather than become stronger. Unacceptable corrosion occurs in prosthesis in which articulating surfaces are both metal. The interface of a polyethylene liner with a metal component usually results in excellent function with satisfactory rates of prosthetic deterioration. Interest has been directed toward porous ingrowth in which the host bone grows into 200-μm canals, leading to firm fixation. Ceramics are more brittle and have been used in selective situations; they are more common in Europe than in the United States and most notably have been used for replacement of the proximal humerus.

Specific anatomical locations have preferential reconstructions dependent on the presence or absence of chemotherapy. The scapula can be removed with impunity. If a small segment around the glenoid and the acromion can be maintained, the shoulder function can be remarkably improved (Fig. 29–9). Even in its absence, the upper extremity has excellent function, although lacking abduction.[12] The proximal humerus is ideally treated with an implant or a vascularized autograft if chemotherapy is used (Fig. 29–10). When no chemotherapy is used, allografts have proved to be the most functional and give the best results. Nonvascularized and vascularized autografts have been used. However, they do not have the same anatomical configuration and, in the long run, they have not led to better results. Resections about the forearm usually involve a single bone. After the resection the remaining bone often can function alone, especially the radius. When reconstruction is necessary, centralization of the remaining bone into the carpus with arthrodesis is preferable. Vascularized autograft with very close anatomical similarity to the distal radius can be used, especially with arthrodesis.

Resections about the pelvis can be in the iliac posterior pelvis, the central pelvis located about the acetabulum, or the pubis.[2, 4, 19, 20] Resections of the pubis and the posterior pelvis often do not need reconstruction. Some surgeons has used autograft to lead to osteosynthesis. Function can be amazingly good even with large resections. Centralized acetabular pelvic resection, however, presents significant problems. The choices include no reconstruction, allowing a girdle stone pseudo-arthrosis (see Fig. 29–3), arthrodesis (see Fig. 29–4), and, last, reconstruction using either an allograft with a total hip replacement or an allograft containing a hip bijoint reconstruction, including the proximal femur as well as the acetabulum (Fig. 29–11). The allograft is ideal when the complete hemipelvis has been resected. It is being used quite successfully in several centers, particularly for chondrosarcomas and other tumors not requiring chemotherapy. If chemotherapy is required, the patient should be treated with an adjuvant program and reconstruction performed following treatment. Resections that involve the proximal femur are best handled with total hip replacement or proximal femoral replacement using artificial implants. These have significantly better function than all other techniques used at this point. Areas about the knee should be divided into those that require part of the joint, half of the joint, or full joint. For those with half a joint, in the absence of chemotherapy an allograft is probably the most efficient (see Fig. 29–7). When half the joint has been removed, allograft and an arthrodesis are of equal advantage; the former allows retention of function but has a significant instability rate. The latter leads to better function but also to a loss of motion about the knee. When the full joint must be resected the best results to date have been obtained with either an artificial implant (see Fig. 29–8) or a creative arthrodesis using vascularized grafts, allografts, or nonviable autografts (turn-up, turn-down procedure). Chemotherapy, however, seriously interferes with this latter alternative and has led to difficulty using allografts and nonviable autografts in this circumstance. Successes have been achieved

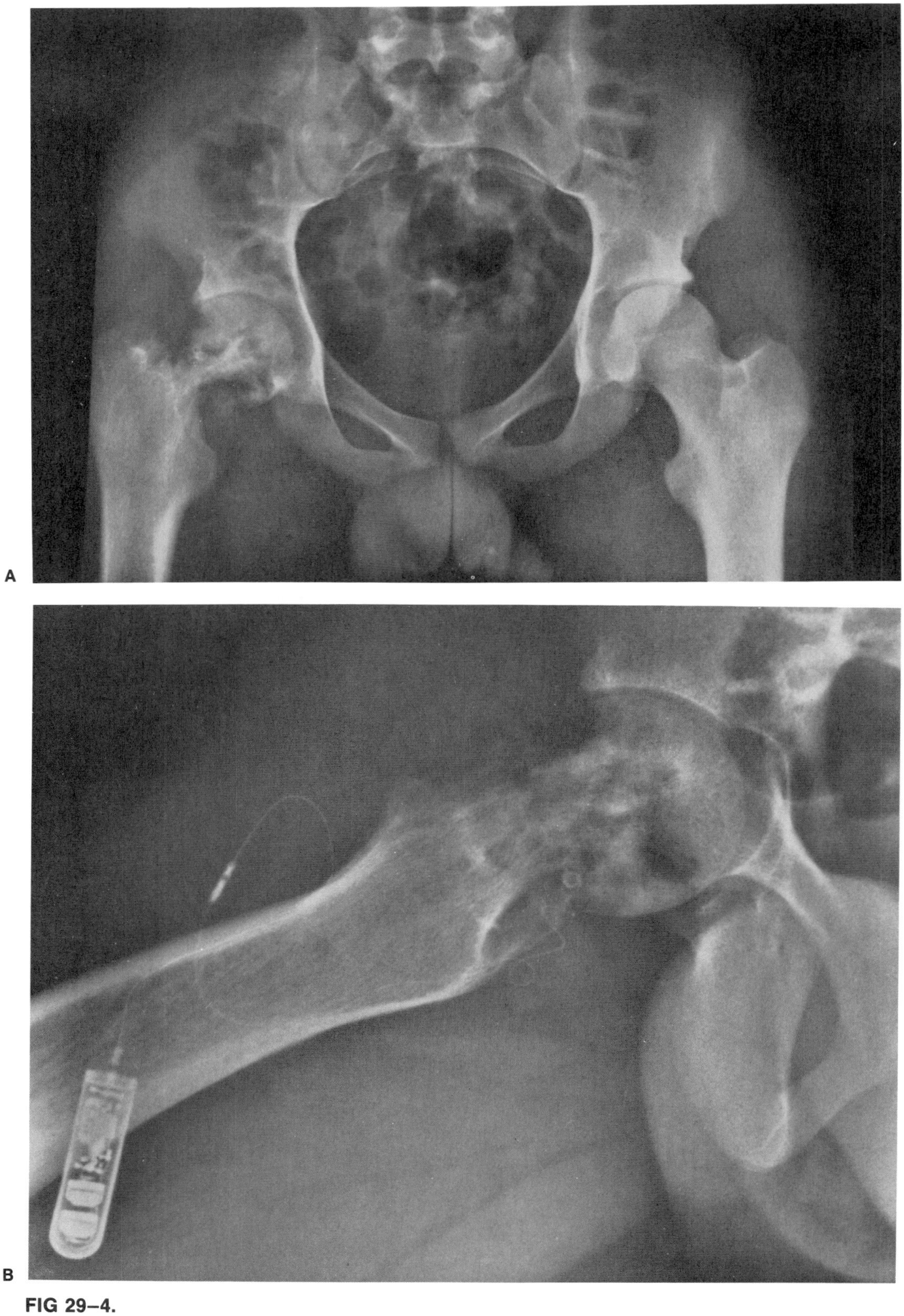

FIG 29–4.

A teenager presented with a pathological fracture of the proximal femur. It was treated unsuccessfully with invasive electricity. At the time of presentation at Memorial Hospital (New York, NY), a diagnosis of underlying high-grade osteogenic sarcoma was made (anteroposterior view, **A,** lateral view, **B**). A bone scan, **C,** demonstrated involvement of the femoral head and acetabulum. The patient was treated with en bloc resection of the proximal femur and acetabulum followed by arthrodesis of the femur to the ischium and iliac wing supplemented by bone graft and stabilized by long plates, **D**.

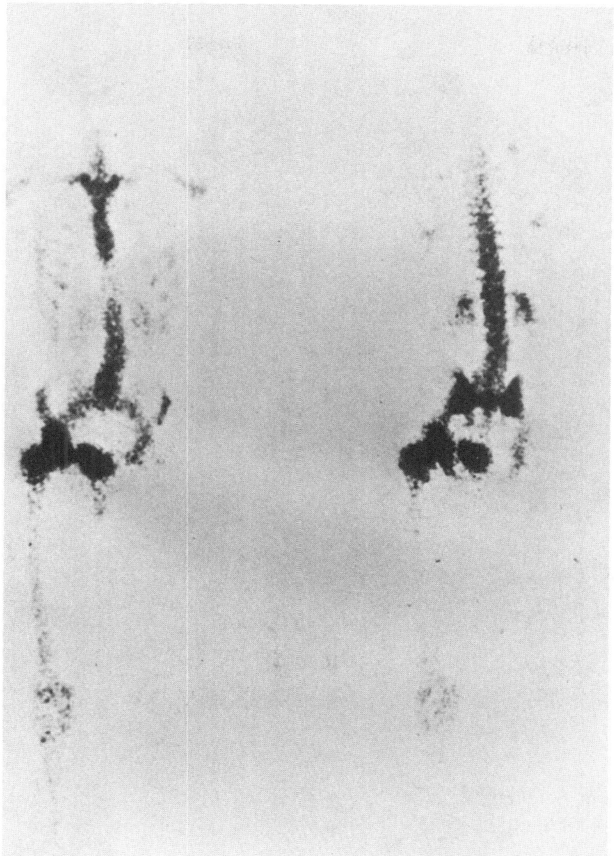

C

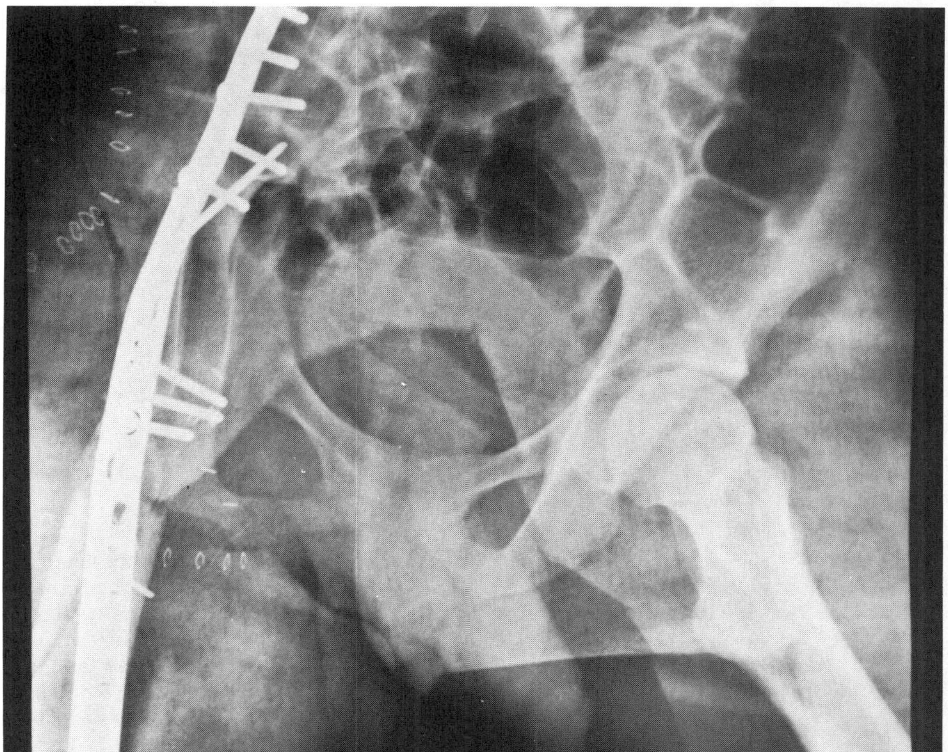

D

FIG 29–4.—*Continued*

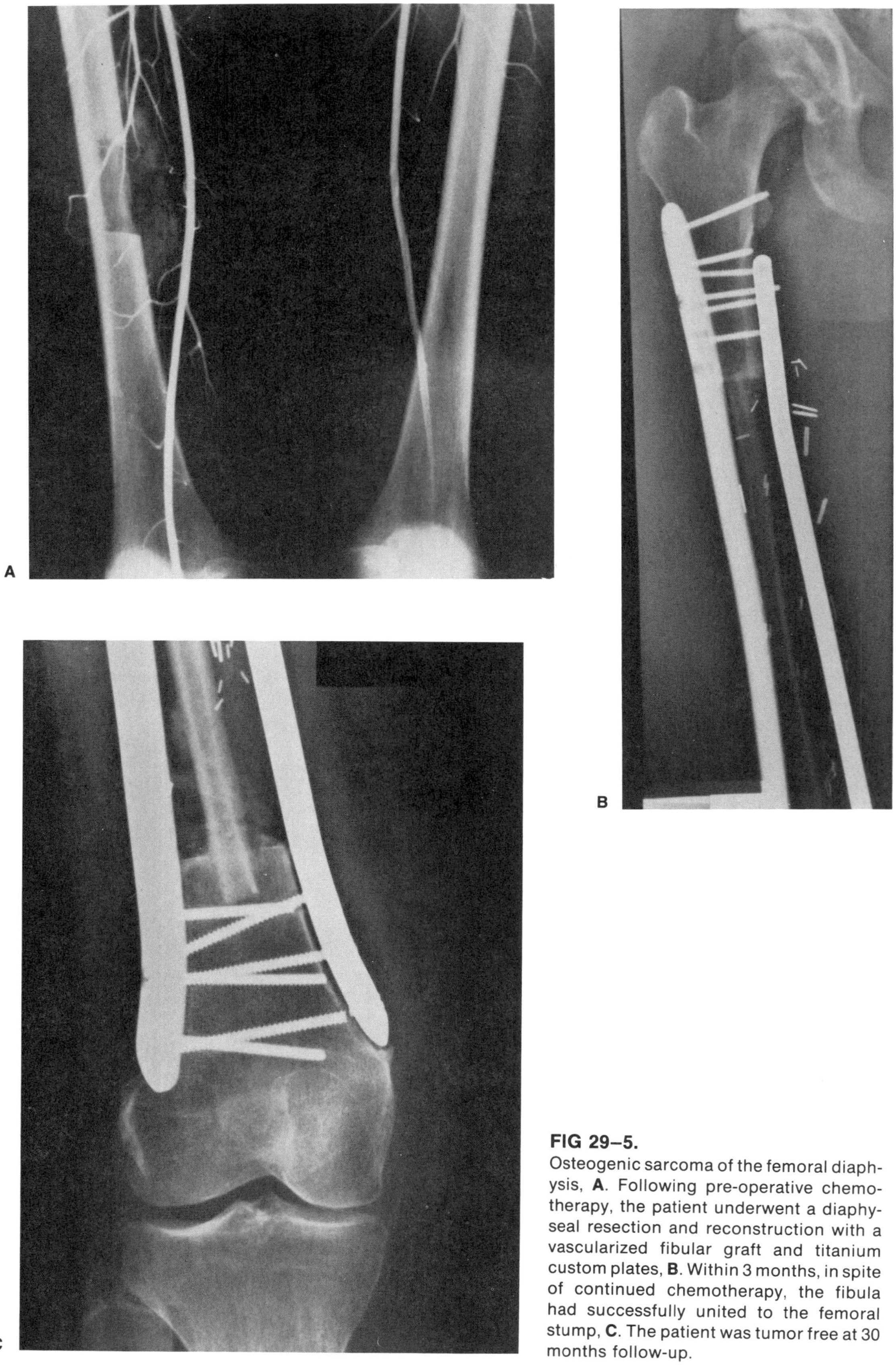

FIG 29–5.
Osteogenic sarcoma of the femoral diaphysis, **A**. Following pre-operative chemotherapy, the patient underwent a diaphyseal resection and reconstruction with a vascularized fibular graft and titanium custom plates, **B**. Within 3 months, in spite of continued chemotherapy, the fibula had successfully united to the femoral stump, **C**. The patient was tumor free at 30 months follow-up.

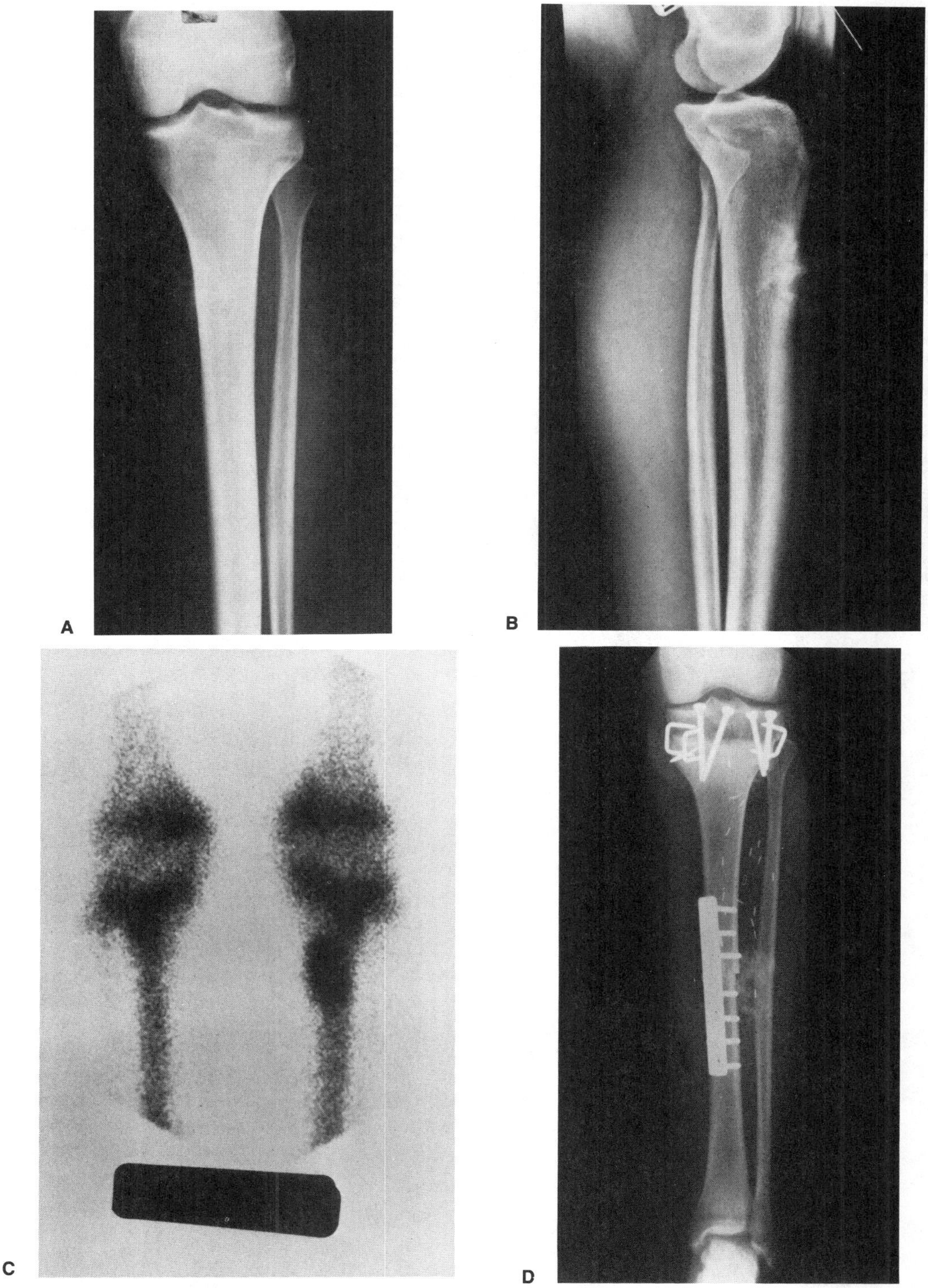

FIG 29–6.
High-grade osteosarcoma of the proximal tibial metaphyseal-diaphyseal junction (anteroposterior view, **A**, lateral view, **B**). A bone scan defined a small, limited lesion **C**. The patient underwent an en bloc resection of the metaphysis and proximal diaphysis. Reconstruction was done with a diaphyseal allograft and internal fixation, **D**. After 4 months, the union was successful.

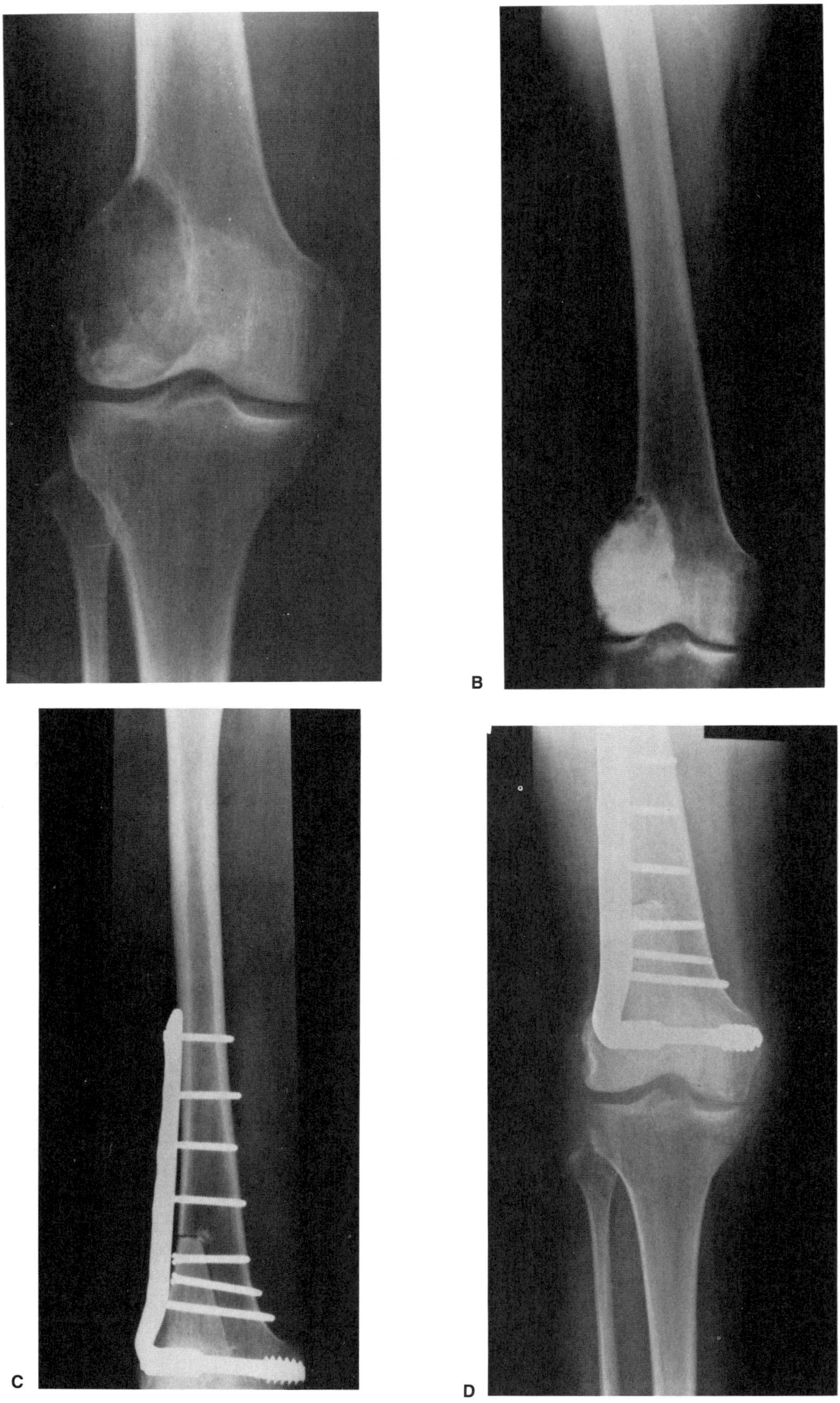

A B C D

FIG 29–7.

A young woman presented with a malignant giant cell tumor of the lateral condyle, **A.** She was initially treated with curettage and cryosurgery, **B,** until an allograft could be obtained. She then underwent hemicondylar resection and reconstruction with an allograft, **C.** Within 2 months, osseous union had been achieved, **D.** The allograft was still functional 30 months later, and the patient was able to play tennis, **E.**

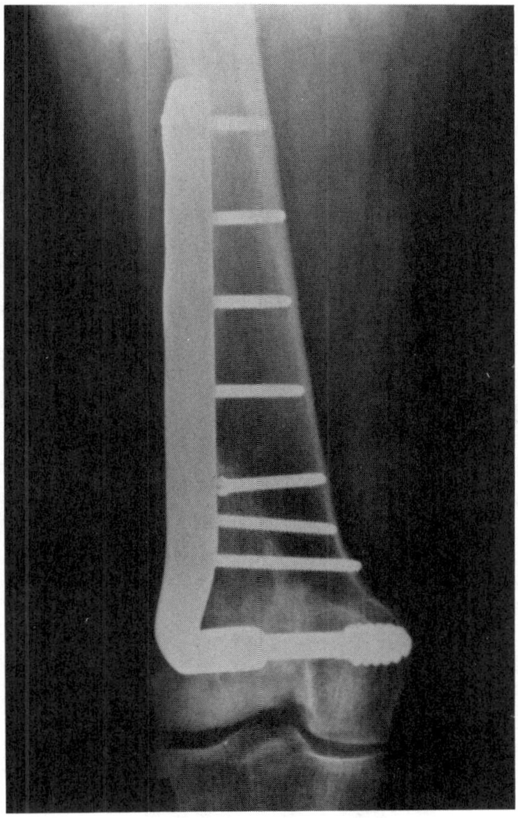

E

FIG 29–7.—*Continued*

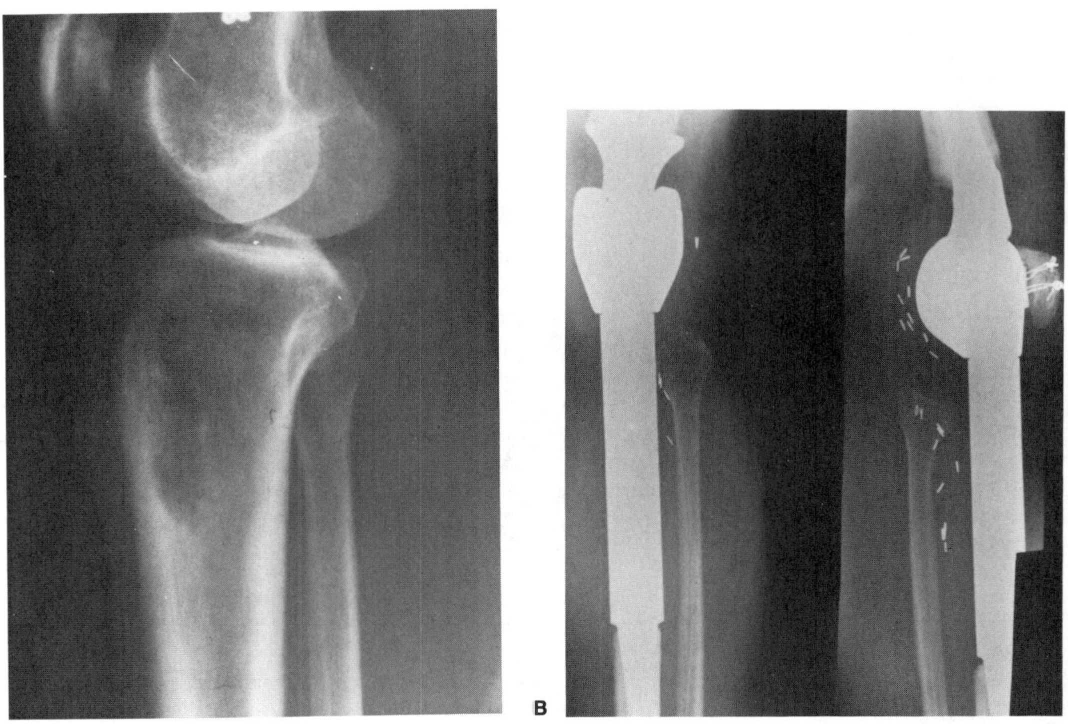

A

B

FIG 29–8.

A young man presented with a malignant fibrohistiocytoma of the proximal tibia, extending anterior to the tibial tubercle, **A.** Following chemotherapy, he had a proximal tibial resection and reconstruction with a BL titanium custom total knee, **B.** To regain active knee extension, the patella was joined to the tibial component through porous ingrowth.

A 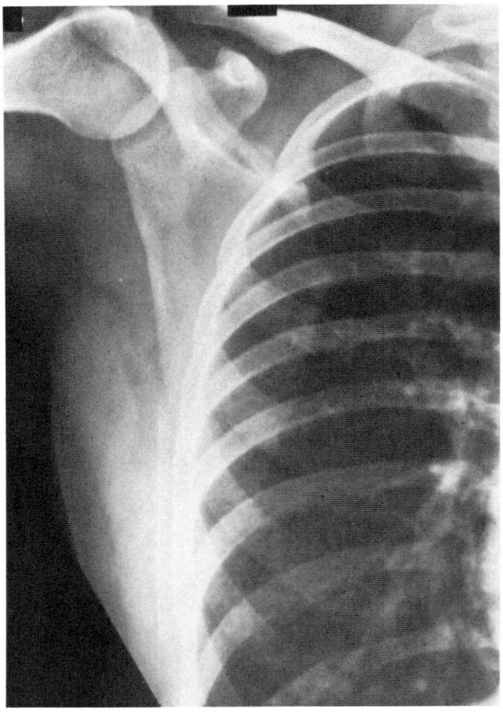

B 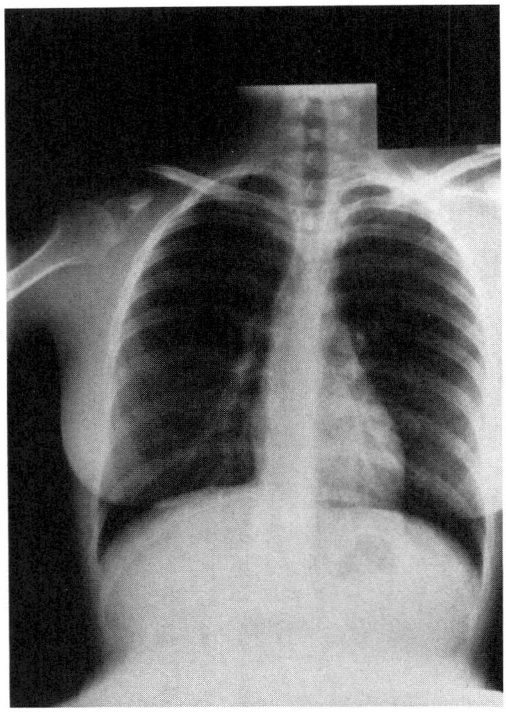

FIG 29–9.
A young woman presented with Ewing's sarcoma of the trapezius and scapula spine, **A.** After chemotherapy, she had a resection of the trapezius and medial 90% of the scapula, **B.** She can abduct her arm over 90° and can comb her hair without difficulty.

with those latter techniques but the complication rates are quite high.

DISCUSSION

It should be noted that this discussion assumes that the patient is skeletally mature. Resections performed in growing children, however, must take into account the problem of continued growth. Successes have been achieved using resection/reduction turniplasty or arthrodesis.[1, 5] Van Ness has used a 180° rotation of the tibia and arthrodesis in the treatment of proximal femoral focal deficiency.[21] This has been applied to tumor patients (Fig. 29–12). Resections about the knee can be accomplished by turning the tibia 180° and using arthrodesis in a shortened position, converting the heel into a pseudoknee. The toes should be retained to optimize function. Patients can then ambulate as if they had a below-knee amputation rather than a high above-knee amputation. The prosthesis that fits below the foot obviously can then be corrected for continued growth of the child. Similar creative surgery has been accomplished for proximal femoral lesions in young children.

FIG 29–10.
Two cases of osteogenic sarcoma of the proximal humerus. A young women presented with an osteosarcoma of the proximal left humerus, **A.** Following pre-operative chemotherapy, she had resection of the proximal 60% of the humerus and shoulder joint, **B.** Reconstruction was done with a titanium proximal humerus. She was tumor free at 36 months and could play the piano. A young male presented with a large humeral osteosarcoma, **C.** He also underwent resection of the tumor but reconstruction was done with a vascularized fibular graft, **D.**

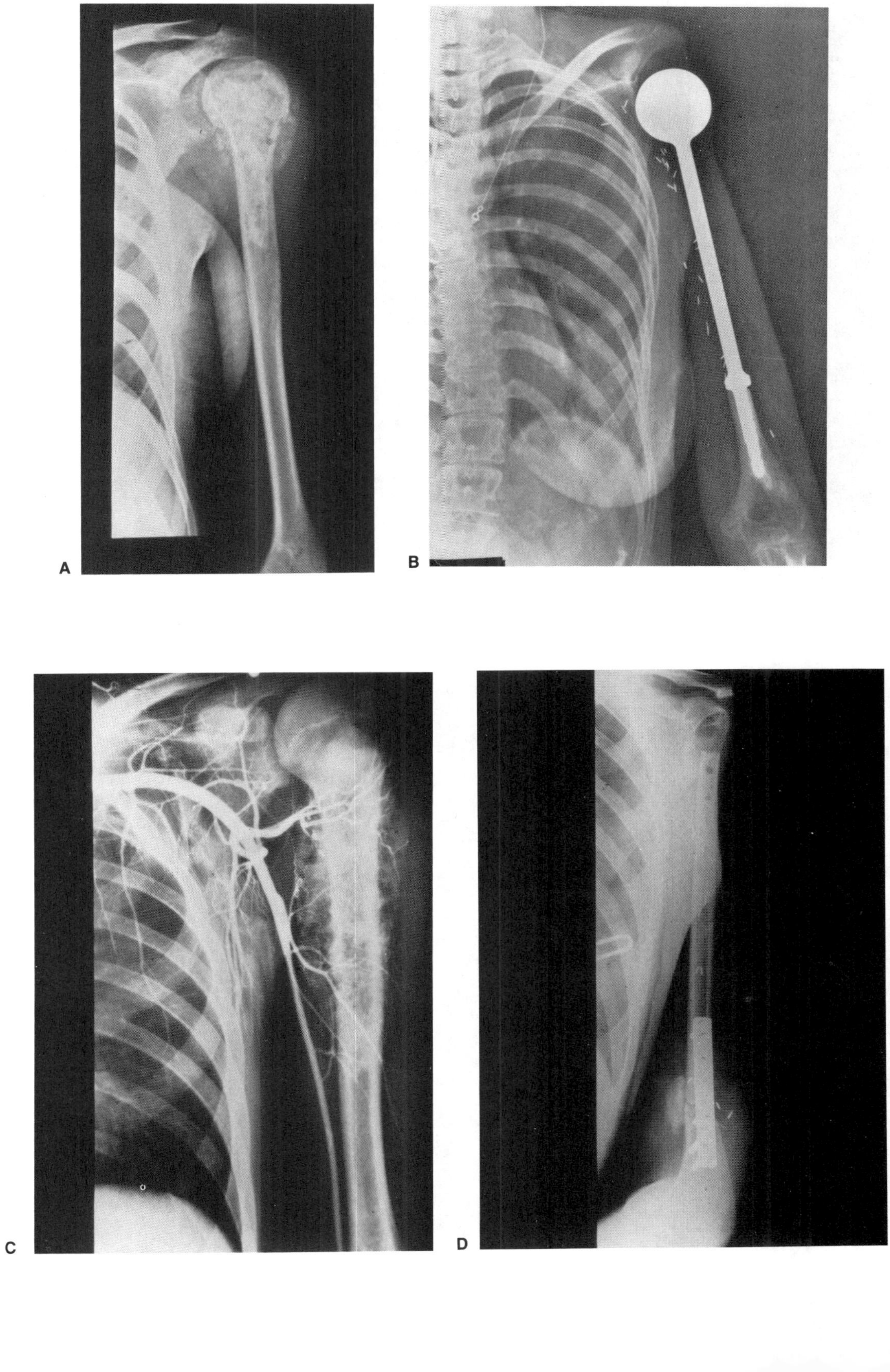
A
B
C
D

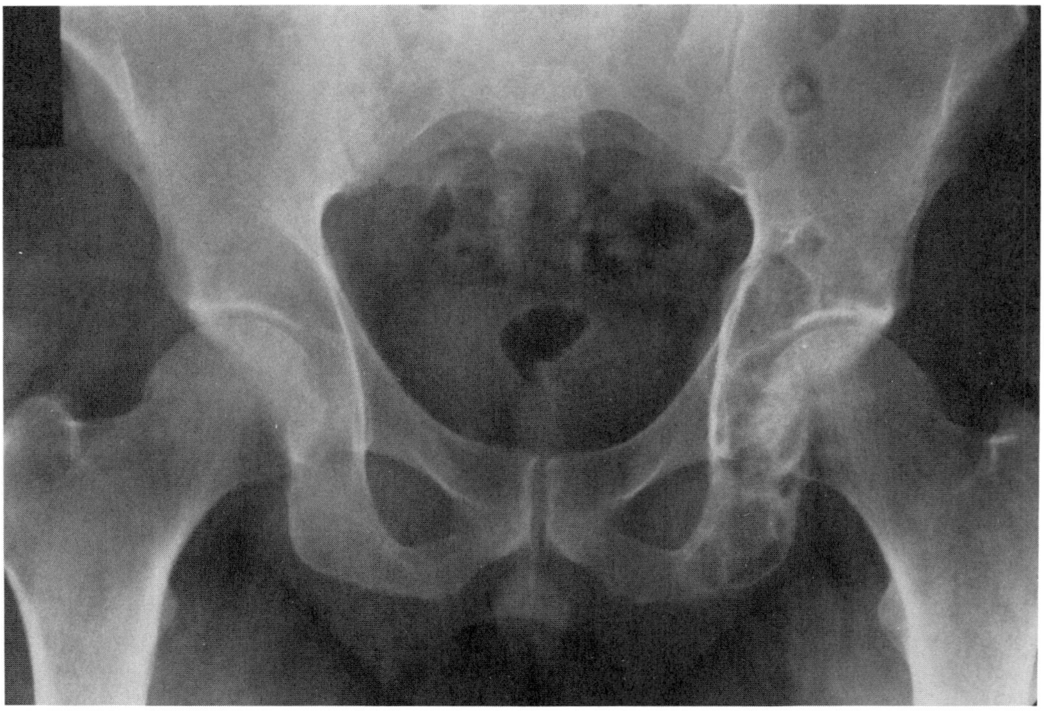

A

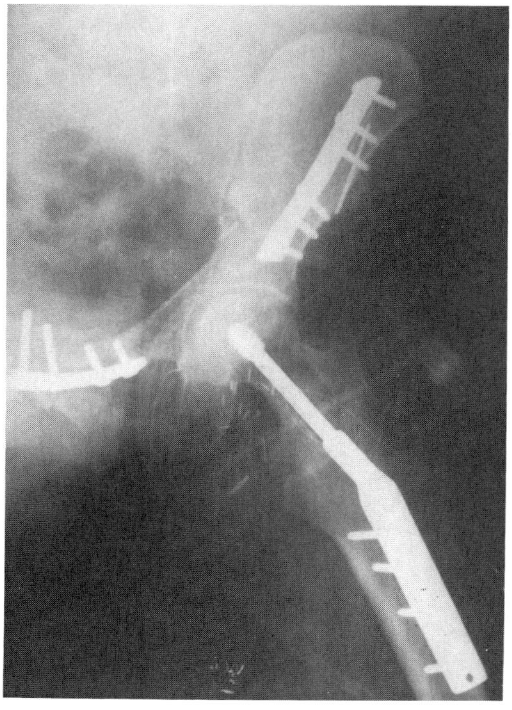

B

FIG 29–11.
A young man had a moderate-grade chondrosarcoma of the peri-acetabulum area, **A.** He underwent an internal hemipelvectomy and reconstruction was done with an allograft, including both the acetabular side and the proximal femur, **B.**

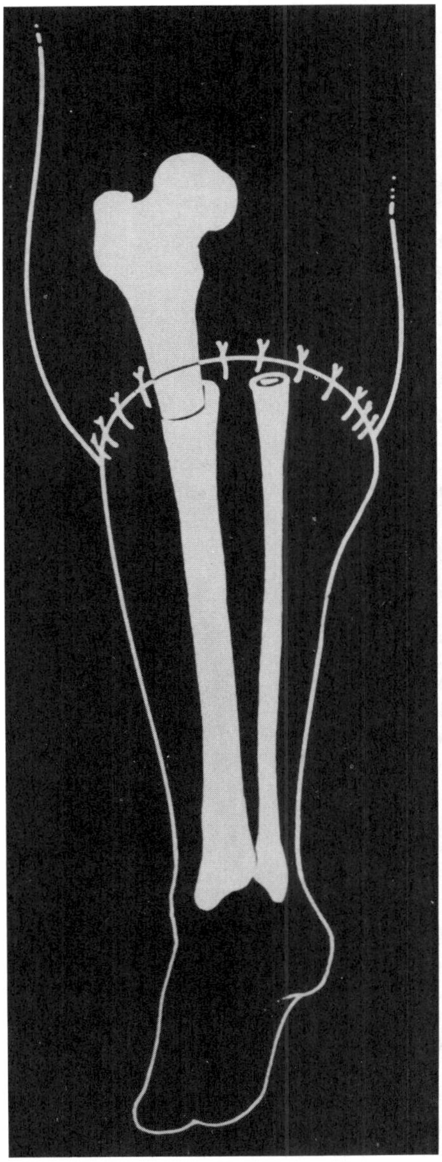

A

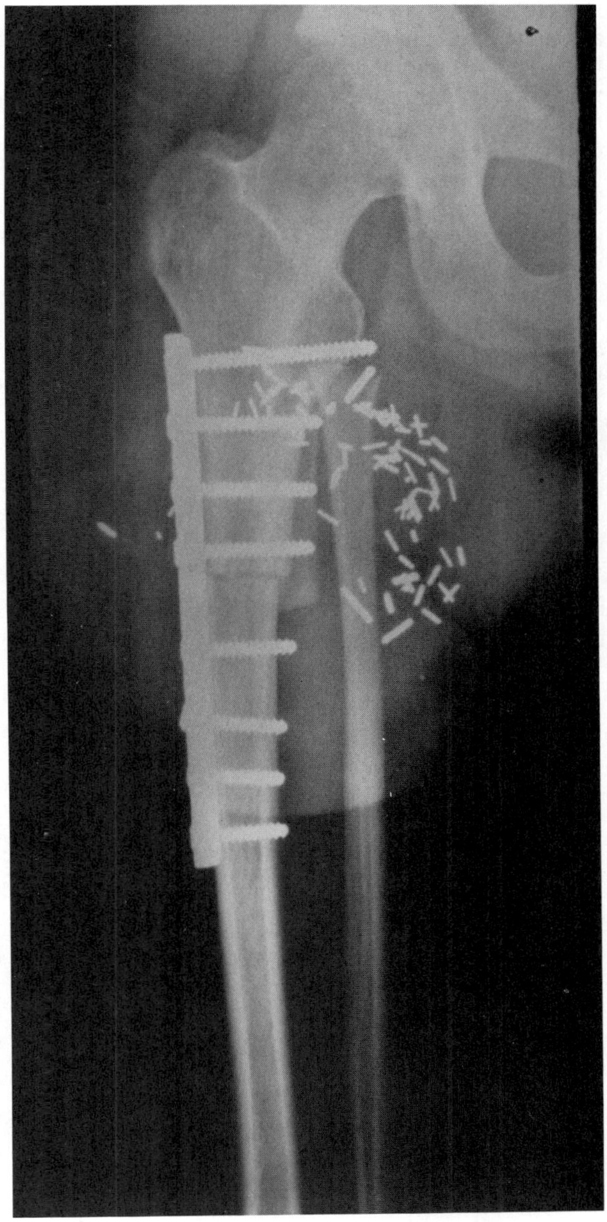

B

FIG 29–12.
A young woman presented with an osteosarcoma of the distal femur. She was treated with a resection of the distal two thirds of the femur and reconstruction was done with a Van Ness turniplasty, **A.** The tibia was rotated 180° and osteosynthesized to the subtrochanteric area of the femur, **B.**

The remaining consideration is the long-term results of these treatments. Autografts have the greatest chance for longevity once union has been achieved and hypertrophy has taken place. Allografts have excellent longevity in two thirds of patients. The biggest problem with implants is progressive loosening and breakage with time. They provide the best quick-fix result and have the poorest long-term success, particularly when correlated with the age of the patient. Psychologically it is always better for the patient to save the limb. Functional studies have been performed to document the advantages of limb salvage versus amputation. Compared to mid thigh amputation, en bloc procedures with artificial implant reconstruction result in superior function, with significantly superior stride length, velocity, lower oxygen expenditure, and use a smaller percentage of aerobic capacity.[12] An exception is a below-knee amputation, which compares favorably with an implant about the ankle due to the difficulty of implant fixation, inadequate musculature, and poor skin coverage. Additional studies are underway at this time to evaluate relative function as related to reconstructive method. As reconstructive techniques improve and analyses of end results become available, we shall be able to provide better advice on treatment choices for our patients.

REFERENCES

1. Kotz R, Salzer M: Rotation-plasty for childhood osteosarcoma of the distal part of the femur. *J Bone Joint Surg* 1982; 64A:959–969.
2. Lane JM: Malignant bone tumors, in Alfonson AE, Gardner E (eds): *The Practice of Cancer Surgery.* New York, Appleton-Century-Crofts, 1982, pp 307–324.
3. Lane JM: Custom prosthetic segmental bone and joint replacement in malignant bone tumor patients, in Choa E, Ivins J (eds): *Tumor Prostheses—The Design and Application,* ch 13. New York, Thieme-Stratton, 1983.
4. Lane JM, Boland PJ: Tumors of bone and cartilage in the practice of surgery, in Goldsmith HS (ed): Philadelphia, Harper and Row, 1983.
5. Hurson BJ, Lane JM: Tumors around the knee, in Insall J (ed): *Surgery of the Knee.* New York, Churchill-Livingston, 1983, pp 791–807.
6. Marcove RC, Lewis MM, Huvos AC: En bloc upper humeral interscapulothoracic resection: The Tikhoff-Linberg procedure. *Clin Orthop Rel Res* 1977; 124:219–228.
7. Rosen G, Caparros B, Huvos AC, et al: Preoperative chemotherapy for osteogenic sarcoma. *Cancer* 1982; 49:1221–1230.
8. Rosenberg SA, Kent SA, Kent H, et al: Prospective randomized evaluation of the role of limb sparing surgery, radiation therapy and adjuvant chemo-immunotherapy in the treatment of adult soft tissue sarcomas. *Surgery* 1978; 84:62–69.
9. Rosenberg SA, Suit HD, Baker LH, et al: Sarcomas of soft tissues and bone, in DeVita VT, Hellman S, Rosenberg SA (eds): *Principles and Practice of Oncology.* Philadelphia, J. B. Lippincott, 1982, pp 1037–1093.
10. Rosenberg SA, Tepper J, Glatstein E, et al: The treatment of soft tissue sarcomas of the extremities. *Ann Surg* 1982; 196:305–315.
11. Shui MH, Castro EG, Hajdu SI, et al: Surgical treatment of 297 soft tissue sarcomas of the lower extremity. *Ann Surg* 1975; 182:597–602.
12. Sim EH, Pritchard DJ, Ivins JC, et al: Total joint arthroplasty: Application in the management of bone tumors. *Mayo Clin Pract* 1979; 54:583–589.
13. Souhami RL: What has adjuvant chemotherapy of osteosarcoma achieved? (discussion paper). *J Soc Med* 1983; 76:943–946.
14. Enneking WF, Spanier SS, Goodman MA: A system for the surgical staging of musculoskeletal sarcoma. *Clin Orthop Rel Res* 1980; 153:106–120.
15. Enneking WF, Shirley PD: Resection arthrodesis for malignant and potentially malignant lesions about the knee using an intramedullary rod and local bone grafts. *J Bone Joint Surg* 1977; 59A:223–235.
16. Enneking WF, Eady JL, Burchardt H: Autogenous cortical bone grafts in the reconstruction of sequential skeletal defects. *J Bone Joint Surg* 1980; 62A:1039–1058.
17. Weiland A, McCormack R: Free vascularized bone grafts in surgery of the upper extremity. *J Hand Surg* 1979; 4:129–143.
18. Mankin HJ, Doppelt SH, Sullivan R, et al: Osteoarticular and intercalary allograft transplantation in the management of malignant tumors of bone. *Cancer* 1982; 50:613–630.
19. Enneking WF, Dunham WK: Resection and reconstruction for primary neoplasm involving the innominate bone. *J Bone Joint Surg* 1978; 60A:731–746.
20. Steel HJ: Partial or complete resection of the hemipelvis: An alternative to hindquarter amputation for peri-acetabular chondrosarcoma of the pelvis. *J Bone Joint Surg* 1978; 60A:719–730.
21. Van Ness CP: Rotationplasty in the treatment of congenital defects of the femur. *J Bone Joint Surg* 1950; 32B:12–16.
22. Otis JC, Lane JM, Hillyer CD: Energy consumption in postoperative osteogenic sarcoma patients, in Choa E, Ivins J (eds): *Tumor Prostheses—The Design and Application,* ch 53. New York, Thieme-Stratton, 1983.

Chapter 30

Reconstructive Surgery After Major Sarcoma Resection

Ted Chaglassian

Joseph Pober

Successful reconstruction of the surgical defect resulting from extensive resection of soft tissue sarcoma is not only essential to the quality of the patient's life, but may also be critical to the effective continued management of the disease.

Soft-tissue sarcomas may occur anywhere in the body, particularly in such areas as the extremities, trunk, head and neck region, and retroperitoneum. The predominant varieties of soft-tissue sarcomas, such as liposarcoma and fibrosarcoma, most frequently affect the lower extremities, usually the medial upper thigh.[1]

The sensitivity of soft-tissue sarcomas to radiation therapy is variable. Although primary radiation therapy is offered for some varieties such as Kaposi's sarcoma,[2] the mode of therapy most often suggested for soft-tissue sarcomas is wide excision. This includes an adequate margin around both the outer pseudocapsule of the sarcoma and any tumor extension along muscle bundles, nerve sheaths, or fascial planes.[3] This extensive surgery may generate a significant soft-tissue defect not amenable to direct closure. Rarely, lymph node involvement, as seen in synovial sarcoma or rhabdomyosarcoma,[1] mandates additional intervention, such as regional lymphadenectomy or radiation therapy. If tumor infiltration is sufficiently extensive or the radiation therapy fails, the situation may anatomically warrant more radical surgery, such as hindquarter or forequarter amputation to prevent ulceration and palliate symptoms.[4] Adjunctive pre- and postoperative radiation therapy and chemotherapy have permitted somewhat more conservative surgery, but have imposed additional reconstructive demands.

It is fundamental to remember that, despite the magnitude of the ablative defect created by curative resection, in no instance should proper treatment be compromised. As a result, the closure after tumor resection often requires the expertise of the plastic and reconstructive surgeon.

The objective of this discussion is to provide a basis for understanding the plastic surgeon's strategies for resolving reconstructive problems. To this end, generally applicable procedures and fundamental principles of reconstructive surgery will be surveyed. In addition, several specific approaches to reconstruction of the sites most frequently affected by soft-tissue sarcomas will be presented, as well as a brief consideration of less frequently affected sites.

GENERAL PRINCIPLES

The reconstructive approach is determined by the nature and location of the surgical defect, as well as the general medical status of the individual. In surgical reconstruction or wound closure, the simplest and most reliable method should be employed to restore viable cutaneous coverage. As a secondary consideration, the method selected should restore useful function and aesthetic structure, while producing a minimal donor site deficit.

When direct closure is not feasible, the sequence of reconstructive options proceeds from grafts, to local flaps, and eventually to distant flaps, including those requiring microsurgical transfer.

SKIN GRAFTS

Skin grafts are indicated for small, stable, well-vascularized soft-tissue defects, including those with exposed fat, cancellous bone, muscle, and fascia. Grafts obviate the need for further alteration of any adjacent structures. They should be harvested observing "no touch" and other oncological principles of surgery to prevent seeding of tumor cells. A separate instrument tray is advised.

Grafts should not be used in areas where they fail to take, fail to supply sufficiently stable structural coverage, or fail to prevent functional impairment. More specifically, the areas where grafts would be undesirable include (1) anesthetic regions of recurrent trauma at bony prominences, (2) wounds that require reopening for further repair of underlying structures, (3) recipient beds with inadequate local capillary circulation, (4) regions where graft contraction would lead to structural (facial feature distraction) or functional (joint contracture) deformity, (5) open wounds over body cavities, such as the abdomen or thorax with exposed perineum or pleura, and (6) large conspicuous regions with composite tissue deficit.

Poor recipient beds for skin graft take include areas of edematous and gelatinous chronic granulation, irradiated areas, exposed fractured cortical bone without periosteum, and vital structures recently repaired. For example, an arterial graft that replaces the resected femoral or brachial artery involved by sarcoma is not ideally suitable for skin grafting. Occasionally, to augment durability of grafted regions, dermal overgrafting or reversed dermal grafts are employed. For a small defect less than 1 to 2 cm in diameter, a composite graft of several tissue components may replace the complex tissue deficit.

FLAPS

All the aforementioned conditions that are effectively contraindications for skin grafts are simultaneously indications for coverage with flaps. In contrast to parasitic grafts, flaps can rely on their own attached vascular supply for nourishment after transfer to the defect. Even when skin grafts may provide viable coverage, often a more stable soft-tissue padding that adds its own vascular supply to the surgical defect is required. This is especially important when considering rehabilitation and further therapy such as radiation therapy or perfusion chemotherapy. This additional blood supply may not only expedite healing of the surgical defect and increase the tolerance of the wound coverage to radiation therapy, but also increases transport of chemotherapeutic agents to the site of resection.

Classification of Flaps

Flaps may be classified into two broad categories: local versus distant (depending on whether the tissue used for coverage lies in proximity to the defect) and random versus axial (depending on the presence of a specific named longitudinal vascular supply (Fig 30–1). The flaps may be further subclassified according to their tissue components (cutaneous, myocutaneous, muscle, fasciocutaneous) and according to the technique of flap transfer. Local flaps can be transferred with peninsula or island cutaneous portions to surgical defects by rotation on a pivot point or advancement. Distant flaps can be transferred directly or indirectly. Distant flaps are directly transferred from or to an extremity. They are often used for reconstruction of certain tumor-free defects. Distant flaps are indirectly transferred in current practice by one-staged microsurgical transplantation of axial flaps.

Microsurgical transfer has supplanted multistaged migrations of tube flaps (Fig 30–2) and three-staged carrier (jump) flap procedures. These techniques have not only been time consuming, but have also been fraught with high morbidity. Even under optimal conditions, these historically traditional techniques require the consumption of additional skin.

In planning multistaged transfer, the original donor skin must be designed larger than the actual dimension of the defect to account for tissue changes such as contraction or scarring that occur in the course of transfer. In addition, recipient defects that are poorly vascularized must be circumferentially enlarged to expose adjacent well-vascularized surrounding tissue. Ultimately, these parasitic multistaged flaps rely on the donor site defect for revascularization. Thus, their lack of efficient skin utilization further limits their appeal and lends greater favor to microsurgical transfer, which requires only exposure of recipient bed vessels for reanastomosis.[5]

Anatomical Considerations in Random Flap Construction

A knowledge of the vascular anatomy of the skin is fundamental to the construction of any flap. If a random flap is constructed in an area of great density of subdermal and dermal vessels, it more reliably contains, within the width of its base, the blood supply capable of nourishing a peninsula of skin. For example, in the facial region, random flaps may have narrow bases (of 1 to 2 cm) because the random subdermal and dermal vessels are closely situated. Moving caudad to the trunk and upper extremities, the concentration of random blood vessels decreases and the flaps, empirically, must be approximately 6 cm wide to maximize the possibility of including sufficient blood supply within the pedicle. Moving further caudad, the density of the cutaneous vasculature decreases further. Therefore, random flaps in the lower extremities need a wider base to assure the inclusion of sufficient blood supply.[6]

The length-to-width ratio of flaps is predominantly determined by the radius of the largest vessel supplying the flap. If a certain region of the skin is supplied by an axial (defined as longitudinal) blood vessel, it has sufficient blood supply for the length of the vessel plus a random extension. The length-to-width ratio of the random portion depends on the radius and concentration of the vessels in the subdermal and dermal plexus. In the lower extremity, the length-to-width ratio of random flaps is 1 : 1. Moving toward the face, it increases to approximately 2 : 1 (Fig 30–3).[6]

There is great heterogeneity in the size and number of vessels supplying the skin even for mirror-image flaps in the same patient. As a

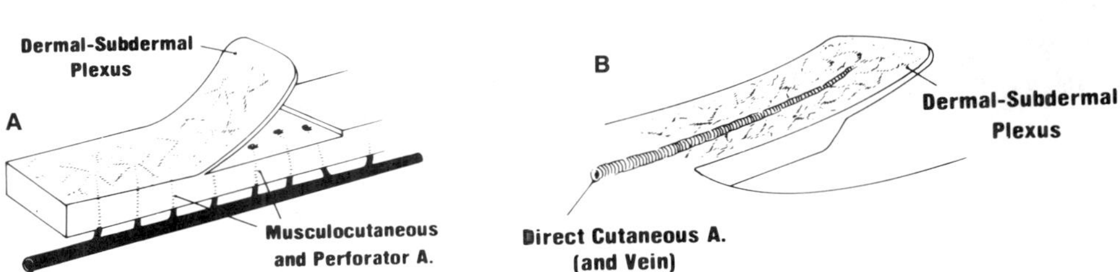

FIG 30–1.
Basic design of random pattern ("old fashicned") flap, **A,** and peninsular axial pattern flap, **B.**

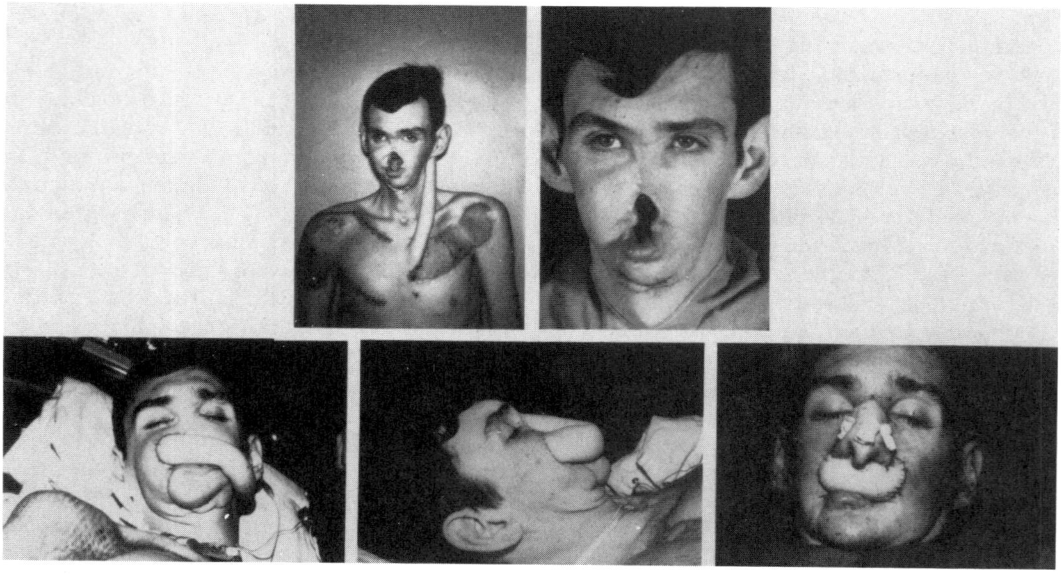

FIG 30–2.
Multistaged nasal reconstruction by means of a tubed flap.

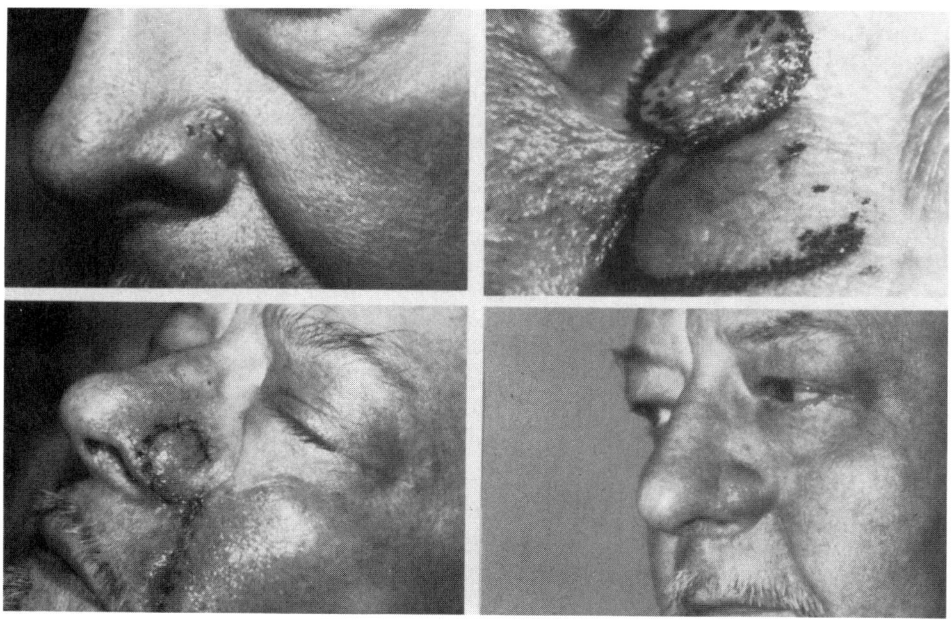

FIG 30–3.
Nasolabial flap.

result, there are no absolute rules governing specifications for flap design that guarantee its survival. Therefore, it is prudent to plan for the risk of partial flap loss with each procedure.[6]

For given regions of the body, a collection of random flaps has been empirically defined with limited length-to-width ratios and optimal locations for the base of the flaps. Flaps should be designed to allow transfer, without tension or kinking, of tissues matched for color, texture, and thickness to the recipient defect. The donor defect left after transfer of the flap should not expose a weight-bearing or frequently contacted area. It should be acceptable to the patient and be amenable to inconspicuous closure, preferably in a primary fashion or with a skin graft.

Planning of a flap design must always be individualized. Any prior local surgical or traumatic procedure (with resultant neurovascular changes) must be considered as well as the overall status of the patient, including vital organ system function. Distal flap necrosis and poor donor site healing are associated with such conditions as diabetes mellitus, arteriosclerotic cardiovascular disease, and prior radiation therapy. The elevation of large flaps produces significant fluid shifts and places demands on the renal and cardiovascular systems.

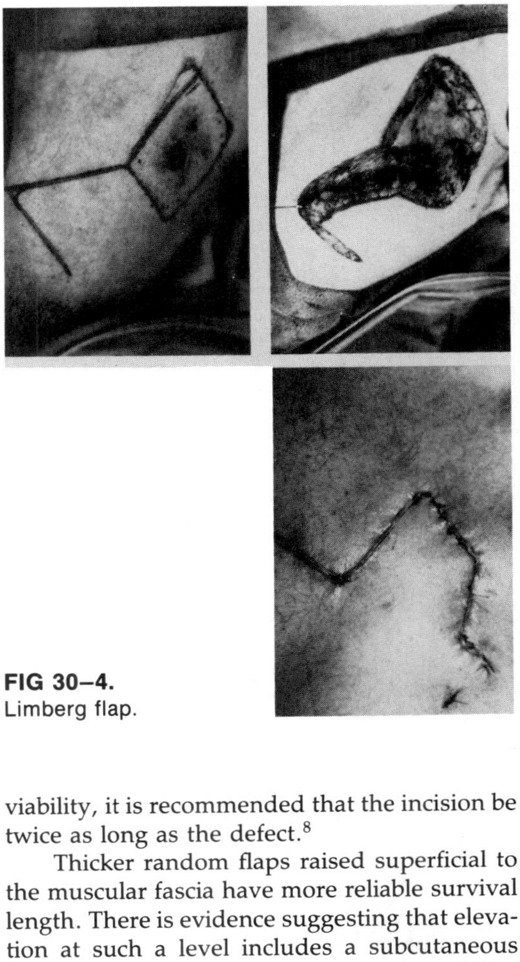

FIG 30–4.
Limberg flap.

Local Random Flaps for Thigh Reconstruction

Wound closure in the thigh is usually accomplished with ease by most surgeons. In certain demanding situations, however, the plastic surgeon's expertise is required to provide strategies to help further expand the general surgical approach to wound closure.

A simple local flap that supplies the needed 1 : 1 ratio for the lower extremity is the Limberg flap (Fig 30–4). It should be within the repertoire of all surgeons because of its versatility and reliability in virtually all parts of the body. When a small defect can be fashioned to resemble a 60° to 120° rhomboid or circle (which is approximated by a hexagonal constellation of three adjoining rhomboids), this flap design will reliably provide coverage.[7]

Another versatile flap, comparable to a 1 : 1 unipedicle flap, is the 2 : 1 bipedicle flap (Fig 30–5). It is suggested to approach defects that approximate a linear ellipse. An incision parallel to the elliptical defect with appropriate undermining creates the flap. To allow wound closure without tension and assure optimal flap viability, it is recommended that the incision be twice as long as the defect.[8]

Thicker random flaps raised superficial to the muscular fascia have more reliable survival length. There is evidence suggesting that elevation at such a level includes a subcutaneous fascial blood supply in addition to the subdermal and dermal plexus.[6]

Distant Random Flaps for Thigh Reconstruction

The cross-leg flap is the traditional distant random flap used for lower extremity coverage. Angiography has demonstrated that the medial calf and lower third of the anterior thigh offer the best blood supply on which to base these flaps.[9] However, these flaps have fallen into disfavor, expecially for reconstruction of the lower extremity following cancer resection. Complications of flap necrosis and infection have been reported in 40% and 28% of patients, respectively.[10] In addition, there are risks associated with the prolonged immobilization required for such flaps, including thrombophlebitis and joint stiffness in the elderly. Another more significant risk of this reconstructive pro-

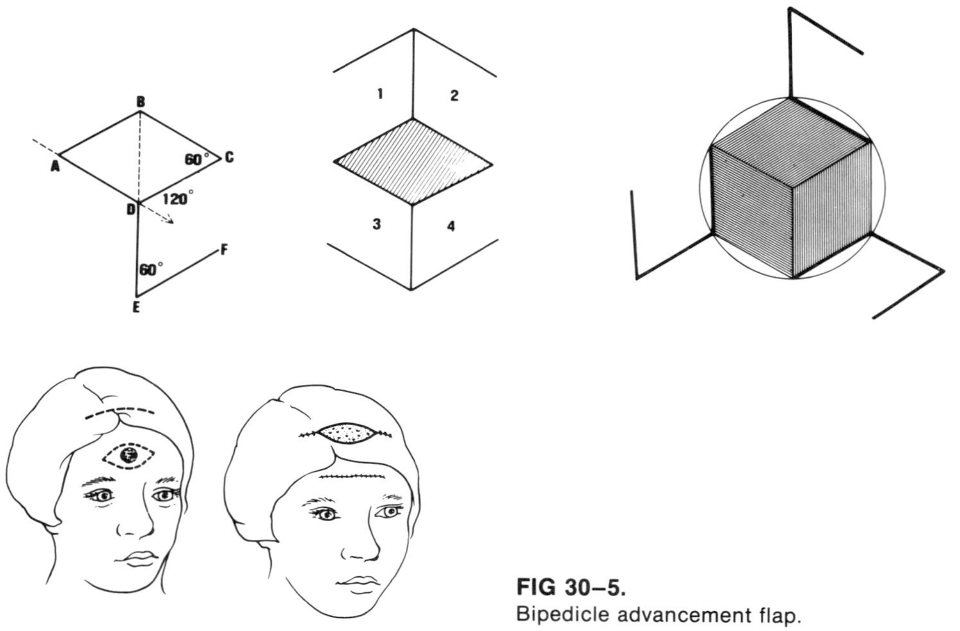

FIG 30–5.
Bipedicle advancement flap.

cedure is the possibility of transfer of residual foci of sarcoma.[11] Therefore, whenever possible, local flaps are suggested for small defects in the thigh and microsurgical transplantation of composite tissue for large defects. These procedures eliminate prolonged immobilization and the risk of tumor spread to a distant body region.

Random Flaps for the Leg

In the leg below the knee, in contrast to the thigh, vascularity and attendant wound healing is extremely poor. Therefore, a random flap is more likely to suffer ischemic distal necrosis and consequently is seldom used for coverage of the tibia. If a random flap is considered, a delay procedure is suggested to extend the length-to-width ratio. Alternatively, creating fasciocutaneous flaps for leg reconstruction offers additional vascular supply to increase the length-to-width ratio.[12]

Axial Cutaneous Flaps: Specific Recommendation for the Lower Extremities

Despite their universal availability, there are several limitations to the use of random flaps: first, their limited length-to-width ratio requires a relatively wide base, restricting the arc of transfer; second, their failure to supply normal sensory innervation to the defect predisposes to recurrent ulceration; finally, their occasional need for delay procedure, especially in indirect transfer as jump flaps, necessitates extended hospitalization.

To overcome some of these difficulties, axial flaps have been introduced. Identified axial cutaneous vessels predominate in the face, around limb girdles, joints, digits, and genitalia. Only a few local axial flaps are available for reconstruction of the thigh and leg. These include the dorsalis pedis, groin, and gluteal thigh flap.

The dorsalis pedis arterial flap has traditionally been used for coverage of defects of the foot and ankle. When designed as an island flap with its pedicle dissected through the extensor retinaculum to the anterior tibial artery, it can be transferred for coverage to the midpretibial area.

Longer flaps such as the groin and gluteal thigh flaps can be transposed locally with a broader arc of rotation about their pivot points. These pivot points are located where their vascular supply first surfaces to a surgically approachable cutaneous or fascial level. For example, in the case of the groin flap, the superficial femoral circumflex artery serves as a pivot point at approximately 3 cm below the midpoint of the inguinal ligament, and for the gluteal thigh flap, the inferior gluteal artery serves as a pivot point 5 cm above the ischial tuberosity. The cutaneous territory of axial flaps is defined by the geometry of their longitudinal vascular supply.

Thus the long axis of the gluteal thigh flap is centered on the posterior thigh midway between the greater trochanter and the ischial tuberosity. It should be recognized that axial flaps may be extended with a contiguous random flap. With respect to the groin flap, a vertical line drawn through the anterior superior iliac spine roughly defines the boundary between its initial axial portion and its random extension.

Axial flaps may also expedite distant indirect transfer of jump flaps. in these transfers, standard tubed random flaps require an initial delay procedure. When the axial groin flap is substituted for the random abdominal tube flap, this initial period of delay before attachment to a wrist carrier may be eliminated.

Peri-operative Management of Axial and Random Flaps

Although flaps are more hardy than skin grafts, they also can suffer ischemic insult and subsequently undergo necrosis. Careful design, gentle flap development, and peri-operative surveillance are crucial to the ultimate viability of the flap. Decreased perfusion of the flaps from pressure by hematoma, tension of the closure, kinking of the vascular pedicle, or peri-operative hypotension all may lead to distal necrosis. These factors must be controlled assiduously.

When local flaps are followed up clinically, axial flaps that have better venous drainage tend to be paler and less edematous than random flaps. If necrosis resulting from an ischemic insult is to occur, axial flaps will progress slowly toward necrosis, whereas random flaps may demonstrate intense pallor rapidly within hours. Marginally viable axial flaps during the first postoperative week may only appear cyanotic and may even display transient periods of apparent improvement before clearly progressing toward necrosis. Often during this slow process the peripheral margins are revascularized at 2 to 5 days from the capillary buds that grow in from the surrounding walls of the surgical defect. Ultimately, therefore, there is a central island of necrosis at the distal extent of the flap, furthest from the source of blood supply.

There is no method to reverse the progression toward necrosis after a critical ischemic period has elapsed. Thus, intra-operative and postoperative monitoring for ischemic changes is crucial before their progression becomes irreversible. Clinical observation at surgery of pallor (ischemia), cyanosis (venous congestion), slow capillary refill, and dark dermal ooze at the incised edge suggests compromised flap viability. The release of any constricting sutures, evacuation of serosanguinous collections, or modification of the flap design must be performed promptly to limit the extent of necrosis. Pink flaps with rapid capillary refill and arterial ooze at the distal incised edge usually remain viable unless a postoperative complication intervenes. Multiple objective methods that attempt to measure the level of circulatory function in flaps (as reflected by the transport of oxygen, red blood cells, carbon dioxide, and heat) have been developed. Intravenous fluorescein infusion is the most commonly used objective method. Employed intra-operatively and postoperatively, it confirms or helps decide questionable adequacy of blood supply, to predict the ultimate viability of a flap.

Postoperatively, prompt drainage of any collection compressing a flap and maintenance of adequate perfusion pressure continues to be critical to flap viability. Experimental pharmacological means for specifically preventing or reversing flap ischemia have met with inconsistent results.

A surgical delay procedure performed prior to flap elevation has reliably increased surviving length of random flaps by 50% to 100%. It may be performed by elevating the intended dimension of a random flap as a bipedicle flap approximately 10 days prior to transfer. Subsequently, over the course of several days, the distal pedicle is transected in stages, continuously monitoring for any possible ischemic changes.

Myocutaneous Flaps

The universality of random flaps is transferred to cutaneous axial flaps by the inclusion of widely available superficial muscles with reliable axial blood supplies. These myocutaneous flaps additionally enable closure of large and deep defects that would not be adequately covered by skin flaps alone. The muscles used for these flaps have been classified according to five patterns of circulation. Muscles with one (type I) or two (type III) vascular pedicles or one dominant and multiple secondary segmental pedicles (type V) entering near their points of attachment have been most frequently used. In contrast, muscles with only minor segmental vascular pedicles (type IV) entering at multiple sites along the course of the muscle belly have a limited range of movement and usefulness. The most common pattern is a combination of dominant and minor vascular pedicles (type II). The location of entry and the number of vascular pedicles are most important in determining the arc of rotation of the muscle or myocutaneous flap and, therefore, in predicting its applicability. The point of entry or rotation is usually at the proximal one third of the muscle. Muscles with two dominant pedicles require both for total survival, each pedicle supplying approximately half of the muscle mass. As with axial skin flaps, muscles and myocutaneous axial flaps require no delay and have specific lengths determined by the geometry of their longitudinal vasculature. Certain myocutaneous flaps have associated sensory nerve supplies that allow for restoration of sensation, which is useful in pressure-bearing areas.

Factors in Selecting Myocutaneous Flaps for Reconstruction of the Lower Extremities

In selection of the most appropriate myocutaneous flap coverage, primary consideration must be given to the reliability of the vascular pedicle in reaching the surgical defect. The defect cannot involve the vascular pedicle of the proposed myocutaneous flap in any detrimental fashion.

As a second consideration, the decision should take into account the restoration of function and structural aesthetics to the resected site. These secondary considerations of function preservation and contour restoration need not, however, compromise the primary goal of wound closure.

FUNCTIONAL PRESERVATION

In situations in which preservation of active joint motion is necessary, special techniques for myocutaneous and muscle flap development have been devised. These include (1) preferentially using the weakest and therefore most expendable synergistic muscle involved in a given particular joint movement, (2) partially preserving the muscle origin and insertion (For example, by splitting the broad and flat origin of the latissimus dorsi and transferring its anteroinferior half while preserving its functionally and structurally more important posterosuperior half), (3) segmentally transposing only one belly of a multilobed muscle, and (4) dissecting the muscle from the tendon without separating the origin or insertion of the muscle.

CONTOUR RESTORATION

For optimal contour restoration, an analysis of the composite nature of the extirpated tissue determines the replacement requirements. In practice, contour restoration for deep soft-tissue defects is accomplished by transfer of myocutaneous flaps and for shallow defects by muscle flaps covered with split-thickness skin grafts.

SPECIFIC RECOMMENDATION: MYOCUTANEOUS FLAPS FOR THIGH RECONSTRUCTION

Specific reconstructive circumstances require that the aforementioned principles be tailored to the individual specific needs. In the thigh, muscle flap coverage is occasionally useful after extensive tumor resection. Many superficial thigh muscles are expendable for ambulatory patients with functional quadriceps and hamstrings. These superficial muscles are suitable for coverage of large defects in this region. For anterior or posterior proximal thigh defects, the primary muscles utilized are the gracilis, tensor fasciae latae, and the vastus lateralis.

The type-II gracilis muscle, as previously mentioned, is an expendable accessory adductor of the medial thigh compartment. Its pivot point is determined by its dominant vascular pedicle, the medial femoral circumflex artery, which enters the muscle approximately 10 cm inferior to its origin on the symphysis pubis (Fig 30–6). The entire length of the gracilis muscle from its origin to its insertion on the medial tibial condyle survives on this dominant pedicle. However, only the ellipse of skin in the proximal two thirds of the thigh overlying the muscle will survive on this blood supply. In addition to reaching the proximal thigh, its arc of rotation can extend to include coverage anteriorly to the abdomen, groin, and genitalia and posteriorly to the ischium, perineum, anus, and buttock. The ellipse of skin undergoes sensory denervation during the course of flap development.

If the major pedicle is divided as a delay procedure, 2 to 3 weeks later the gracilis muscle

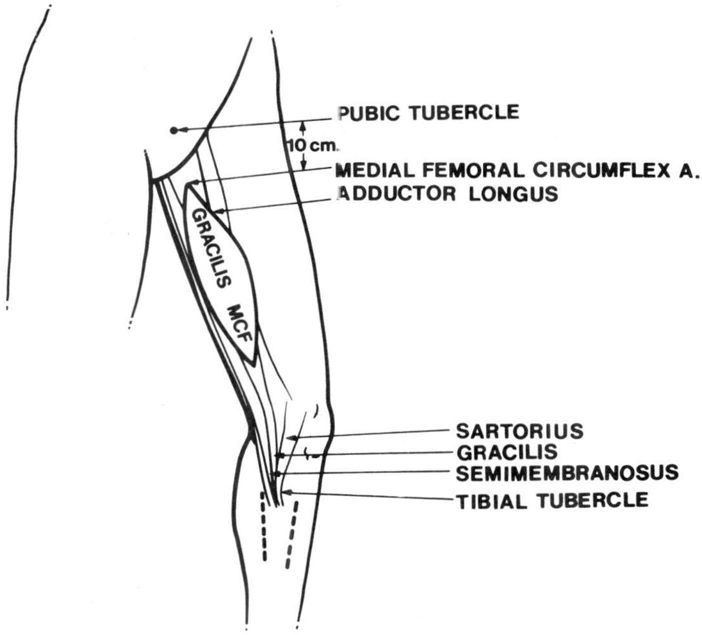

FIG 30–6.
Gracilis myc cutaneous flap.

can be based on its inferior minor pedicles from the superficial femoral artery and be employed to cover the knee anteriorly and posteriorly. The donor defect (usually less than 6 cm wide) is amenable to primary closure and is inconspicuous.

Similarly, the tensor fasciae latae (Fig 30–7) is an expendable adductor and medial rotator of the thigh. Its consistent type I vascular supply is especially useful for lower-extremity reconstruction. Its short and broad muscle portion originates from the anterior iliac spine and from its transferable osseous territory, the iliac crest. It extends 12 to 15 cm inferiorly to insert on the iliotibial tract. Approximately 8 cm inferior to the anterior superior iliac spine, its vascular pedicle, the lateral femoral circumflex artery enters the muscle to serve as the pivot point for the flap. Although the muscle is short, its cutaneous territory is four times larger, extending almost to the level of the knee. Therefore it has a wide arc of rotation, providing coverage not only to the proximal thigh but also to the abdomen, groin, and perineum anteriorly and to sites of pressure ulcers posteriorly such as the sacrum, ischium, and trochanteric region. The donor defect (often 8 cm wide) can usually be closed primarily. If a wide tensor fasciae latae myocutaneous flap is elevated, occasionally a split-thickness skin graft is required over the exposed underlying muscle to close the donor site.

For closure of small defects, in the superior half of the thigh the sartorius and gracilis muscles are used, whereas in the inferior half of the thigh the vastus medialis and vastus lateralis muscles are used. Posteriorly, the semimembranosus and semitendinosus muscles provide additional options for wound coverage. In marginally ambulatory patients with limited quadriceps and hamstring function, free flaps should be used to preserve the remaining musculoskeletal function. Transfer of the entire rectus femoris, gluteus maximus, or biceps femoris produces difficulty in ambulation. The preservation techniques mentioned should be considered when these flaps are developed. In a paraplegic patient, all superficial muscles are expendable, except those that provide some joint stability.

SPECIFIC RECOMMENDATIONS FOR MYOCUTANEOUS FLAP COVERAGE FOR THE LEG

In contrast to the thigh, the superficial muscles in the leg are less expendable and there is less soft-tissue bulk available to cover the superficial osseous surfaces.

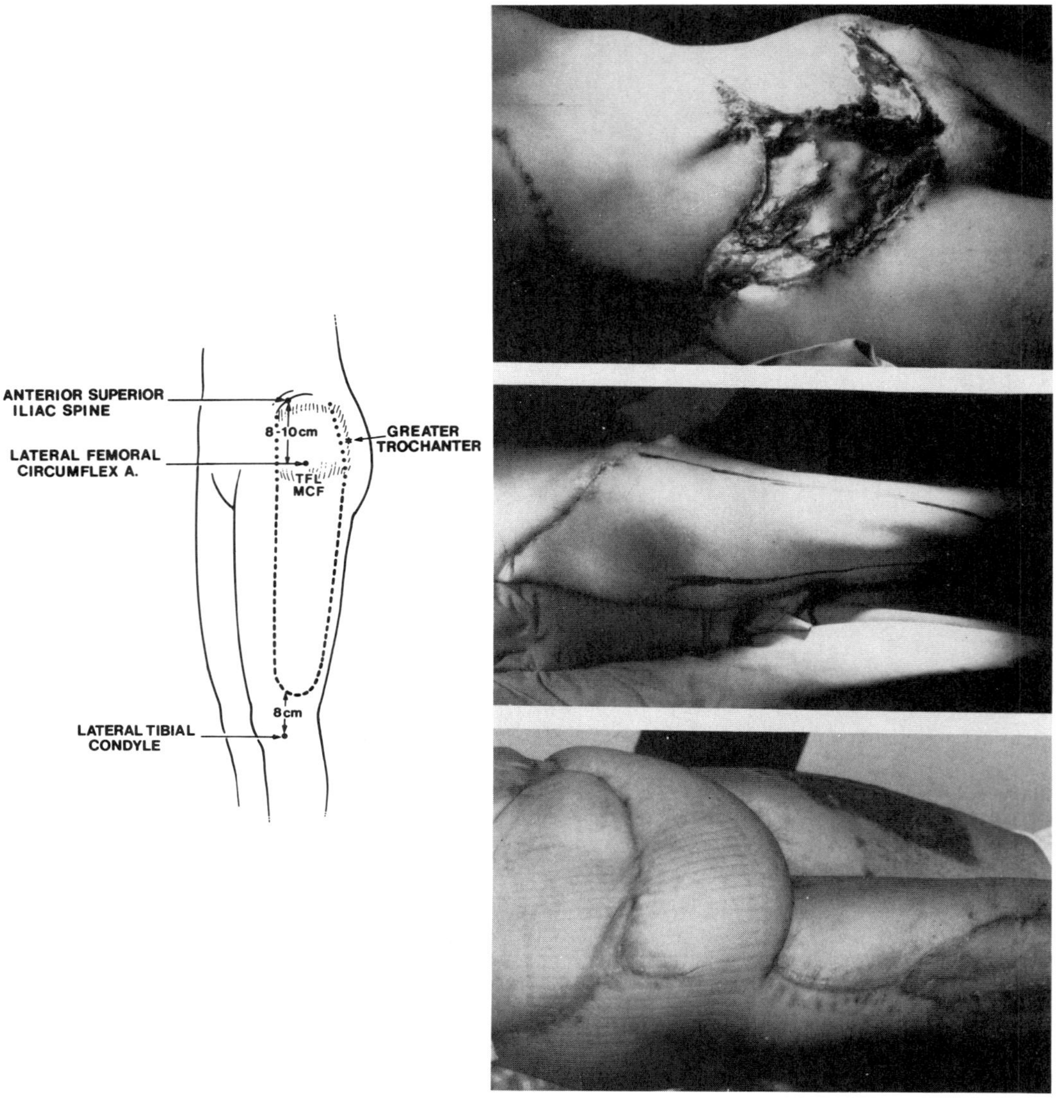

FIG 30–7.
Tensor fasciae latae neurovascular myocutaneous flap.

By convention, the leg is divided into the proximal, middle, and lower thirds for purposes of reconstruction. The myocutaneous flap preferred for the proximal third of the leg is the medial gastrocnemius flap. The broad, long belly of the medial gastrocnemius with a single (type I) proximal neurovascular pedicle is most reliable. By sparing the lateral head, no functional deficit is incurred. Other available options for soft-tissue coverage for this region include the lateral gastrocnemius, soleus, and tibialis anterior muscles. Although no ambulatory deficit is suffered with transfer of the soleus, there may be some loss of the venous pump mechanism. In contrast, the tibialis anterior is an important muscle in dorsiflexion. It should be considered as a last resort for coverage of the proximal third of the leg, and a function-preservation technique is suggested. For example, the tibialis anterior may be developed as a bipedicle flap to retain its function.

For reconstruction of defects in the middle third of the leg, in addition to either the medial or lateral gastrocnemius myocutaneous flaps, the proximally based soleus has frequently been used. Supplied by the peroneal and proximal posterior tibial arteries, the proximal soleus muscle can be reliably transferred to cover anterior leg defects. Other muscle flaps (flexor digitorum longus, tibialis anterior, extensor hallucis longus, and flexor hallucis longus) employed in the reconstruction of the middle third are useful only for small defects that exceed the territorial range of the proximally based soleus muscle flap. It should be recognized that although the flexor digitorum longus is expendable, the tibialis anterior, flexor hallucis longus, and extensor hallucis longus are not, especially in the athletic patient.

FREE FLAPS

Defects in the distal one third of the leg are not readily amenable to closure by local myocutaneous flaps, Muscular flaps, such as the peroneus brevis, flexor digitorum longus, and distally based soleus, have occasionally been employed for closure of wounds in this region. However, these flaps have had a failure rate higher then that reported for microsurgical free-flap transfer. With appropriate selection of free flaps (latissimus dorsi, tensor fasciae latae, gracilis, and other axial flaps) and end-to-side arterial anastomosis in nontraumatized beds, success rates of greater than 95% have been reported with microvascular transplantation. The free myocutaneous flaps usually require staged excision of excess bulk, whereas free muscular flaps covered with split-thickness skin grafts eliminate this need and produce a minimal cutaneous donor site defect.

Functional preservation techniques are also valuable in the development of myocutaneous flaps for free transfer. For example, in developing the latissimus dorsi myocutaneous flap for microsurgical transplantation, it is recommended that, if feasible, only the anterior branch of the thoracodorsal artery be used for transfer of the antero-inferior half of the latissimus dorsi. This permits functional preservation of its posterosuperior half with its attendant neurovascular supply.

In sarcoma of the thigh, local resection with adequate margins in three dimensions often requires sacrifice of major neurovascular structures. This places the entire limb distal to the resection in jeopardy. Narrow margins near these vital structures often lead to a high rate of tumor recurrence. Accordingly, soft-tissue sarcomas such as fibrosarcoma, liposarcoma, and rhabdomyosarcoma extensively involving the thigh, hip, and buttock provide frequent indication for hemipelvectomy. Closure of the resulting defect, especially with pre-operative radiation therapy, may pose some challenge.

The hindquarter amputation has traditionally been closed with a posterior gluteal thigh flap (when tumor is confined to the anterior thigh and hip) and with an anterior thigh flap (when the buttock region is involved). In patients with previous radiation therapy or with division of the common iliac artery, high rates of skin necrosis requiring flap debridement and skin grafting have been reported. However, when curative resection permits salvage of the hypogastric artery and its inferior gluteal branch, closure with the gluteal thigh flap has been found to be reliable. It can be rapidly performed and has remained the closure of choice when there is no further evidence of disease. To provide for flap sensation, the gluteal thigh flap can be designed with the inclusion of the posterior femoral cutaneous nerve of the thigh.[13]

In other curative hindquarter amputations where the femoral vessels and anterior thigh muscles are salvaged, the quadriceps myocutaneous flap provides reliable, sensate coverage. This flap adapts well to the hemipelvectomy prosthesis and affords solid support to the abdominal viscera.[14] The rectus abdominus myocutaneous flap based on the inferior epigastric artery has also been described to provide an alternative for closure. In hemipelvectomy in which curative resection dictates wide margins and requires sacrifice of the common iliac artery, a delayed contralateral tubed axial thoraco-epigastric flap, based on the opposite superficial epigastric artery,[15] has been used effectively. Free flaps provide other options for coverage. In select instances, precise replacement of ablated tissue deficiencies with vascularized free muscle and bone transfer, as well as microvascular grafts, may also offer an alternative to amputation. However, the indications for extensive microsurgical reconstruction of the lower extremity in cancer patients have yet to be defined. Retaining the lower extremity with intact proprioception and protective sensibility offers some advantage in certain cases. For example, a child who may require minimal bone shortening or a bilateral amputee suffering loss of both lower extremities may be reasonable candidates for such microsurgical reconstruction. However, even in patients with a favorable prognosis these advantages should be weighed against those offered by a form-fitting prosthesis and the time required to recover from extended, multistaged procedures.

SPECIFIC RECOMMENDATIONS FOR INFREQUENTLY INVOLVED SITES

The Breasts

Very rarely, the breast is involved by sarcoma. The most common variety is cystosarcoma phyllodes. The malignant variant is present in 10% of cases. The usual treatment for both malignant and benign forms is simple mastectomy, because axillary metastasis is very uncommon.

Reconstruction is easily accomplished by the introduction of a submuscular implant through the mastectomy scar or an inframammary fold incision. Occasionally a myocutaneous flap such as the latissimus dorsi or rectus abdominus is employed.

Head and Neck

Soft-tissue sarcomas of the head and neck are particularly rare. However, the defect resulting from extensive resection is conspicuously mutilating and often requires a myocutaneous flap for coverage. The pectoralis major myocutaneous flap (type V) has become the standard in these cases (Fig 30–8). Its range extends to the level of the midface for head and neck reconstruction, including orbital, intraoral, esophageal, and pharyngeal regions. The pectoralis major myocutaneous flap has also been reported to serve as a carrier of the fifth rib for mandibular reconstruction, although with variable reliability. Transposition through the neck is easily accomplished via a subcutaneous, supraclavicular tunnel in the patient who has undergone a radical neck dissection.[16]

The pivot point at which the dominant thoraco-acromial artery enters is medial to the pectoralis minor. Clinically, it is found approximately in the midclavicular region or medial to the deltopectoral groove. If the flap is elevated deep to the rectus fascia, its cutaneous territory extends beyond the limits of the muscle to the costal margin. The functional loss of some adduction and medial rotation of the arm is well tolerated when this flap is used for transfer.

Designing a traditional Bakamjian deltopectoral flap in conjunction with the pectoralis major myocutaneous flap offers an additional option for head and neck closure or, alternatively, can serve as a defensive back-up (Fig. 30–9). For intra-oral defects, this combination permits the pectoralis major island myocutaneous flap to line the oral cavity and the deltopectoral flap to provide cutaneous coverage.

SUMMARY

The nature and location of the surgical defect after wide excision of soft-tissue sarcoma determine the reconstructive approach. The simplest method should always be considered

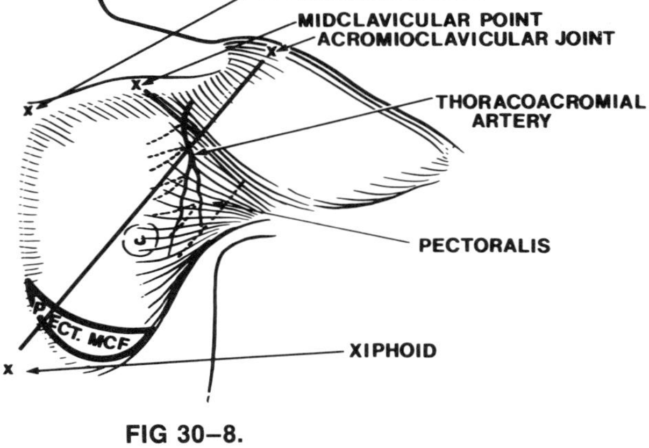

FIG 30–8.
Pectoralis major myocutaneous flap.

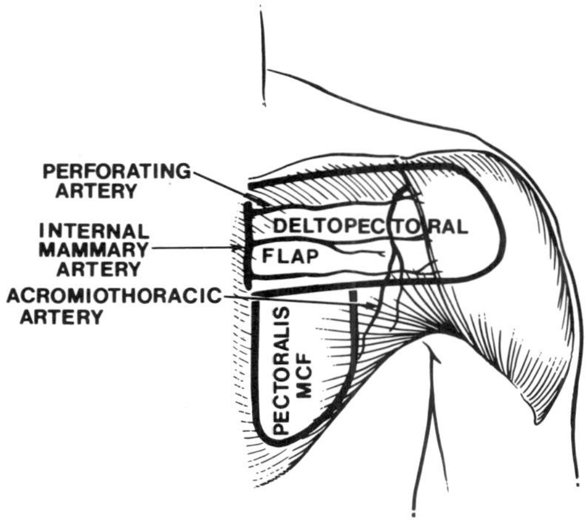

FIG 30–9.
Outline of combined pectoralis major myocutaneous and deltopectoral flaps.

at the outset. A wide range of reconstructive strategies is available, permitting the closure of even very extensive, disfiguring defects. Thus, curative therapy should not be compromised by this consideration.

REFERENCES

1. Morton DL: Soft tissue sarcomas, in Holland JF, Frei E III (eds): *Cancer Medicine.* Philadelphia; Lea & Febiger, 1973, pp 1845–1861.
2. Davis J: Kaposi's sarcoma: Present concept of clinical course in treatment. *NY State J Med* 1968; 68:2067–2073.
3. Shiu MH, Castro EB, Hajdu SI, et al: Surgical treatment of 297 soft tissue sarcomas of the lower extremity. *Ann Surg* 1975; 182:597–602.
4. Pack GT, Ariel IM: Tumors of the soft somatic tissues, in Hoeber PB (ed): *Treatment of Cancer and Allied Diseases.* New York; Paul B. Hoeber, Inc., 1958.
5. Converse JM, McCarthy JG, Brauer RD, et al: Transplantation of skin grafts and flaps, in *Reconstructive Plastic Surgery.* Philadelphia, W. B. Saunders, 1977, pp 152–239.
6. Pearl RM, Johnson D: The vascular supply to the skin: An anatomical and physiologic reappraisal—part II. *Ann Plast Surg* 1985; 11:196–205.
7. Skiles MS, Chaglassian T: A simple geometric flap for the closure of skin defects. *Surg Gynecol Obstet* 1979; 149:249–251.
8. Crawford BS: The repair of defects of the lower limbs, using a local flap. *Br J Plast Surg* 1957; 10:32.
9. Stark RB: The cross-leg flap procedure. *Plast Reconstruct Surg* 1952; 9:173.
10. Dawson RLG: Complications of the cross-leg flap operation. *Proc R Soc Med* 1972; 65:627.
11. Sherman JE, Urmacher C, Lane J, et al: The use of cross-leg flap in malignancy: Realization of a potential complication. *Plast Reconstruct Surg* 1981; 67:230–233.
12. Barclay TL, Cardoso E, Sharpe DT, et al: Repair of leg injuries with fasciocutaneous flaps. *Br J Plast Surg* 1982; 35:127–132.
13. Hurwitz DJ, Swartz WM, Mathes SJ: Gluteal thigh flap: Reliable, sensate flap for closure of buttock and perineal wounds. *Plast Reconstruct Surg* 1981; 68:521–530.
14. Larson DL, Ling MD: The quadriceps musculocutaneous flap: A reliable, sensate flap for the hemipelvectomy defect. *Plast Reconstruct Surg* 1983; 72:347–353.
15. Didolkar MS, Baffi RR, Bakamjian VY: Use of a tube thoracoepigastric flap to cover the defect from a hindquarter amputation. *Plast Reconstruct Surg* 1978; 61;112–114.
16. Ariyan S: The pectoralis major myocutaneous flap: A versatile flap for reconstruction in the head and neck. *Plast Reconstruct Surg* 1979; 63:73–81.

SUGGESTED BASIC READING LIST

Rudolph R, Fisher JC, Ninnemann JL: *Skin Grafting.* Boston, Little Brown & Co., 1979.

Grabb WC, Myers MB (eds): *Skin Flaps.* Boston, Little Brown & Co., 1975.

Mathes SJ, Nahai F: *Clinical Atlas of Muscle and Musculocutaneous Flaps.* St. Louis, C. V. Mosby, 1979.

Chapter 31

Cryosurgery for Cytoreduction of Soft-Tissue Sarcomas

George F. Muschler

Cryosurgery is the surgical use of extreme cold to cause selective tissue death. It was first introduced into the modern operating room for neurosurgical applications by Goldstein and Hess[1] and in 1963 by Cooper[2] with the development of a closed cryosurgery probe. Since then the utility of cryosurgery has been documented in many areas, including the treatment of many skin lesions, head and neck tumors, and carcinoma of the cervix and prostate.[3] Applications in the treatment of benign bone tumors, metastatic lesions, and both chondrosarcoma and osteosarcoma have been documented by Marcove[4–8] and others.[9–13] However, there are few reported cases of cryosurgical treatment of soft-tissue sarcomas in the literature,[7] and no clear role for cryosurgery has been established. This chapter reviews the basic physiology and technique of cryosurgery and attempts to define situations in which it may have value in the treatment of soft-tissue sarcomas.

PHYSIOLOGY OF CRYOSURGICAL CYTOTOXICITY

Frostbite provides a common example of freeze-induced tissue necrosis. However, cold temperatures alone do not always result in tissue death. In fact, living cells and tissues are routinely frozen in tissue culture laboratories and tissue banks for the purpose of cell preservation and storage. An understanding of the factors that determine whether preservation or destruction results from freezing is critical if cryosurgery is to be used effectively.

Two major factors are thought to be responsible for freeze injury. These are intracellular dehydration, and cell membrane and organelle rupture by formation of intracellular ice crystals. Both mechanisms can be intuitively grasped by considering Meryman's description of the freezing process as "nothing more than the removal of pure water from solution and its isolation into biologically inert foreign bodies, the ice crystals."[14, 15] Other mechanisms may play a role, including electrolyte and osmotic imbalance, protein denaturation,[14, 15] and microvascular thrombosis.[16–20]

The physiology of freezing has been extensively studied in cell suspensions, and in a variety of tissues. From this work we know that the viability of cells exposed to freezing depends on multiple factors, including the rate of freezing,[14, 20, 21] the temperature of freezing,[21, 22] the thawing time,[22, 24] the number of freezing cycles[14, 21–23, 25] the presence of tissue ischemia,[21, 24] and the presence of cryopreservatives such as glycerol[25] or dimethyl sulfoxide (DMSO).[14, 15, 23, 26–29]

When a tissue is cooled below −3°C, nucleation of ice crystals takes place. When freezing rates are slow, relatively few nucleation sites form and these tend to be located in the extracellular matrix. As the temperature drops, more and more free water is added to the growing crystals, which can become many times larger than the surrounding cells. When the tissue temperature falls to −10°C, as much as 90% of the free water present in the specimen is frozen, resulting in profound dehydration of the surrounding matrix and cells. A further drop in temperature results in dramatic dehydration down to −130°C, below which further crystallization does not take place.

With rapid freezing the tissue may be supercooled to as low as −20°C before crystallization is initiated. Under these conditions many more nucleation sites are initiated and they occur in a homogeneous pattern, both in the extracellular matrix and intracellularly. As a result, rapid freezing produces many more but smaller ice crystals that are more evenly distributed between the intracellular and extracellular compartments. Once frozen, if the temperature is kept below −70°C the ice crystals formed in a animal tissue remain fairly stable.

Thawing is also an important determinant of ultimate cell viability, due to the recrystallization that occurs during thawing. Recrystallization is a process by which existing crystals become modified by constant thawing and refreezing, with the net result that small crystals are progressively fused into larger ones, which are more stable. This same process is responsible for the growth we see in frozen condensation on a window pane. Recrystallization occurs rapidly at temperatures near the freezing point, but will occur to some degree at any temperature over −130°C. If crystals are present only in the extracellular matrix, recrystallization may represent little added insult to cells. However, if significant intracellular crystallization has been produced by rapid freezing, the growth of intracellular crystals can be lethal, resulting in membrane and organelle rupture. This effect is enhanced, the longer recrystallization is allowed to proceed.

If tissue is refrozen, several factors seem to enhance the killing efficacy of the second freeze. With repeated freezing, the rate of freezing is enhanced (possibly due to microvascular thrombosis of regional blood flow), there is much greater intracellular crystal formation, and the duration of thawing is prolonged. These factors make multiple freeze cycles a highly effective means of enhancing local cell injury.

Ischemia induced by local vessel occlusion or local epinephrine infiltration may also enhance tissue necrosis. This may be due in part to the increased freezing rate and prolonged thawing time due to loss of regional blood flow, as well as to some direct ischemic effect.

Experiments using several animal tumor models have documented the reliability of cryosurgery.[21, 22, 25] These studies indicate that cure rates for small tumors approach 100% when optimal cryosurgery is applied alone and without excision. They also highlight the potential for high local failure rates when an optimal freezing environment is not maintained.

Overall, based on theory and experimental evidence, optimal technique for cytotoxic cryosurgery should involve rapid freezing of the treatment area to or near −90°C and then slow and complete thawing. Irrigation should not be used to speed thawing so that recrystallization can be maximized. At least three freeze cycles should be administered and, when possible, regional circulation should be occluded during the freeze.

There have as yet been no investigations to evaluate the cryosensitivity of various cell types. Similarly, we have no experimental data on potentially important variables such as large tumor size, or the effect of blood flow through large vessels within or adjacent to a tumor. Both are likely to decrease tumor cell killing by altering freezing rates or thawing times.[30]

EFFECT OF CRYOSURGERY ON BLOOD VESSELS

The effect of cryosurgery on normal tissue adjacent to the area of tumor treatment must be carefully considered. There have been many studies reporting the physiological effect of cryosurgery on major blood vessels.[16, 17, 29, 31–34] Even when major blood vessels are frozen solid by techniques designed to optimize tissue necrosis, they withstand cryosurgery injury and maintain their function as a fluid conduit despite regional cell necrosis.

Following cryogenic injury, the frozen intraluminal blood thaws relatively quickly, undergoes cytolysis, and is washed away along with the endothelial lining cells.[16, 34] The internal elastic lamina shows little change, however. Degeneration in smooth muscle cells and the external elastic lamina is evident by the first week. This is followed by a regenerative process that results in re-endothelialization and healing of the vessel wall with some thickening and fibrosis by 5 weeks.[34]

There appear to be few sequelae of freezing large vessels. Thrombosis, aneurysm formation, or late vessel rupture are rare. Minor degrees of calcification, bone formation, cartilaginous metaplasia, atherosclerotic changes, and rarely stenosis of the vessel wall have been reported.[16] In fact, the major risk of freezing large vessels seems to be the acute risk of injury during the time that a vessel is frozen, because movement can fracture a frozen vessel like a glass rod.

Vessel injury is less likely if flow is maintained during a freeze[33]; however, given the goal of optimal freeze technique and the low morbidity of vessel freezing, there appears to be no reason to risk compromise of the freezing technique in an effort to limit vessel injury.

The effect of cryosurgery on blood vessels is highly dependent on vessel size. In contrast to large vessels, vessels under 1.0 to 1.5 mm in diameter are severely affected by cryosurgery,[16, 20] particularly the endothelium of capillaries and venules. Following freezing of these vessels, flow becomes acutely diminished and complete thrombosis of the local microcirculation occurs in 10 to 60 minutes.[17–19]

EFFECT OF CRYOSURGERY ON PERIPHERAL NERVES

Nerves also do surprisingly well following a freezing injury. Although there is a period of lost function, lesions are in general partly or completely reversible. This is illustrated by experience with elective anesthetic cryosurgery of intercostal nerves following thoracic surgery, where predictable recovery is seen by 6 to 12 months.[35–37]

A dense loss of function for all fibers of a peripheral nerve results following any therapeutic freeze, although large, myelinated motor fibers are most sensitive and the small nociceptor C fibers are least sensitive to injury. Provided the nerve is not fractured or cut, Wallerian degeneration takes place with renervation of both motor and sensory function.[38] Recovery can be followed clinically by an advancing Tinel's sign. The time to recovery is dependent on the distance from the injury site to the effector site, and can be estimated at approximately 25 mm/month. Even lower extremities with dense cryogenic injuries to the sciatic nerve can be expected to recover brace-free function with time.[39]

TECHNIQUES OF CRYOSURGERY

Cryosurgery can be applied by several different techniques. In "closed" methods, a cannulated metal probe is cooled by circulating liquid nitrogen (Fig 31–1). The probe is then applied directly to the tissue to be frozen. The nitrogen gas produced by evaporation is vented outside the operative field and never comes in direct contact with the treated tissue. The area of treatment can be controlled by selection among the variety of probe sizes and designs that are commercially available. While this method offers the surgeon the greatest precision in controlling the freeze, its use is limited to small anatomical sites. When large or highly contoured areas are encountered, particularly sites over about 5 cm^2 in area, probes usually cannot conform to the site for efficient heat conduction. The rate of heat exchange is also limited by the size of the probe and the throughput of liquid nitrogen. Usually no more than 2 to 3 cm of frost penetration can be accomplished regardless of the length of probe application.

One must remember that although the tissue may be visibly frozen, this does not indicate freezing to an optimal killing temperature of −90°C or below. Because the probe temperature is generally warmer than liquid nitrogen (about −160°C vs. −196°C) and the edge of the freeze

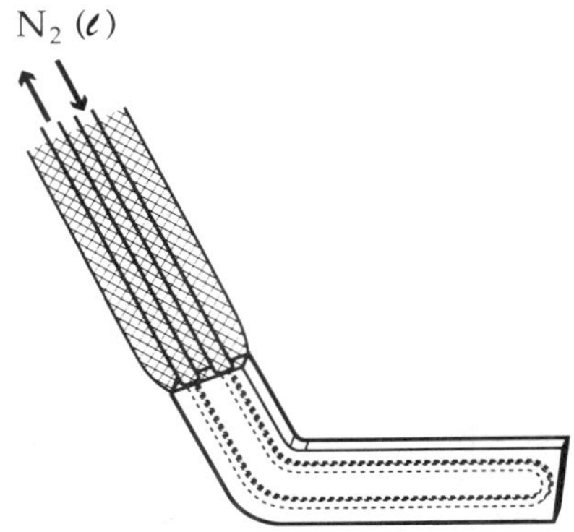

FIG 31–1.
Closed cryosurgery probe.

can be considered to be 0°C, only about half of the frost depth and diameter should be considered optimally treated.

There are several methods of "open" application of liquid nitrogen, meaning that the liquid nitrogen comes in direct contact with the treated tissue. These include use of a liquid spray (Fig 31–2), direct pouring of liquid nitrogen into a dependent cavity (Fig 31–3), or open application of liquid nitrogen that is contained in an instrument such as a funnel (Fig 31–4).

The use of a spray gun can be effective in accomplishing a dense but superficial freeze over a large surface area, even on the under side of a surface, as shown in Figure 31–2. This can be versatile, although the temperature of the freeze and the depth of penetration cannot be known with confidence. Selection of an appropriate spray nozzle is an important variable. Nozzles vary in shape, spray volume, spray area, and spray density.

Open methods are necessary when large volumes of tissue are involved. These techniques are powerful. The rate of heat extraction is vastly increased by the improved contact and conduction between the treated tissue and liquid nitrogen. The depth of freezing is dependent on the duration of application and the blood flow in local tissues. Frost depths up to 5 cm or more can usually be obtained. Even large vessels, such as the superficial femoral artery, can be frozen solid by this method, although they are usually resistant to freezing due to warm inflowing blood.

Judging the penetration of freezing can be difficult. Unless separate probes are used to monitor local tissue temperature, the surgeon must rely on two general assumptions to assess the depth and temperature of freezing. The first is that the shape of the frozen volume of tissue is roughly spherical, so the depth of the freeze will approximate the radius of the frost around the liquid nitrogen source. In general, this will be an overestimate and the true depth will be

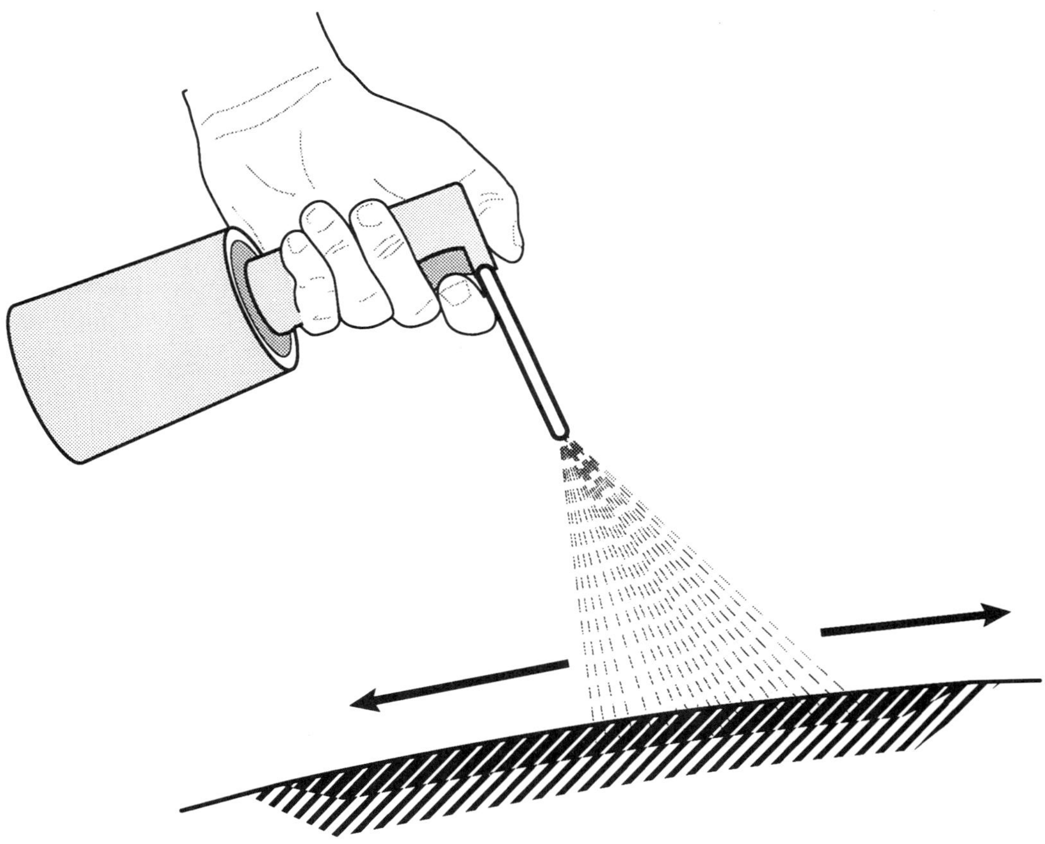

FIG 31–2.
Open spray technique.

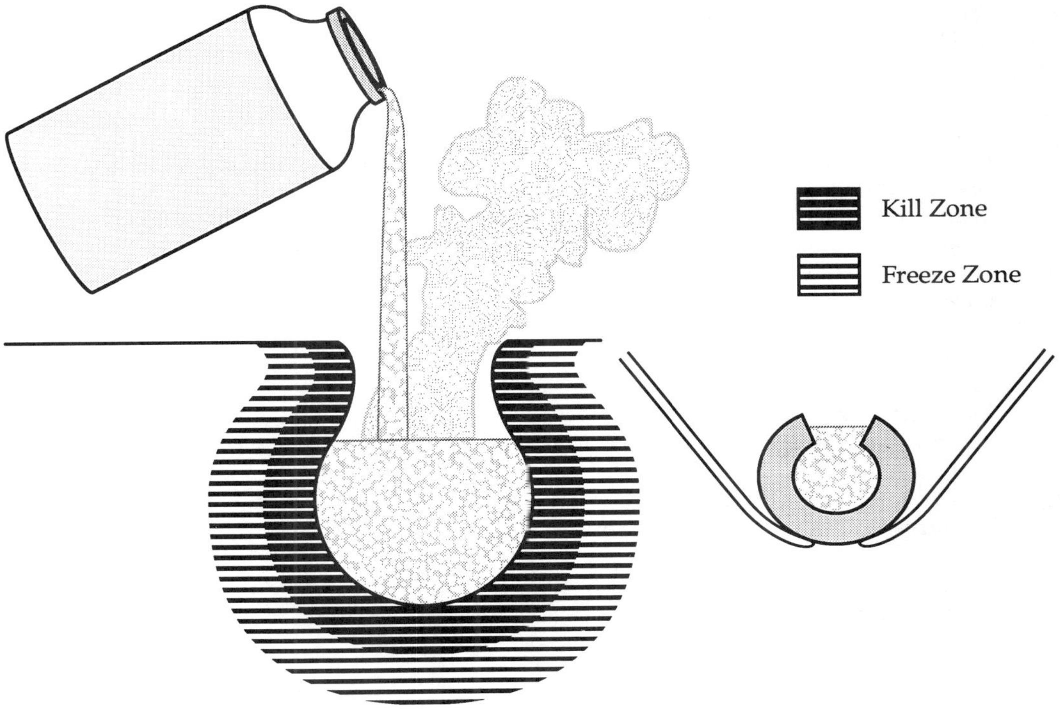

FIG 31–3.
Open pour technique (note distinction between the freeze zone and kill zone). Smaller figure on the right illustrates a cross-section through a long bone in which the open pour technique is being used. Surrounding soft tissue is protected from freeze injury by retractors that isolate the freeze area.

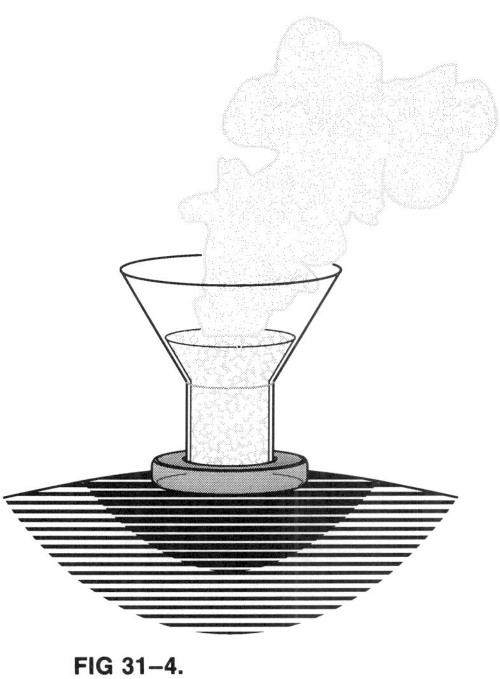

FIG 31–4.
Open pour technique using funnel.

less because the rate of warming from surrounding tissues is more rapid than warming from room air. The true shape of the freeze is likely to be more spoon shaped than spherical. In some cases the depth of freezing can be judged quite acccurately by direct palpation. The second assumption is that there will be essentially a linear gradient of temperature from the liquid nitrogen source (−196°C) and the frost edge (0°C) Therefore, if −90°C is the approximate target temperature for an adequate freeze, the margin of treated tissue lies about halfway between the site of application and the frost margin.

One other technical point warrants mention. Because the rate of freezing is so important and the rate of cooling decreases at points distant to the cold source, the largest possible surface contact area between the target tissue and cold source should be sought. For this reason funnels with diameters up to 4 cm are frequently used. If the target area is larger than 6–8 cm in diameter, multiple freezing sites should be used.

POTENTIAL ROLE FOR CRYOSURGERY OF SOFT-TISSUE SARCOMAS

Cryosurgery is of course only one of several tools for the selective ablation or necrosis of tumor tissue, and any potential role for cryosurgery must be considered in light of the existing armament of surgical adjuvants: intra-operative radiation, brachytherapy, external beam radiation, hyperthermia, and chemotherapy. Local application of distilled H_2O, hydrogen peroxide, or phenol can also be added to this list.

External beam radiation and brachytherapy are well-established methods that deliver a fairly homogeneous therapeutic dose of radiation to a large tissue volume and are well suited to settings in which the entire operative field is at risk. Cryosurgery does not have a role in this setting.

Cryosurgery may have a role, however, when a specific tissue area or volume at risk can be defined. In this setting cryosurgery has the highly desirable attributes of producing a high density of necrosis in the treated site while allowing tissues not at risk to be selectively spared. Cryosurgery does not require a specially equipped operating room as is needed for delivery of intraoperative radiation. It is significantly more flexible in terms of targeting, and it is not associated with a risk of induced malignancies. Furthermore, the use of cryosurgery does not preclude the use of radiation therapy or chemotherapy.

The anatomical and clinical settings of surgery for soft-tissue sarcomas are highly varied. Even when computed tomography (CT) and magnetic resonance imaging (MRI) studies make extensive pre-operative planning possible, the surgeon must rely heavily on intra-operative judgment for selection of an appropriate margin of resection. Defining an adequate or optimal margin or excision based on intra-operative observations is difficult. It is possible, however, to propose situations in which cryosurgery may have value (Box 31–1). These can be divided into four groups: treatment of an area of high risk prior to dissection, treatment of an area of known tumor prior to dissection, treatment of an area of known tumor prior to intralesional dissection, treatment of an area of high risk after dissection, and treatment of an area of known contamination. Figure 3–5 illustrates some of these potential settings.

BOX 31–1.

EXAMPLES OF INDICATIONS FOR USE OF CRYOSURGERY

- Pretreatment of a high-risk area (before dissection)
  - Major nerve or vessel at the tumor margin
  - Neurosarcoma arising from the major nerve
  - Tumor with intimate contact on bone
- Pretreatment of known tumor site
  - Planned intralesional excision where tumor spill may be limited by prior freezing
  - Planned intralesional excision where bleeding may be controlled by freezing during the excision[39]
- Treatment of high-risk area
  - Site of suspected marginal or intralesional excision Treatment of known tumor contamination
  - Contained site of contamination

COMPLICATIONS

The use of cryosurgery may be accompanied by several potential risks that are critical for the surgeon to anticipate (Box 31–2). Open techniques are associated with the most risk, but many of the same complications are possible with closed technique procedures as well. The surgeon must remember that frozen arteries,

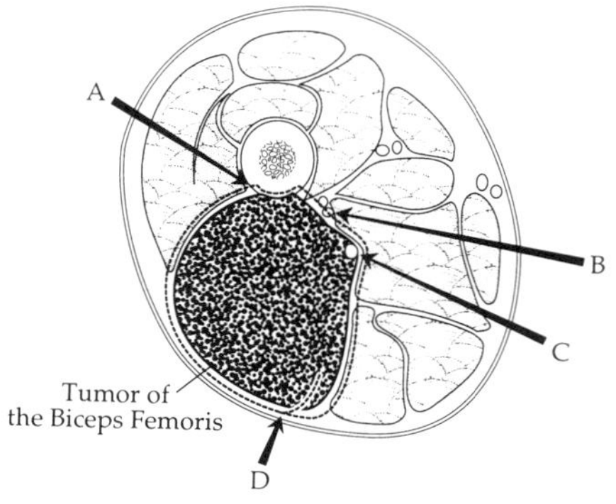

FIG 31–5.
Potential sites for use of cryosurgery, because of high risk for local recurrence following surgical resection. **A,** subperiosteal margin on bone; **B,** margin between tumor and major blood vessel; **C,** margin between tumor and nerve; **D,** previous biopsy site, an area of known tumor contamination.

BOX 31–2.

CRYOSURGERY COMPLICATIONS

Skin necrosis
Cryogenic nerve injury
Nerve or vessel fracture
Aneurysm formation
Bone necrosis and late fracture
Seroma
Nitrogen emboli

veins, and nerves will break if moved, so assistants must be carefully instructed to avoid changing the position of retractors or repositioning a limb during a freeze. The surgeon must be careful to insulate the skin from the frozen area. Skin should be observed at all times and irrigated frequently with warm saline. The frozen fog alone, which rises from the wound during a large freeze, can be enough to freeze exposed skin. Inadvertent freezing of a major nerve is also a concern. In some cases, a nerve at risk can be isolated and protected or monitored using a nerve stimulator or separate temperature probe.

If the funnel technique is used, the base of the funnel must be carefully sealed using a ring of saline-soaked Gelfoam (Upjohn, Kalamazoo, MI), which freezes quickly to seal the base. Limiting the volume of free liquid nitrogen in the funnel serves to limit the risk of any mishap. Should the funnel become dislodged or leak, however, it is important to have on the surgical field a large syringe or basin of warm saline that can quickly quench any spill. Attempts to use the surgical suction to control a spill of liquid nitrogen will quickly freeze any water in the suction tubing and waste valuable time.

Surgeons treating soft-tissue sarcomas will rarely if ever find situations in which a cavity technique is the method of choice. This technique is almost exclusively limited to treatment of bone lesions following curettage. If this technique is used, however, it is critical that the surgeon ensure a free path of escape for nitrogen gas from the wound. Marcove reported one early experience in which the opening to a cavity in the tibia undergoing cryosurgery became blocked, resulting in almost immediate intraoperative death, presumably from massive fat and nitrogen emboli.[7]

The local tissue necrosis that accompanies cryosurgery predisposes to several potential complications. Necrosis of bone may result in late fracture, particularly if the entire bone and intramedullary cavity are frozen intra-operatively. Tissue necrosis also predisposes the patient to seroma formation and infection, particularly when large surface areas are involved.

CONCLUSION

Cryosurgery represents an additional experimental tool in the armanent of the surgical oncologist. The surgeon must have a firm grasp of the physiological basis of this technique to use it effectively. It is important to remind ourselves that there is no established track record of efficacy for cryosurgery in the treatment of soft-tissue sarcomas. Efficacy in treatment of benign bone lesions and carcinomas may not be transferable to sarcomas in which the cell morphology, extracellular matrix, and anatomical setting are so different. The success of cryosurgery is highly technique dependent, as shown in in vivo animal studies and as illustrated by Marcove's experience in treating giant cell tumors of bone with cryosurgery. Marcove's initial series of 25 patients had a local recurrence rate of 28%. The next 25 had a recurrence rate of 12%. Only after experience had been gained in 50 cases did the local recurrence rate fall to its current level of 2%.[7]

At the present time cryosurgery should be used cautiously in selected settings where its potential contribution is additive to conventional therapy.

REFERENCES

1. Goldstein RS, Hess PW: Cryosurgical treatment of cancer. *Vet Clin N Am* 1977; 7:51–64. February, 1977.
2. Cooper IS: Cryogenic surgery: A new method of destruction or extirpation of benign or malignant tissues. *N Engl J Med* 1963; 268:743–749.
3. Gage AA: Cryosurgery for cancer. Comp Ther 1984; 10:61–69.
4. Marcove RC, Miller TR: The treatment of primary and metastatic localized bone tumors by cryosurgery. *Surg Clin N Am* 1969; 49:421–430.

5. Marcove RC, Weis LD, Vaghaiwalla MR, et al: Cryosurgery in the treatment of giant cell tumors of bone. *Cancer* 1978; 41:957–969.
6. Marcove RC, Stovell PB, Huvos AG, et al: The use of cryosurgery in the treatment of low and medium grade chondrosarcoma. *Clin Orthopaed* 1977; 122:147–156.
7. Marcove RC: A 17-year review of cryosurgery in the treatment of bone tumors. *Clin Orthopaed* 1982; 163:231–234.
8. Marcove RC, Searfoss RC, Whitemore WF, et al: Cryosurgery in the treatment of bone metastases from renal cell carcinoma. *Clin Orthopaed Rel Res* 1977; 127:220–227.
9. Popescu V, Spirescu JE: Bone resection, extra-corporal cryotherapy and immediate reimplantation in the treatment of mandibular tumours. *J Max Fac Surg* 1980; 8:8–16.
10. Huvos AG, Marcove RC, Erlandson RA, et al: Chondroblastoma of bone: A clincopathologic and electron microscopic study. *Cancer* 1972; 29:760–771.
11. Biesecker JL, Marcove RC, Huvos AG, et al: Aneurysmal bone cysts: A clinicopathologic study of 66 cases. *Cancer* 1970; 26:615–625.
12. Cummings CW, Leipzig B: Replacement of tumor-involved mandible by cryosurgically devitalized autograft. *Arch Otolaryngol* 1980; 106:252–254.
13. Gartsman GM, Ranawat CS: Treatment of osteoid osteoma of the proximal phalanx by use of cryosurgery. *J Hand Surg* 1984; 2:275–277.
14. Meryman HT: Mechanics of freezing in living cells and tissues. *Science* 1956; 124:515–521.
15. Meryman HT: Physical limitations of the rapid freezing method *Proc R Soc B* 1957; 147:452–459.
16. Gage AM, Montes M, Gage AA: Freezing the canine thoracic aorta in situ. *J Surg Res* 1979; 27:331–340.
17. Zacarian SA, Stone D, Clater M: Effects of cryogenic temperatures on microcirculation in the golden hamster cheek pouch. *Cryobiology* 1970; 7:27–39.
18. Rabb JM, Renaud ML, Brandt PA, et al: Effect of freezing and thawing on the microcirculation and capillary endothelium of the hamster cheek pouch. *Cryobiology* 1974; 11:508–518.
19. Bowers WD Jr, Hubbard RW, Daum RC, et al: Ultrastructural studies on muscle cells and vascular endothelium immediately after freeze-thaw injury. *Cryobiology* 1973; 10:9–21.
20. Giampapa VC, Oh C, Aufses AH: The vascular effect of cold injury. *Cryobiology* 1981; 1:49–54.
21. Neel HB III, DeSanto LW: Cryosurgical control of cancer: Effects of freeze rates, tumor temperatures, and ischemia. *Ann Otol* 1973; 82:716–723.
22. Neel HB III, Riggle GC, Myers RS, et al: Apparatus modifications for experimental cryogenic surgery of cancer. *Cryobiology* 1971; 8:501–505.
23. Zacarian SA: Cryo corner: The observation of freeze-thaw cycles upon cancer-cell suspensions. *J Dermatol Surg Oncol* 1977; 3:173–174.
24. Myers RS, Hammond WG, Ketcham AS: Cryosurgery of experimental tumors. *J Cryosurg* 1969; 2:5, 225–229.
25. Leibo SP, Farrant J, Mazur P, et al: The effects of freezing in marrow stem cell suspensions. Interaction of cooling and warming rates in the presence of PVP, sucrose or glycerol. *Cryobiology* 1970; 6:315–332.
26. Lenz H, Noack W: Electrophysiological and morphological investigations on the sciatic nerve of rabbits after cryosurgery with and without cryoprotective agents. *Min Med* 1974; 65:3658–3663.
27. Smith AU: Survival of frozen chondrocytes isolated from cartilage of adult mammals. *Nature Lond* 1965; 205:782.
28. Smith AU: Organ preservation for transplantation, in Kopow AM Jr, Abouna GJM, Humphries AL Jr (eds): Boston, Little, Brown & Co., 1924.
29. Tomford WW: Cryopreservation of articular cartilage, in Friedlaender GF, Manking HJ, Sell KW (eds): *Osteochondral Allografts* Boston, Little, Brown & Co., 1983.
30. Ganz H: Experiments on cryosurgery of tumors at the great blood vessels in the neck. *Min Med* 1974; 65:3645–3647.
31. McIntosh GS, Hobbs KEF, O'Reilly PO: In situ freezing of the pancreas and portal vein in the pig. *Cryobiology* 1985; 22:183–190.
32. Holman WL, Ikeshita M, Ungerleider RM, et al: Cryosurgery for cardiac arrhythmias: Acute and chronic effects on coronary arteries." *Am J Cardiol* 1983; 51:149–155.
33. Feldmann VH, Martin H, Unger RR, et al: Zum Kryoeffekt an der aorta abdominalis und der arteria iliaca des kaninchens. *Z Exp Chirurg* 1977; 10:69–74.
34. Cooper IS, Samra K, Wisniewska K: Effects of freezing on major arteries. *Stroke* 1971; 2:471–482.

35. Miles TS, Hribar D: Recovery of function after cryosurgical lesions of peripheral nerves in rats. *Neurosci Lett* 1981; 24:285–288.
36. Nelson KM, Vincent RG, Bourke RS, et al: Intraoperative intercostal nerve freezing to prevent post-thoracotomy pain. *Ann Thorac Surg* 1974; 18:280–285.
37. Crynitz S, Schroder M: Intraoperative cyrolysis of intercostal nerves in thoracic surgery. *Scand J Thorac Cardiovasc Surg* 1986; 20:85–87.
38. Myers RR, Powell HC, Heckman HM, et al: Biophysical and pathological effects of cryogenic nerve lesion. *Ann Neurol* 1981; 10:478–485.
39. Marcove R: Personal communication. New York, 1987.

PART 4

Treatment: Radiation Therapy

Chapter 32

Pre- and Postoperative Radiation Therapy

Herman D. Suit

Henry J. Mankin

William C. Wood

Karl H. Proppe

RATIONALE FOR COMBINING RADIATION AND SURGERY

The efficacy of radiation combined with surgery is under investigation for tumors of many anatomical sites. There is a powerful rationale for the use of this combined approach; radiation at moderate dose levels is highly effective in eradication of tumor that has infiltrated on a microscopic basis beyond the visible or palpable lesion into adjacent and grossly normal tissue. Such radiation should therefore decrease local treatment failure secondary to tumor that has extended beyond the confines of the surgical margin.

There are two classes of clinical problems for which this combined approach should yield important gains. First, there are several situations for which currently employed radical surgery is highly effective in achieving local control, but is associated with major cosmetic and functional loss. That loss does not result from resection of the obvious primary tumor but from the resection of large volumes of adjacent and grossly normal tissues in order to eradicate the regional microscopic extensions of tumor. For those sites, the combination of radiation and a conservative surgical procedure should achieve a local control rate comparable to that for radical surgery, but with a much greater preservation of anatomy and function and a superior cosmetic result. This is the general situation for sarcomas of soft tissue, which are the subject of this chapter. In addition, this clearly applies to the popular use of excisional biopsy and radiation as treatment of early-stage breast cancer.

Second, for a few anatomical sites, even radical surgery alone is associated with a high local failure rate, such as in treatment for carcinoma of the rectosigmoid, locally advanced carcinoma of the urinary bladder, or carcinoma at several sites within the upper respiratory and digestive passage. By combining radiation with the radical surgery, the local failure rate should be reduced. Here, the gain would be entirely in terms of improved local control and, if anything, less favorable functional or cosmetic results.

That the combined modality approach is effective in the treatment of patients with sarcomas of soft tissue is evident from data (Tables 32–1 and 32–2)[1] showing patterns of failure in patients treated by surgery alone or by the combined modality approach (irrespective of adjuvant chemotherapy).[2–4] The local failure rate for 464 patients with sarcomas of soft tissue treated by radical resectional surgery or amputation at four institutions was 18.1%.[1] In comparison, a series of 416 patients treated by relatively *conservative* surgery followed by radiation in the amount of ≥6,000 cGy at three centers had a local failure rate of 18.3%.[1] There is no suggestion that the two groups of sarcomas were comparable with respect to tumor size, histological type, or histological grade. However, the results can be taken as an indication that there is no major difference in the rate of local control or distant metastases in patients treated by radical surgery or by the more conservative combined modality procedure. Most of the published data regarding the efficacy of this combined modality approach for the treatment of sarcoma of soft tissue are based on radiation given *postoperatively* to patients who had less than classic radical resectional surgery.[1, 5–10] There are more limited data on the efficacy of other strategies, that is, radiation administered pre-operatively followed by conservative surgery,[1, 11, 12] intra-arterial Adriamycin (doxorubicin) and radiation (350 cGy × 10) followed by resection,[13, 14] or resection and intra-operative interstitial therapy.[15–17]

At the Massachusetts General Hospital, Boston, we have employed radiation given pre-operatively or postoperatively and conservative surgery in the management of 170 patients with operable sarcoma of soft tissue.[1, 18, 19] An analysis of this experience is discussed below, along with a brief review of related work in other centers.

SEQUENCING OF RADIATION AND SURGERY

Before proceeding to our results, we will consider the theoretical merits of using radiation pre-operatively or postoperatively. For radiation administered *pre-operatively*, the treatment volume is designed to cover only the grossly evident tumor and the adjacent tissues suspected of microscopic involvement. This treatment volume is almost always smaller than that treated when radiation is given postoperatively. In that situation, the treatment volume must cover not only the tissues suspected of being involved by tumor but all tissues handled at surgery, including the site of the drain wound, even though this may be remote from the tumor bed. Second, the tumor is usually smaller at surgery following pre-operative radiation; this facilitates the performance of a planned conservative resection. Third, for radiation administered pre-operatively, the surgery will usually be performed by a surgeon who is part of a multidisciplinary team, with interest in and experience with this group of uncommon tumors. Involvement of the whole multidisciplinary team is beneficial both in terms of the diagnostic work-up and development of the treatment strategy. There is better communication be-

TABLE 32–1.
Patterns of Treatment Failure in Patients With Soft-Tissue Sarcomas Treated by Radical Resection or Amputation*

Center/(Percentage of total number of patients)	Number of Patients	Follow-Up (yr)	Local Failure Plus Distant Metastasis	Distant Metastasis
Memorial Hospital[3]	297	5–24	54	100
Goteberg[4]	97†	3–23	9	31
University of Florida[5]	54‡	2–19	21	12
National Cancer Institute[6]	16	1–7	0	3
Pooled data	464	1–24	84 (18.1%)	146 (31.5%)

* *Data from Suit HD, Mankin JH, Wood WC, et al:* Cancer *1985; 55:2659–2667.*
† *Eighty-seven patients were not included in the analysis (patients presenting with distant metastasis not given).*
‡ *Fourteen patients were treated for localized disease but were not included in the analysis.*

TABLE 32–2.
Patterns of Failure in Patients Treated by Conservative Surgery and Postoperative Irradiation for Sarcoma of Soft Tissue*,†

Center/(Percentage of total number of patients)	Number of Patients	Follow-Up (yr)	Local Failure Plus Distant Metastases	Distant Metastases
M. D. Anderson[7]	279‡	5–16	59	73
National Cancer Institute[6]	27	1–7	4	2
Massachusetts General Hospital[1]	110	1–11	13	19
Pooled data	416	1–16	76 (18.3%)	94 (22.6%)

* *Data from Suit HD, Mankin JH, Wood WC, et al:* Cancer *1985; 55:2659–2667.*
† *Dose level ≥6,000 cGy in 6 wk or its equivalent; extremity lesions only.*
‡ *Status at 5 yr.*

tween the operating surgeon and the radiation therapist. Also through this approach there is the opportunity to include intra-operative radiation as a convenient treatment to boost the radiation dose to the tumor bed (with minimum irradiation of uninvolved tissues). Fourth, because the radiation inactivates virtually all the tumor cells (>0.999), the need for resection of a wide margin of normal tissue around the tumor is diminished. Finally, there is much less likelihood at the time of surgery of autotransplanting the tumor into the surgical wound, or causing distant metastases to be established due to viable tumor cells being dislodged into vascular spaces.

There are, of course, advantages for radiation administered *postoperatively:* (1) the pathologist is given the entire (unirradiated) tumor specimen for determination of the histological type and grade; (2) the exact extent of the tumor can be accurately determined by intra-operative inspection and palpation; and (3) there is no delay in surgery, and for some patients this is a psychological advantage.

There is not in our judgment, however, any medical gain by immediate surgery instead of initiating treatment with radiation. In those patients in whom there is a delay in wound healing following surgery, the residual tumor cells may increase in number. Thus, the longer the delay between surgery and the start of radiation, the greater the number of tumor cells that must be inactivated by the radiation. If there is a major delay in wound healing, there may indeed be reappearance of palpable tumor in the surgical wound. This is usually a disaster. Radiation administered pre-operatively means no delay in the start of radiation. It is unlikely that there will be a delay in the performance of surgery as a consequence of the radiation reaction, provided the total radiation dose is in the range of 5,000–5,600 cGy and the radiation therapist employs a shrinking field technique.

EXPERIENCE AT MASSACHUSETTS GENERAL HOSPITAL

At the Massachusetts General Hospital, 170 stage M0 patients with operable sarcoma of soft tissue were treated by a combination of radiation and surgery during the period September 1971 to August 1982.[1] The results were analyzed December 1983.

Of these, 110 were treated by surgery and postoperative radiation and 60 by radiation followed by conservative surgery. For postoperative radiation therapy the dose was 6,000 to 7,000 cGy, with most patients receiving 6,600 to 6,800 cGy. Details of radiation treatment included an immobilization device, wedge-compensator filters, individually shaped fields, two or more fields per day, bolus on the scar for the first 5,000 cGy, and the shrinking field technique.[20] Treatment was delivered as 180 to 200 cGy/day. For patients receiving Adriamycin chemotherapy before or after, but not during, the radiation therapy the dose was reduced by 10% to 12%.

The basic technique was the same for patients treated pre-operatively, and the dose carried to approximately 5,600 cGy. After a delay of 2.5 to 3 weeks, a conservative resection was performed. In some patients, a further 1,000 to 1,200 cGy was administered intra-operatively by interstitial or electron-beam technique. For those situations where this was not convenient, small field external-beam techniques directed to the tumor bed (defined by clips placed at resection margins) were used to administer a final

1,000 to 1,200 cGy by fractionated radiation. The results from this experience, according to American Joint Commission (AJC) stage, are shown in Tables 32–3 and 32–4, and according to size in Table 32–5. These tables present causes of failure and 5-year actuarial local control and survival results. There is an important difference between the two groups of patients in the distribution of tumor size and grade; the fractions of tumors <50 mm in the post- and pre-operative groups were 0.53 and 0.16, respectively. Also, the fractions of patients with stages IIB, IIIB–IVA in the post- and pre-operative groups were 0.43 and 0.73, respectively. There were some patients who were treated by excisional biopsy and postoperative radiation for small lesions around the knee, elbow, and ankle. These patients have done well and make the postoperative radiation series not comparable with the pre-operative series in terms of gravity of the clinical problems. A comparison of local control results for the two groups versus size in Table 32–5 shows 0.78 for the largest tumor size, that is, >150 mm in diameter treated by pre-operative radiation, as compared with 0.61 for the postoperative group (the difference is not significant, $P > 0.05$).

A pertinent consideration is, of course, how successful can salvage treatment be for patients with local failure? There have been, among the total of 170 patients, 19 with local failure ± distant metastasis and 36 patients with distant metastasis alone. Of the 19 patients who had local failure, six had distant metastasis before or at diagnosis of local failure. Thus, 13 patients were diagnosed as local failure and no radiographically evident metastatic disease. One of these was a frail 79-year-old female who was not a candidate for salvage surgery. The remaining 12 patients were subjected to a salvage procedure, 11 surgical and one radiation. Of these 12, seven had no evidence of disease at 1 to 3½ years after treatment. All but one of the 12 has achieved local control. Although in two patients two salvage surgical procedures were necessary, both of these patients were alive and free of disease at >18 months.

INTRA-ARTERIAL ADRIAMYCIN, RADIATION, AND RESECTION

The experience of Eilber and associates[14] at the University of California at Los Angeles in the treatment of patients with intermediate to high-grade sarcomas, particularly on extremities, by administering intra-arterial Adriamycin (30 mg/m^2 per 24 hours for 3 consecutive days) followed by 3,500 cGy in 10 fractions and then surgery, has been impressive. Of 96 patients treated for stage M0 disease and followed for 3 to 84 months, there have been only three local failures.[11] The local control rate will certainly be of great interest as the observation period of these patients is extended and 5-year actuarial figures are derived. This approach does appear,

TABLE 32–3.

Current Status and 5-yr Actuarial Local Control and Survival Results in 110 Patients with Sarcomas of Soft Tissue According to AJC Stage Following Treatment by Conservative Surgery and Postoperative Radiation at Massachusetts General Hospital*,†

Stage	Number of Patients	Status					5-yr Actuarial	
		NED	LF	LF + DM	DM	ID	LC	Survival
IA	8	8	0	0	0	0	1.00	1.00
IB	14	13	0	0	0	1	1.00	0.92
IIA	18	12	3	0	1	2	0.71	0.80
IIB	22	11	3	2	5	1	0.74	0.63
IIIA	23	17	0	0	5	1	1.00	0.76
IIIB	22	10	2	2	8	0	0.74	0.55
IIIC–IVA	3	2	1	0	0	0	0.50	1.00
Total	110	73	9	4	19	5	0.84 (0.74–0.90)‡	0.73 (0.63–0.81)‡

* *Data from Suit HD, Mankin JH, Wood WC, et al:* Cancer *1985; 55:2659–2667.*
† *NED = no evidence of disease; LF = local failure; DM = distant metastasis; ID = died of intercurrent disease; LC = local control.*
‡ *Ninety-five percent confidence limits on weighted average.*

TABLE 32–4.
Current Status and 5-yr Actuarial Local Control and Survival Results in 60 Patients With Sarcoma of Soft Tissue According to AJC Stage Following Treatment by Pre-Operative Radiation and Conservative Surgery at Massachusetts General Hospital*,†

Stage	Number of Patients	Status					5-yr Actuarial	
		NED	LF	LF + DM	DM	ID	LC	Survival
IB	7	5	1	1	1	0	0.67	0.80
IIA	3	2	0	0	1	0	1.00	1.00
IIB	17	12	0	0	5	0	1.00	0.66
IIIA	6	5	0	1	0	0	0.83	0.75
IIIB	24	10	1	2	9	2	0.80	0.42
IIIC–IVA	3	2	1	0	1	0	1.00	1.00
Total	60	36	3	4	17	2	0.86 (0.73–0.94)‡	0.62 (0.45–0.76)‡

** Data from Suit HD, Mankin JH, Wood WC, et al:* Cancer *1985; 55:2659–2667.*
† NED = no evidence of disease; LF = local failure; DM = distant metastasis; ID = died of intercurrent disease; LC = local control.
‡ Ninety-five percent confidence limits on weighted average.

however, to be a highly attractive alternate to radical surgery alone.

RESECTION AND INTERSTITIAL THERAPY (BRACHYTHERAPY)

The technique of interstitial radiation therapy for sarcomas has been described in reports from several centers.[15–17, 21, 22] The general approach has been resection of the primary tumor and then implantation of the tumor bed. Radiation dose has been given either by the implant technique alone, or by implantation combined with external beam. Results for some tumor situations have been good, especially for primary lesions, and time for treatment is much shorter than for external beam radiotherapy. Further experience with this approach is needed to improve skill in patient selection, and in judging the scope of the implant and dose level to avoid wound complications.

INTRA-OPERATIVE RADIATION THERAPY

The Massachusetts General Hospital and several other institutions have begun pilot studies of intra-operative radiation therapy (IORT) delivered at the time of surgery, usually to the retroperitoneum.[23, 24] A single high dose is di-

TABLE 32–5.
Actuarial Local Control Results at 5 yr for Soft-Tissue Sarcoma According to Tumor Size in Patients Treated by Postoperative or by Pre-Operative Radiation*

Size (mm)	Postoperative		Pre-Operative	
	Number of Patients	Local Control	Number of Patients	Local Control
<25	16	0.74	3	1.00
26–50	42	0.90	7	0.86
51–100	32	0.86	24	0.85
101–150	11	0.89	9	1.00
>150	9	0.61	17	0.78
Total	110	0.84 (0.74–0.90)†	60	0.86 (0.73–0.94)†

** Data from Suit HD, Mankin JH, Wood WC, et al:* Cancer *1985; 55:2659–2667.*
† Ninety-five percent confidence limits on weighted average.

rected to an unresectable retroperitoneal sarcoma, or to the tumor bed following resection, after moving the bowel away from the field. The incidence of radiation enteritis can thereby be reduced, although the technique may cause fibrosis of the ureter, major vessels, and nerves. Investigators at the National Cancer Institute[25] randomized 35 patients with resectable retroperitoneal soft-tissue sarcomas between IORT and postoperative external beam radiation. With a minimum follow-up of 15 months, no difference was found in actuarial disease-free survival or overall survival.

COMPLICATIONS

The complications associated with pre-operative radiation plus or minus intra-arterial chemotherapy are not trivial.[13] In our practice, the pre-operative radiation dose has been scaled down from 5,600–6,000 cGy to 5,000–5,200 cGy. The radiation dose given intra-operatively or postoperatively directly to the tumor bed has been increased so that the total dose to the tumor bed remains at 6,600 to 6,800 cGy. Eilber and associates have scaled the pre-operative radiation dose from 3,500 cGy to 1,750 cGy. These changes will surely result in some reduction of the treatment-related morbidity. The points of interest, of course, are the extent to which treatment-related morbidity is reduced and whether excellent local control results will continue to be achieved. In our experience, wound-healing delay produced by pre-operative radiation has been seen most prominently in older patients, particularly those who are obese, and especially for lesions in the upper thigh. These have been three patients with thigh sarcomas and three patients with sarcomas in the knee region who required skin grafting to facilitate wound healing. One patient of the 60 had an unplanned amputation. This patient was a 67-year-old male who had a hemangiopericytoma involving almost all of the anterior compartment. The leg was thin; the skin was fragile and atrophic. The full anterior compartment was opened. Unfortunately, wound healing did not occur. No tumor was found in the specimen. The patient is free of disease at this time following amputation. Although it is true that had he been treated by surgery alone initially the procedure would have been amputation, the result is still disappointing. This type of result does point out that in some anatomical sites in the elderly patient the combined approach will be difficult. For the patient with predicted problems, there may be a gain in performing a myocutaneous graft at resection. We have done this in two difficult cases with excellent results (see Ref. 26 for a description of one of these).

Of our 60 patients receiving pre-operative radiation therapy, nine with lesions of the proximal extremity had a planned amputation, but stump recurrence was judged to be almost a certainty because of the close margins. Nonetheless, of these nine patients, there have been no local treatment failures and no wound-healing delays.

OCCULT METASTATIC TUMOR

The results from several centers (see Tables 32–1 and 32–2) demonstrate the major and largely unsolved problem of occult metastatic disease in stage M0 patients who have large and intermediate- to high-grade sarcomas. The efficacy of adjuvant chemotherapy, even with protocols featuring Adriamycin, has not been established. We conducted a clinical trial of adjuvant Adriamycin chemotherapy (90 mg/m^2 q 3 weeks × 5, or a total dose of 450 mg/m^2), but we were not able to show a gain.[27] There is an obvious need for sustained efforts to develop a successful strategy against occult metastatic disease by use of techniques that do not produce major morbidity in a high proportion of patients.

SUMMARY

In summary, the experience accumulated in several centers provides strong supporting evidence for the use of the combined modality therapy, that is, radiation and conservative surgery, in the treatment of a high proportion of patients with sarcoma of soft tissue. Our experience with radiation administered pre-operatively indicates that this is an effective strategy in achieving local control of the primary tumor, particularly for large tumors. This therapeutic strategy should be subjected to much more intensive investigation, with special efforts directed toward reducing treatment-related morbidity. Major efforts should also be directed toward utilization of new approaches to reduce the impact of metastatic sarcoma.

REFERENCES

1. Suit HD, Mankin JH, Wood WC, et al: Preoperative, intraoperative, and postoperative in the treatment of primary soft tissue sarcoma. *Cancer* 1985; 55:2659–2667.
2. Suit HD, Russell WO, Martin RG: Sarcoma of soft tissue: Clinical and histopathologic parameters and response to treatment. *Cancer* 1975; 35:1478–1483.
3. Shiu MH, Castro EB, Hajdu SI, et al: Surgical treatment of 297 soft tissue sarcomas of the lower extremity. *Ann Surg* 1975; 182–597.
4. Markhade G, Angervall L, Stener B: A multivariate analysis of the prognosis after surgical treatment of malignant soft-tissue tumors. *Cancer* 1982; 49:1721–1733.
5. Simon MA, Enneking WF: The management of soft-tissue sarcomas of the extremities. *J Bone Joint Surg* 1976; 58-A:317.
6. Rosenberg SA, Tepper J, Glatstein E, et al: The treatment of soft tissue sarcomas of the extremities. *Ann Surg* 1982; 196:305–315.
7. Lindberg RD, Martin RG, Romsdahl MM, et al: Conservative surgery and postoperative radiotherapy in 300 adults with soft-tissue sarcomas. *Cancer* 1981; 47:2391–2397.
8. Leibel SA, Tranbaugh RF, Wara WM, et al: Soft tissue sarcoma of the extremities: Survival and patterns of failure with conservative surgery and postoperative irradiation compared to surgery alone. *Cancer* 1982; 50:1076–1083.
9. Suit H, Goitein M, Munzenrider J, et al: Evaluation of the clinical applicability of proton beams in definitive fractionated radiation therapy. *Int J Radiat Oncol Biol Phys* 1982; 8:2199–2205.
10. Karakousis CP, Emrich LJ, Vesper DS: Soft-tissue sarcomas of the proximal lower extremity. *Arch Surg* 1989; 124:1297–1300.
11. Atkinson L, Garvan JM, Newton NC: Behavior and management of soft connective tissue sarcomas. *Cancer* 1963; 16:1552–1562.
12. Lindberg RD, Martin RG, Romsdahl MM, et al: Conservative surgery and radiation therapy for soft tissue sarcomas, in *Management of Primary Bone and Soft Tissue Tumors.* Chicago and London, Year Book Medical Publishers, 1977, pp 289–298.
13. Morton DL, Eilber FR, Weisenburger TH, et al: Limb salvage using preoperative intraarterial Adriamycin and radiation therapy for extremity soft tissue sarcomas. *Aust NZ J Surg* 1978; 48:56–59.
14. Eilber FR, Morton DL, Eckhardt J, et al: Limb salvage for skeletal and soft tissue sarcomas: Multidisciplinary preoperative therapy. Unpublished data.
15. Collins JE, Paine CH, Ellis F: Treatment of connective tissue sarcomas by local excision followed by radioactive implant. *Clin Radiol* 1976; 27:39–41.
16. Mills EED, Hering ER: Management of soft tissue tumors by limited surgery combined with tumor bed irradiation using brachytherapy and supplementary teletherapy. *Br J Radiol* 1981; 54:312–317.
17. Shiu MH, Turnbull AD, Dattatreyudu N, et al: Control of locally advanced extremity soft tissue sarcomas by function-saving resection and brachytherapy. *Cancer* 1984; 53:1385–1392.
18. Willett CG, Schiller AL, Suit HD, et al: The histologic response of soft tissue sarcoma to radiation therapy. *Cancer* 1987; 60:1500–1504.
19. Suit HD, Mankin HJ, Wood WC, et al: Treatment of the patient with stage M_0 soft tissue sarcoma. *J Clin Oncol* 1988; 6:854–862.
20. Rosenberg SA, Suit HD, Baker LH, et al: Sarcomas of the soft tissue and bone, in DeVita V, Hellman S, Rosenberg S (eds): *Cancer: Principles and Practice of Oncology,* 1st ed. Philadelphia, J. B. Lippincott, 1982, pp 1036–1093.
21. Schray MF, Gunderson LL, Sim FH, et al: Soft tissue sarcoma. Integration of brachytherapy, resection, and external irradiation. *Cancer* 1990; 66:451–456.
22. Clarke DH, Martinez A: An overview of brachytherapy in cancer management. *Oncology* 1990; 4:39–54.
23. Gunderson LL, Shipley WU, Suit HD, et al: Intraoperative irradiation. A pilot study combining external beam photons with "boost" dose intraoperative electrons. *Cancer* 1982; 49:2259–2266.
24. Sindelar WF, Hockstra HJ, Kinsella TJ: Surgical approaches and techniques in intraoperative radiotherapy for intra-abdominal, retroperitoneal, and pelvic neoplasms. *Surgery* 1988; 103:247–256.
25. Kinsella TJ, Sindelar WF, Lack E, et al: Preliminary results of a randomized study of

adjuvant radiation therapy in resectable adult retroperitoneal soft tissue sarcomas. *J Clin Oncol* 1988; 6:18–25.

26. Malt RA, Suit HD: Multimodal treatment of myxosarcoma of the shoulder, in Malt RA, Moncure AC, Ottinger LW (eds): *Complex Operations at the Massachusetts General Hospital*. Philadelphia, W. B. Saunders, 1983, pp 246–259.

27. Antman K, Suit HD, Amato D, et al: Preliminary results of a randomized trial of adjuvant adriamycin for sarcomas: Lack of apparent difference between treatment groups. *J Clin Oncol* 1984; 2:601–608.

Chapter 33

Hyperthermia and Radiation Therapy

Jae Ho Kim

Successful clinical application of radiation therapy for cancer makes use of the sensitivity differential between cancer and normal tissues. In most instances, however, any intrinsic differential radiosensitivity exists only within a narrow range. Over the past decades, various physical, biological, and chemical strategies have been used to widen this difference and improve the effectiveness of radiation therapy. Many approaches have been used to this end, including radiosensitizers and protectors, use of high linear energy transfer radiation such as neutrons, helium ions, and negative pi mesons and, more recently, the use of hyperthermia in conjunction with conventional radiation therapy.

Attempts to use heat in the treatment of cancer date back many years. Busch, in 1866, described the complete disappearance of a sarcoma of the face following prolonged fever produced by erysipelas infection. W. B. Coley[1] of Memorial Hospital (New York, NY) deliberately injected cancer patients with bacterial toxins and obtained documented, complete tumor regression and long-term survival. Although striking cures have been recorded for different types of cancers, the toxins were rarely standardized biologically, and the effects were inconsistent. Warren[2], in 1925, combined hyperthermia with conventional radiotherapy and reported on radiosensitizing effects of heat.

Thereafter, there were only sporadic reports of hyperthermia research until the biological evidence of selective thermosensitivity of cancer cells was more fully appreciated. During the past two decades, there has been a dramatic renewal of interest in the use of heat as a new modality in the treatment of cancer, mainly due to the detailed studies and better understanding of the biology of hyperthermia. In particular, optimism has been raised that hyperthermia in combination with radiation therapy and/or chemotherapy can improve the therapeutic efficacy of conventional therapeutic modalities.

BIOLOGICAL CONSIDERATIONS

Thermosensitivity of Cancer Cells

The difference in heat sensitivity between tumor and normal tissues was first shown by Crile,[3] using sarcoma 180 implanted in the foot of a mouse. Crile showed that while the tumor could be destroyed by exposure to temperatures of 44°C for 30 minutes, 200 minutes of exposure was required to damage the healthy foot. Further studies on the difference in heat sensitivity between cells of normal tissue origin and malignant cells were carried out by Chen and Heidelberger[4] using chemically induced transformed prostatic cells in culture. They reported that higher thermosensitivity appeared to be an integral part of the characteristics of malignant cells. Levine and Robbins[5] similarly showed a differential thermosensitivity of normal and malignant cells in culture. They suggested that the differential thermosensitivity of normal and malignant cells might be a result of the varying growth states of cell populations, that is, the contact-inhibited versus non–contact-inhibited state. A study by Giovanella et al.[6] also showed that, in explanted human melanoma cells, thermosensitivity was related to malignancy of the cell strain as evaluated by tumor formation in nude mice. Using human embryonic fibroblasts transformed by oncogenic virus, Kase and Hahn[7] and Hahn[8] initially showed that the transformed cells exhibited an increased heat sensitivity relative to the parental nontransformed cells in their exponential growth phase. However, more recent studies by Hahn with virally transformed 10 T-1/2 mouse fibroblasts showed no differential heat sensitivity between nontransformed and transformed cells. Therefore, at the present time the observations on the differential thermosensitivity between cells of normal tissue origin and malignant cells in culture may be controversial, when the microenvironment of cell culture conditions is rigorously controlled to be similar between the cells of tumor and normal tissue.

Modifying Factors

There is now clear evidence that some of the factors associated with the microenvironment of the tumor tissues strongly modify the thermosensitivity of cancer cells. The significant factors that modify the thermosensitivity of mammalian cells, including cancer cells, are growth rates, cell cycle phases, cellular acidity, ambient oxygen concentration, and the nutritional status of cells.

Earlier cell culture studies with synchronized cells demonstrated that thermosensitivity markedly varied within the division cycle of cells.[9, 10] That is, cells in S phase are more heat sensitive than cells in other phases of the cycle, in contrast to the radiation response, because cells in S phase are more radioresistant. Concerning effects of heat on the progression through the cell cycle and the division delay, heat produces much longer division delays than an X-ray dose producing a similar amount of cell killing. These long division delays would induce a partial accumulation of cells in the G_2 phase of the cycle.[11, 12] Some evidence also exists that heat treatment of in vivo tumors recruits noncycling plateau-phase cells into the proliferating compartment.[13]

In addition to the age-response function of thermosensitivity, pH has been found to be a potent hyperthermic modifier in a variety of cellular systems. The pH-sensitizing effect is thought to be particularly significant in that many solid tumors contain interstitial fluid with a pH below 7.0.[14, 15] Increased aerobic glycolysis and the impairment of exchange of metabolic products increases the hydrogen ion concentration in the extracellular space of tumor tissues. At 37°C, cell proliferation occurs over a wide range of pH in a variety of normal and transformed cells in culture. However, cells at low pH (< 7.0) have a dramatically increased response to hyperthermia. Overgaard,[16] Gerweck,[17] and Hofer and Mivechi[18] have quantified this pH-sensitizing effect as a function of elevated temperatures. Sensitization to hyperthermia is apparent at temperatures above 41°C, proportional to decreasing pH, although this sensitizing effect is most pronounced at temperatures that are only moderately lethal at normal pH.[19]

The thermosensitivity of hypoxic tumor cells becomes important mainly because hypoxic cells are radioresistant and, to some measure, resistant to certain cytotoxic agents. The initial cell culture studies showed that hypoxic cells were exquisitely heat sensitive relative to well-oxygenated cells.[20–22] However, subsequent studies with hypoxic cells at neutral pH showed no difference in the thermosensitivity of cells between aerobic and hypoxic states.[22, 23] Therefore, at the present time the thermosensitivity of cells in aerobic and hypoxic conditions is regarded as similar. On the other hand, Kim et al.[24] have shown that hypoxic cells undergoing glucose deprivation have dramatically enhanced thermosensitivity, even at neutral pH.

Combined Hyperthermia and Radiation

Data obtained from cell culture studies have provided quantitative information that may be useful in the therapeutic approach by combination hyperthermia and radiation. Hyperthermia at temperatures above 41°C kills mammalian cells and enhances radiation sensitivity, with the degree of killing and radiosensitization proportional to the temperature changes. Several cellular mechanisms are involved in the enhancement of radiation effects by hyperthermia. Studies have shown that postirradiation hyperthermia inhibits the sublethal recovery process in Chinese hamster cells.[25] These effects were clearly shown at temperatures that do not affect cell viability by heat alone. Heat has also been shown to be an effective inhibitor of repair of potentially lethal damage in various mammalian cells.[26] Studies with synchronized cell systems have shown that the sequential treatment of radiation immediately followed by hyperthermia resulted in an enhanced cell killing throughout the cell cycle, with a marked synergism occurring in cells in S phase.[27–30] The above studies have clearly delineated that hyperthermia and radiation are quite complementary with respect to cytotoxicity.

An important observation regarding the combination of hyperthermia and radiation is that heat significantly enhances the killing of the radioresistant hypoxic tumor cell population. Hypoxic tumor cells are known to be highly radioresistant. Gray et al.[31] provided experimental evidence to show that hypoxic cells are usually three times more resistant to X-rays than are oxygenated cells. This ratio between the radiosensitivity of hypoxic cells and oxic cells is known as the oxygen enhancement ratio (OER). The reduction in OER was first reported by Robinson et al.[32] for X-irradiated bone marrow cells subsequently assayed by the spleen colony method. In their studies, the OER was reduced from 2.5 to 1.3 by a 43°C hyperthermic treatment for 2 hours immediately after X-irradiation.[33] The work of Durand[34] also showed that the hypoxic cells at the center of tumor spheroids were selectively killed and radiosensitized by hyperthermia.

The major criticism of the foregoing observations on the reduced OER was the ill-defined status of cell culture conditions of hypoxia with respect to pH and nutritional status. Because the experimental induction of hypoxia by means of heavy cell density (more than 10^6 cells/mL) is invariably associated with changes in the nutritional status of the culture, that is, the glucose concentration and cellular acidity, the apparent heat sensitivity of hypoxic cells may not necessarily be a direct reflection of the ambient oxygen concentration. It soon became apparent that the pH of the culture medium modified the thermal sensitivity of the cells under aerobic and hypoxic conditions. In addition to the pH, the nutritional status of the cell culture was also shown to modify the thermal sensitivity of cells. Even though some in vivo tumor tissues might exist in a hypoxic, low-pH, nutrient-deprived microenvironment, one must define what specific factors, if any, are responsible for the observed reduction in OER by heat. Kim et al.[35] have shown that, under the conditions of glucose deprivation and hypoxia, the OER of HeLa cells was reduced from 3.0 to 2.0.

Studies of combined X-irradiation and hyperthermia with in vivo tumor systems have also shown that heat sensitizes tumors to X-irradiation in a large number of laboratory investigations.[36] However, heat was also found to sensitize many normal tissues when combined with X-irradiation.[37] It is, therefore, important to be able to assess the thermal sensitization in both tumor and normal tissue to evaluate the therapeutic gain. To quantitate the enhancement of radiation effects by heat, two parameters are employed, and defined as follows:

$$\text{Thermal enhancement ratio (TER)} = \frac{\text{dose required to give a specified level of damage without heat}}{\text{dose to give the same level of damage with heat}}$$

$$\text{Therapeutic gain factor (TGF)} = \frac{\text{TER of tumor}}{\text{TER of normal tissue}}$$

A survey of the published literature on the TER of tumor shows that TER values vary widely; the magnitude of the TER depends on the temperature, sequence of the combined therapy, and type of tumor used.[38, 39] In general, the maximum TER was obtained when heat was delivered immediately before, during, and after X-irradiation.[40, 41] However, in most tissues studied (mostly skin), TER values of normal tissues are equally enhanced compared to tumor, so that changes in the therapeutic gain factor are either very small or marginal. Others have suggested an improved TGF may be obtained with a time interval of 2 to 6 hours between application of X-rays and heat.[42] Studies with low-dose-rate irradiation (e.g., 40 cGy/hr) and hyperthermia indicate that the TGF may be significantly improved at lower temperatures and reduced total radiation dose.[43–45]

LOCAL AND REGIONAL HYPERTHERMIA

The clinical application of hyperthermia in the treatment of cancer can be grouped into two approaches, that is, systemic hyperthermia and regional or localized hyperthermia. Conceptually, systemic hyperthermia is a more desirable approach because the treatment could affect both local and metastatic lesions. However, host tolerance for systemic hyperthermia is a major limiting factor at the present time. The maximum tolerable systemic temperature is less than 42°C. In contrast, the tissue tolerance for localized hyperthermia can be much higher (up to 45°C). However, heating deep-seated tumors in humans by external means requires much information on phenomena such as the bioheat mechanism, mode of heat absorption, and interaction of tissue with the external source. These considerations make the physics of hyperthermia extremely complex. Most clinical studies of hyperthermia are directed toward the combination of localized hyperthermia and radiation therapy.

Technology of Heating Systems

At the present time, there are basically two distinct physical approaches for heating deep-seated human tumors: electromagnetism and ultrasound. Each of these has its advantages and disadvantages (Table 33–1). Depending on the anatomical site and tumor volume, different forms of physical energy can be employed.

Ultrasound Heating

Electrical excitation of piezo-electric crystals results in the generation of mechanical pressure waves that may be transmitted to tissue through a coupling medium and dissipated as heat. Ultrasound at the frequencies of 0.5 to 3 MHz, when focused, has the potential for noninvasive selective heating of a target volume at depth. The existing ultrasound technology permits heating of various superficial tumors, up to about 7 cm in diameter and 3 cm in depth, by means of single-plane transducers. Because absorption in tissue is proportional to frequency, the depth of penetration can be improved by lowering the ultrasound frequency.[46, 47]

The main advantage of ultrasound heating is that the energy of the beam can be focused at a specified depth and volume of tissue. The presence of inhomogeneities of tissues (e.g., air in the lung, bone) causes reflections of the waves and interfaces, making ultrasound unsuitable for specific body cavities or organs. Another potential advantage of the ultrasound system is its penetration of focused beams into the

TABLE 33–1.
Local Regional Heating Systems

Systems	Frequencies (MHz)	Depth of Heating (cm)	Localization	Remarks
Radiofrequency				
Capacitive	13.56; 27.12	3–6	Regional heating	Excessive heating of fatty tissue
Inductive	27.12	3–6	Regional heating	Potential deep heating
Wave	Below 100	6–8	Regional heating	Annular phased array
Microwave				
High frequencies	915; 2,450	2–4	Localized	Shielded rooms
Low frequencies	400	3–6	Regional	Shielded rooms
Ultrasound				
Single-plane transducer		3–4	Focused	Interface problems from tissue inhomogeneities (e.g., bone, air)
Multiple-plane transducer	0.5–3	4–6	Focused	
Scanning focused transducer	0.5–3	4–6	Focused	

body. Several innovative focusing devices are being developed to improve the depth of heating. With the use of special scanning focused ultrasound techniques, Lele and Parker[48] were able to obtain an excellent homogeneous isotherm profile from 2 to 7.5 cm in depth. The system developed by Hynynen et al.[49] has unique capabilities in that it incorporates a commercial diagnostic ultrasound scanner with higher energy therapeutic transducers.

Radiofrequency Heating

The term *radiofrequency* (RF) *hyperthermia* covers a variety of techniques in which the elevation of temperature is induced by electromagnetic power at frequencies in the range of 1 to 100 MHz, most commonly at 13.56 and 27.17 MHz, two frequencies reserved for medical use. The techniques most frequently used are usually referred to as capacitive (di-electric) and inductive heating. In the capacitive method, a circuit conducts current from an RF generator to a region of the body via electrodes (capacitor plates). These are usually parallel to and placed on the surface of the region. Because the conductivity of muscle is much greater than that of fat, capacitive heating produces a preferential heating of the fatty tissue. The problem of overheating subcutaneous fat can be overcome by cooling the skin during the entire course of treatment and/or just prior to it. The depth of penetration may be improved in several ways. In the capacitive method, as the size of the applicators is increased, the heated region grows both in diameter and in depth. One such approach is the use of multiple sets of electrodes, each pair being energized only while the others are switched off. The switching is done at a fast rate and each pair "cross-fires" at the tumor.[50]

In the inductive modality, by contrast, there is no preferential heating of the fatty tissue relative to muscle and bone. For superficial tumors, single applicators, for example the "pancake"-type applicator, have been used to treat tumors at depths up to 3 cm. As an approach to the heating of bulky deep-seated tumors, Storm et al.[51] developed a magnetic loop induction system (Magnetrode) that consists of a concentric single-turn, self-resonant, noncontact coil with built-in impendence-matching circuitry operating at 13.56 MHz. One disadvantage of this system is that the magnetic field cannot be localized to the region of the tumor; therefore selective heating of the tumor is dependent on selectively diminished blood perfusion in the tumor. Corry and Jabboury[52] developed another inductive RF system that uses solenoidal and coaxial paired electrodes mounted on a specially designed treatment head to achieve improved localization and energy deposition. Von Ardenne and Kruger[53] describe moving two large coils in opposite planes parallel to the body, but this technique also becomes one of regional heating.

Microwave Heating

Because the technology for microwave sources is well known, these sources have been used in many clinical trials. Microwaves at 433, 915, and 2,450 MHz have produced noninvasive localized hyperthermia of large areas of surface tissues.[54, 55] Because of the physical limitations of a single microwave applicator, local heating in tumors with a depth of more than 3 cm from the skin is difficult. This problem of lack of penetration by microwaves is improved to some extent by employing lower-frequency microwave sources (e.g., 400 MHz) with multiple wave guides in a phase array, in an attempt to improve depth of heating and to focus more energy within the deeper tumors.[56]

Interstitial Hyperthermia

Interstitial hyperthermia involves implantation of a set of electrodes within the tumor volume to induce highly localized hyperthermia. The advantages of interstitial hyperthermia over hyperthermia applied via external heating sources would include (1) greater sparing of normal tissue, especially the overlying skin areas within the thermal field, (2) greater control of the heat distribution within the tumor, and (3) adaptability with conventionally used interstitial radioactive implant techniques.

The power source of interstitial hyperthermia may be either microwaves (915 MHz) or radiofrequency currents. The RF hyperthermia is produced through resistive heating caused by RF electric currents driven between pairs of electrically connected arrays of stainless steel implant guides.[57] The optimum range of RF frequency is 0.1 to 1.0 MHz. Microwave interstitial hyperthermia may be produced through the use of coaxial microwave antennas inserted in Teflon catheters implanted in the tumor volume. One advantage of interstitial hyperthermia is its compatibility with invasive thermometry. The placement of multisensor probes within the implanted volume through needle guides would yield an adequate thermal map of the target volume. A new approach to interstitial hyperthermia investigates a technique called *hysteresis heating*. In this technique, a bolus of small (1 μm) ceramic particles is directly injected into the tumor and an applied magnetic field of 50 KHz heats the ceramic particles, which, in turn, conductively heat the surrounding tissue.

Clinical Studies

Localized Hyperthermia

Superficial cancers of various histologies, including soft-tissue sarcoma and malignant melanoma, provide certain advantages for the study of clinical hyperthermia, especially in combination with radiotherapy. Superficial tumors are readily accessible to inspection, biopsy, and other quantitative assays, facilitating assessment of the therapeutic effects. Most importantly, it is reasonably easy to heat superficial tumors to a target temperature in a consistent manner with currently available hyperthermia systems.

The results of all published studies employing external beam radiation therapy and radiotherapy plus hyperthermia for treatment of superficial cancers have been summarized by Meyer[58] and updated by Overgaard.[59] Considering the range of tumors, study designs, and investigators, the studies have been surprisingly consistent in showing a therapeutic advantage of the combined modality over radiation alone. In general, complete response rates obtained with radiation plus hyperthermia (Fig 33–1) were more than double the complete responses obtained with the same radiation given alone (Table 33–2).

Kim et al.[60, 61] and Valdagni et al.[62] analyzed various factors influencing the therapeutic outcome of the combined treatment. Some of the important factors identified were the time and sequence of the combined modality, time-dose radiation fractionation schedules, tumor volume and hyperthermia parameters, including thermal dose, number of heat treatments, and quality of hyperthermia. At the present time, patients with multiple cutaneous lesions of malignant melanoma and soft-tissue sarcoma will obtain beneficial palliation with the combined treatment of radiation and hyperthermia.

Interstitial Hyperthermia

The clinical data accrued so far by the combined use of interstitial hyperthermia and interstitial brachytherapy have been consistently superior to those achieved by external heating

A 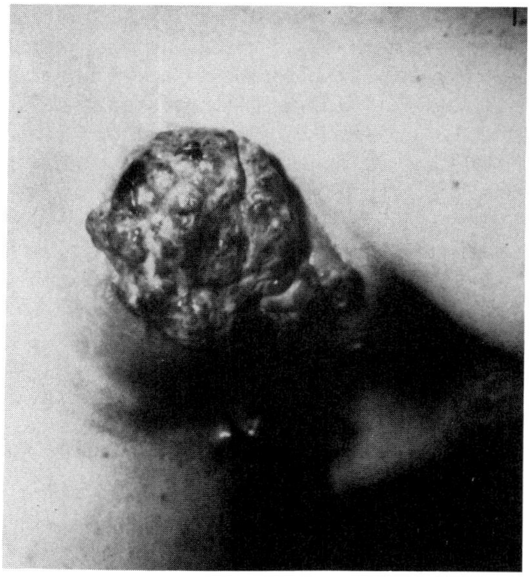 B 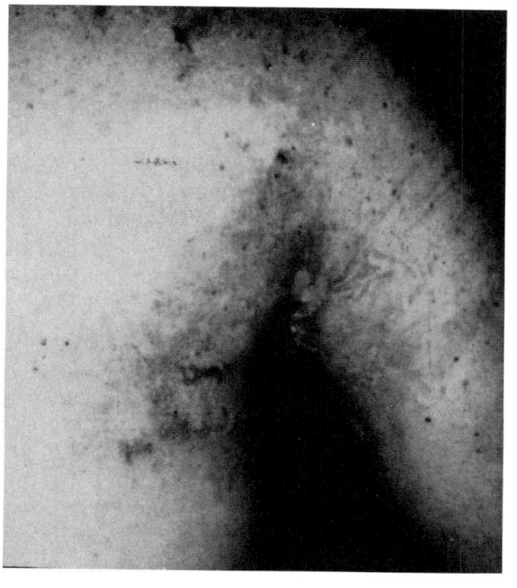

FIG 33–1.
A, a recurrent malignant melanoma in the axilla before treatment. **B,** complete regression of the mass after a combination of hyperthermia and radiation therapy. Note a minimal normal skin reaction.

TABLE 33–2.
Tumor Response After Combination Hyperthermia and Radiation Therapy*

Histological Type	Number of Patients	Complete Response: Radiation Therapy	Complete Response: RF + Radiation Therapy	Median Follow-Up (mo)
Malignant melanoma	38	11/32	31/38	15
Mycosis fungoides	15	3/12	12/15	36
Lymphoma cutis	6	2/6	5/6	26
Breast cancer	10	4/9	9/10	9
Chondrosarcoma	3	0/2	3/3	9
Others	14	4/12	9/14	9
Total	86	24/73 (33%)	69/86 (80%)	

* *Most lesions were heated with RF inductive mode (27.12 MHz) for 45 to 60 min before irradiation. A few bulky lesions were heated with an RF conductive unit (13.56 MHz). Radiation dose level was the same between radiation therapy alone versus RF plus radiation therapy. The trial was of internal control type for patients wth melanomas, mycosis fungoides, and lymphoma cutis.*[62]

techniques for superficial cancers.[45, 63] The reason for the superior results is most likely due to an improved heat distribution and increased minimum tumor temperature within the target tissue. Although the results with the combined interstitial treatments have been quite impressive, many technical and biological problems concerning equipment development and the sequence and timing of the two modalities remain. At the present time, interstitial treatment is the effective therapeutic modality in localized lesions, particularly in recurrent tumors that have been previously irradiated.[64]

Regional Hyperthermia

Most clinical studies in U.S. medical centers have been carried out with microwave systems using an annular phased array approach. In contrast, in Japan a device that operates as an 8-MHz radiofrequency capacitive system has been used for regional hyperthermia.

Heating from the annular phased array could be achieved in slightly more than 50% of the patients, which is often more effective in heating centrally for pelvic tumors.[65] In the abdomen, however, no consistent heating could be achieved, mainly due to systemic heating and the pain associated with increased power deposition. A similar experience was obtained with RF capacitive heating, that is, tumors in the head and neck, lower abdomen, and pelvis could be heated better than tumors in the upper abdomen. In particular, greater heating efficacy was shown in patients with large, hypovascular tumors, and with subcutaneous fat measuring less than 1.5 cm thick.[66] In general, the acute tolerance to regional hyperthermia has been remarkably good, and the side effects were usually limited to pain in the region of heating. Hyperthermia by annular phased array seems more stressful to the patient because of systemic elevation of the temperature relative to the RF capacitive heating.

The clinical results with the above devices are limited to date. A multicenter phase I study using an annular phased array showed that the overall response rate was 27% (95 of 353), with a 2-year survival rate of 41% and a median survival of 71 weeks. It should be noted that only 50% of the treated patients achieved a degree of regional hyperthermia and that an even smaller proportion reached a meaningful level of hyperthermia. Experience with RF capacitive heating shows an overall response rate of 63% (25 of 40). Of the 40 tumors treated, 15% exhibited complete response. Interestingly, although more than 50% of the tumors heated did not regress completely, they have shown no evidence of recurrence and have a computed tomography appearance showing a low-density area, indicating varying degrees of liquefaction within the heated region.

SYSTEMIC HYPERTHERMIA

The difficulties in achieving uniform thermal distribution within the tumor volume, localizing the target tissue, and the inhomogeneity of tissue components that are encountered with local or regional hyperthermia become minimal when systemic hyperthermia is employed to heat both primary and metastatic cancers.

Various methods have been used to induce systemic hyperthermia. Historically, microbes or proteins (e.g., mixed bacterial toxins) have been injected intramuscularly or intravenously to induce fever. Because of individual variations and the inability to regulate the temperature in a predictable manner, this approach currently is not being widely used. The most common approach currently involves the use of a device to insulate the body surface and raise the body temperature by an external heating method. The methods include coating the patients with paraffin, initiating hot-air breathing, using water blankets, and adding external heat by a microprocessor-controlled feedback, lukewarm water suit.[67, 68] The third means of inducing whole-body hyperthermia uses an extracorporeal heating device, developed by Parks et al.[69] A Dacron femoral arteriovenous shunt is placed in the anterior aspect of the thigh, and the blood is heated with an extracorporeal circuit heat exchanger. More recently, Robins et al.[70] attempted to achieve whole-body hyperthermia by means of a radiant heat device.[70] No significant alterations of hematological or biochemical parameters have been observed with the radiant heat device.

Phase I studies of systemic hyperthermia have shown that whole-body temperatures of 41.5 to 42°C could be safely sustained for several hours without producing irreversible toxicity. The most commonly observed acute toxicities include nausea, vomiting, diarrhea, posthyperthermia fever as high as 41°C, and occasionally seizures and peripheral neuropathy. All these symptoms are reversible within several days. Due to the increased metabolic rate induced by hyperthermia, a profound cardiovascular stress is produced. Bull et al.[68] have shown that cardiac rate increased with each degree rise of temperature, with a maximum cardiac rate reaching 160 ± 90 beats/min at 41.8°C. Therefore, to be eligible for systemic hyperthermia patients should be able to withstand a high-output cardiac state during temperature induction and maintenance phase on systemic heating.

The overall response rate from heat alone has varied with different investigators. No particular histological types of tumors are known to respond better than others to systemic hyperthermia. Because of transitory response and known synergistic interaction between heat and other treatment modalities, investigators have attempted to combine systemic hyperthermia with either localized radiation therapy or chemotherapy. Studies by Gerad et al.[71] using doxorubicin, cyclophosphamide, and whole-body hyperthermia indicate that complete or partial responses can be obtained in patients with advanced liposarcoma or leiomyosarcoma. A detailed evaluation of combined heat and other modalities is not yet available, but the important questions of sequencing the heat and drug or radiation, and frequency of hyperthermia, should be thoroughly explored.

REFERENCES

1. Coley WB: The treatment of inoperable sarcoma with the mixed toxins of erysipelas and *Bacillus prodigiosus:* Immediate and final results in one hundred and forty cases. *JAMA* 1989; 31:389–395, 456–465.
2. Warren SL: Preliminary study of the effect of artificial fever upon hopeless tumor cases. *AJR* 1925; 33:75.
3. Crile G: Selective destruction of cancers after exposure to heat. *Ann Surg* 1962; 156:404–414.
4. Chen TT, Heidelberger C: Quantitative studies on malignant transformation of mouse prostate cells by carcinogenic hydrocarbons in vitro. *Int J Cancer* 1969; 4:166–178.
5. Levine EM, Robbins EB: Differential temperature sensitivity of normal and cancer cells in culture. *J Cell Comp Physiol* 1980; 76:373–380.
6. Giovanella BC, Stehlin JS, Yim SO: Correlation of the thermosensitivity of cells to their malignant potential. *Ann NY Acad Sci* 1980; 335:206–214.
7. Kase C, Hahn CM: Differential heat response of normal and transformed human cells in tissue culture. *Nature Lond* 1975; 255:228–229.
8. Hahn GM: Comparison of the malignant potential of 10 T-1/2 cells and transformants with their survival responses to hyperthermia and to amphotericin B. *Cancer Res* 1980; 40:3763–3767.
9. Gerweck LE, Gillette EL, Dewey WC: Killing of Chinese hamster cells in vitro by heating under hypoxic or aerobic conditions. *Eur J Cancer* 1974; 10:691–693.
10. Kim SH, Kim JH, and Hahn EW: The enhanced killing of irradiated HeLa cells in

synchronous culture by hyperthermia. *Radiat Res* 1976; 66:337–345.

11. Kal HB, Hatfield M, Hahn GM: Cell cycle progression of murine sarcoma cells after x-irradiation or heat shock. *Radiology* 1975; 117:215–217.
12. Sapareto SA, Hopwood LE, Dewey WC, et al: effects of hyperthermia on survival and progression of Chinese hamster ovary cells. *Cancer Res* 1978; 38:393–400.
13. Dickson JA, Calderwood SK: In vivo hyperthermia of Yoshida tumor induces entry of non-proliferating cells into cycle. *Nature Lond* 1976; 263:772–774.
14. Naeslund J, Swenson KE: Investigations of the pH of malignant tumors in mice and humans after the administration of glucose. *Acta Obstet Gynecol Scand* 1953; 32:359–367.
15. Ashby BS: pH studies in human malignant tumors. *Lancet* 1966; 2:312–315.
16. Overgaard J: Influence of extracellular pH on the viability and morphology of tumor cells exposed to hyperthermia. *J Natl Cancer Inst* 1976; 56:1243–1250.
17. Gerweck LE: Modification of cell lethality of elevated temperatures: The pH effect. *Radiat Res* 1972; 70:224–235.
18. Hofer KG, Mivechi NF: Tumor cell sensitivity to hyperthermia as a function of extracellular and intracellular pH. *J Natl Cancer Inst* 1980; 65:621–625.
19. Gerweck LE: Effect of microenvironmental factors on the response of cells to single and fractionated heat treatments. *Natl Cancer Inst Monogr* 1982; 61:19–26.
20. Schulman N, Hall EJ: Hyperthermia: The effect on proliferative and plateau phase cell culture. *Radiology* 1974; 113:297–309.
21. Kim SH, Kim JH, Hahn EW: Enhanced killing of hypoxic tumor cells by hyperthermia. *Br J Radiol* 1975; 48:872–874.
22. Gerweck LE, Richardo B, Jennings M: The influence of variable oxygen concentration of the response of cells to heat or x-irradiation. *Radiat Res* 1981; 85:314–320.
23. Bass H, Moore JL, Coakley WT: Lethality in mammalian cells due to hyperthermia under oxic and hypoxic conditions. *Int J Radiat Biol* 1978; 33:57–67.
24. Kim SH, Kim JH, Hahn EW, et al: Selective killing of glucose and oxygen deprived HeLa cells by hyperthermia. *Cancer Res* 1980; 40:3459–3462.
25. Ben-Hur E, Elkind MM, Bronk BV: Thermally enhanced radioresponse of cultured Chinese hamster cells. *Radiat Res* 1974; 58:38–51.
26. Dewey WC, Freeman ML, Raaphorst GP, et al: Cell biology of hyperthermia and radiation, in Meyn RE, Withers R (eds): *Radiation Biology in Cancer Research,* Raven, 1980, pp 585–619.
27. Li GC, Evans RC, Hahn GM: Modification and inhibition of repair of potentially lethal x-ray damage by hyperthermia. *Radiat Res* 1976; 67:491–501.
28. Murthy AK, Harris JR, and Belli JA: Hyperthermia and radiation response of plateau phase cells. *Radiat Res* 1977; 70:241–247.
29. Gerweck LE, Gillette EL, Dewey WC: Effect of heat and radiation on synchronous Chinese hamster cells: Killing and repair. *Radiat Res* 1975; 64:611–613.
30. Dewey WC, Sapareto SA, Betten DA: Hyperthermic radiosensitization of synchronous Chinese hamster cells: Relationship between lethality and chromosomal aberrations. *Radiat Res* 1978; 76:48–59.
31. Gray LH, Conger AD, Ebert M, et al: The concentration of oxygen dissolved in tissues at the time of irradiation as a factor in radiotherapy. *Br J Radiol* 1953; 26:638–648.
32. Robinson JE, Wizenberg MJ, McCready WA: Combined hyperthermia and radiation suggest an alternative to heavy particle therapy for reduced oxygen enhancement ratio. *Nature Lond* 1974; 251:521–522.
33. Kim SH, Kim JH, Hahn EW: The radiosensitization of hypoxic tumor cells by hyperthermia. *Radiology* 1975; 114:727–728.
34. Durand RE: Effect of hyperthermia and/or irradiation in multicell spheroid systems. *Proc Int Symp Cancer Therapy by Hyperthermia and Radiation.* Chicago, American College of Radiology, 1975, pp 101–103.
35. Kim JH, Kim SH, Hahn EW: Hypoxic cell radiosensitization by moderate hyperthermia and glucose deprivation. *Radiat Res* 1983; 93:416–420.
36. Thrall DE, Gerweck LE, Gillette EL, et al: Response of cells in vitro and tissue in vivo to hyperthermia and x-irradiation. *Adv Radiat Biol* 1976; 6:211–226.
37. Stewart FA, Denekemp J: Combined x-rays and heating: Is there a therapeutic gain?, in Streffer C (ed): *Cancer Therapy by Hyperthermia and Radiation.* 1978; 249–250.
38. Hahn EW, Alfieri AA, Kim JH: The significance of fractionation regimens in radiation and combined hyperthermia using a murine fibrosarcoma. *Cancer* 1978; 42:2596–2599.

39. Overgaard J: Simultaneous and sequential hyperthermia and radiation treatment of an experimental tumor and its surrounding normal tissue in vivo. *Int J Radiat Oncol Biol Phys* 1980; 6:1507–1517.

40. Overgaard J: Influence of sequence and interval on the biological response to combined hyperthermia and radiation. *Natl Cancer Inst Monogr* 1982; 61:325–332.

41. Alfieri AA, Hahn EW, Kim JH: The relationship between the time of fractionated and single doses of radiation and hyperthermia on the sensitization of an in vivo mouse tumor. *Cancer* 1975; 36:893–903.

42. Stewart FA, Denekamp J: The therapeutic advantage of combined heat and x-rays on a mouse fibrosarcoma. *Br J Radiol* 1978; 51:307–316.

43. Hall EJ, Harisiadis L, Sung D, et al: Hyperthermia and low dose rate irradiation. *Radiology* 1978; 129:195–198.

44. Moorthy CR, Hahn EW, Kim JH, et al: Improved response of a murine fibrosarcoma to interstitial radiation when combined with hyperthermia. *Int J Radiat Oncol Biol Phys,* 1984; 10:1528–1533.

45. Manning MR, Cetas TC, Gerner EW: Interstitial thermoradiotherapy. *Natl Cancer Inst Monogr* 1982; 61:357–360.

46. Marmor JB, Pounds D, Hahn GM: Treatment of superficial human neoplasms by local hyperthermia induced by ultrasound. *Cancer* 1979; 43:196–205.

47. Corry PM, Barlogie B, Tilchen EJ, et al: Ultrasound induced hyperthermia for the treatment of human superficial tumors. *Int J Radiat Oncol Biol Phys* 1982; 8:1225–1229.

48. Lele PP, Parker KJ: Temperature distributions in tissues during local hyperthermia by stationary or steered beams of unfocused or focused ultrasound. *Br J Cancer* 1982; 45:108–121.

49. Hynynen K, Roemer R, Anhalts D, et al: A scanned, focused, multiple transducer ultrasonic system for localized hyperthermia treatments. *Int J Hyperthermia* 1987; 3:21.

50. LeVeen HH, Ahmed N, Piccone VA, et al: Radiofrequency therapy: Clinical experience. *Ann NY Acad Sci* 1980; 335:362–371.

51. Storm FK, Harrison WH, Elliott RS, et al: Normal tissue and solid tumor effects of hyperthermia in animal models and clinical trials. *Cancer Res* 1979; 39:2245–2251.

52. Corry PM, Jabboury K: Magnetic induction hyperthermia with transaxial coils. Proc 5th Int. Symp. Hyperthermia and Oncology, in *Hyperthermic Oncology,* vol II. New York, Taylor & Francis, 1988, pp 595–597.

53. Von Ardenne M, Kruger W: The use of hyperthermia within the frame of cancer multistep therapy. *Ann NY Acad Sci* 1980; 335:356–361.

54. Cheung AY, Golding WM, Samaras GM: Direct contact applicators for microwave hyperthermia. *J Microwave Power* 1981; 16:151–161.

55. U R, Noell KT, Woodward KT, et al: Microwave induced local hyperthermia in combination with radiotherapy for human malignant tumors. *Cancer* 1980; 45:638–646.

56. Gibbs FA: Clinical evaluation of a microwave/radiofrequency system (BSD Corporation) for induction of local and regional hyperthermia. *J Microwave Power* 1981; 16:185–192.

57. Kim JH, Antich P, Ahmed S, et al: Clinical experience with radiofrequency hyperthermia. *J Microwave Power* 1981; 16:193–197.

58. Meyer JL: The clinical efficacy of localized hyperthermia. *Cancer Res* 1984; 44(suppl): 4745S–4751S.

59. Overgaard J: The current and potential role of hyperthermia in radiotherapy. *Int J Radiat Oncol Biol Phys* 1989; 16:535–541.

60. Kim JH, Hahn EW, Ahmed SA, et al: Clinical study of the sequence of combined hyperthermia and radiation therapy of malignant melanoma, in Overgaard J (ed): *Hyperthermic Oncology,* vol 1. London and Philadelphia, Taylor & Frances, 1984.

61. Kim JH, Hahn EW, Ahmed S: Combination hyperthermia and radiation therapy for malignant melanoma. *Cancer* 1982; 50:478–482.

62. Valdagni R, Anichetti M, Parvi G: Radical radiation alone versus radical radiation plus microwave hyperthermia for N_3 (TNM-UICC) neck nodes: A prospective randomized clinical trial. *Int J Radiat Oncol Biol Phys* 1988; 15:13–18.

63. Emami B, Perez CA, Leybovich L, et al: Interstitial thermoradiotherapy in treatment of malignant tumors. *Int J Hyperthermia* 1987; 3:107–110.

64. Lam K, Astraham M, Langholz B, et al: Interstitial thermoradiotherapy for recurrent or persistent tumors. *Int J Hyperthermia* 1988; 4:259–263.

65. Petrovich Z, Langholz B, Gibbs FA, et al: Regional hyperthermia for advanced tumors: A clinical study of 353 patients. *Int J Radiat Oncol Biol Phys* 1989; 16:601–610.

66. Hiraoka M, Shiken J, Akuta K, et al: Radiofrequency capacitive hyperthermia for deep-seated tumors. II. Effects of thermoradiotherapy. *Cancer* 1987; 60:128–134.

67. Larkin J, Edwards W, Smith D, et al: Systemic thermotherapy: Description of a method and physiologic tolerance in clinical subjects. *Cancer* 1977; 40:3155–3159.

68. Bull JM, Less D, Schuette W, et al: Whole body hyperthermia: A phase I trial of a potential adjuvant to chemotherapy. *Ann Intern Med* 1979; 90:317–323.

69. Parks LC, Minabary D, Smith DP, et al: Treatment of far advanced bronchogenic carcinoma by extracorporeally induced systemic hyperthermia. *J Thorac Cardiovasc Surg* 1979; 78:883–892.

70. Robins HI, Wynn MM, Carlson SK, et al: Clinical use of a radiant heat device for whole body hyperthermia. 4th Ann. Meet. Int. Clin. Hyperthermia Society. London, England, June, 1982.

71. Gerad H, VanEcho DA, Whitacre M, et al: Doxorubicin, cyclophosphamide, and whole body hyperthermia for treatment of advanced soft tissue sarcoma. *Cancer* 1984; 53:2585–2591.

PART 5

Treatment: Chemotherapy

Chapter 34

Chemotherapy for Unresectable Soft-Tissue Sarcomas

Peter P. Sordillo

ADRIAMYCIN

The use of effective chemotherapy in adults with unresectable soft-tissue sarcomas dates to the discovery of the antineoplastic activity of doxorubicin (Adriamycin) in the early 1970s. Before this time, impressive responses were seen in children with embryonal rhabdomyosarcoma given combinations of vincristine, actinomycin D, and cyclophosphamide (VAC),[1-3] but adults with soft-tissue sarcomas responded infrequently to chemotherapy. Clinical benefit was achieved in less than 10% to 15% of adults with these tumors, and few patients attained long-lasting remission.[4, 5]

In 1970, Bonadonna et al.[6] published the results of a study in Milan documenting the activity of Adriamycin against a wide variety of cancers, including soft-tissue sarcomas. Of 50 patients with soft-tissue sarcomas treated with Adriamycin according to a variety of schedules, 11 had partial responses (22%).* Although the median duration of response was only 3 months and there were no complete responders, this 22% response rate was encouraging, especially because many of the patients had been pretreated with other chemotherapeutic drugs. The activity of Adriamycin in patients with these tumors was subsequently confirmed by investigators in the United States. Blum,[7] summarizing the results of five early trials in the United

* A *partial* response (PR) is generally defined as an at least 50% decrease in the size of all tumor masses, lasting at least 1 month. A *complete* response (CR) is the complete disappearance of all tumor masses, lasting at least 1 month. Partial or complete responses are considered *major* responses. Decreases in tumor size of less than 50% (*minor* responses) are considered less useful when evaluating the activity of a single drug or drug combination.

States, found a 34% response rate in 130 patients with soft-tissue sarcomas. It was clear from these studies that the activity of Adriamycin in these tumors exceeded any other chemotherapeutic agent, and chemotherapy with Adriamycin alone or in combination quickly became standard therapy for adults with metastatic soft-tissue sarcoma.

Other studies of Adriamycin as a single agent have also confirmed its activity in this group of tumors (Tables 34–1).[8–13] Most of these studies have shown response rates to Adriamycin of at least 25%, although a few studies have reported a response rate as low as 13%.[9, 11, 13] The range of response rates seen may be accounted for by several factors. Older age, poor performance status, and prior treatment all decrease the chance of obtaining a response to chemotherapy.[14–17] Young adults with embryonal rhabdomyosarcoma respond well to chemotherapy, whereas certain types of sarcomas such as malignant schwannoma, leiomyosarcoma of the gastrointestinal tract, mixed mesodermal sarcoma, and extra-osseous osteogenic sarcoma appear to respond more poorly to chemotherapy than sarcomas as a whole, so inclusion of a disproportionate number of patients with these kinds of tumors could change the response rate.[17–25]

Most importantly, the response to Adriamycin may depend on the dose schedule used.[15] Indeed, another major conclusion of these early studies was that there appeared to be a sharp dose-response curve to Adriamycin, with 60 to 90 mg/m² more effective than lower doses of this drug. The sharp dose-response curve with Adriamycin had been noted in animal and tissue culture studies,[26–28] and clinical studies in patients with sarcomas appeared to confirm this observation.[5, 12, 20, 29] O'Bryan et al.[12] noted a higher response rate with higher doses of Adriamycin both in "good-risk" patients with sarcomas receiving 45, 60, or 75 mg/m² and "poor-risk" patients given 25 or 50 mg/m² (Table 34–2). The difference in response rate was not as marked for patients in the study by O'Bryan et al. with other types of cancer, especially in those with breast cancer (for whom 45 mg/m² may be as good as higher doses); however, the authors also noted that almost two thirds of the complete responses for the entire group occurred in patients receiving 75 mg/m². In another study, Schoenfeld et al.[5] reported a 27% major response rate in patients with sarcomas receiving Adriamycin at 70 mg/m² every 3 weeks, but only a 19% response rate when Adriamycin was given (in addition to cyclophosphamide and vincristine) at a dose of 50 mg/m² every 3 weeks. Similarly, combinations in which the Adriamycin was given at intervals of 5 to 6 weeks rather than every 3 weeks have also generally resulted in poor response rates.[30–32]

Wheeler and associates[33] have explored the use of high-dose Adriamycin (120 mg/m² every 3 weeks) in patients with a variety of tumors. The use of doses this high was based on pilot work by Nagel,[34] who found that doses of 120 to 240 mg/m² of Adriamycin could be administered to patients with proper supportive care.[34] Also of note in the study by Nagel was the fact that responses could be achieved with these doses in patients who had previously failed with conventional doses of Adriamycin. In the study by Wheeler et al. the response rate, excluding

TABLE 34–1.
Responses to Adriamycin in Patients with Soft-Tissue Sarcomas*

Dose	Number of Patients	CR	PR	MRR (%)	Ref.
70 mg/m²	66	4	14	27	5
Variety of dosage schedules	50	0	11	22	6
60–90 mg/m² q3 wk	130†	0	44	34	7
75 mg/m² q3 wk	38	1	9	26	8
20 mg/m²/day for 3 days q3 wk	88‡	2	12	16	9
0.4 mg/kg days 1, 2, 3, 8, 9, 10, then weekly	36‡	3	11	39	10
0.4 mg/kg days 1, 2, 3, 8, 9, 10; then twice weekly	41	1	6	17§	11
25–75 mg/m² q3 wk (dose response)	82‡	1	22	28	12
20–25 mg/m²/day for 3 days q3 wk	15	0	2	13	13

** CR = complete response; PR = partial response; MRR = major response rate = (CR + PR)/total number of patients.*
† Summary of data from five studies. A few patients were treated according to other schedules.
‡ Patients with bone sarcomas excluded.
§ Randomized study against three other combinations. Response rate without cross-overs was 22%.

TABLE 34–2.
Comparative Study of Different Doses of Adriamycin in Patients with Sarcomas, Showing a Better Response With Higher Doses[12]

Dose	Number of Patients†	CR & PR	MRR† (%)
Good-risk patients			
75 mg/m² q3 wk	41	15	37
60 mg/m² q3 wk	10	2	20
45 mg/m² q3 wk	28	5	18
Poor-risk patients			
50 mg/m² q3 wk	9	1	11
25 mg/m² q3 wk	10	0	0

** Includes bone sarcomas.*
† MRR = major response rate.

that of patients with malignant melanoma, was 58% with 21% complete responses, and there were three major responses in seven evaluable patients with soft-tissue sarcomas. Although increased toxicity was noted with this regimen, it deserves more exploration. These studies also provide further evidence of a dose-response curve to Adriamycin in patients with soft-tissue sarcomas, and emphasize the importance of using adequate doses of this agent when the drug is given in multidrug combinations. Currently, patients with soft-tissue sarcomas should receive Adriamycin at doses of at least 60 to 75 mg/m² every 3 weeks. In addition, because patients who do not respond to low does may respond to higher doses,[33, 34] treatment with higher doses of Adriamycin should be considered in patients who have previously received doses less than 60 mg/m².

Adriamycin Cardiotoxicity

The activity of Adriamycin patients with soft-tissue sarcomas significantly exceeds the activity of any other single agent. However, the enthusiasm over the discovery of the activity of Adriamycin in soft-tissue sarcomas has been tempered by several facts. Although 20% to 30% of patients have major responses to Adriamycin, the majority of patients do not respond, and most of the responses are partial rather than complete responses. The use of Adriamycin in these and other patients is also limited by its cardiotoxicity. With increasing cumulative doses of this drug, greater number of patients experience clinical symptoms of congestive heart failure.[35–42] With the widespread use of Adriamycin, this has become a well-known clinical entity, and there is now a voluminous literature on the subject.

Signs of Adriamycin cardiotoxicity can appear suddenly and may be followed by rapidly progressive heart failure leading to death. Presenting symptoms include sudden onset of shortness of breath, edema of the legs, unexplained fatigue, or a nonproductive cough.[43–45] Patients with the sudden onset of severe congestive heart failure tend to have the worst prognosis.[37] Treatment consists of digitalis and diuretics, bed rest, and, of course, discontinuation of Adriamycin.[37, 44] Aggressive therapy is warranted because patients with mild congestive heart failure (CHF) may recover.[37, 39, 40] Supraventricular and ventricular arrhythmias may also occur, frequently acutely after a bolus injection of Adriamycin; however, these are usually transient and do not signify the development of cardiomyopathy.[43–45] Pathologically, damage to the myocardium results in the appearance of mild edema, progressing to myocyte vacuolization, perivascular fibrosis, severe edema, and myocytolysis.[44–46] On electron microscopy, the normal myocardial ultrastructure is markedly disrupted, showing a distinct loss of contractile elements including a drop out of the myofibrils, distention of the sarcoplasmic reticulum, and degeneration of elements of the tubular system and mitochondria.[46]

Patients can experience cardiotoxicity at any total dose level, but the risk of cardiomyopathy sharply increases in patients who have received cumulative doses of more than 500 mg/m². Minow et al.[45] have reported that 9% of patients who received total doses of between 500 and 550 mg/m² of Adriamycin developed clinical evidence of cardiomyopathy, whereas 20% of patients receiving 550 to 600 mg/m² and 41% of those receiving more than 600 mg/m² developed this complication.[45]

It has also been reported that concurrent administration of other chemotherapeutic agents (including cyclophosphamide, mitomycin C, and actinomycin D), a history of previous mediastinal irradiation, advanced age, and possibly other factors may predispose to Adriamycin cardiotoxicity.[41, 42, 44–51] Therefore, most clinicians now arbitrarily limit total doses of Adriamycin to 450 to 550 mg/m². The dose and schedule by which Adriamycin is given are also important. The high-dose bolus schedule, may be more cardiotoxic than a weekly low-dose schedule.[41, 50, 52, 53]

Several methods have been designed to try

to monitor and prevent the development of cardiomyopathy, including serial measurements of ECG voltage,[45, 47] echocardiography,[40, 54, 55] and systolic time-interval determinations.[35, 40, 56] However, none of the above methods has proven consistently reliable for monitoring the hearts of individuals receiving Adriamycin.[57–60] Serial chest X-rays and cardiac enzyme determinations have also proven not to be useful in predicting the development of Adriamycin cardiomyopathy.[43, 47, 56, 61] The use of serial endomyocardial biopsy[35, 38, 41, 49, 58, 62] and radionuclide cineangiography[38, 39, 63–65] is more promising in monitoring individuals receiving Adriamycin. These tests should be used when available. The latter methods are not only more accurate in predicting congestive heart failure, but appear to be more sensitive in detecting the early changes caused by Adriamycin cardiotoxicity.[38, 39] With the availability of these techniques, studies have shown that Adriamycin cardiotoxicity at cumulative doses of 450 to 550 mg/m^2 is a much more frequent complication than previously thought; one half of these patients will have asymptomatic Adriamycin cardiomyopathy at these doses.[39, 65]

Adriamycin Combinations

Because of its cardiotoxicity, Adriamycin cannot be used for maintenance therapy. Because most patients receive 50 to 75 mg/m^2 every 3 weeks, the total duration of treatment with Adriamycin even for complete responders can usually be only 6 to 9 months. As would be expected, this length of treatment is generally insufficient to produce cure or long-lasting remission, and many patients who do achieve a complete response will suffer a relapse just a few months after discontinuing Adriamycin.

Despite these limitations, it is clear that the discovery of the activity of adriamycin against soft-tissue sarcomas was the first step in finding a successful drug treatment for these patients. Over the last 10 years, further work has proceeded in three directions. One approach has been to try to improve the response rate and duration of response by adding other "conventional" drugs to Adriamycin to form multidrug combinations. A second approach has been to modify the dose schedule or method of administration of Adriamycin, or to test new derivatives of Adriamycin in an attempt to increase response rates or to decrease cardiotoxicity. The third approach has been to continue to search for new agents that might have activity against this type of tumor.

Much of the early work in developing Adriamycin combinations was done at M. D. Anderson Hospital, Houston, TX, under the direction of Gottlieb et al.[20] (Table 34–3). The M. D. Anderson group had been studying 5-(3,3-dimethyl-1-triazeno)-imidazole-4-carboxamide (DTIC) and had observed one complete response and eight partial responses using this agent in 53 patients with soft-tissue sarcomas, for a response rate of 17%.[66] DTIC causes severe nausea and vomiting, and many investigators do not agree that the response rate to DTIC is this high. However, because Adriamycin and DTIC appeared to be synergistic in animal tumors,[67, 68] and because a phase I trial had shown only a minimal increase in toxicity with the combination compared with Adriamycin alone,[69] a large multi-institution study of the combination was conducted. Not only did the major response rate increase to 42% with the Adriamycin-DTIC combination (46% if patients with bone sarcomas and mesotheliomas are excluded) compared with 31% in the previous study at M. D. Anderson Hospital with Adriamycin alone, but the complete response rate increased from 4% to 11% (14% for soft-tissue sarcomas only). Equally important was the fact that the median survival of responders increased from 8 months to more than 16 months with the combination. The subsequent addition of vincristine to these two drugs did not appear to add much, giving the same 42% response as the two-drug combination, although there was a slight increase in the response rate when patients with bone sarcomas and mesotheliomas were excluded, and a higher percentage of patients appeared to have stable rather than progressive disease. However, with the addition of cyclophosphamide (CYVADIC), the major response rate improved to 55% (61% for soft-tissue sarcomas only) and the complete response rate to 14%.[20]

This combination appeared to be a major advance, and for some time it was hoped that further manipulations of the CYVADIC combination and the addition of other drugs would result in higher response rates and longer survivals. This has not happened, and the use of combination chemotherapy has several disadvantages over the use of Adriamycin alone. DTIC, particularly, causes severe nausea and vomiting, as do many of the other drugs used with Adriamycin; side effects not seen with

TABLE 34–3.
Development of the CYVADIC Combination[20]

Protocol	Dose (mg/m²)	Schedule*	Number of Patients†	CR	PR	MRR (%)	MRR in Patients with Soft-Tissue Sarcoma Only (%)
Adriamycin alone	75	Day 1	49	2	13	31	29
Adriamycin +	60	Day 1	218	25	67	42	46
DTIC (ADIC)	250	Days 1–5					
Adriamycin +	60	Day 1	107	9	36	42	50
DTIC +	250	Days 1–5					
vincristine (VADIC)	1.5‡	Days 1 and 5					
Adriamycin +	50	Day 1	136	19	56	55	61
DTIC +	250	Days 1–5					
vincristine +	1.5‡	Days 1 and 5					
cyclophosphamide (CYVADIC)	500	Day 1					

** Doses repeated every 3 wk.*
† Bone sarcomas and mesotheliomas included.
‡ Top dose, 2 mg.

Adriamycin alone, such as neuropathy (vincristine) and hemorrhagic cystitis (cyclophosphamide), may occur with combination therapy (Table 34–4). As noted previously, the simultaneous use of other chemotherapeutic agents may also increase the risk of Adriamycin cardiomyopathy. Perhaps most important, there are additional myelosuppressive effects when multiple chemotherapeutic agents are used, resulting in more frequent episodes of sepsis and bleeding in patients receiving combination therapy. There is also the theoretical disadvantage that one may have to reduce the dose of the most active drug, Adriamycin, because of the myelosuppressive effects of the other drugs in the combination.

For these and other reasons, the substitution or addition of other drugs to the CYVADIC combination has not increased the response rate. Indeed, other investigators have not been able to produce the same response rate to CYVADIC as that seen by Gottlieb et al.[20] Rather than the 55% to 60% first suggested, most investigators report response rates of 35% to 50% (Table 34–5).[70–74] Although a few other investigators have reported response rates to CYVADIC outside this range, these studies involved only small numbers of patients.[75, 76] In addition, re-evaluation of the first CYVADIC study reclassified several of the partial responders as "no change," thus lowering the response rate seen from 55% to 47%.[16]

Despite this, CYVADIC does appear superior to Adriamycin alone, not only because the 35% to 50% response rate exceeds the 20% to 30% response rate seen with Adriamycin alone,

TABLE 34–4.
Common Side Effects of Chemotherapeutic Agents Used in Patients with Soft-Tissue Sarcomas

Agent	Effect
Adriamycin	Leukopenia, thrombocytopenia, alopecia, nausea and vomiting, mucositis, tissue necrosis at injection site, cardiomyopathy
Cyclophosphamide	Leukopenia, thrombocytopenia, alopecia, nausea and vomiting, hemorrhagic cystitis, cardiomyopathy (usually with very high doses only), pulmonary fibrosis (rare).
Vincristine	Leukopenia, alopecia, neuropathy, constipation, tissue necrosis at injection site
DTIC	Leukopenia and thrombocytopenia (generally modest), severe nausea and vomiting
Methotrexate	Leukopenia, thrombocytopenia, mucositis, diarrhea, renal failure, pulmonary fibrosis (rare), hepatitis
Actinomycin D	Leukopenia, thrombocytopenia, alopecia, severe nausea and vomiting, tissue necrosis at injection site, mucositis

TABLE 34–5.
Results of Trials with CYVADIC Combinations in Patients With Soft-Tissue Sarcomas

Author	Number of Evaluable Patients	CR	PR	MRR (%)
Gottlieb et al.[20]	112	18	50	61*
Karakousis et al.[70]	41	3	8	27
Pinedo et al.[71]	60	8	14	37
Schmidt et al.[72]	11	3	2	45
Benjamin et al.[23, 73]	229	27	80	47
Rodriguez et al.[75, †]	27	6	12	66
Giuliano et al.[76]	20	2	1	15
Bui et al.[74]	23	3	9	52

* *Later re-evaluation of these results by Yap et al.*[16] has reduced the response rate to 50%.
† Some patients treated with intensified doses and in a protected environment with prophylactic antibiotics.

but also because of the 10% to 15% complete response rate to CYVADIC (compared with less than 5% for Adriamycin) and the longer survival of responders to the combination.

However, we may have reached the maximum response rate that can be achieved by adding agents with marginal activity to Adriamycin. For example, actinomycin D is an active agent against embryonal rhabdomyosarcoma in children and appears to have some minor activity against soft-tissue sarcomas in adults as well,[77, 78] but no additive antitumor effect is seen when this drug is combined with Adriamycin. Replacement of DTIC in the CYVADIC combination with actinomycin D (CYVADACT) gave only a 36% response rate compared with a 47% response rate with CYVADIC in a randomized trial.[18, 73] Another study adding actinomycin D to Adriamycin gave a response rate of only 28%, similar to the response rate to Adriamycin alone.[79] Likewise, the addition of actinomycin D to a number of Adriamycin-based combinations generally gave response rates of only 20% to 30% (Table 34–6).[17–19, 31, 32, 73, 79, 80–83] Indeed, the addition of actinomycin D to combinations containing Adriamycin, cyclophosphamide, and DTIC, which might be expected to give response rates at least as good at CYVADIC, has instead generally given *poorer* response rates.[19, 32, 80, 82] Whether the poorer response rates seen with these combinations are due to the added myelosuppressive activity of actinomycin D, necessitating reduction of the dose of adriamycin, or to an antagonism between actinomycin D and Adriamycin, as suggested by several investigators,[20, 82] is unclear. The use of actinomycin D in drug combinations that lack Adriamycin has also proved to be of no major value in patients with sarcomas (Table 34–7).[1, 4, 5, 11, 17, 78, 84, 85]

Methotrexate has been reported to have activity against soft-tissue sarcomas, with both low-dose[17, 86–88] and high-dose regimens requiring citrovorum factor rescue (Table 34–8).[89–91] Although response rates to methotrexate as high as 25% to 40% have been reported in small series of patients,[17, 89, 90] some studies show no activity for methotrexate with either the high- or low-dose regimen.[92–94] As with actinomycin D, attempts to increase the response rate to chemotherapy by adding this drug to Adriamycin-

TABLE 34–6.
Response to Chemotherapy Combinations Containing Both Adriamycin and Actinomycin D In Adults With Soft-Tissue Sarcomas Showing Lack of an Additive Effect

Combination*	Number of Evaluable Patients	CR	PR	MRR (%)
VCR-CTX-MTX-ADR-Act D[17]	40	2	9	27
VCR-CTX-ADR-ACT D (CYVADACT)[18, 73]	224	25	55	36
ADR-Act D-DTIC[18, 83]	98	9	15	24
VCR-CTX-MTX-CTIC-ADR-ActD[19]	232	13	33	20
VCR-MTX-DTIC-CLB-ADR-Act D[31]	48	3	10	27
VCR-MTX-ADR-Act D[31]	34	4	11	44
CTX-DTIC-ADR-Act D[32]	29	0	6	21
ADR-Act D[79]	21	2	4	28
CTX-DTIC-ADR-Act D[80]	20	0	4	20
VCR-ADR-Act D[81]	15	0	3	20
CTX-DTIC-ADR-Act D[82]	23	1	2	13

* *VCR = vincristine; CTX = cyclophosphamide; MTX = methotrexate; CLB = chlorambucil; DTIC = dacarbazine; ADR = adriamycin; Act D = actinomycin D.*

TABLE 34–7.
Drug Combinations With Actinomycin D but Without Adriamycin In Adults With Soft-Tissue Sarcomas

Combination*	Number of Evaluable Patients	CR	PR	MRR (%)
VCR-Act D-CTX (VAC)[4]	61	1	4	8
VCR-Act D-CTX[5] (VAC)	63	1	6	11
Act D-L-PAM[11]	25	0	1	4
Act D-L-PAM-VCR[11]	26	0	0	0
Act D-L-PAM-Cycloleucine[1]	25	0	0	0
CTX-5FU-VCR-Act D-MTX[17]	14	3	1	28
Act D-CLB[78]	40	0	5	13
Act D-CLB-MTX[78]	40	0	8	20
VCR-Act D-CTX (VAC)[84]	15	0	2	13
Methyl CCNU-Act D[85]	29	1	0	3

** VCR = vincristine; CTX = cyclophosphamide; L-PAM = phenylalanine mustard; 5 FU = 5-fluorouracil; MTX = methotrexate; Act D = actinomycin D; CLB = chlorambucil.*

based combinations have been unsuccessful. Lynch et al.,[95] for example, treated 36 patients with soft-tissue sarcomas with CYOMAD, a combination of moderately high-dose methotrexate (250 mg/m^2) and citrovorum factor rescue with a modified CYVADIC regimen. The response rate was a disappointing 25%, less than that seen with CYVADIC alone. Other combinations of methotrexate and Adriamycin-based regimens have also resulted in poorer response rates than the best reported for CYVADIC.[17, 19, 30, 31, 84, 96, 97]

A number of other agents including chlorambucil and streptozotocin have been added to adriamycin-based regimens, again with no increase in response rate.[31, 98] There has been one report of a 49% response rate (three CR and 17 PR in 41 patients) from a combination using methyl CCNU (semustine) and Adriamycin.[99] This is somewhat surprising, considering the lack of activity of methyl CCNU as a single agent: five responses among 85 patients (6%) in two published studies.[4, 100] Two other studies using methyl CCNU in combination have also failed to confirm its activity. Yap et al.[85] studied the combination of methyl CCNU and actinomycin D and reported only one response in 29 patients (3%), and Magill et al.[31] studied the combination of methyl CCNU, Adriamycin, and vincristine and reported only a 26% response rate, no different from the activity reported with Adriamycin alone.

Vindesine sulfate (DVA) is a drug of the *Vinca* alkaloid class that has attracted interest because of its activity in a wide range of human cancers, including carcinomas of the lung, breast, and esophagus.[101, 102] Interest in the use of this drug in patients with soft-tissue sarcomas

TABLE 34–8.
Activity of Methotrexate as a Single Agent In Adults With Soft-Tissue Sarcoma

Dose	Number of Evaluable Patients	CR	PR	MRR (%)
Variety of schedules[17, 87, 88]	52	6	7	25
0.2 mg/kg[86] on days 1, 2, 3, 4, 6, 8, 10, 12. Repeat course on day 42	19	0	2	11
4 g/m^2 with CF[89, *]	13	3	0	23
50–300 mg/kg with CF[90]	11	0	5	45
"High-dose" with CF[91, †]	26	—	—	20
25–250 mg/m^2 with CF[92]	9‡	0	0	0
2–4 g/m^2 with CF[93]	18	1	0	6
40 mg/m^2 without CF[94]	33	0	0	0

** CF = citrovorum factor.*
† Review of three previous studies.
‡ Includes bone sarcomas.

was prompted by reports of the effectiveness of vindesine against human tumors heterotransplanted into nude mice,[103] and of some minor activity of vindesine against sarcomas in phase I and II trials, especially among previously untreated patients.[104, 105] Brenner et al.[106] combined this agent with Adriamycin and cyclophosphamide. The major response rate to this combination was only 35% (48% in previously untreated patients). This is no better than the response rate seen with CYVADIC. However, the 19% CR rate and 16 month survival of responders in this study compare favorably with the results seen with CYVADIC, and suggest it may be possible to substitute other agents for DTIC in an Adriamycin-based regimen, thus reducing the severe nausea and vomiting caused by combinations including this agent.

Illustrative Case Report

A 62-year-old whtie man was well until September 1980, when a mass developed in the soft tissue over his left scapula, and in November 1980 he underwent resection of a 3.5 × 3.5-cm-high-grade fibrosarcoma. One month later, he presented to Memorial Sloan-Kettering Cancer Center, New York, NY, with a possible recurrence at the same site. He was treated with radical, wide, soft-part resection with removal of a large block of muscle, including portions of the trapezius and the latissimus dorsi. Fibrosarcoma was present in the specimen. Pathological margins were free of tumor. Adjuvant chemotherapy was recommended but refused by the patient.

The patient did well until 7 months later, when he was found to have multiple pulmonary metastases on chest radiograph. In August 1981 he was started on chemotherapy with a combination of Adriamycin (60 mg/m^2), cyclophosphamide (600 mg/m^2), and vindesine (3 mg/m^2), all on day 1, and vindesine (3 mg/m^2) again on day 8, with cycles repeated every 3 weeks. Response to chemotherapy was complete, with disappearance of the lung nodules on chest X-ray. He was continued on chemotherapy with this combination until February 1982, when Adriamycin was discontinued because the cumulative Adriamycin dose had reached 540 mg/m^2 and he had evidence of decreased cardiac function on a gated blood pool study. The patient was continued on vindesine and cyclophosphamide. Three months after discontinuing Adriamycin, however, recurrent disease was documented on chest X-ray. He began a short course of VP16 (etoposide), and then metoprine, without response.

The patient was subsequently seen by a thoracic surgeon who performed multiple wedge resections of metastatic tumor nodules in both lungs. The patient was treated postoperatively with a combination of actinomycin D and methotrexate. His lungs remained clear; however, in January 1983, brain metastases developed without evidence of disease elsewhere. He had some temporary improvement with whole-brain radiation therapy, but died in March 1983, with progressive neurological dysfunction secondary to brain metastases.

New Methods of Using Adriamycin

Despite the apparent increase in response rate with combination therapy, only 10% to 12% of patients achieve complete responses, the duration of response in most patients is short, and many patients who do achieve a complete response suffer relapse shortly after reaching the maximum dose of Adriamycin.[107, 108] A number of researchers have focused their efforts on finding methods of improving the response rate or decreasing the cardiotoxicity of Adriamycin. As noted previously, high-dose Adriamycin (120–240 mg/m^2) has been studied in a few patients with some promising results.[33, 34] Besides the increased toxicity with these high doses, however, this approach has the disadvantage that patients reach their maximum cumulative dose of Adriamycin in only a short period of time. Very high-dose chemotherapy may be of use, nevertheless, in conjunction with autologous bone marrow transplantation, and this approach deserves investigation.[109]

A major area of research has been the administration of Adriamycin by continuous infusion.[110–115] Studies of a variety of schedules have suggested that a 96-hour infusion apparently is less cardiotoxic than a 24- to 48-hour or 6-hour infusion.[111–113] Patients receiving a 96-hour infusion have been able to tolerate cumulative doses of over 1000 mg/m^2 of Adriamycin without developing evidence of cardiomyopathy on endomyocardial biopsy.[113] The administration of Adriamycin by continuous infusion, if the response rate is as good as by bolus, may be especially useful for patients achieving a complete response who could take Adriamycin for longer periods to prevent relapse. It may also permit a longer period of administration of Adriamycin in adjuvant therapy programs.

Considerable research has been performed over the last several years on the use of Adriamycin as a radiosensitizing agent. This was based on work in experimental systems showing a synergistic effect of irradiation and relatively small doses of Adriamycin.[116–119] Clinical studies of a variety of malignant tumors appear to confirm this observation,[119, 120] as have two studies in patients with soft-tissue sarcomas.[115, 121] In one study,[121] six CR and 12 PR were seen in 29 evaluable patients with soft-tissue sarcomas (62%) who received five bolus injections of Adriamycin (20 mg/m^2 on day 1 and 10 mg/m^2 on days 8, 15, 22, and 29), each 90 minutes prior to a dose of 580 rads of external radiotherapy once a week for 5 weeks (total, 2,900 rads). In another study,[115] patients received Adriamycin (12 mg/m^2/day) by continuous infusion over 120 hours every 3 to 4 weeks and concomitant radiation therapy of 150 rads/day for 5 days. The authors reported three CR and two PR in five patients with sarcomas. Both of these regimens were accompanied by only mild to moderate toxicity, although the usefulness of this treatment was complicated by the short duration of responses in both studies, often because of progression of lesions outside the irradiated area. This approach may be beneficial, however, in selected patients with limited extent of disease or in conjunction with a multimodality program of therapy.

The efficacy of intra-arterial Adriamycin has also been studied by a number of investigators. Administration of Adriamycin in this manner rather than intravenously is based on the concept that perfusing a tumor with a high concentration of this agent will cause higher drug uptake by the tumor cells. Several early trials described the use of intra-arterial Adriamycin in patients with soft-tissue or skeletal sarcomas.[122–125] Shah et al.[125] reported five PR in eight patients receiving intra-arterial Adriamycin infusion. Other investigators have reported higher response rates with intra-arterial Adriamycin than are seen when given intravenously (although these studies all involve small numbers of patients).[122–131] However, the major use of this therapy has been pre-operatively as part of a multidisciplinary program, together with radiation therapy or immunotherapy and limb-sparing surgery.[126–131] With this multidisciplinary approach, limb salvage is possible in a high percentage of patients. Local failure rates in patients receiving this combined modality therapy have been quite low.

Two other novel methods designed to reduce the cardiotoxicity of Adriamycin are under study. There have been several reports on the use of Adriamycin complexed with DNA in patients with a variety of tumors.[132–135] Theoretically, these complexes might be preferentially taken up by tumor cells, which have increased pinocytotic activity, while being excluded from heart muscle cells, thus allowing Adriamycin to be administered with less risk of developing cardiomyopathy.[135] There have also been several reports of animal studies suggesting that Adriamycin cardiotoxicity might be prevented or reversed by treatment with a free-radical scavenger, such as *N*-acetyl cysteine or α-tocopherol,[136–138] although a study in 11 patients with soft-tissue sarcomas failed to confirm this theory.[139] Both of these approaches deserve further investigation, however.

Adriamycin Derivatives

One of the most important areas of research has been the effort to develop derivatives of Adriamycin that are less cardiotoxic or more effective than the parent drug. Numerous Adriamycin derivatives have been synthesized by chemical modification in the C-4 position in the chromophore, or the C-4′ position of the aminosugar.[140] Several have been reported to be less cardiotoxic in experimental systems.[141–145] Most of these agents have not yet been thoroughly evaluated, but several under investigation may retain the antitumor activity of Adriamycin while causing less cardiotoxicity (Table 34–9). One of the first drugs to be studied was carminomycin, an anthracycline developed in the Soviet Union. Carminomycin was originally reported to give a 27% response rate in 48 patients with sarcomas, comparable to the response rate seen with Adriamycin, as well as a 19% minor response rate while showing less cardiotoxicity.[146] However, a randomized study comparing this drug with Adriamycin carried out by the European Organization for Research and Treatment Against Cancer (EORTC) group showed the definite superiority of Adriamycin with its 26% response rate versus the 3% response rate for carminomycin.[8, 94]

4′-Epi-Adriamycin (epirubicin), the 4′-epimer of Adriamycin, has been studied in patients with a wide variety of cancers.[147] In 43 patients with soft-tissue sarcomas treated with

TABLE 34–9.
Activity of Adriamycin Derivatives in Patients With Soft-Tissue Sarcomas

Drug	Total Number of Patients	CR	PR	MRR (%)
Carminomycin[146]	48	—	—	27
Carminomycin[8, 94, *]	33	0	1	3
4′-Epi-Adriamycin[147, †]	43	1	8	21
4′-Demethoxydaunorubicin[149]	22	0	1	5
4′-Demethoxydaunorubicin[150] (previously untreated patients)	18	0	1	6
Duborimycin[151]	23	0	1	4

** Randomized trial versus Adriamycin.*
† Summary of data from six studies.

this drug from a number of centers, there have been one CR and eight PR (21% response rate).[147] Studies with other tumors also indicate that 4′-epi-Adriamycin may be less cardiotoxic than Adriamycin,[147] although this needs to be confirmed in a larger number of patients.

4′-Demethoxydaunorubicin has been reported to be more active than Adriamycin in experimental systems.[142, 148] Raymond et al.[149] reported the results of a trial of this drug in 22 patients with soft-tissue sarcomas, 19 of whom had been pretreated with other drugs. Only one partial response was noted in the 22 patients (5%), and in addition, evidence of cardiotoxicity was seen. Studies of this agent in patients who had received no prior chemotherapy have likewise shown no significant activity.[150] Another anthracycline, duborimycin, was studied in 23 patients with bone and soft-tissue sarcomas.[151] One partial response was seen (4%). Aclacinomycin A, rubidazone, quelamycin, and detorubicin have also been studied in small numbers of patients with sarcomas[108]; however, the number of patients treated with each of these compounds is too small to draw any conclusions concerning their activity in this tumor.

NEW DRUG STUDIES

The administration of Adriamycin by continuous infusion or the discovery of an effective noncardiotoxic Adriamycin derivative may lengthen the duration of response by allowing patients to remain on anthracycline treatment for longer periods of time, and may even allow some patients who would only be partial responders to achieve a complete response. However, these methods are unlikely to help the majority of patients who do not respond to anthracyclines. To improve response rates significantly for patients with soft-tissue sarcomas, new agents with activity against the tumor are needed. Numerous agents have been tested over the last 10 years, but no agent with activity as great as that of Adriamycin in these tumors has been discovered. Nevertheless, this remains the most important area of chemotherapeutic research in patients with these tumors.

Stewart et al.[108] have published an excellent review of drug studies in patients with soft-tissue sarcomas in the 1970s.[108] More recently, a large number of additional compounds have been studied. As with Adriamycin, considerable interest has been focused on finding new derivatives of established drugs. For example, a number of new *Vinca* alkaloids, nitrosoureas, alkylating agents, antifolates, and derivatives of cisplatin are under development and some show significant promise as potential antitumor agents.

Antifolates

Several antifolates, in addition to methotrexte, have been tested in patients with sarcomas. Baker's antifol and N^6-benzyladenosine-5-monophosphate have not shown activity,[152–154] but metoprine, a new lipid-soluble antifolate does appear to have some minor activity. Alberto et al.[155] reported one partial response in 15 patients heavily pretreated with metoprine,[155] and Magill et al.[156] obtained two complete responses, two partial responses, and seven minor responses in 47 pretreated patients. It was hoped a higher response rate would be achieved with metoprine in previously untreated patients; however, only one CR was found in a subsequent study of 23 previously untreated patients.[157] Nevertheless, the minor activity seen with this drug and the responses reported with both high- and low-dose methotrexate[17, 86–91] have led to the testing of new antifolates.

Vinca Alkaloids

Because of the demonstrated activity of vincristine in embryonal rhabdomyosarcoma in children and suggestions of its activity in adults with soft-tissue sarcomas,[158–160] a number of *Vinca* alkaloids and other plant products have been tested (Table 34–10). Additional interest in this family of drugs is due to their different mechanism of action (compared with anthracyclines, antifolates, etc.) and the platelet-sparing effect of many of these compounds,[102, 160, 161] making them particularly attractive for combination chemotherapy. Studies report that vindesine has minor activity in patients with soft-tissue sarcomas.[103–105] Other than that reported for vincristine and vindesine, however, little activity has been seen with this class of compounds. VP-16-213 (etoposide), a semisynthetic podophyllotoxin, appeared to have no activity in patients with soft-tissue sarcomas in several different studies,[162–165] although this drug appeared to be quite active in patients with Kaposi's sarcoma and acquired immune deficiency syndrome (AIDS).[166] Likewise, VM-26 appears to be of no value in the treatment of patients with sarcomas.[162, 163] Maytansine, a naturally occurring ansa macrolide with antimitotic properties similar to those of the *Vinca* alkaloids, has also been tested extensively in patients with sarcomas via a variety of dose schedules,[167–171] but no activity in this tumor has been seen. In another study, no responses were seen among 30 patients receiving Velban (vinblastine) or vindesine by continuous infusion.[172]

Cisplatin

Cisplatin (CPDD) has attracted considerably interest because of its activity in a wide variety of cancers, including osteogenic sarcoma.[173, 174] Karakousis et al.[175] obtained three major responses in 13 patients with soft-tissue sarcomas, including two of seven patients receiving high dose CPDD (100 mg/m^2) and mannitol diuresis. However, studies with both high-dose[176, 177] and low-dose[178, 179] regimens have failed to confirm this observation (Table 34–11). Samson et al.[178] observed only three major responses in 42 patients (7%) receiving 15 mg/m^2/day of CPDD for 5 days. Likewise, Brenner et al.[176] reported only two partial responders among 34 pretreated patients (6%) taking CPDD at 120 mg/m^2. Follow-up studies in previously untreated patients have also shown only two responses in 26 patients (8%).[180] A number of cisplatin, derivatives, some without the severe nephrotoxicity of cisplatin, are currently being evaluated in other types of cancer,[181, 182] but none of these compounds has been thoroughly tested in patients with sarcoma. Another heavy metal compound, gallium nitrate, an anhydrous salt of gallium, despite suggestions of activity against sarcomas in early phase I trials,[183, 184] has been shown to be inactive in subsequent phase II studies.[184, 185]

Nitrosoureas

Nitrosoureas have generated interest because of their activity in lymphomas and other tumors.[186] As mentioned previously, methyl CCNU was reported to produce a 49% response rate when combined with Adriamycin,[99] although subsequent studies have not been able to confirm the effectiveness of methyl CCNU.[4, 31, 85, 100] Other nitrosoureas, such as BCNU (carmustine) and CCNU (lomustine), have been reported to have activity,[18, 187, 188] although in most cases these drugs have not been adequately studied. One trial of CCNU, however, showed only two partial responses in 20 patients with this tumor (10%).[10] Chlorozotocin,

TABLE 34–10.
Activity of *Vinca* Alkaloid Drugs in Adults With Soft-Tissue Sarcomas

Drug	Number of Evaluable Patients	CR	PR	MRR (%)
Vincristine[106]	14	0	2	14
Vindesine[104, 105]	49	1	4	10
Vindesine[172]—continuous infusion	15	0	0	0
Velban[172]—continuous infusion	15	0	0	0
VP-16-213[163–165]	71	0	2	3
VM-26[163]	20	0	0	0

TABLE 34–11.
Trials of Cisplatin in Patients With Soft-Tissue Sarcomas

Dose	Patients	CR	PR	MRR (%)
1 mg/kg[175]	6	1	0	16
100 mg/m^2 [175]	7	1	1	28
120 mg/m^2 [176]	34	0	2	6
110–120 mg/m^2 [177]	17	0	0	0
15 mg/m^2 for 5 days[178]	42	0	3	7
20 mg/m^2 for 4 days[179]	8	0	0	0
120 mg/m^2 [180]	26	0	2	8

a water-soluble nitrosourea, was initially reported to have some activity in patients with sarcomas, but this has not been confirmed in subsequent phase II trials.[189–191] A number of newer nitrosoureas with activity comparable to or greater than that of these compounds in animal systems have been developed.[192, 193] Most have not been evaluated at all in patients with sarcomas, or only in small numbers of heavily pretreated patients, so the activity of these compounds is not known.[108]

Alkylating Agents

Alkylating agents have not been shown to have much activity in adults with soft-tissue sarcomas. Cyclophosphamide is definitely an active drug in children with embryonal rhabdomyosarcoma,[2, 82, 187] and it appears to have some minor activity as a single agent in adults with soft-tissue sarcomas as well.[194, 195] A number of alkylating agents, including hexamethylmelamine,[187, 196, 197] yoshi 864,[198] dianhydrogalactitol,[199] and prednimustine,[200] a prednisolone ester of chlorambucil, have been studied in phase II trials. None of these agents has shown activity against soft-tissue sarcomas. There was a suggestion of minor activity against these tumors with dibromodulcitol, as shown by five responses in 42 patients.[201] However, a more recent trial of this agent produced only one partial response in 45 patients (2%).[167] Most other alkylating agents have not been studied in sufficient numbers of patients with sarcomas to draw conclusions as to their activity.

Antitumor Antibiotics

Among antitumor antibiotics, pyrazofurin,[202, 203] piperazinedione,[204, 205] and neocarzinostatin[108, 206] have been shown to be inactive. Azotomycin has been reported to have some activity, with five responses reported in 25 patients from three separate studies,[207–209] although the severe nausea and vomiting and the other side effects seen will limit the effectiveness of this drug even if its activity is confirmed.[208]

Other New Agents

Miscellaneous agents including methylglyloxal-bis(guanylhydrazone) (methyl-GAG),[210, 211] cycloleucine,[9, 10, 212, 213] 4′-(9-acrydinylamino)-methanesulfon-*m*-anisidide (*m*-AMSA),[215–217] cytembena,[217, 218] anguidine,[219] diglycoaldehyde,[220] mitoxantrone,[221] *N*-phosphonacetyl-L-aspartate (PALA),[222] lonidamine,[224] 5-azacytidine,[10] and razoxane,[167, 224] have also been tested. Only cycloleucine at a dosage of 300 mg/kg/day for 8 days showed any activity, with 14 of 88 patients in three studies (16%) achieving partial responses (Table 34–12).[9, 10, 212] However, treatment with cycloleucine at this dosage was accompanied by severe toxicity, including marked thrombocytopenia and severe central nervous system depression.[9] Razoxane, although having no activity alone, may have value as a radiosensitizing agent.[224–226]

Many other agents have been tested only in phase I trials, which usually include only a few patients with soft-tissue sarcomas.[108] Because of the rarity of this type of tumor, only a limited number of agents can be studied in phase II trails against this disease. Prescreening of drugs against human sarcomas heterotransplanted into nude mice[103, 227] or utilizing a human tumor-cloning system[228] may aid in the selection of the most promising chemotherapeutic agents for evaluation in phase II trials.

TABLE 34–12.
Phase II Trials of Cycloleucine in Patients With Soft-Tissue Sarcomas

Dose	Number of Evaluable Patients	CR	PR	MRR (%)
200 mg/kg/day for 8 days[9]	51	0	3	6
300 mg/kg/day for 8 days[9]	51	0	7	14
300 mg/kg/day for 8 days[10]	9	0	0	0
300 mg/kg/day for 8 days[213]	28*	0	7	25
40–52 g/m^2 [214]	14	0	0	0

* *Includes responses in six of 14 patients with leiomyosarcoma.*

Ifosfamide

There have been several promising reports concerning the activity of ifosfamide, an oxazaphosphorine similar to cyclophosphamide, in patients with soft-tissue sarcomas. Scheulen et al.[229] reported two complete responses and three partial responses in 16 patients (30% major response rate). Likewise, Stuart-Harris et al.[230] noted six complete responses and nine partial responses in 42 patients, a 38% response rate. Niederle et al.[231] reported three complete responses and 14 partial responses in 57 patients (30%) who received either ifosfamide alone or ifosfamide with cisplatin; the response rate to ifosfamide alone in this study was not reported. Other reports[232] of the activity of ifosfamide in smaller numbers of patients with this tumor have also appeared. Further studies of ifosfamide in patients with sarcomas are certainly warranted, both as a single agent and in combination with Adriamycin.

SUMMARY

The only drug with major activity in adult patients with soft-tissue sarcomas is Adriamycin, and Adriamycin alone or in combination must be regarded as standard therapy for patients with these tumors. The combination of DTIC, cyclophosphamide, and vincristine with Adriamycin (CYVADIC) may increase the response rate in these patients from the 20% to 30% seen with Adriamycin alone to perhaps 35% to 50%. However, the addition of drugs such as methotrexate, actinomycin D, or other agents to an Adriamycin-based combination has not only been ineffective in increasing the response rate but has, in fact, generally given lower response rates than those seen with CYVADIC. Most authors think there is a sharp dose-response curve for Adriamycin, with 75 mg/m^2 being more effective than 45 mg/m^2. Doses of at least 60 to 75 mg/m^2 of Adriamycin every 3 weeks should be used when possible. The potential for Adriamycin cardiotoxicity, usually at cumulative doses greater than 450 to 550 mg/m^2, significantly limits the use of Adriamycin over long periods of time. Work has focused on increasing the response rate or decreasing the cardiotoxicity of Adriamycin by administering it in 72- to 96-hour continuous infusion, or through development of new, less cardiotoxic Adriamycin derivatives. It is too early to tell how successful these approaches will be, although it does appear that the 96-hour continuous infusion method of administration will prove less cardiotoxic than bolus injection.

The other major area of chemotherapy research for patients with these tumors is the evaluation of new agents. A number of new nitrosoureas, antifolates, *Vinca* alkaloids, alkalating agents, and other drugs are currently under study. Although many of these drugs have been tested in patients with soft-tissue sarcomas over the last several years without positive results, the search for new agents is probably the most important approach by which chemotherapy for patients with these tumors will ultimately be improved.

ACKNOWLEDGMENTS

The author wishes to thank Dr. R. B. Golbey for helpful comments and suggestions, and Ms. E. Abel for excellent secretarial assistance.

REFERENCES

1. Donaldson SS, Castro JR, Wilbur JR, et al: Rhabdomyosarcoma of the head and neck in children: Combination treatment by surgery, irradiation, and chemotherapy. *Cancer* 1973; 31:26–35.
2. Pratt CB: Response of childhood rhabdomyosarcoma to combination chemotherapy. *J Pediatr* 1969; 74:791–794.
3. Jaffe N, Filler RM, Farber S, et al: Rhabdomyosarcoma in children: Improved outlook with a multidisciplinary approach. *Am J Surg* 1973; 125:482–487.
4. Creagan ET, Hahn RG, Abmann DL, et al: A comparative clinical trial evaluating the combination of Adriamycin (NSC-123127), imidazole carboxamide (NSC-45388), vincristine (NSC-67574), the combination actinomycin-D (NSC-3053), cyclophosphamide (NSC-26271), vincristine and a single agent, methyl CCNU (NSC-95441) in advanced sarcomas. *Cancer Treat Rep* 1976; 60:1385–1386.
5. Schoenfeld DA, Rosenbaum C, Horten J, et al: A comparison of adriamycin versus vincristine and Adriamycin and cyclophosphamide versus vincristine, actinomycin-D and cyclophosphamide for advanced sarcoma. *Cancer* 1982; 50:2757–2762.
6. Bonadonna G, Monfardini S, DeLena M, et al: Phase I and preliminary phase II evaluation of Adriamycin (NSC-123127). *Cancer Res* 1970; 30:2572–2582.
7. Blum RH: An overview of studies with adriamycin (NSC-123127) in the United States. Part 3. *Cancer Chemother Rep* 1975; 6:247–251.
8. Mouridsen HT, Bramwell V, Mulder JH, et al: Adriamycin vs. carminomycin in advanced soft tissue sarcomas: A preliminary analysis of the EORTC soft tissue and bone sarcoma group. Paper presented at 3rd NCI-EORTC symposium of new drugs in cancer therapy. Brussels, October, 1981.
9. Savlov ED, MacIntyre JM, Knight E, et al: Comparison of doxorubicin with cycloleucine in the treatment of sarcomas. *Cancer Treat Rep* 1981; 65:21–27.
10. Mitts DL, Gerhardt H, Armstrong DM, et al: Chemotherapy for advanced soft tissue sarcomas: Results of phase I and II cooperative studies. *Tex Med* 1979; 75:43–47.
11. Cruz AB Jr, Thames EA Jr, Aust JB, et al: Combination chemotherapy for soft-tissue sarcomas: A phase III study. *J Surg Oncol* 1979; 11:313–323.
12. O'Bryan RM, Baker LH, Gottlieb JE, et al: Dose response evaluation of Adriamycin in human neoplasia. *Cancer* 1977; 39:1940–1948.
13. Creagan ET, Hahn RG, Ahmann DL, et al: A clinical trial of adriamycin (NSC-123127) in advanced sarcomas. *Oncology* 1977; 34:90–91.
14. Pinedo HM, Vendrik CPJ, Staquet M, et al: EORTC randomized trial for metastatic soft-tissue sarcoma. *Eur J Cancer* 1978; 13:765–771.
15. Pinedo HM, van Oosterom AT: Treatment of advanced soft-tissue sarcomas in adults: Past, present and future, in van Oosterom AT, et al (eds): *Therapeutic Progress in Ovarian Cancer, Testicular Cancer and the Sarcomas.* The Hague, Martinus Nijhoff, Leiden Univ Holland, Kluwer Academic, 1980, pp 425–438.
16. Yap BS, Baker LH, Sinkovics J: Cyclophosphamide, vincristine, adriamycin and DTIC (CYVADIC) combination chemotherapy for treatment of advanced sarcomas. *Cancer Treat Rep* 1980; 64:93–98.
17. Wiltshaw E, Harmer CL, McKinna JA: Soft-tissue sarcoma: Treatment of advanced disease in the Royal Marsden Hospital, in van Oosterom AT, et al (eds): *Therapeutic Progress in Ovarian Cancer, Testicular Cancer and the Sarcomas.* The Hague, Martinus Nijhoff, Leiden Univ Holland, Kluwer Academic, 1980, pp 413–424.
18. Rosenberg SA, Suit HD, Baker LH, et al: Sarcomas of the soft tissue and bone, in DeVita VT Jr, Hellman S, Rosenberg SA (eds): *Cancer: Principles and Practice of Oncology.* Philadelphia, J. B. Lippincott, 1982, pp 1036–1093.
19. Presant CA, Lowenbraun S, Bartolucci AA, et al: Metastatic sarcomas: Chemotherapy with adriamycin, cyclophosphamide, and methotrexate alternating with actinomycin D, DTIC, and vincristine. *Cancer* 1981; 47:457–465.
20. Gottlieb JA, Baker LH, O'Bryan RM, et al: Adriamycin (NSC-123127) used alone or in combination for soft tissue and bony sarcomas. Part 3. *Cancer Chemother Rep* 1975; 6:271–282.
21. Sordillo P, Chapman R, Hajdu S, et al: Lymphagiosarcoma. *Cancer* 1981; 48:1674–1679.
22. Sordillo P, Helson L, Hajdu SI, et al: Malignant schwannoma—clinical characteristics, survival and response to therapy. *Cancer* 1981; 47:2503–2509.

23. Benjamin RS, Baker LH, O'Bryan RM, et al: Advances in the chemotherapy of soft tissue sarcomas. *Med Clin N Am* 1977; 61:1039–1043.
24. Sordillo P, Hajdu SI, Magill GB, et al: Extraosseous osteogenic sarcoma: Review of 48 patients. *Cancer* 1983; 51:727–734.
25. Kruger G, Cheng E, Magill G, et al: Chemotherapy of leiomyosarcoma of the intestinal tract. *Proc Am Soc Clin Oncol* 1983; 23:235.
26. Goldin A, Johnson RK: Experimental tumor activity of adriamycin (NSC-123127). *Cancer Chemother Rep* 1975; 6:137–145.
27. Barranco SC, Gerner EW, Burk KH, et al: Survival and cell kinetics effects of Adriamycin on mammalian cells. *Cancer Res* 1973; 33:11–16.
28. Drewenko B, Gottlieb JA: Survival kinetics of cultured human lymphoma cells exposed to Adriamycin. *Cancer Res* 1973; 33:1141–1145.
29. Blum RH, Corson JM, Wilson RE, et al: Successful treatment of metastatic sarcomas with cyclophosphamide, Adriamycin, and DTIC (CAD). *Cancer* 1980; 46:1722–1726.
30. Bryant BM, Wiltshaw E: Results of the Royal Marsden Hospital second soft tissue sarcoma schedule (STS II) chemotherapy regimen in the management of advanced sarcoma. *Cancer Treat Rep* 1980; 64:689–692.
31. Magill GB, Golbey RB, Krakoff JH: Chemotherapy combinations in adult sarcomas. *Proc Am Soc Clin Oncol* 1977; 18:332.
32. Creagan ET, Edmonson JH, Hahn RG, et al: A preliminary study of cyclophosphamide (NSC-26271), Adriamycin (NSC-123127), imidazole carboxamide (NSC-45388), and actinomycin D (NSC-3053) with or without MER-BCG in patients with advanced sarcomas. *Med Pediatr Oncol* 1978; 4:85.
33. Wheeler RH, Ensminger WD, Thrall JH, et al: High dose doxorubicin: An exploration of the dose response curve in human neoplasia. *Cancer Treat Rep* 1982; 66:493–498.
34. Nagel GA: Tumortherapie mit Adriamycin in hohen Dosen, in Ghrone M, Fetzen J, Maier M (eds): *Ergebnisse der Adriamycin Therapie*. Berlin, Springer-Verlag, 1975, pp 119–123.
35. Friedman MA, Bozdeck MD, Billingham ME, et al: Doxorubicin cardiotoxicity, serial endomyocardial biopsies and systolic time intervals. *JAMA* 1978; 240;1603–1606.
36. Bristow MR, Billingham ME, Mason JW, et al: Clinical spectrum of anthracycline cardiotoxicity. *Cancer Treat Rep* 1978; 62:873–879.
37. Hag M, Legha S, Choksy J, et al: Natural history of Adriamycin-induced congestive heart failure in adults. *Proc Am Soc Clin Oncol* 1983; 2:231.
38. Chawla SP, Mann G, Benjamin RS, et al: Monitoring of Adriamycin cardiotoxicity beyond the conventional limits of 500 mg/m^2. *Proc Am Assoc Cancer Res* 1983; 24:134.
39. Dresdale A, Bonow RO, Wesley R, et al: Prospective evaluation of doxorubicin-induced cardiomyopathy resulting from postsurgical adjuvant treatment of patients with soft tissue sarcomas. *Cancer* 1983; 52:51–61.
40. Goorin AM, Borow KM, Goldman A, et al: Congetive heart failure due to Adriamycin cardiotoxicity. *Cancer* 1981; 47:2810–2816.
41. Torti FM, Bristow MR, Howes AE, et al: Endomyocardial biopsy evidence of reduced cardiotoxicity of doxorubicin delivered on a weekly schedule. *Proc Am Soc Clin Oncol* 1983; 2:26.
42. McDonald IG, Hobson ER: A comparison of the relative value of noninvasive techniques—echocardiography, systolic time intervals and apex cardiography—in the diagnosis of primary myocardial disease. *Am Heart J* 1974; 88:454–462.
43. Lefrak EA, Pitha J, Rosenheim S, et al: A clinicopathologic analysis of Adriamycin cardiotoxicity. *Cancer* 1973; 32:302–314.
44. Cortes EP, Lutman G, Wanka J, et al: Adriamycin (NSC-123127) cardiotoxicity: A clinicopathologic correlation. Part 3. *Cancer Chemother Rep* 1975; 6:215–225.
45. Minow RA, Benjamin RS, Gottlieb JA: Adriamycin (NSC-123127) cardiomyopathy—an overview with determination of risk factors. Part 3. *Cancer Chemother Rep* 1975; 6:195–201.
46. Olson HM, Young DM, Prieur DJ, et al: Electrolyte and morphologic alterations of myocardium in Adriamycin-treated rabbits. *Am J Pathol* 1974; 77:439–454.
47. Minow RA, Gottlieb JA: Adriamycin cardiotoxicity. *Ann Intern Med* 1975; 82:855–857.
48. Buzdar AU, Legha SS, Tashima CK, et al: Adriamycin and mitomycin C: Possible synergistic cardiotoxicity. *Cancer Treat Rep* 1978; 62:1005–1008.
49. Bristow MR, Mason JW, Billingham ME, et

al: Doxorubicin cardiomyopathy: Evaluation by phonocardiography, endomyocardial biopsy, and cardiac catherization. *Ann Intern Med* 1978; 88:168–175.

50. Von Hoff DD, Layard MW, Basa P, et al: Risk factors for doxorubicin induced congestive heart failure. *Ann Intern Med* 1979; 91:710–717.
51. Kushner JP, Hansen VL, Hammar SP: Cardiomyopathy after widely separated courses of Adriamycin exacerbated by actinomycin-D and mithramycin. *Cancer* 1975; 36:1577–1584.
52. Weiss AJ, Metter GE, Fletcher WS, et al: Studies on Adriamycin using a weekly regimen demonstrating its clinical effectiveness and lack of cardiac toxicity. *Cancer Treat Rep* 1976; 60:813–822.
53. Praga C, Beretta G, Vigo PL, et al: Adriamycin cardiotoxicity: A survey of 1273 patients. *Cancer Treat Rep* 1979; 63:827–834.
54. Ewy GA, Jones SE, Friedman JJ, et al: Noninvasive cardiac evaluation of patients receiving Adriamycin. *Cancer Treat Rep* 1978; 62:915–922.
55. Bloom KR, Bini RM, Williams CM, et al: Echocardiography in Adriamycin cardiotoxicity. *Cancer* 1978; 41:1265–1269.
56. Rinehart J, Lewis RP, Balcerak SP: Adriamycin cardiotoxicity in man. *Ann Intern Med* 1974; 81:475–478.
57. Henderson IC, Sloss LJ, Jaffe N, et al: Serial studies of cardiac functions in patients receiving Adriamycin. *Cancer Treat Rep* 1978; 62:923–929.
58. Mason JW, Bristow MR, Billingham ME, et al: Invasive and noninvasive methods of assessing Adriamycin cardiotoxic effects of man: Superiority of histologic assessment using endomyocardial biopsy. *Cancer Treat Rep* 1978; 62:857–864.
59. Friedman MJ, Ewy GA, Jones SE, et al: 1-year follow-up of cardiac status after Adriamycin therapy. *Cancer Treat Rep* 1979; 63:1809–1816.
60. Weaver SK, Fulkerson PK, Lewis RP, et al: A paucity of chronic electro-cardiographic changes with Adriamycin therapy. *J Electrocardiol* 1978; 11:233–238.
61. Kafkas P, Papqevanglou G, Kanaginu T, et al: Frequency of electrocardiographic alterations in patients with leukemia: Statistical analysis of 480 cases. *Ann Clin Res* 1973; 5:23–26.
62. Billingham M, Bristow M, Mason J, et al: Endomyocardial biopsy findings in Adriamycin treated patients. *Proc Am Assoc Cancer Res* 1976; 17:281.
63. Alexander J, Dainiak N, Berger HJ, et al: Serial assessment of doxorubicin cardiotoxicity with quantitative radionuclide angiocardiography. *N Engl J Med* 1979; 300:278–283.
64. Kennedy JW, Sorensen SG, Ritchie JL, et al: Radionuclide angiography for the evaluation of anthracycline therapy. *Cancer Treat Rep* 1978; 62:941–943.
65. Gottdiener JS, Mathieson DJ, Borer JS, et al: Doxorubicin cardiotoxicity: Assessment of late left ventricular dysfunction by radionuclide cineangiography. Part 1. *Ann Intern Med* 1981; 94:430–435.
66. Luce JK, Thurman WG, Isaacs BL, et al: Clinical trials with the anti-tumor agent 5-(3,3-dimethyl-1-triazeno)imidazole-4-carboxamide (NSC-45388). *Cancer Chemother Rep* 1970; 54:119–124.
67. Griswold DP, Laster WR JR, Schabel FM Jr: Therapeutic potentiation by Adriamycin and 5-(3,3-dimethyl-1-triazeno)imidazole-4-carboxamide (NSC-45388) against B16 melanoma, C3H breast carcinoma, Lewis lung carcinoma and leukemia L1210. *Proc Am Assoc Cancer Res* 1973; 14:15.
68. Goldin A: Some factors influencing the chemotherapeutic effectiveness of Adriamycin, in Carter SK, DiMarco A, Ghione M, et al (eds): *International Symposium on Adriamycin*. New York, Springer-Verlag, 1972, pp 64–74.
69. Gottlieb JA, Baker LH, Quagliana JM, et al: Chemotherapy of sarcomas with a combination of Adriamycin and dimethyl triazeno imidazole carboxamide. *Cancer* 1972; 30:1632–1638.
70. Karakousis CP, Rao U, Parks HC: Combination chemotherapy (CYVADIC) in metastatic soft tissue sarcomas. *Eur J Cancer Clin Oncol* 1982; 18:33–36.
71. Pinedo HM, Vendrik CPJ, Bramwell VHC, et al: Reevaluation of the CYVADIC regimen for metastatic soft-tissue sarcomas. *Proc Am Soc Clin Oncol* 1979; 20:346.
72. Schmidt M, Sodomann CP, Gropp C, et al: Treatment of metastasizing soft-tissue sarcoma with a uniform combination chemotherapy of cyclophosphamide, vincristine, Adriamycin and DTIC. *D Med Wschr* 1978; 103:1204–1206.
73. Benjamin RS, Gottlieb JA, Baker LH, et al: CYVADIC vs. CYVADACT — A randomized trial of cyclophosphamide (CY), vincristine (V) and Adriamycin (A) plus either

dacarbazine (DIC) or actinomycin-D (DACT) in metastatic sarcoma. *Proc Am Assoc Cancer Res* 1976 17:256.

74. Bui B, Chauvergne J, Durand M, et al: Palliative chemotherapy for adult soft tissue sarcomas with cyclophosphamide-vincristine-Adriamycin-dacarbazine (CYVADIC). *Bull Cancer (Paris)* 1981; 68:1–5.
75. Rodriquez V, Bodey GP, Freireich EJ: Increased remission rate and prolongation of survival in patients with soft tissue sarcomas treated with intensive chemotherapy on a protected environment — prophylactic antibiotic programme (PEPA). *Proc Am Soc Clin Oncol* 1977; 18:320.
76. Giuliano AE, Larkin KL, Eilber FR, et al: Failure of combination chemotherapy (CYVADIC) in metastatic soft-tissue sarcomas: Implications for adjuvant studies. *Proc Am Soc Clin Oncol* 1978; 19:359.
77. Livingston RB, Carter SK: *Single Agents in Cancer Therapy*. New York, IFI/Plenum, 1970.
78. Golbey R, Li MC, Kaufman RF: Actinomycin in the treatment of soft part sarcomas. James Ewing Society Scientific Program (Abstr.), 1968.
79. Brenner DE, Chang P, Wiernik PH: Doxorubicin and dactinomycin therapy for advanced sarcomas. *Cancer Treat Rep* 1981; 65:231–236.
80. Dalley DN, Levi JA, Nesbitt RA et al: Cyclical combination chemotherapeutic regimen in adult soft tissue sarcoma. *Cancer Clin Trials* 1981; 4:163–165.
81. Douglas HO Jr, Karakousis C: Alternating administration of Adriamycin (NSC-123127) and vincristine (NSC-67574)-actinomycin D (NSC-3053) in advanced sarcomas. *Cancer Chemother Rep* 1975; 59:1045–1047.
82. Pinedo HM, Kenis Y: Chemotherapy of advanced soft-tissue sarcomas in adults. *Cancer Treat Rev* 1977; 4:67–86.
83. Baker L, Benjamin R, Fine G, et al: Combination chemotherapy in the management of disseminated soft-tissue sarcomas — A Southwest Oncology Group Study. *Proc Am Soc Clin Oncol* 1979; 20:378.
84. Beretta G, Fraschini P, Tedeschi L: Chemotherapy of soft tissue sarcomas. *Oncology* 1980; 37 (suppl 1):92–96.
85. Yap BS, Benjamin RS, Burgess MA, et al: A phase II evaluation of methyl CCNU and actinomycin D in the treatment of advanced sarcomas in adults. *Cancer* 1981; 47:2807–2809.
86. Andrews N, Wilson W: Phase II study of methotrexate (NSC-740) in solid tumors. *Cancer Chemother Rep* 1967; 51:471–474.
87. Subramanian S, Wiltshaw E: Chemotherapy of sarcoma — a comparison of three regimens. *Lancet* 1978; 1:683–686.
88. Wiltshaw E: Methotrexate in treatment of sarcomata. *Br Med J* 1967; 2:142–145.
89. Karakousis C: High dose methotrexate in metastastic sarcomas. *Proc Am Soc Clin Oncol* 1978; 19:401.
90. Isacoff WH, Eilber F, Tabbarah H, et al: Phase II clinical trial with high dose methotrexate therapy and citrovorum factor rescue. *Cancer Treat Rep* 1978; 62:1295–1304.
91. Von Hoff DD, Rozencweig M, Louie AC, et al: "Single" agent activity of high dose methotrexate with citrovorum factor rescue. *Cancer Treat Rep* 1978; 62:233–235.
92. Ambinder EP, Perloff M, Ohnuma T, et al: High dose methotrexate followed by citrovorum factor reversal in patients with advanced cancer. *Cancer* 1979; 43:1177–1182.
93. Karakousis CP, Rao U, Carlson M: High-dose methotrexate as secondary chemotherapy in metastatic soft-tissue sarcomas. *Cancer* 1980; 46:1345–1348.
94. Bonadonna G, Santoro A: Bone and soft tissue sarcomas, in Pinedo HM (ed): *Cancer Chemotherapy* 4. New York, Elsevier, 1982, pp 373–396.
95. Lynch G, Magill GB, Sordillo P, et al: Combination chemotherapy of advanced sarcomas in adults with "CYOMAD" (S7). *Cancer* 1982; 50:1724–1727.
96. Lowenbraun S, Moffit S, Smalley R, et al: Combination chemotherapy with Adriamycin, cyclophosphamide and methotrexate (ACM) in metastatic sarcomas. *Proc Am Soc Clin Oncol* 1977; 18:286.
97. Kaufman JH, Catane R, Douglass HO Jr: Combined Adriamycin, vincristine and methotrexate in advanced adult soft-tissue sarcoma. *NY State J Med* 1977; 77:742–743.
98. Chang P, Wiernik PH: Combination chemotherapy with Adriamycin and streptozotocin. *Clin Pharmacol Ther* 1976; 20:605–610.
99. Rivkin SE, Gottlieb JA, Thigpen T, et al: Methyl CCNU and Adriamycin for patients with metastatic sarcomas — A Southwest Oncology Group Study. *Cancer* 1980; 46:446–451.
100. Tranum BP, Haut A, Rivkin SE, et al: A

phase II study of methyl CCNU in the treatment of solid tumors and lymphomas in the Southwest Oncology Group. *Cancer* 1974; 35:1148–1153.

101. Gralla RJ, Raphael BG, Golbey RB, et al: Phase II evaluation of vindesine in patients with non-small cell carcinoma of the lung. *Cancer Treat Rep* 1979; 63:1343–1346.

102. Smith IE, Hedley DW, Powles TJ, et al: Vindesine: A phase II study on the treatment of breast carcinoma, malignant melanoma, and other tumors. *Cancer Treat Rep* 1978; 62;1427–1433.

103. Sordillo PP, Hajdu SJ, Magill GB, et al: Effect of desacetyl vinblastine amide (DVA) against human sarcomas heterotransplanted in nude mice. *Cancer Clin Trials* 1980; 3:391–394.

104. Banerjee TK, Ousley JL, Mazza JJ, et al: Vindesine response in a phase II trial in malignant tumors. *Proc Am Soc Clin Oncol* 1983; 2:225.

105. Sordillo PP, Magill GB, Gralla RJ: Phase II evaluation of vindesine sulfate in patients with advanced sarcomas. *Cancer Treat Rep* 1981; 65:515–516.

106. Brenner J, Magill GB, Wissel P, et al: Chemotherapy of patients with advanced soft tissue sarcoma with DVA (vindesine sulfate), Adriamycin and cyclophosphamide (DAC). *Cancer* 1983; 52:1142–1145.

107. Yap BS, Sinkovic JG, Benjamin RS, et al: Survival and relapse patterns of complete responders in adults with advanced soft tissue sarcomas. *Proc Am Assoc Cancer Res* 1979; 20:352.

108. Stewart DJ, Benjamin RS, Baker LH, et al: New drugs for the treatment of soft tissue sarcomas, in van Oosterom AT, et al (eds): *Therapeutic Progress in Ovarian Cancer, Testicular Cancer and the Sarcomas*. The Hague, Martnius Nijhoff, 1980, pp 453–480.

109. Kaizer H, Leventhal BG, Santos GW, et al: The use of cryopreserved autologous bone marrow-lethal chemoradiotherapy in the treatment of selected pediatric malignancies. *Proc Am Assoc Cancer Res* 1978; 19:402.

110. Benjamin R, Legha S, Mackay B, et al: Reduction of Adriamycin cardiac toxicity using a prolonged continuous intravenous infusion. *Proc Am Assoc Cancer Res* 1981; 22:179.

111. Legha S, Benjamin R, Ewer M, et al: Reduction of Adriamycin cardiotoxicity by continuous IV infusion: The effect of duration of infusion on cardiotoxicity. *Proc Am Assoc Cancer Res* 1982; 23:127.

112. Green MD, Speyer JS, Blum R, et al: The effect of 6 hour infusions of Adriamycin (ADR) on toxicity. *Proc Am Soc Clin Oncol* 1983; 2:26.

113. Benjamin RS, Chawla SP, Ewer MS, et al: Cardiac toxicity of high-cumulative-dose Adriamycin by rapid or 24-96 hour continuous infusion. *Proc Am Soc Clin Oncol* 1983; 2:40.

114. Hortobagyi G, Frye D, Blumenschein G, et al: FAC with Adriamycin by continuous infusion for treatment of advanced breast cancer. *Proc Am Soc Clin Oncol* 1983; 2:105.

115. Rosenthal CJ, Bhutiani I, Rotman MC, et al: Efficacy of Adriamycin by continuous infusion and concurrent radiation therapy for recurrent and metastatic sarcoma. *Proc Am Soc Clin Oncol* 1983; 2:238.

116. Durand RE: Adriamycin: A possible indirect radiosensitizer of hypoxic tumor cells. *Radiology* 1976; 119:217–222.

117. Schaeffer J, El-Mahdi AM: Combination Adriamycin-radiation treatment of pulmonary tumors in mice. *Oncology* 1981; 38:35–38.

118. Bistrovic M, Nagy B, Maricic Z, et al: Interaction of Adriamycin and radiation in combined treatment of mouse L-cells. *Eur J Cancer* 1978; 14:411–414.

119. Watring WG, Byfield JE, Lagasse LD, et al: Combination Adriamycin and radiation therapy in gynecologic cancers. *Gynecol Oncol* 1974; 2:518–526.

120. Kolaric K, Maricic Z, Roth A, et al: Adriamycin alone and in combination with radiotherapy in the treatment of inoperable esophageal cancer. *Tumori* 1977; 63:485–491.

121. Sordillo PP, Magill GB, Schauer PK, et al: Preliminary trial of combination therapy with Adriamycin and radiation in sarcomas and other malignant tumors. *J Surg Oncol* 1982; 21:23–26.

122. DiPietro S, Depalo G, Gennari L, et al: Cancer chemotherapy by intraarterial infusion with Adriamycin. *J Surg Oncol* 1973; 5:521–530.

123. Haskell CM, Eilber ER, Morton DL: Adriamycin (NSC-123127) by arterial infusion. *Cancer Chemother Rep* 1975; 6:187–189.

124. Haskell CM, Silverstein MJ, Ranzel D, et al: Multimodality cancer therapy in man: A pilot study of Adriamycin by arterial infusion. *Cancer* 1974; 33:1485–1490.

125. Shah P, Baker LH, Vaitkevicius VK: Preliminary experiences in intra-arterial

Adriamycin. *Cancer Treat Rep* 1977; 61:1565–1567.

126. Karakousis CP, Lopez R, Catane R, et al: Intra-arterial Adriamycin in the treatment of soft tissue sarcomas. *J Surg Oncol* 1980; 13:21–27.
127. Morton DL, Eilber FR, Weisenburger TH, et al: Limb salvage using preoperative intra-arterial Adriamycin and radiation therapy for extremity soft tissue sarcomas. *Aust N Z J Surg* 1978; 48:56–59.
128. Weisenburger TH, Eilber FH, Grant TT, et al: Multidisciplinary "limb salvage" treatment of soft tissue and skeletal sarcomas. *Int J Radiat Oncol Biol Phys* 1981; 7:1495.
129. Morton DL, Eilber FR, Townsend CM Jr, et al: Limb salvage from a multidisciplinary treatment approach for skeletal and soft tissue sarcomas of the extremity. *Ann Surg* 1976; 184:268–278.
130. Guiliano AE, Eilber FR, Morton DL: Limb salvage by multimodality management of locally recurrent soft tissue sarcoma. *Proc Am Soc Clin Oncol* 1982; 1:179.
131. Azzarelli A, Quagliuolo V, Audisio RA, et al: Intra-arterial Adriamycin followed by surgery for limb sarcomas: Preliminary report. *Eur J Cancer Clin Oncol* 1983; 19:885–890.
132. Rozencweig M, Kenis Y, Atassi G, et al: DNA-Adriamycin complex: Preliminary results in animals and man. Part 3, *Cancer Chemother Rep* 1975; 6:131–136.
133. Langlet A, Pye I, Lie SO: Decreased cardiac toxicity of Adriamycin and daunorubicin when bound to DNA. *Acta Pharmacol Toxicol* 1974; 35:379–385.
134. Trouet A, Deprez-de Campeneere D, DeSmeldt-Malengreu M, et al: Experimental leukemia chemotherapy with a "lysosomotrophic" Adriamycin-DNA complex. *Eur J Cancer* 1974; 10:405–411.
135. Hall SW, Benjamin RS, Burgess MA, et al: Doxorubicin-DNA complex: A phase I clinical trial. *Cancer Treat Rep* 1982; 66:2033–2037.
136. Doroshow JH, Locker GY, Myers CE: The enzymatic defense of the mouse heart against reactive oxygen metabolite. *J Clin Invest* 1980; 65:128–135.
137. Sonneveld P: Effect of alpha tocopherol on the cardiotoxicity of Adriamycin in the rat. *Cancer Treat Rep* 1978; 62:1033–1036.
138. Myers CE, McGuire W, Young R: Adriamycin amelioration of toxicity by alpha tocopherol. *Cancer Treat Rep* 1976; 60:961–962.
139. Dresdale AR, Barr LH, Bonow RO, et al: Prospective randomized study of the role of *N*-acetyl cysteine in reversing doxorubicin-induced cardiomyopathy. *Am J Clin Oncol* 1982; 5:657–683.
140. Arcamone F, Penco S, Vigevani A, et al: Synthesis and antitumor properties of new glycosides of daunomycinone and adriamycinone. *J Med Chem* 1975; 18:703–707.
141. Zbinden G, Brandle E: Toxicologic screening of daunorubicin (NSC-82151), Adriamycin (NSC-123127), and their derivatives in rats. *Cancer Chemother Rep* 1975; 59:707–715.
142. Casazza AM, Bellini O, Savi G, et al: Antitumor activity and cardiac toxicity of 4′-deoxydoxorubicin (4′-deoxy-DX) in mice. *Proc Am Assoc Cancer Res* 1981; 22:267.
143. Villani F, Piccinini F, Favalli L: Anthracycline analogs: Correlation between calcium turnover in guinea pig atria and cardiotoxicity in humans, in Nelson JD, Grossi C (eds): *Current Chemotherapy and Infectious Disease*, Washington, D.C., American Society of Microbiology, 1980, pp 1696–1698.
144. Unverferth DV, Balzerak SP, Neidhart JA: Cardiac evaluation of aclacinomycin (ACLAC) and dihydroxyanthracenedione (DHAD). *Proc Am Assoc Cancer Res* 1982; 23:135.
145. Casazza AM, DiMarco A, Bonadonna G, et al: Effects of modifications in position 4 of the chromophore or in position 4′ of the aminosugar, on the antitumor activity of daunorubicin and doxorubicin, in Cooke ST, Reich SD (eds): *Anthracyclines: Current Status and New Developments*. New York, Academic Press, 1980, pp 404–430.
146. Perevodchikova NI, Lichinitser MR, Gorbunova VA: Phase I clinical study of carminomycin: Its activity against soft tissue sarcomas. *Cancer Treat Rep* 1977; 61:1705–1707.
147. Ganzina F: 4′-Epi-doxorubicin, a new analogue of doxorubicin: A preliminary overview of preclinical and clinical data. *Cancer Treat Rev* 1983; 10:1–22.
148. Salmon SE, Liu RM, Casazza AM: Evaluation of new anthracycline analogs with the human tumor stem cell assay. *Cancer Chemother Pharmacol* 1981; 6:103–110.
149. Raymond V, Magill GB, Welt S, et al: 4-Demethoxydaunorubicin (DMDR) in advanced soft tissue sarcomas (STS). *Proc Am Soc Clin Oncol* 1983; 2:235.
150. Magill GB: Personal communication.
151. Chauvergne J, Carton M, Berlie J, et al:

Essai de chimiotherapie anticancereuse par la duborimycine. *Bull Cancer* 1976; 63:41–57.

152. Rodriguez V, Gottlieb J, Burgess MA, et al: Phase I studies with Baker's antifol (BAF) (NSF 139105). *Cancer* 1976; 38:690–694.

153. Thigpen JT, O'Bryan RM, Benjamin RS, et al: Phase II trial of Baker's antifol in metastatic sarcoma. *Cancer Treat Rep* 1977; 61:1485–1487.

154. Catane R, Kaufman JH, Nime FA, et al: Phase I study of N^6-benzyladenosine-5′ monophosphate. *Cancer Treat Rep* 1978; 62:1371–1373.

155. Alberto P, DeJager RL, Brugarolas A, et al: Phase II study of diamino-dichlorophenyl-methylpyrimidine with folinic acid protection and rescue. *Proc Am Assoc Cancer Res* 1979; 20:323.

156. Magill GB, Brenner J, Sordillo P, et al: Phase II trials of metoprine (DDMP) in pretreated adults with advanced soft tissue sarcomas. *Proc Am Assoc Cancer Res* 1982; 23:22.

157. Welt S, Magill GB, Sordillo PP, et al: Metoprine therapy of advanced sarcomas in previously untreated adults. *Proc Am Assoc Cancer Res* 1983; 24:149.

158. Selawry OS, Holland JF, Wolman IJ: Effect of vincristine (NSC-67574) on malignant solid tumors in children. *Cancer Chemother Rep* 1968; 52:497–499.

159. Korbitz BC, Davis HL Jr, Ramirez G, et al: Low doses of vincristine (NSC-67574) for malignant disease. *Cancer Chemother Rep* 1969; 53:249–254.

160. Holland JF, Scharlau C, Gailani S, et al: Vincristine treatment of advanced cancer: A cooperative study of 392 cases. *Cancer Res* 1973; 33:1258–1264.

161. Rossof AH, Chandra G, Walter J, et al: Phase II trial of vindesine (desacetyl vinblastine amide sulfate, VND) in advanced metastatic cancer. *Proc Am Asoc Cancer Res* 1979; 20:146.

162. Bleyer WA, Chard RL, Krivit W, et al: Epipodophyllotoxin therapy of childhood neoplasia: A comparative phase II analysis of VM-26 and VP 16-213. *Proc Am Assoc Cancer Res* 1978; 19:373.

163. Radice PA, Bunn PA Jr, Ihde DC: Therapeutic trials with VP-16-213 and VM-26: Active agents in small cell lung cancer, non-Hodgkin's lymphomas and other malignancies. *Cancer Treat Rep* 1979; 63:1231–1239.

164. Welt S, Magill GB, Sordillo PP, et al: Phase II trial of VP-16-213 in adults with advanced soft tissue sarcomas. *Proc Am Soc Clin Oncol* 1983; 2:234.

165. Santoro A, Bonfante V, Bonadonna G: Phase II study of etoposide (VP-16) in malignant lymphomas and solid tumors. Paper presented at the International Symposium on New Drugs for Cancer Therapy in the Eighties. Rome, 10-11 April, 1981.

166. Laubenstein LF, Krigel RL, Hymes KB, et al: Treatment of epidemic Kaposi's sarcoma with VP 16-213 (Etoposide) and a combination of doxorubicin, bleomycin and vinblastine (ABV). *Proc Am Soc Clin Oncol* 1983; 2:228.

167. Borden EC, Ash A, Enterline HT, et al: Phase II evaluation of dibromodulcitol, ICRF-159, and maytansine for sarcomas. *Am J Clin Oncol* 1982; 5:417–420.

168. Edmonson JH, Hahn RG, Creagan ET, et al: Phase II study of maytansine in advanced sarcomas. *Cancer Treat Rep* 1983; 67:401–402.

169. Wasserman P: Maytansine in advanced sarcomas. *Proc Am Soc Clin Oncol* 1981; 22:524,

170. Eagan RT, Ingle JN, Rubin J, et al: Early clinical study of an intermittent schedule for maytansine (NSC-153858): Brief communication. *J Natl Cancer Inst* 1978; 60:93–96.

171. Blum RH, Kahlert T: Maytansine: A phase I study of an ansa macrolide with antitumor activity. *Cancer Treat Rep* 1978; 62:435–438.

172. Yap BS, Benjamin RS, Plager C, et al: A randomized study of continuous infusion vindesine versus vinblastine in adults with refractory metastatic sarcomas. *Am J Clin Oncol* 1983; 6:235–138.

173. Ochs JJ, Freeman AJ, Douglass HO, et al: Cis chlorodiammineplatinum (II) in advanced osteogenic sarcoma. *Cancer Treat Rep* 1978; 62:239–245.

174. Rosen G, Nireberg A, Caparros B, et al: Cis-diamminedichloroplatinum (II) in metastatic osteogenic sarcoma, in Croke ST, Carter S (eds): *Current Status and New Developments with Cisplatin*. New York, Academic Press, 1980, pp 465–475.

175. Karakousis CP, Holtermann OA, Holyoke ED: Cis-dichlorodiammineplatinum (II) in metastatic soft tissue sarcomas. *Cancer Treat Rep* 1979; 63:2071–2075.

176. Brenner J, Magill GB, Sordillo PP, et al:

Phase II trial of cisplatin (CPDD) in previously treated patients with advanced soft tissue sarcoma. *Cancer* 1982; 50:2031–2033.

177. Bramwell VHC, Brugarolas A, Mouridsen HT, et al: EORTC phase II study of cisplatin in CYVADIC-resistant soft tissue sarcoma. *Eur J Cancer* 1979; 15:1511–1513.

178. Samson MK, Baker LH, Benjamin RS, et al: Cis-dichlorodiammineplatinum (II) in advanced soft tissue and bony sarcomas: A Southwest Oncology Group Study. *Cancer Treat Rep* 1979; 63:2027–2029.

179. Sarna G, Skinner DG, Smith RB, et al: Cis-diamminedichloroplatinum (II) alone and in combination in the treatment of testicular and other malignancies. *Cancer Treat Rep* 1980; 64:1077–1082.

180. Brenner J: Personal communication.

181. Lee FH, Canetta R, Issell BF, et al: New platinum complexes in clinical trials. *Cancer Treat Rev* 1983; 10:39–51.

182. Sternberg CN, Cheng E, Sordillo PP, et al: Preliminary phase II trial of 1,2-diaminocyclohexane-(4-carboxyphthalato)platinum (II) (DACCP) in colorectal carcinomas. *Proc Am Soc Clin Oncol* 1983; 2:36.

183. Brown J, Santos E, Rosen G, et al: Phase I study of gallium nitrate in patients with advanced cancer. *Proc Am Assoc Cancer Res* 1979; 19:198.

184. Samson MK, Fraile RJ, Baker LH, et al: Phase I-II clinical trial of gallium nitrate (NSC-15200). *Cancer Clin Trials* 1980; 3:131–136.

185. Saiki JH, Baker LH, Stephens RL, et al: Gallium nitrate in advanced soft tissue and bone sarcomas: A Southwest Oncology Group Study. *Cancer Treat Rep* 1982; 66:1673–1674.

186. Weiss RB, Issell BF: The nitrosoureas: carmustine (BCNU) and lomustine (CCNU). *Cancer Treat Rev*. 1982; 9:313–330.

187. Wasserman TH, Comis RL, Goldsmith M, et al: Tabular analysis of the clinical chemotherapy solid tumors. *Cancer Chemother Rep* 1975; 6:399–419.

188. Slavik M: Clinical studies with nitrosoureas in various solid tumors. *Cancer Treat Rep* 1976; 60:795–800.

189. Sordillo P, Magill GB, Gralla RJ: Chlorozotocin: Phase II evaluation in patients with advanced sarcomas. *Cancer Treat Rep* 1981; 65:513–514.

190. Mouridsen HT, Bramwell VHC, Lacave J, et al: Treatment of advanced soft tissue sarcoma with chlorozotocin: A phase II trial of the EORTC soft tissue and bone sarcoma group. *Cancer Treat Rep* 1981; 65:509–512.

191. Talley RW, Samson MK, Brownlee RW, et al: Phase II evaluation of chlorozotocin in advanced human cancers. *Eur J Cancer* 1981; 17:337–343.

192. Habs M, Reinbold H, Eisenbrand G, et al: Antitumor activity of new nitrosoureas on Yoshida sarcoma ascites cells implanted into the colon wall of rats. *J Cancer Res Clin Oncol* 1981; 101:285–302.

193. Zeller WJ, Eisenbrand G, Fiebig HH: Examination of four newly synthesized 2-chloroethylnitrosoureas in comparison with BCNU, CCNU, MeCCNU, chlorozotocin and hydroxyethyl-CNU in preterminal rat leukemia-L 5222. *J Cancer Res Clin Oncol* 1979; 95:43–49.

194. Bergsagel DE, Levin WC: A preliminary clinical trial of cyclophosphamide. *Cancer Chemother Rep* 1960; 8:120–134.

195. Korst DR, Johnson D, Frenkel EP, et al: Preliminary evaluation of the effect of cyclophosphamide on the course of human neoplasms. *Cancer Chemother Rep* 1960; 7:1–12.

196. Borden EC, Larson P, Ansfield FJ, et al: Hexamethylmelamine treatment of sarcomas and lymphomas. *Med Pediatr Oncol* 1977; 3:401–406.

197. Blum RH, Livingston RB, Carter SK: Hexamethylmelamine: A new drug with activity in solid tumors. *Eur J Cancer* 1973; 9:195–202.

198. Altman SJ, Metter GE, Nealon TF, et al: Yoshi 864 (l-propanol, 3,3′-iminodi-, dimenthanesulfonate ester, hydrochloride): A phase II study in solid tumors. *Cancer Treat Rep* 1978; 62:389–395.

199. Thigpen JT, Samson MK: Phase II trial of dianhydrogalactitol in advanced soft tissue and bony sarcomas: A Southwest Oncology Group Study. *Cancer Treat Rep* 1979; 63:553–555.

200. Karakousis CP, Didolkar MS, Ambrus JL, et al: Prednimustine in advanced soft tissue sarcomas. *Cancer Treat Rep* 1982; 66:201–202.

201. Mischler NE, Earhart RH, Carr B, et al: Dibromodulcitol. *Cancer Treat Rev* 1979; 6:191–204.

202. Gralla RJ, Sordillo PP, Magill GB: Phase II evaluation of pyrazofurin in patients with metastatic sarcoma. *Cancer Treat Rep* 1978; 62:1573–1574.

203. Cormier WJ, Hahn RG, Edmonson JH, et al: Phase II study of advanced sarcoma: Randomized trial of pyrazofurin versus a combination of cyclophosphamide, doxorubicin and cis-dichlorodiammineplatinum (II) CAP. *Cancer Treat Rep* 1980; 64:655–658.

204. Benjamin RS, Keating MJ, Valdivieso M, et al: Phase I-II study of piperazinedione in adults with solid tumors and acute leukemia. *Cancer Treat Rep* 1979; 63:939–943.

205. LaGasse L, Thigpen T, Morrison F: Phase II trial of piperazinedione in treatment of advanced endometrial carcinoma, uterine sarcoma nad vulvar carcinoma. *Proc Am Assoc Cancer Res* 1979; 20:388.

206. Griffin TW, Comis RL, Lokich JJ, et al: Phase I and preliminary phase II study of neocarzinostatin. *Cancer Treat Rep* 1978; 62:2019–2025.

207. Weiss AJ, Ramirez G, Grage T, et al: Phase II study of azotomycin (NSC-56654). *Cancer Chemother Rep* 1968; 52:611–614.

208. Chang P, Wiernik PH: Phase II study of azotomycin in sarcomas. *Cancer Treat Rep* 1977; 61:1719.

209. Sooriyaarachchi GS, Ramirez G, Roley EL, et al: Hemangiopericytoma of the uterus. *J Surg Oncol* 1978; 10:399–406.

210. Warrell RP Jr, Burchenal JH: Methylglyloxal-bis(guanylhydrazone) (methyl-GAG): Current status and future prospects. *J Clin Oncol* 1983; 1:52–65.

211. Welt S, Magill GB, Sordillo PP, et al: A phase II study of methyl-GAG (methylglyloxal-bis(guanylhydrazone)) in patients with advanced sarcomas. *Proc Am Assoc Cancer Res* 1982; 23:146.

212. Aust JB, Andrews NC, Schroeder JM, et al: Clinical note: Phase II study of 1-aminocyclopentanecarboxylic acid (NSC-1026) in patients with cancer. *Cancer Chemother Rep* 1970; 54:237–241.

213. Baker LH, Fraile RJ, Samson MK: Phase II evaluation of cycloleucine in the treatment of patients with disseminated sarcomas. *Cancer Treat Rep* 1981; 65:358–359.

214. Sordillo P, Magill GB, Gralla RJ, et al: Phase II evaluation of 4′-(9-acridinylamino)-methanesulfon-*m*-anisidide (m-AMSA) in patients with advanced sarcomas. *Cancer Treat Rep* 1980; 64:1129–1130.

215. Yap BS, Plager C, Benjamin RS, et al: Phase II evaluation of AMSA in adult sarcomas. *Cancer Treat Rep* 1981; 65:341–343.

216. Sordillo P, Helson L, Lesser M: Evaluation of 4′-(9-acridinylamino)-methanesulfon-*m*-anisidide (m-AMSA) (NSC 249992) on human tumors in nude mice. *Cancer Clin Trials* 1980; 3:385–389.

217. Baker LH, Samson MK, Izbicki RM: Phase I and II evaluation of cytembena in dessem-inated epithelial cancer and sarcomas. *Cancer Treat Rep* 1976; 60:1389–1391.

218. Matejovsky Z: Effects of cytembena in the treatment of malignant musculoskeletal tumors. *Neoplasma* 1971; 18:473–480.

219. Thigpen JT, Vaughn C, Stuckey WJ: Phase II trial of anguidine in patients with sarcomas unresponsive to prior chemotherapy: A Southwest Oncology Group Study. *Cancer Treat Rep* 1981; 65:881–882.

220. Vosika GJ, Briscoe K, Carey RW, et al: Phase II study of diglycoaldehyde in malignant melanomas and soft tissue sarcomas. *Cancer Treat Rep* 1981; 65:823–825.

221. Smith IE: Mitoxantrone (Novantrone): A review of experimental and early clinical studies. *Cancer Treat Rev* 1983; 10:103–115.

222. Bramwell V, van Oosterom A, Mouridsen HT, et al: *N*-(Phosphonacetyl)-L-aspartate (PALA) in advanced soft tissue sarcoma: A phase II trial of the EORTC soft tissue sarcoma group. *Eur J Cancer Clin Oncol* 1982; 18:81–84.

223. Magill GB: Personal communication.

224. Dyment PG, Starling KA, Land VJ, et al: ICRF-159 (razoxane) in the treatment of pediatric solid tumors: A Southwest Oncology Group Study. *Cancer Treat Rep* 1979; 63:1397–1398.

225. Hellman K, Ryall RDH, MacDonald E, et al: Comparison of radiotherapy with or without razoxane (ICRF 159) in the treatment of soft tissue sarcomas. *Cancer* 1978; 41:100–107.

226. Rhomberg WJ: Radiotherapy combined with ICRF-159 (NSC 129943). *Int J Radiat Oncol Biol Phys* 1978; 4:121–126.

227. Sordillo P, Helson C, Lesser ML, et al: Effects of phase I and II chemotherapeutic agents against human lymphomas heterotransplanted in nude mice. *Oncology* 1983; 40:15–17.

228. Von Hoff DD, Clark GM, Stogdill BJ, et al: Prospective clinical trial of a human tumor cloning system. *Cancer Res* 1983; 43:1926–1931.

229. Scheulen MF, Niederle N, Bremer K, et al: Efficacy of ifosfamide in refractory malig-

nant diseases and uroprotection by MESNA: Results of a clinical phase II study with 151 patients. *Cancer Treat Rev* 1983; 10(A):93–101.

230. Stuart-Harris R, Harper PG, Kaye SB, et al: High-dose ifosfamide by infusion with MESNA in advanced soft tissue sarcoma. *Cancer Treat Rev* 1983; 10(A):163–164.

231. Niederle N, Scheulen MF, Cremer M, et al: Ifosfamide in combination chemotherapy for sarcoma and testicular carcinomas. *Cancer Treat Rev* 1983; 10(A):129–135.

232. Hilgard P, Herdrich K, Brade W: Ifosfamide—current aspects and perspectives. *Cancer Treat Rev* 1983; 10(A):183–192.

Chapter 35

Regional Chemotherapy by Isolation-Perfusion

Charles M. McBride*

A phrase currently in vogue in surgical oncology is "limb-sparing procedure." Until the late 1950s, most patients with soft-tissue sarcomas were treated by a major amputation. Subsequently, the concept of regional block dissection of muscle groups was developed, and adjuvant radiation therapy and regional chemotherapy was a natural evolution from this procedure. Regional chemotherapy by isolation-perfusion was developed in New Orleans in the mid-1950s[1] and has been used for the treatment of soft-tissue sarcomas of the limbs at the M. D. Anderson Cancer Center, Houston, TX, since the early 1960s. Regional chemotherapy permits a lesser dissection than required by a radical en bloc approach. For some parts of the limb, regional chemotherapy usually produces fewer undesirable side effects than when the area is treated with adjuvant radiation therapy (i.e., for tumors around the foot and ankle). Although regional chemotherapy by intra-arterial infusion is a more common form of therapy for soft-tissue sarcomas of the limbs today, the higher concentration of chemotherapeutic agent obtainable by isolation-perfusion seems to confer a survival advantage on these patients over other forms of therapy.[2]

* Deceased.

M. D. ANDERSON SERIES

In an effort to reduce the necessity for major amputations, 109 perfusions were performed on 105 patients with soft-tissue sarcomas of the limbs at the M. D. Anderson Cancer Center between January 1960 and August 1983. In most instances, the chemotherapeutic agents used were L-phenylalanine mustard and actinomycin D, and the perfusion was followed by local excision of the lesion 6 weeks later. The distribution of the patients by sex and involved limb is given in Table 35–1. Twenty-nine percent of these patients had liposarcoma, 17% unclassified sarcoma, 10% fibrosarcoma, 10% synovial sarcoma, 8% malignant fibrous histiocytoma, 7% angiosarcoma, 5% neurofibrosarcoma, 5% clear cell sarcoma of tendon sheath; 8% had other sarcomas such as rhabdomyosarcoma, leiomyosarcoma, extraskeletal osteogenic sarcoma, extraskeletal chondrosarcoma, and epithelioid sarcoma. Only one fifth of these sarcomas had been graded histologically, and of these more than 50% were high grade. Table 35–2 shows the raw survival statistics for these patients with different types of sarcoma as related to lesion size (≥5 cm in diameter versus <5 cm in diameter). The distribution by age and sex of the patients with sarcomas of the limbs is given in Figure 35–1.

TABLE 35–1.
Sarcoma Patient Distribution by Sex and Limb Involved

	Sex	
Limb	Males (57%)	Females (43%)
Arm	28%	24%
Leg	72%	76%

METHOD OF ISOLATION-PERFUSION

The selection of drug dosage for an individual depends on three factors: local tissue tolerance (i.e, a fair-skinned patient does not tolerate as high a dose of drug as a dark-skinned patient), leak of the drug into the systemic circulation during isolation-perfusion, and size of the patient. In the series of patients reported here, the median dose of L-phenylalanine mustard used in the leg was 1.3 mg/kg, and the median dose of actinomycin D was 0.3 mg/kg. In the arm, the median dosage of L-phenylalanine mustard was 0.7 mg/kg and for actinomycin D it was 0.02 mg/kg. Both drugs were given sequentially at the beginning of the perfusion, which normally lasted 1 hour. Iliac dissections and perfusions were performed on 50% of the patients; 27% had axillary perfusions, 14% had femoral perfusions, and 9% had popliteal perfusions.

Leakage of drug into the systemic circulation was monitored by placing a scintillation counter over the ventricular blood mass, injecting radioiodinated serum albumin into the pump circuit, and monitoring for appearance of this isotope in the systemic circulation.[3] The dissection was checked and the tourniquet adjusted until the rate of leakage from the perfusion circuit was such that it would not exceed 15% during the 1-hour period. When this was established, the drugs were injected into the isolation-perfusion circuit.

RESULTS

The survival curves for the 105 sarcoma patients, uncorrected for age at diagnosis or cause of death, are given in Figure 35–2. Of the patients with soft-tissue sarcomas of the limbs, 88 had at least 5 years of follow-up; the status of their disease at that time is given in Table 35–3. The regional recurrence rate for these patients was 19%; an additional 22% had developed systemic metastases by that time. Of the patients who developed regional recurrence during the 5 years following isolation-perfusion, 53% were salvaged by retreatment via such modalities as local re-excision, major amputation, radiation therapy, or a combination of these. Only 5% of those developing systemic metastases before local failure were alive at 5 years.

The high doses of drugs necessary with this technique to obtain local control of soft-tissue sarcomas in the limbs may result in complications. As seen in Table 35–4, 10% of the patients subsequently required amputation, either for recurrent disease (six patients) or due to complications from the perfusion itself (four patients). Only one patient in this series died within 30 days of the perfusion, and this was from a pulmonary embolus.

Of the patients followed for 5 years, 82 were thought at the time of treatment by isolation-perfusion to have localized tumors only. Of these, 50 were treated for the initial primary tumor, whereas 32 were treated for locally recurrent tumor that had been treated previously and had recurred up to a maximum of six times. No significant difference was detected between the survival of these two groups of patients following treatment. The survival of the 33 patients whose tumor masses were ×5 cm in diameter, however, was better than that of the 54 patients whose tumors were ≥5 cm in diameter ($p = 0.04$).

Because most soft-tissue sarcomas grow within a compression capsule, a surgeon who is seldom called on to treat this disease will "shell out" the tumor. The frequency of this form of inadequate initial treatment of the primary sarcoma makes these tumors among the most difficult to control. The time to gain local control of sarcomas is at the time of initial therapy.[4]

In the series of patients reported here, the regional recurrence rate of 19% after initial therapy compares favorably with reports of trials using other modalities from this institution,[5] the 29% reported in another series,[6] and the 39% reported by an earlier group.[7] The patients in these other series were treated by radical surgical therapy; some patients were included, however, whose primary site of tumor origin was not in the limbs. Although the series of patients reported here is small, the results suggest that survival rates for patients with recurrent sarcoma of the limbs when treated by isolation-

TABLE 35–2.
Survival by Tumor Type for Patients With Sarcomas of the Limbs Treated by Isolation-Perfusion

Type	Survival						Total Number of Patients Treated
	1 year		5 year		10 year		
	Lesion <5 cm	Lesion ≥5 cm	Lesion <5 cm	Lesion ≥5 cm	Lesion <5 cm	Lesion ≥5 cm	
Liposarcoma	8/8	18/20	4/5	11/19	4/5	9/18	(28)
Unclassified sarcoma	5/7	12/13	4/6	6/11	3/5	5/10	(20)
Fibrosarcoma	5/5	4/5	5/5	4/5	5/5	1/4	(10)
Synovial sarcoma	4/4	6/6	3/4	3/5	2/4	2/5	(10)
Malignant fibrous histiocytoma	5/5	4/4	1/1	2/3	1/1	0/1	(9)
Angiosarcoma	3/4	3/3	1/4	2/3	0/3	1/3	(7)
Neurofibrosarcoma	3/3	4/4	3/3	0/3	3/3	0/2	(7)
Clear cell sarcoma of tendon sheath	5/5	—	5/5	—	3/4	—	(5)
Other soft-tissue sarcomas*	—	8/8	—	3/6	—	2/5	(8)

* *Rhabdomyosarcomas, leiomyosarcomas, extraskeletal osteogenic sarcomas, extraskeletal chondrosarcomas, and epithelioid sarcomas.*

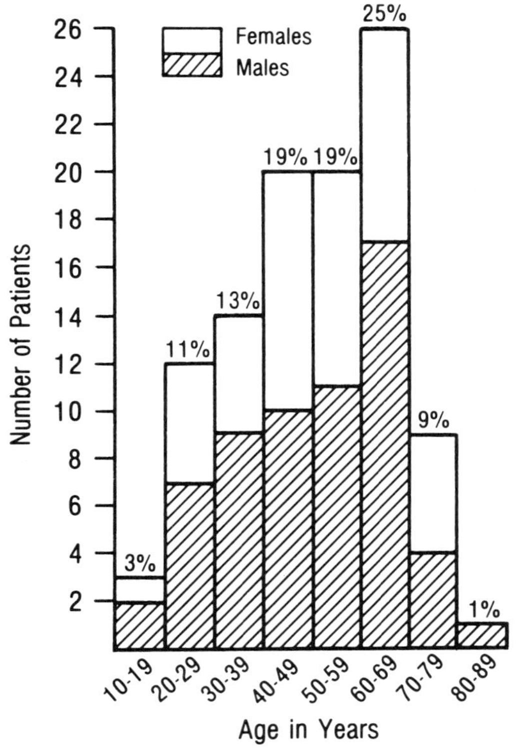

FIG 35–1.
Distribution by age and sex of 105 patients with sarcomas of the limbs.

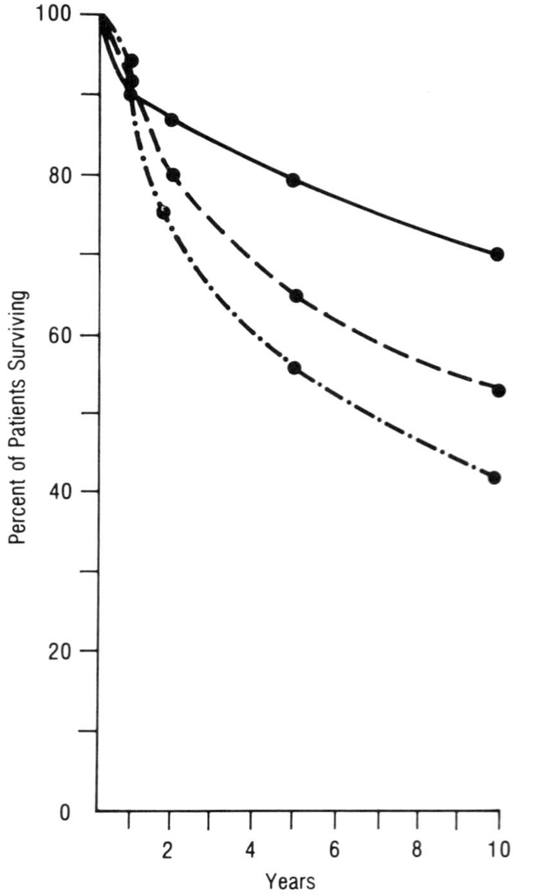

FIG 35–2.
Raw survival curve for 105 patients with soft-tissue sarcomas of the limbs.—, patients with lesions <5 cm in diameter; ---, all patients;-·-, patients with lesions ≥5 cm in diameter.

perfusion may be similar to that for patients treated by isolation-perfusion for a primary lesion.

Differences in numerical distribution of the various histological types of sarcomas in various series of patients may affect the reported control rates. As suggested previously, however,[8, 9] the histological type of sarcoma may not be as im-

TABLE 35–3.
Status at 5 Years of 88 Patients With Soft-Tissue Sarcomas of the Limbs

Status	Number (Percentage) of Patients
Alive, no evidence of disease	57 (65%)
Dead of disease	25 (28%)
Determinant cases at 5 years	82 (93%)
Dead, documented intercurrent disease	4 (5%)
Lost to follow-up	2 (2%)

TABLE 35–4.
Complications Resulting From 109 Perfusions in 105 Patients

Complication	Number (Percentage) of Patients
Death (pulmonary embolus)	1 (1%)
Subsequent amputation	10 (10%)
Edema of limb	5 (5%)
Major skin slough	2 (2%)
Major wound infection	1 (1%)

portant as other considerations, such as size of the tumor mass, which would appear to be the most important. The age distribution of the patients treated by isolation-perfusion for soft-tissue sarcomas of the limbs is similar to that in a series reported from the M. D. Anderson Cancer Center[4] and also in a series reported in 1962.[10] Because this is a retrospective study, it is impossible to state what factors other than treatment may have contributed to the overall 10-year survival rate of 53%, which is slightly better than that previously reported.[7, 10, 11]

Fifty-three percent of patients who failed initial therapy are salvaged by retreatment. This suggests that even when initial control is not obtained by regional chemotherapy, the tumor may be controlled by an alternative treatment. Although the group of patients reported here had a 10% amputation rate, this compares favorably with most reported series for soft-tissue sarcomas of the limbs. It is similar to the amputation rate (12%) reported by Klaase et al.[12] in patients with sarcomas who had isolation-perfusion with doxorubicin (Adriamycin). The surgical mortality of just under 1% is expected of any group of patients having operations of similar magnitude.

A regional recurrence rate of 75% following simple excisional surgery, or 70% following radiotherapy alone, clearly indicates that radical surgical resection, or a combination of these therapies, should be the minimal treatment for soft-tissue sarcomas of the limbs. Although a major amputation is no longer the treatment of choice for primary soft-tissue sarcomas, a decision to amputate may be based on involvement of vital anatomical structures by the sarcoma or by increased aggression by the tumor with each local recurrence. Our patients with recurrent sarcomas did as well as those with intact primary sarcomas when treated by isolation-perfusion, which is a more encouraging result than suggested previously.[1]

CONCLUSION

No absolute guidelines have been established as to the best therapy for soft-tissue sarcomas of the limbs. Constant re-evaluation of anticancer techniques and agents is necessary to ensure the best form of treatment. Adjuvant chemotherapy by isolation-perfusion treats all of the tissues involved primarily by soft-tissue sarcomas arising in the limbs and makes it possible to reduce the extent of surgical resection necessary to obtain control of the disease. It is a safe procedure that has been used in patients ranging in age from 11 to 80 years. Isolation-perfusion with L-phenylalanine mustard and actinomycin D provides an acceptable rate of regional control for patients with soft-tissue sarcomas of the limbs and is not associated with a higher incidence of systemic metastases than are other forms of treatment.

REFERENCES

1. Ryan RF, Winblad JN, Krementz ET, et al: Treatment of malignant neoplasms with chemotherapeutic agents utilizing a pump-oxygenator: Techniques and early results. *Bull Tulane Med Fac* 1958; 17:133–143.
2. McBride CM: Regional chemotherapy for soft tissue sarcomas, in Martin RG, Ayala AG (eds): *Management of Primary Bone and Soft Tissue Tumors*. Chicago, Year Book Medical Publishers, 1977, pp 353–360.
3. Stehlin JS Jr, Clark RL, Dewey WC: Continuous monitoring of leakage during regional perfusion. *Arch Surg* 1961; 83:943–949.
4. Clark RL, Martin RG, White FC, et al: Clinical aspects of soft tissue tumors. *Arch Surg* 1957; 74:859–870.
5. Suit HD, Martin RG, Russell WO: Sarcoma of soft tissue: Clinical histopathological parameters and response to treatment. *Cancer* 1975; 1478–1483.
6. Cantin J, McNeer GP, Chu FC, et al: The problem of local recurrence after treatment of soft tissue sarcoma. *Ann Surg* 1968; 168:47–53.
7. Pack GT, Ariel I: End results in the treatment of sarcoma of the soft somatic tissues, in Pack GT, Ariel IM (eds): *Tumor of the Soft Somatic Tissues: A Clinical Treatise*. New York, Paul B. Hoeber, 1958, pp 779–796.
8. McBride CM: Sarcomas of the limbs: Results of adjuvant chemotherapy using isolation-perfusion. *Arch Surg* 1974; 109:304–308.
9. Suit HD, Russell WO: Radiation therapy of soft tissue sarcomas. *Cancer* 1975; 36:759–764.
10. Shieber W, Graham P: An experience with sarcomas of the soft tissue in adults. *Surgery* 1962; 52:295–298.

11. Martin RG, Butler JJ, Albores-Saavedra J: Soft tissue tumors: Surgical treatment and results, in Cumley RW (ed): *Tumors of Bone and Soft Tissue*. Chicago, Year Book Medical Publishers, 1965, pp 333–347.

12. Klaase JM, Kroon BBR, Benckhuijsen C, et al: Results of regional isolation perfusion with cytostatics in patients with soft tissue tumors of the extremities. *Cancer* 1989; 64:616–621.

Chapter 36

Tourniquet Infusion Chemotherapy

Constantine P. Karakousis

In the past, a substantial number of patients with soft-tissue sarcomas of the extremities have been treated with amputation. In one large series, the rate of amputation was 43%.[1] Following amputation, the rate of local control was satisfactory, with a local recurrence rate of 7% to 8%.[1,2] Patients treated with wide excision or compartmental resection had a local recurrence rate of 28% to 36%.[1,2] Following simple local excision the local recurrence rate was 65% to 90%.[2,3]

In the past decade, increasing effort to achieve limb salvage in patients with sarcomas of the extremities has been made through the use of combinations of treatment modalities.

Regional chemotherapy was initially used in 1950[4] and has been used fairly extensively for liver tumors, primary or metastatic, that are not amenable to resection.[5] The rationale of regional chemotherapy is that the first passage of a drug given intra-arterially will be through the capillaries supplying the tumor, before the drug is mixed with and diluted in the circulating blood volume. A higher drug concentration may therefore be expected in the regional tissues.

The proportion of a drug given intra-arterially that is actually absorbed in the region supplied by the artery has not been studied extensively, and the proportion may not be the same for the various drugs that have been used in regional chemotherapy. In a few studies, comparable plasma levels were found following either intra-arterial or intravenous chemotherapy.[6] The clinical evidence indicates that the portion of the drug retained in the regional tissues cannot be a substantial portion of the total dose, because the systemic toxicity is not appreciably different between regional and systemic chemotherapy for a given drug and dose. As a corollary, the total dose that can be tolerated by the bone marrow or other normal tissues sensitive to the drug is also not appreciably different using these two modes of administration. Drug levels might be low in the regional tissues following intra-arterial chemotherapy because high blood flow rate through the patent artery would tend to (1) dilute the infused drug and (2) carry the drug through the capillaries and into the veins too fast for it to diffuse through the capillary membrane into the interstitial tissue.

Using an experimental dog model, we injected Adriamycin (doxorubicin hydrochloride) at 1 mg/kg into the canine femoral artery as a bolus injection while blood samples from the jugular vein were obtained at frequent intervals. High plasma levels of the drug were noted (Fig. 36–1). Biopsy specimens of the gastrocnemius muscle of the treated extremity 1 hour following drug injection showed no detectable levels of Adriamycin. Temporary occlusion of the femo-

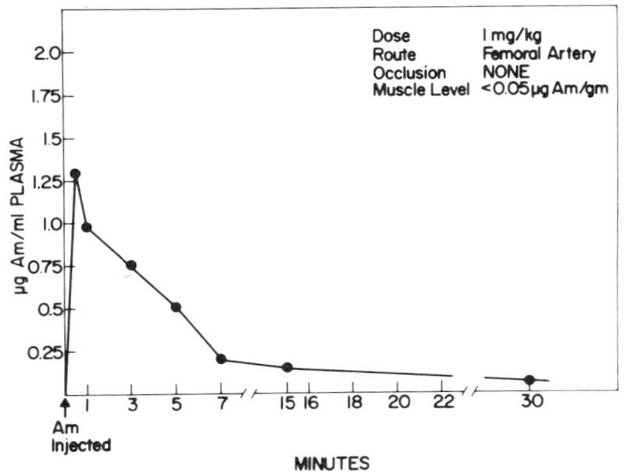

FIG 36–1.
Injection of Adriamycin (Am, 1 mg/kg) in the canine femoral artery is followed by high plasma levels (in jugular vein blood samples), which decline 15 minutes later. One hour later, no Adriamycin is detectable in biopsy specimens of the gastrocnemius muscle of the treated extremity.

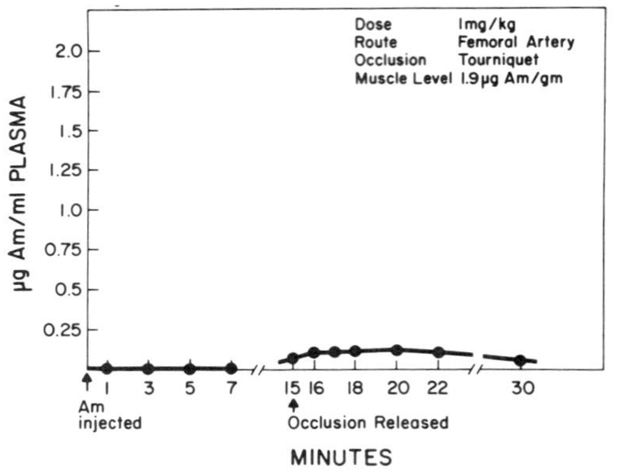

FIG 36–2.
Injection of Adriamycin (Am, 1 mg/kg) into the canine femoral artery distal to a tourniquet. Following release of the tourniquet, only low plasma levels of the drug were detectable in jugular vein blood.

ral artery only and injection of drug distal to the occlusion gave similar results, due to shunting of the Adriamycin into the systemic circulation through proximal thigh branches of the femoral artery. External application of a tourniquet on the proximal thigh and injection of the same dose of Adriamycin distal to the tourniquet produced high tissue levels of Adriamycin in the gastrocemius muscle (1.9 μg/g tissue). As expected, during the 15-minute occlusion period with the tourniquet no Adriamycin was detectable in the peripheral plasma, but after release of the tourniquet low levels of the drug were detectable (Fig 36–2). Furthermore, significant skin ulcerations appeared in extremities treated with the tourniquet infusion method, whereas intra-arterial injection of the same dose of Adriamycin without tourniquet occlusion produced no skin changes.[7]

In our preliminary experience with patients, tourniquet infusion resulted in high degrees of histological tumor necrosis and evidence of regression in a variety of tumors.[8] Further experience confirmed the effectiveness of this method in a variety of tumors.[9] It also became apparent that the tourniquet need not be applied for more than 5 minutes to achieve high drug levels in the regional tissues and correspondingly low leak of drug into the systemic circulation (Fig 36–3). Our experience in patients with soft-tissue sarcomas treated with this method is reported below.

MATERIALS AND METHODS

Because a space of about 8 cm is required below the groin crease or the axilla for the application of an external tourniquet, only tumors

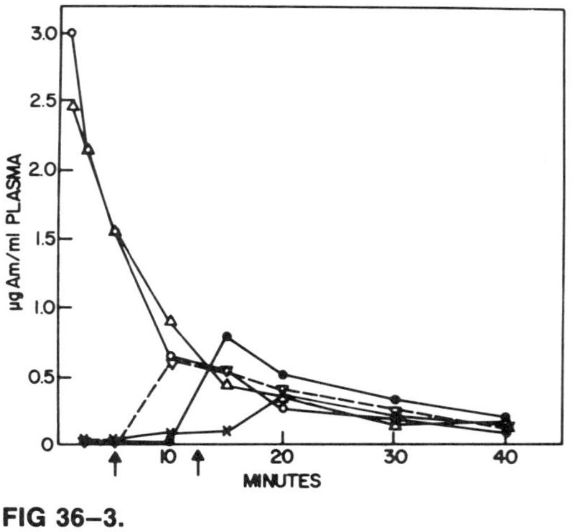

FIG 36–3.
Injection of 20 mg of Adriamycin (Am) in the femoral artery of patients without application of a proximal tourniquet produces high systemic plasma drug levels (○, △), while injection of this amount with the tourniquet applied for as short a time as 3 minutes results in low plasma Adriamycin levels following release of the tourniquet (▽, ●, ×).

located below the middle third of the thigh or middle of the arm are amenable to this method of treatment.

The percutaneous intra-arterial catheter is placed using fluoroscopic control, and the tip is guided to the desired level in the artery, marked previously on the skin. It is connected to an apparatus providing a slow drip of heparinized saline solution (3,000 IU of heparin in 500 mL of normal saline); the rate is controlled with a Sorenson valve. A three-way stopcock is placed between the arterial catheter and the Sorenson valve. The patient returns to the ward and a peripheral intravenous line is started to provide a continuous drip of heparin (10,000 IU every 12 hours). The peripheral heparin is given to avoid clot formation around the catheter. Prior to each application of the tourniquet, a bolus intravenous injection of 5,000 IU of heparin is given. The tourniquet is then applied so that the distal margin of the cuff is clearly above the tip of the catheter. A second tourniquet may then be applied below the tumor, if the distal extremity is not to be treated. The tourniquet may be a standard tourniquet used in the operating room or a regular blood pressure cuff (preferably, narrow cuffed to easily fit above the tip of the catheter).

Because there is minimal variation in the size of adult extremities, we routinely use 20 mg of Adriamycin for each dose. Each 10 mg of the drug is diluted in 50 mL of normal saline in a 50-mL syringe. The tourniquet is then inflated above systolic pressure, and the first 50 mg of the drug is injected over 1 minute. The proximal cuff pressure is decreased to the level of the mean arterial pressure, and the remaining 50 mL of the drug is injected over 1 minute. The tourniquet is left in place for an additional 3 minutes and then released. The only pain associated with this procedure is the pressure exerted by the cuff and some burning sensation due to the drug. Most patients tolerate this without any sedation.

The catheter is left indwelling, and the treatment is repeated the next day. On the third day, another treatment is given, the peripheral intravenous heparin is discontinued, and the catheter is removed. Although most patients have been treated with three daily injections, a few received only two injections because they developed a marked drug-induced erythema. Wide surgical resection of the tumor was performed within 1 week of this treatment.

RESULTS

Patient data are shown in the Table 36–1. Of 13 patients treated, with a mean follow-up period of 32 months (range, 9 to 69 months), there was one local recurrence. Of the 11 patients with localized tumor, pulmonary metastases subsequently developed in two.

This treatment was given to patients with large proximal tumors, or tumors located in the distal extremity where it was clear that no or minimal margin could be obtained surgically (Figs. 36–4 and 36–5). High levels of Adriamycin were measured in the tumor tissue using a fluorometric assay.[10]

Three patients with multiple lesions from Kaposi's sarcoma of the lower extremity were also treated with this method. In all three, the tumor underwent complete regression. In two of these patients, a small number of lesions reappeared after 18 and 16 months, respectively, and regressed when treated with intralesional vinblastine. Vinblastine was used several times for the management of recurrent lesions; both patients were disease free for 49 and 26 months, respectively, from the time of diagnosis of their disease. The third patient underwent complete regression of a plantar lesion, and remained disease free 6 months later.

Five patients with squamous cell carcinoma were treated with the above method. One of them with lesions of the hand and in-transit lesions in the forearm had complete regression of these lesions; when he died 8 months later of progression of pulmonary metastases, the original lesions still had not recurred. A second patient with squamous cell carcinoma extensively involving the anterior aspect of the knee was treated with the tourniquet infusion method, followed by simple surgical excision and skin graft. She was well 50 months later. Another patient was in-transit lesions in the forearm, arising from the hand, had progression of these lesions following one course of treatment. Two patients with squamous cell carcinoma of the ankle arising in a chronic stasis ulcer had greater than 50% regression after one course of treatment. One of these patients had a relapse, which was managed with amputation. The other patient is still being treated.

Two patients with bone tumors were treated using the tourniquet infusion method. One of them, a girl with one osteogenic sarcoma of the proximal tibia, was given three courses of chemotherapy by the tourniquet infusion

TABLE 36–1.

Patients With Soft-Tissue Sarcoma Treated With Tourniquet Infusion of Adriamycin and Subsequent Surgical Resection

Patient Number	Sex	Age (yr)	Histological Classification	Location	Local Recurrence	Systemic Recurrence	Follow-Up (mo)	Present Status*
1	F	45	Liposarcoma	(L) Thigh	0	0	36	AND
2	F	27	Neurofibrosarcoma	(R) Thigh	Yes	0	38	AND
3	M	32	Liposarcoma	(R) Calf	0	0	69	AND
4	F	52	Malignant fibrohistiocytoma	(L) Ankle	0	0	55	AND
5	M	20	Myogenic sarcoma	(R) Calf	0	Yes	44	AWD
6	M	35	Recurrent liposarcoma	(R) Calf	0	0	35	AND
7	M	40	Liposarcoma	(R) Thigh	0	0	38	AND
8	F	21	Neurofibrosarcoma	(R) Thigh	0	0	25	AND
9	F	50	Fibrosarcoma	(L) Leg	0	0	13	AND?
10	F	75	Liposarcoma	(R) Forearm	0	0	9	AND
11	M	56	Malignant fibrohistiocytoma	(L) Leg + (L) inguinal metastasis	0	Yes	27	DWD
12	M	37	Hemangiopericytoma	(L) Foot + pulmonary metastasis	0	Pulmonary metastasis	14	DWD
13	M	65	Leiomyosarcoma	(L) Knee, recurrent	0	Pulmonary metastasis	15	DWD

** AND = alive, no disease; DWD = died with disease; AWD = alive with disease.*

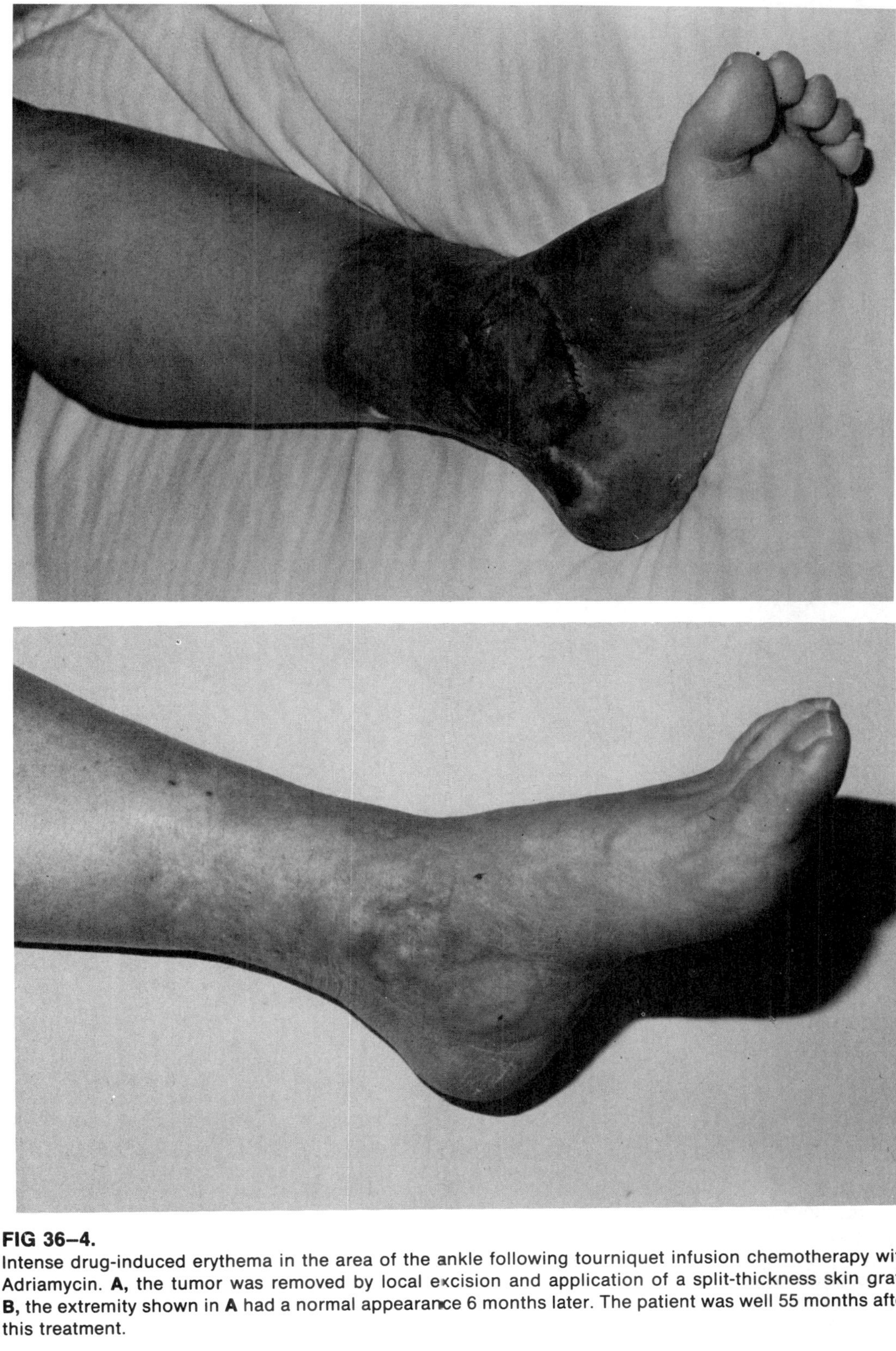

A

B

FIG 36–4.
Intense drug-induced erythema in the area of the ankle following tourniquet infusion chemotherapy with Adriamycin. **A,** the tumor was removed by local excision and application of a split-thickness skin graft. **B,** the extremity shown in **A** had a normal appearance 6 months later. The patient was well 55 months after this treatment.

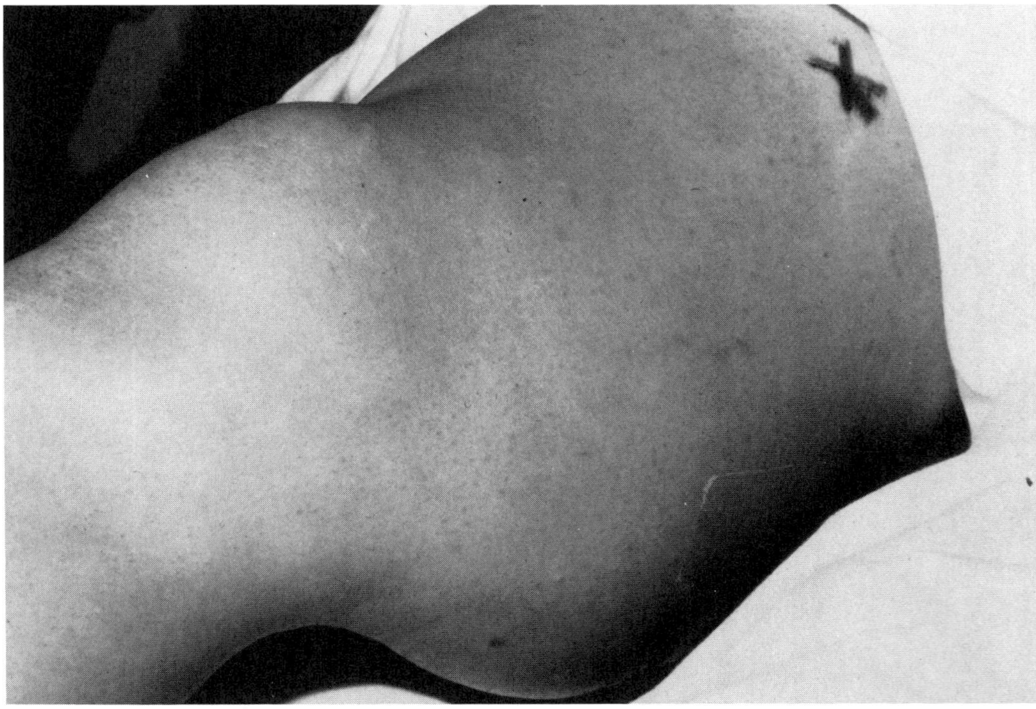

A

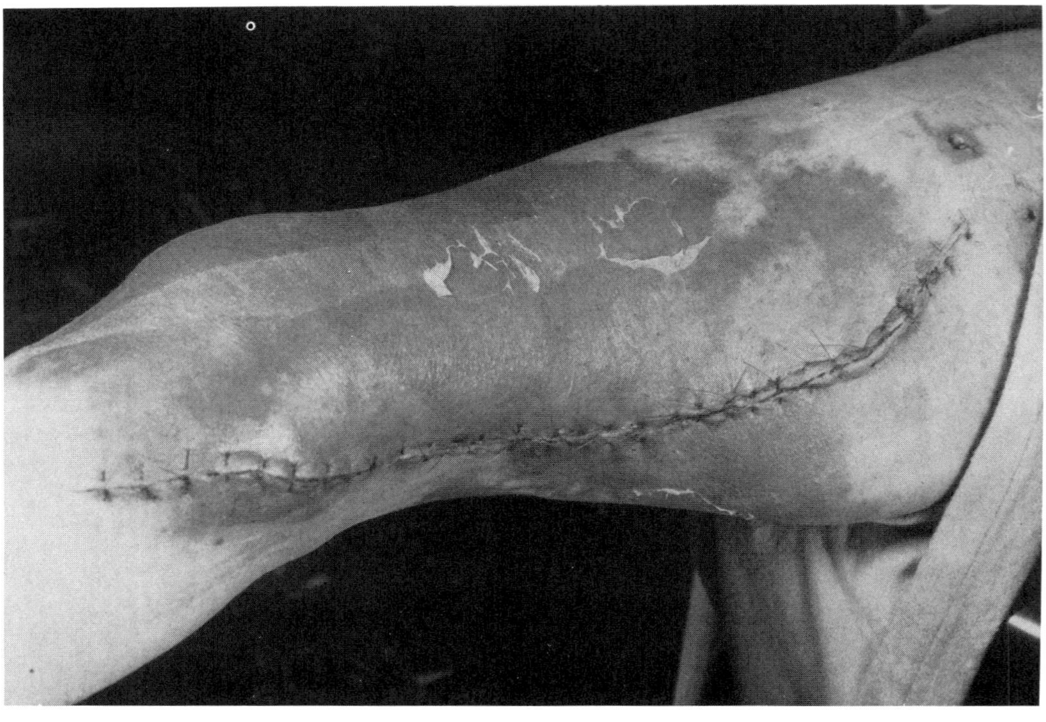

B

FIG 36–5.

A, large, bulging liposarcoma in the lower right medial thigh. The mark on the skin indicates the position of the tip of the catheter. Early erythema after the first injection of Adriamycin was limited to the area of the tumor by application of a below-the-knee tourniquet during each treatment. **B,** the same extremity, following resection of the liposarcoma. Skin changes, including areas of blistering, were evident. **C,** the same extremity, 6 months later. The patient was well 38 months after this treatment, and skin erythema and blisters had disappeared.

C 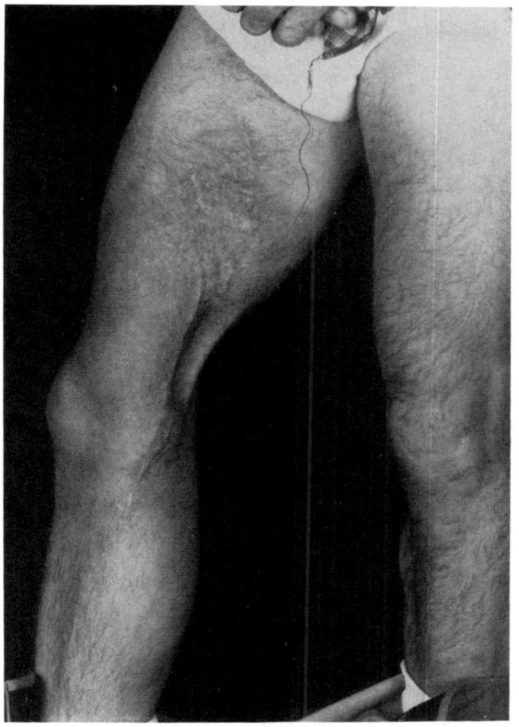

FIG 36–5.—*Continued*

method, then another biopsy was performed. In the repeat biopsy specimens there was osteoid surrounded by fibrous and hyalinized cells, but no histological trace of tumor cells in the entire specimen. The second patient, who had histologically proved metastatic renal cell carcinoma in the distal femur, had no evidence of tumor in biopsy specimens from the same area of the bone following three courses of treatment.

Several patients with recurrent melanoma of the extremity were treated using Adriamycin with the tourniquet infusion method. Following regional chemotherapy, their lesions were excised, then the patients were observed. Of seven patients with stage IIIA melanoma (in-transit metastases) with a mean follow-up period of 19.3 months (range, 4 to 38 months), five patients had no further regional recurrence and remain alive and well, whereas two patients had recurrence both locally and systemically. Of 13 patients with stage IIIAB melanoma (in-transit lesions plus regional lymph node metastases) treated by node dissection, intra-arterial chemotherapy and excision of the in-transit lesions, nine patients later had further in-transit lesions as well as hematogenous metastases, two patients had hematogenous metastases only, and one patient remains alive and well. Three patients with hematogenous metastases were given palliative treatment using tourniquet infusion to in-transit lesions involving an extremity. One patient showed complete regional regression, which lasted until her death from systemic melanoma 2 years later, whereas the other two patients showed no objective regression.

DISCUSSION

Regional chemotherapy has been based on the rationale that the drug concentration in tissues supplied by the infused artery should be higher than can be achieved by systemically administered chemotherapy. A variable that has not been thoroughly studied is the rate of drug infusion. Is there an optimal infusion rate, that is, a rate that will provide the highest drug concentration in the tumor tissue for a given dose of the drug?

Temporarily stopping or slowing the arterial flow while the venous outflow is occluded by an externally applied tourniquet increases significantly the tissue concentration of the infused drug. In the canine model, tourniquet infusion provided mean tissue levels of Adriamycin, actinomycin D, and melphalan comparable to hyperthermic isolation perfusion.[9] Advantages of the tourniquet infusion method are as follows: (1) the placement of the arterial catheter is percutaneous and does not require an operation; (2) it may be repeated as frequently as desired; (3) it is possible to treat only a portion of the extremity; and (4) systemic toxicity is reduced because the doses required are well below those tolerated systemically.

Drawbacks of the tourniquet method compared with hyperthermic isolation-perfusion are as follows: (1) tourniquet infusion may be used only for tumors located below the middle of the thigh because the tourniquet must be applied above the tip of the catheter; and (2) drug distribution in tissues is often spotty when using tourniquet infusion, although distribution can be improved with appropriate manipulation of the tip of the catheter and infusion of additional drug solution.

The tourniquet infusion method needs to be studied further not only in relation to improving drug distribution, but also with drugs other than Adriamycin. Local hyperthermia may also increase drug concentration and susceptibility of the tumor. This method was developed in the laboratory with the intention of using it in the treatment of soft-tissue sarcomas of the extremities, because another technique (hyperthermic isolation-perfusion) was already an effective treatment in the management of recurrent melanoma of the extremities. The choice of Adriamycin was based on its effectiveness against sarcomas. Because the technique and dosages were already worked out for Adriamycin, we also used this agent in patients with melanomas.

Our preliminary experience with tourniquet infusion in combination with resection for limb salvage has been satisfactory; there has been only one local recurrence among 13 patients with soft-tissue sarcomas so treated. We have not used this method in more patients because we had already embarked on a program of adjuvant postoperative radiation for soft-tissue sarcomas resected with inadequate margins. Our results from the combination of surgical excision plus postoperative radiation are encouraging,[11] and similar good results have been reported by other authors.[12] Because of the efficacy of surgery plus adjuvant radiation in achieving local control, there has not been strong clinical pressure to develop alternatives. There are clinical situations, however, where regional chemotherapy would be clearly preferable to radiation (multiple tumor lesions that cannot be easily encompassed in one radiation field, or where the tumor involves half or more of the circumference of the extremity). In these cases the field is too extensive for radiation, or the risk of complications from circumferential radiation is prohibitively high.

In patients with soft-tissue sarcomas requiring surgery plus adjuvant treatment using chemotherapy or radiation for limb salvage, a large tumor mass is often present, and complete regression using regional chemotherapy alone cannot be expected. There are ischemic areas in the large tumor masses that do not receive adequate amounts of drug. Repeated courses of tourniquet infusion chemotherapy would likely increase drug toxicity in normal tissues, and if a clinical regression did occur it would remain indeterminate whether destruction of the tumor was complete. For these reasons, we have used the tourniquet infusion method *pre-operatively* to destroy microscopic residual tumor around the macroscopic mass, therefore increasing the chance of local control even with narrower surgical margins.

Encouraging results have been obtained with other tumors. Three patients with Kaposi's sarcoma had complete regression, which in two lasted 18 and 16 months. In a patient with osteogenic sarcoma of the tibia, tissue obtained by curettage of the involved area of the bone six weeks following tourniquet infusion chemotherapy contained no trace of tumor. There has been no long-term follow-up yet in this patient.

Our experience with the tourniquet infusion method for in-transit malignant melanoma lesions has been more ambiguous. This treatment was given to destroy microscopic disease in the lymphatic system, and the in-transit lesions were surgically removed following the infusion. Of seven patients with in-transit lesions, five remain disease free after a mean follow-up of 19 months. Of 13 patients with in-transit lesions plus lymph node metastases, other in-transit lesions and distant metastases developed in nine, indicating that the tourniquet infusion method using Adriamycin was ineffective in eradicating microscopic melanoma in the lymphatic system. It appears that this method, using Adriamycin, is not as effective as standard hyperthermic isolation-perfusion for recurrent melanoma.[13] Clearly, experience with other drugs more specific for melanoma is needed. A preliminary study in Europe produced encouraging results in treating recurrent melanoma with decarbazine (DTIC)[14] by tourniquet infusion.

CONCLUSIONS

Tourniquet infusion chemotherapy is a method of regional chemotherapy for extremity tumors that uses a proximal tourniquet to decrease arterial flow, while the venous outflow is totally occluded. With Adriamycin as the chemotherapeutic agent, this method, in combination with surgical resection of the gross tumor, appears promising in the management of extremity soft-tissue sarcomas.

REFERENCES

1. Shiu MH, Castro EG, Hajdu SI, et al: Surgical treatment of 297 soft tissue sarcomas of the lower extremity. *Ann Surg* 1975; 182:597–602.
2. Abbas JS, Holyoke ED, Moore R, et al: The surgical treatment and outcome of soft tissue sarcoma. *Arch Surg* 1981; 116:765–769.
3. Cadman NL, Soule EH, Kelly PJ: Synovial

sarcoma: An analysis of 134 tumors. *Cancer* 1965; 18:613–627.

4. Cleveland JC, Johns DG, Farnham G, et al: Arterial function of dichloromethotrexate in cancer of the head and neck: A clinicopharmacologic study. *Curr Top Surg Res* 1969; 1:113.
5. Sullivan RD, Zurek WZ: Chemotherapy for liver cancer by protracted ambulatory infusion. *JAMA* 1965; 194:481–486.
6. Didolkar MS, Kanter PM, Baffi BR, et al: Comparison of regional versus systemic chemotherapy with adriamycin. *Ann Surg* 1978; 187:332–336.
7. Karakousis CP, Kanter PM, Lopez R, et al: Modes of regional chemotherapy. *J Surg Res* 1979; 26:134–141.
8. Karakousis CP, Rao U, Holtermann OA, et al: Tourniquet infusion chemotherapy in extremities with malignant lesions. *Surg Gynecol Obstet* 1979; 149:481–490.
9. Karakousis CP, Kanter PM, Park HC, et al: Tourniquet infusion versus hyperthermic perfusion. *Cancer* 1982; 49:850–858.
10. Schwartz HS: A fluorometric assay for daunomycin and Adriamycin in animal tissues. *Biochem Med* 1973; 7:396–404.
11. Karakousis CP, Johnson RR: Adjuvant radiation in soft tissue sarcomas, in Salmon SE, Jones SE (eds): *Adjuvant Therapy of Cancer III*. Grune & Stratton, 1981, pp 211–216.
12. Rosenberg SA, Tepper J, Glatstein E, et al: The treatment of soft-tissue sarcomas of the extremities: Prospectives randomized evaluation of (1) limb-sparing surgery plus radiation therapy compared with amputation and (2) the role of adjuvant chemotherapy. *Ann Surg* 1982; 196:305–315.
13. Stehlin JS Jr: Hyperthermic perfusion for melanoma of the extremities: Experience with 165 patients, 1967 to 1979. *Ann NY Acad Sci* 1980; 335:352–355.
14. Ingvar C, Erichsen C, Stridbeck H, et al: Tourniquet infusion chemotherapy in locally advanced malignant melanoma and Kaposi sarcoma on the lower extremities. *Proceedings of the 13th International Congress of Chemotherapy*, Verlag H. Egermann, August 28–September 2, 1983, Vienna, Part 246, pp 43–46.

Chapter 37

Combined Modality Treatment: Limb-Sparing Surgery Plus Radiation Therapy and Adjuvant Chemotherapy

Henry A. Briele
Michael J. Walker
John A. Greager
Donald K. Wood
William F. Lindsey
Tapas K. Das Gupta

INTRODUCTION

The management of malignant mesenchymal tumors has undergone considerable change in recent years. The hitherto accepted dictum of radical operation or radical radiation therapy is no longer considered the prima facie mode of treatment; rather, judicious conservatism, with the appropriate combination of surgery and radiation therapy for management of the primary tumors and chemotherapy for eradication of micrometastases, has become the guiding principle.[1-11] Although this multimodal treatment program is highly desirable, because it probably will improve the overall disease-free survival and salvage a number of limbs, it is imperative that its proper role be established and that our initial enthusiasm should not cloud good clinical judgment.

To gain a proper perspective on the evolution of combined modality therapy it is desirable to trace the history of the development of each individual form of treatment used in the management of soft-tissue sarcomas. In this evolutionary scale, surgical treatment was the first form utilized.

SURGERY

The established practice of radical surgery was based on the poor results of limited local excision of the primary tumors. [12–17] Analysis of the data generated by various authors[12–14, 16, 18, 19] showed that the more radical the excision of the primary tumor, the lower the incidence of local recurrence with wide soft-tissue resection.[12, 15, 18, 19] Abbas et al.[12] found that the incidence of local recurrence was 65% after limited local excision, 36% after wide resection, and 8% after amputation. Based on these and other historic observations, the concept of major amputation for control of primary soft-tissue sarcomas of the extremities was derived.[12–15, 17–19] Because the lower extremity is the most common site for adult soft-tissue sarcomas, the proper treatment of these tumors has generated the highest amount of controversy. In 1975, Shiu et al.[17] stated that major amputation or disarticulation offers the surest means of eradication of a soft-tissue sarcoma in terms of obtaining the widest margin of resection. In their retrospective series from Memorial Sloan-Kettering Cancer Center (New York, New York), they found the incidence of local recurrence after resection to be 28%, but after a major amputation, only 7%.

In another prospective evaluation of surgical treatment of soft-tissue sarcomas performed by a single group at the University of Illinois (Chicago), the overall incidence of local recurrence following both soft-tissue resection and amputation was 8%.[12, 20]

It appears, therefore, that judiciously applied regional surgical treatment in itself can bring the incidence of local recurrence down to an acceptable minimum. The factors that influence distant dissemination, however, are dependent on the size, histological type, grade, more, in a number of patients control of the primary tumor is not synonymous with control of metastases. It becomes clear, at least in sarcomas of the extremities, that although amputation is a useful mode of treatment it cannot be equated with cure; hence an alternative form of management, with preservation of a functional limb, must be sought.

RADIOTHERAPY

Clinical trials of radiation therapy as a primary treatment of soft-tissue sarcomas have in the past been disappointing, with local tumor control achieved in fewer than 5% of patients.[21, 22] However, with the advent of megavoltage equipment, a sufficient number of soft-tissue sarcoma patients have been treated and results have been encouraging enough to warrant a growing optimism. There is now adequate clinical experience to state that radiation therapy does control certain forms of primary soft-tissue sarcomas.[4, 21, 22] Additionally, the beneficial role of radiation therapy in the palliative management of patients with soft-tissue sarcomas has been adequately demonstrated and is now in general use.[4, 21, 22] Pre-operative irradiation appears to sterilize well-oxygenated tumor cells located on the periphery of the neoplasm, thereby rendering the tumor more amenable to conservative excision. It is now generally accepted that a combination of conservative surgery and radiation therapy at radical dose levels can control certain sarcomas and avoid deformity or loss of limb.

The concept has evolved that microscopic tumors can be controlled with doses of radiation that allow good cosmetic and functional results, thereby avoiding disabling operations. This is founded on the biological principle that effective "log kill" of well-oxygenated microscopic tumor can be achieved using a moderate radiation dose, such as 4,500 to 5,000 cGy. The problem of radiation resistance by hypoxic tumor cells at the center of the mass is circumvented by subsequent surgical resection.

Based on this operational hypothesis, Suit et al.[23] described the Massachusetts General Hospital (Boston) experience with 36 soft-tissue sarcoma patients who were treated by *pre-operative* radiation therapy followed by conservative surgery. In 33 of these patients, the tumors were greater than 5 cm. The radiation dose was 5,000 to 6,000 cGy (200 cGy, five times a week), followed in approximately 3 weeks by conservative excision; a booster dose to the tumor bed was given intra-operatively or postoperatively. Local control was achieved in 31 of 33 patients (follow-up periods ranged from 3 months to 8 years). Although this was an uncontrolled and inconclusive study, it pointed out the need for further investigation of the role in pre-operative radiation therapy.

Simultaneously with Suit et al.,[23] Lindberg et al.[24] described the beneficial role of *postoperative* radiation therapy for 300 patients treated at the M. D. Anderson Cancer Center (Houston, Texas). These authors reported absolute 2- and 5-year survival rates of 74% and 61%, respectively, and an overall local recurrence rate of

22%. Lindberg et al.[24] emphasized that radical dose radiation therapy after conservative local excision was as effective as radical surgery, that is, a major amputation.

CHEMOTHERAPY

Despite reasonable control of local disease, however, distant metastases are common in most high-grade soft-tissue sarcomas. Drugs have been used in an attempt to eradicate widespread recurrences. The most commonly used chemotherapeutic agents in soft-tissue sarcomas prior to 1970 were cyclophosphamide, actinomycin D, and vincristine, given alone or in combination. In 1970, Jacobs[25] reviewed several individual series and found that 56 of 238 patients (23.5%) had shown an objective response to these drugs. However, when the childhood cases of rhabdomyosarcoma were eliminated the response rate was found to be only 18% (32 of 179 cases), and only a small number of long-term remissions was reported.

In 1969, DiMarco et al.[26] reported encouraging results in initial trials with Adriamycin (doxorubicin) in the treatment of soft-tissue sarcomas. These data were later confirmed by Benjamin et al. in 1973.[27] Definite activity was also noted during the initial investigations with 5-(3,3-dimethyl-1-triazeno)imidazole-4-carboxamide (DTIC), a synthetic congener of the naturally occurring purine precursor 5- (or 4)-aminoimidazole 4-(or 5)-carboxamide.[28] During initial single-agent trials with Adriamycin and DTIC, response rates of 29% and 15%, respectively, were achieved at most centers.[20] Gottlieb et al.[29, 30] later found that DTIC lengthened the duration of remission. In 1974, they reported that of 200 evaluable patients with all types of soft-tissue and bone sarcomas, 22 showed a complete response and 63 a partial response (overall rate, 42.5%).

A review of the published data on chemotherapy of adult soft-tissue sarcomas suggests, although the conclusions are sometimes too optimistic, that Adriamycin at present constitutes the most effective single agent and that the addition of DTIC probably improves the response rate duration of response, or both, in a reasonable number of patients. In 1977, Pinedo and Kenis[31] reviewed the literature on chemotherapy of advanced soft-tissue sarcomas in adults and expressed the then generally held view that the most effective regimen was a combination of cyclophosphamide, vincristine, Adriamycin, and DTIC.[31] It appears that there is a definite place for chemotherapy in the management of metastatic soft-tissue sarcomas in both adults and children. Based on these observations, several attempts have been made to evaluate the role of a single agent or multiple agents as adjuvant chemotherapy in the treatment of primary soft-tissue sarcomas in both children and adults.

The most significant influence of adjuvant chemotherapy has been in the management of childhood rhabdomyosarcomas. Today, a combination of conservative surgery, supplemental radiation therapy, and adjuvant chemotherapy is the accepted method of management of all childhood rhabdomyosarcomas.[32–43] Hays[44] has summarized the pertinent findings of cancer study groups in the United States. These groups studied a total of 750 children from 1972 to 1978. Patients were divided into four clinical groups on the basis of (1) extent of disease at the time of diagnosis and (2) the surgical procedure performed. Each patient was then randomly assigned to one of two chemotherapy arms. Among 67 children in clinical group (stage) I, the use of radiation therapy failed to improve the survival rate. Between 92% and 96% of the children were alive with local recurrence rates of 3.7% and 5.5%, respectively, at the time of Hays' report. In clinical group II, 73% of 110 patients showed no evidence of disease, and 82% were still alive in 1978. Although these spectacular results have not been achieved with other histological types of sarcoma, attempts are being made to apply these same therapeutic principles to fibrosarcomas,[44] synovial sarcomas,[44] and other skeletal sarcomas.[20]

Reports that adjuvant chemotherapy provides some success in the management of childhood sarcomas led Das Gupta et al.[18] to initiate a prospective study to determine the effect of chemotherapy as an adjuvant to surgery in the initial treatment of adult primary soft-tissue sarcomas. The results were compared with those obtained in a group of patients with similar histological types of primary sarcoma treated by surgery alone. The chemotherapy regimen consisted of Adriamycin, 60 mg/m^2 intravenously on day 1, and DTIC, 250 mg/m^2 on days 1 through 5. The cycle was repeated every 22 days. The total dose of Adriamycin was 500 mg/m^2; the DTIC was continued for 1 year. The adjuvant chemotherapy group consisted of 113 patients (group I), and the concurrent surgical resection group consisted of 144 patients (group II). In group I, 53 tumors were T_1 and 50 were T_2; 67 of the tumors were grade III, and 46 were grade IV. In group II, 65 had T_1 and 79 had T_2 tumors; 82 tumors were grade III and 62 were grade IV. The anatomical location and histological types were similar in both groups. Eighty-seven (77%) of the 113 patients in group I lived disease free for 2 years, compared with 59% of the 144 treated by resection alone. Of the patients eligible for 5-year survival analysis, 74% were disease free in the adjuvant chemotherapy group compared with 50% in the surgically treated group. The incidence of local recurrence was about the same in both groups. From a histological standpoint, malignant fibrous histiocytomas and myogenic sarcomas appeared to benefit most from use of the two-drug regimen; the least favorable response was in liposarcomas and fibrosarcomas. Since then, several other studies[1–3, 10, 21, 45] with various chemotherapy combinations[1–3, 21, 45] have shown that although proof of absolute efficacy of adjuvant chemotherapy was lacking, the burgeoning evidence is in keeping with the initial data reported from the University of Illinois.[18]

COMBINED MODALITIES

In adults, the lower extremity is the most frequent site of development of soft-tissue sarcomas, followed by the upper extremity; therefore an attempt to salvage a limb by the use of all three methods of treatment described above has become one of the most important considerations in the management of soft-tissue sarcomas. It is in these anatomical sites that the role of combining all three treatment modalities has become the major objective. Several authors have obtained data suggesting that the combined modality treatment can indeed salvage a tumor-bearing limb without jeopardizing the disease-free interval. In 1976, Morton et al.[16] reported that multimodality management of extremity skeletal and soft-tissue sarcomas with pre-operative Adriamycin and radiation therapy, radical resection, and postoperative chemotherapy or chemo-immunotherapy resulted in preservation of a functional extremity in 13 of 14 patients. The disease-free interval varied between 4 and 34 months. These authors concluded that the results of the combined modality approach were significantly better than those obtained by one method alone.

Rosenberg et al.[46] reported the results of their prospective randomized study of 43 adults with extremity soft-tissue sarcomas. The study was conducted as follows: Between May 1975 and April 1981, 43 adult patients with high-grade soft-tissue sarcomas of the extremities were assigned randomly to receive either amputation at or above the joint proximal to the tumor, including all involved muscle groups, or to receive a limb-sparing resection plus adjuvant radiation therapy. The limb-sparing resection group received wide local excision followed by 5,000 cGy to the entire anatomical area at risk for local spread and 6,000 to 7,000 cGy to the tumor bed. Both randomization groups received postoperative chemotherapy with doxorubicin (maximum cumulative dose, 550 mg/m^2), cyclophosphamide, and high-dose methotrexate. Twenty-seven patients were assigned randomly to receive limb-sparing resection and radiotherapy, whereas 16 had amputation only (randomization was 2:1). There were four local recurrences in the limb-sparing group and none in the amputation group ($P = 0.06$, generalized Wilcoxon test). However, there were no differences in disease-free survival rates (71% and 78% at 5 years; $P = 0.75$) or overall survival rates (83% and 88% at 5 years; $P = 0.99$) between the limb-sparing group and the amputation treatment groups. Multivariate analysis indicated that the only correlate of local recurrence was the final margin of resection. Patients with positive margins of resection had a higher likelihood of local recurrence than those with negative margins ($P < 0.0001$), even when postoperative radiotherapy was used.

The simultaneous prospective randomized study by these investigators[46] of postoperative chemotherapy in 65 patients with high-grade soft-tissue sarcoma of the extremities revealed better results in those receiving chemotherapy compared with those who did not, in 3-year continuous disease-free rates (92% vs. 60%; $P = 0.0008$) and in overall survival (95% vs. 74%; $P = 0.04$). The authors concluded that the combination of limb-sparing surgery, radiation therapy, and adjuvant chemotherapy was successful as treatment in the great majority of adult patients with soft-tissue sarcomas of the extremity.

We have been conducting a similar study at the University of Illinois.[47] Our present analyzable data are based on 42 patients. Forty-two consecutive patients with a high-grade soft-tissue sarcoma of an extremity were treated pre-operatively with concomitant intra-arterial infusion of Adriamycin (10 mg/m^2 daily for 10 days) and radiotherapy (2,500 cGy in ten fractions in 2 weeks). Two weeks later, an en bloc resection was performed. Depending on surgical specimen findings, additional postoperative radiotherapy was given, bringing the total dose to a continuous schedule equivalent of between 5,000 cGy in 5 weeks and 6,000 cGy in 6 weeks. A functionally intact limb was preserved in 40 patients (96%). Local recurrence developed in one patient (3%). The actuarial overall survival at 3 years was 70% and the disease-free survival was 65%.[48]

The extent of tumor necrosis in previously untreated surgical specimens has been reported to be between 5% and 12%. Pre-operative radiation therapy in a dose of 5,000 to 6,000 cGy results in minimal or moderate histological changes in the surgical specimen in 47% of patients.[47] Using a moderate pre-operative radiation dose of 2,500 cGy given in ten fractions together with intra-arterial Adriamycin, we have observed extensive tumor necrosis in 41% and no residual tumor in 28%. These findings suggest that the constant presence of Adriamycin during radiation therapy has an additive effect, perhaps by sensitizing the tumor to the radiation.

In view of the excellent local control, the functional integrity of the treated extremities, and the minimal long-term complication rate, we think that in patients undergoing compartmental or muscle group excision with clear surgical margins, the cumulative radiation dose should be limited to 5,000 cGy in 5 weeks or its equivalent. Radiation doses of 6,000 cGy in 6 weeks are recommended only for patients with either microscopically positive resection margins or with incomplete resections.

CONCLUSION

Combined modality treatment of soft-tissue sarcomas is here to stay. Combining more than one form of treatment does provide a better end result, frequently without sacrifice of the tumor-bearing limb. The question that remains unanswered is whether there is an absolute need to combine all three forms, or whether a combination of two would provide similar results; for example, whether adequate excision along with adjuvant chemotherapy would provide an end result similar to that achieved with surgery, irradiation, and chemotherapy. There are some data[20] to suggest that in small tumors, supplemental radiation therapy probably does not add a great deal to the ultimate outcome.

Each method has its own drawbacks and side effects. Inadequate surgery may result in increased local recurrence. The disability induced by amputation has been detailed during the last decade. However, certain types of sarcomatous conditions, for example, aggressive fibromatosis or neurofibrosarcoma, are not overtly radiosensitive; in patients with these tumors, amputation frequently is the safest method of local treatment. Today, the prosthetic industry is well developed, and outright rejection of amputation in such selected instances is unwarranted. Similarly, there are certain histological types of sarcomas that do not respond satisfactorily to presently available agents, even when some of these drugs are administered by means of continuous 24-hour infusion. To use adjuvant chemotherapy in patients with such tumors is not logical.

In summary, a large number of adult patients with soft-tissue sarcomas will fare better with combined modality treatment. It is imperative, however, that the selection of methods of treatment be based on careful scrutiny of histological type, grade, and location of the tumors.

REFERENCES

1. Antman KH, Corson J, Greenberger J, et al: Multimodality therapy in the management of angiosarcoma of the breast. *Cancer* 1982; 50:2000–2003.
2. Sordillo PP, Magill GB, Schauer PK, et al: Preliminary trial of combination therapy with Adriamycin and radiation in sarcomas and other malignant tumors. *J Surg Oncol* 1982; 21:23–26.
3. Rosen G, Juergens H, Caparros B, et al: Combination chemotherapy (T-6) in the multidisciplinary treatment of Ewing's sarcoma. *Natl Cancer Inst Monogr* 1981; 56:289–299.
4. Perez CA, Tefft M, Nesbit ME Jr, et al: Radiation therapy in the multimodal management of Ewing's sarcoma of bone: Report of the intergroup of Ewing's sarcoma study. *Natl Cancer Inst Monogr* 1981; 56:263–271.
5. Kaufman JJ, Gelbard M: Leiomyosarcoma of renal vein and inferior vena cava. *Urology* 1981; 18:173–176.
6. Middleton AW Jr, Elman AJ, Stewart JR, et al: Combined modality therapy with conservation of organ function in childhood geni-

tourinary rhabdomyosarcoma. *Urology* 1981; 18:42–46.

7. Ransom JJ, Pratt CB, Hustu HO, et al: Retroperitoneal rhabdomyosarcoma in children: Results in multimodality therapy. *Cancer* 1980; 45:845–850.
8. King DR, Clatworthy HW Jr: The pediatric patient with sarcoma. *Semin Oncol* 1981; 8:215–221.
9. Mandard AM, Chasle J, Manard JC, et al: The pathologist's role in a multidisciplinary approach for soft part tissue sarcoma: A reappraisal (39 cases). *J Surg Oncol* 1981; 17:69–81.
10. DeVita VT Jr, Henney JE, Weiss RB: Advances in the multimodal primary management of cancer. *Adv Intern Med* 1980; 26:115–129.
11. Cruz AB Jr, Thames EA Jr, Aust JB, et al: Combination chemotherapy for soft-tissue sarcomas: A phase III study. *J Surg Oncol* 1979; 11:313–323.
12. Abbas JS, Holyoke ED, Moore R, et al: The surgical treatment and outcome of soft-tissue sarcoma. *Arch Surg* 1981; 116:765–769.
13. Cantin J, McNeer GP, Chu FC, et al: The problem of local recurrence after treatment of soft tissue sarcoma. *Ann Surg* 1968; 168:47–53.
14. Castro GG, Hajdu S II, Fortner JG: Surgical therapy of fibrosarcoma of the extremities: A reappraisal. *Arch Surg* 1973; 107:284–286.
15. Eilber FR, Mirra JJ, Grant TT, et al: Is amputation necessary for sarcomas? *Ann Surg* 1980; 192:431–438.
16. Morton DL, Eilber FR, Townsend CM Jr, et al: Limb salvage from a multidisciplinary treatment approach for skeletal and soft tissue sarcomas of the extremity. *Ann Surg* 1976; 184:268–278.
17. Shiu MH, Castro EB, Hajdu S, et al: Surgical treatment of 297 soft-tissue sarcomas of the lower extremities. *Ann Surg* 1975; 182:597–602.
18. Das Gupta TK, Patel M, Chaudhuri PK, et al: The role of chemotherapy as an adjuvant to surgery in the initial treatment of primary soft tissue sarcomas in adults. *J Surg Oncol* 1982; 19:139–144.
19. Pritchard DJ, Soule EH, Taylor WF, et al: Fibrosarcoma: A clinicopathological and statistical study of 199 tumors of soft tissues of extremities and trunk. *Cancer* 1974; 33:888–897.
20. Das Gupta TK: *Tumors of the Soft Tissues.* East Norwalk, Appleton-Century-Crofts, 1983.
21. Suit HD: Soft tissue sarcomas (excluding rhabdomyosarcoma): Radiotherapy applications. *Natl Cancer Inst Monogr* 1981; 56:245–249.
22. Liebner EJ: Radiation therapy. In: Das Gupta, TK. *Tumors of the Soft Tissues.* East Norwalk Appleton-Century-Crofts, 1983, pp 271–308.
23. Suit HD, Proppe KH, Mankin HJ, et al: Preoperative radiation therapy for sarcoma of soft tissue. *Cancer* 1981; 47:2269–2274.
24. Lindberg RD, Martin RG, Romsdahl MM, et al: Conservative surgery and postoperative radiotherapy in 300 adults with soft-tissue sarcomas. *Cancer* 1981; 47:2391–2397.
25. Jacobs EM: Combination chemotherapy of metastatic testicular germinal cell tumors and soft part sarcomas. *Cancer* 1970; 25:324–332.
26. DiMarco A, Gaetani M, Scarpinato B: Adriamycin (NSC-123-127): A new antibiotic with antitumor activity. *Cancer Chemother Rep* 1969; 53:33–37.
27. Benjamin RS, Riggs CE Jr, Bachur NR: Pharmacokinetics and metabolism of Adriamycin in man. *Clin Pharmacol Ther* 1973; 14:592–600.
28. Gottlieb JA: Combination chemotherapy for metastatic sarcoma. *Cancer Chem Rep* 1974; 58:265–270.
29. Gottlieb JA, Baker LH, Quagliana JM, et al: Chemotherapy of sarcomas with a combination of Adriamycin and dimethyltriazenoimidazole carboxamide. *Cancer* 1972; 30:1632–1638.
30. Gottlieb JA, Benjamin RS, Baker LH, et al: Role of DTIC (NSC-45388) in chemotherapy of sarcomas. *Cancer Treat Rep* 1976; 60:199–203.
31. Pinedo HM, Kenis Y: Chemotherapy of advanced soft-tissue sarcomas in adults. *Cancer Treat Rev* 1977; 4:67–86.
32. Pinkel D: Curability of childhood cancer. *JAMA* 1976; 235:1049–1050.
33. D'Angio G: Pediatric cancer in perspective: Cure is not enough. *Cancer* 1975; 35:866–870.
34. Jaffe N, Filler RM, Farber S, et al: Rhabdomyosarcoma in children: Improved outlook with a multidisciplinary approach. *Am J Surg* 1973; 125:482–487.
35. Ragab AH, Vietti TJ, Perez CA, et al: Malignant tumors of the soft tissues, in Sutow

WW, Vietti TJ, Fernbach W (eds): *Clinical Pediatric Oncology*. St. Louis, C. V. Mosby, 1973, pp 450–472.

36. D'Angio GH, Evans A: Soft tissue sarcomas, in Bloom GJ, et al (eds): *Cancer in Children*. New York, Springer-Verlag, 1975, pp 217–241.
37. Jenkin RDT: Rhabdomyosarcoma in childhood, in Godden OJ (ed): *Cancer In Childhood*. Toronto, Ontario Cancer Treatment and Research Foundation, 1972, pp 157–165.
38. Sutow WW, Lindberg RD, Gehan EA, et al: Three-year relapse-free survival rates in childhood rhabdomyosarcoma of the head and neck. *Cancer* 1982; 49:2217–2221.
39. Raney RB Jr, Zimmerman RA, Bilaniuk LT, et al: Management of craniofacial sarcoma in childhood assisted by computed tomography. *Int J Radiat Oncol Biol Phys* 1979; 5:529–534.
40. Raney RB Jr, Ragab AH, Ruymann F, et al: Soft-tissue sarcoma of the trunk in childhood. *Cancer* 1982; 49:2612–2616.
41. Ghavimi F, Exelby PR, D'Angio GJ, et al: Combination therapy of urogenital embryonal rhabdomyosarcoma in children. *Cancer* 1973; 32:1178–1185.
42. Johnson DG: Trends in surgery for childhood rhabdomyosarcoma. *Cancer* 1975; 35:916–920.
43. Pratt CB, Husto HO, Fleming ID, et al: Coordinated treatment of childhood rhabdomyosarcoma with surgery, radiotherapy, and combination chemotherapy. *Cancer Res* 1972; 32:606–610.
44. Hays DM: The management of rhabdomyosarcoma in children and young adults. *World J Surg* 1980; 4:15.
45. Perloff M, Holland JF: Surgical adjuvant chemotherapy. *Annu Rev Med* 1977; 28:475–488.
46. Rosenberg SA, Tepper J, Glatstein E, et al: The treatment of soft-tissue sarcomas of the extremities. *Ann Surg* 1982; 196:305–314.
47. Mantravadi RVP, Trippon MJ, Patel MK, et al: Limb salvage in extremity soft-tissue sarcoma: Combined modality therapy. *Radiology* 1984; 152:523–526.
48. Kaplan EL, Meier P: Nonparametric estimation from incomplete observations. *J Am Statist Assoc* 1958; 53:457–481.

Index

D

E

F

G

N

O

P

Q

R

S

T

U

V

W